Neuroradiology

Volume 1

Neuroradiology

Volume 1

Edmund H. Burrows, M.Rad., D.M.R.D., F.R.C.R.

Consultant Neuroradiologist, Wessex Neurological Centre,
Southampton University Hospitals; Honorary Clinical
Senior Lecturer, University of Southampton; Honorary
Civilian Consulting Radiologist to the Royal Naval Hospital, Haslar, Gosport
President, British Society of Neuroradiologists

and

Norman E. Leeds, M.D., F.A.C.R.

Head, Neuroradiology Section, Montefiore Hospital and Medical
Center; Professor of Radiology, Albert Einstein College of
Medicine of Yeshiva University, Bronx, New York
Past President, American Society of Neuroradiology

Churchill Livingstone
New York, Edinburgh, London, and Melbourne   1981

© Churchill Livingstone Inc. 1981

Distributed in the United Kingdom by Churchill Livingstone, Robert Stevenson House, 1-3 Baxter's Place, Leith Walk, Edinburgh EH1 3AF and by associated companies, branches and representatives throughout the world.

First published 1981
Printed in USA

ISBN 0-443-08016-x

7 6 5 4 3 2 1

Library of Congress Cataloging in Publication Data

Burrows, Edmund H
    Neuroradiology.

    Bibliography: p.
    Includes index.
    1. Nervous system — Radiography. 2. Diagnosis, Radioscopic. I. Leeds, Norman E., 1928-
joint author. II. Title. [DNLM: 1. Nervous system — Radiography. 2. Nervous system — Radiography — Problems. WL 141 B972n]
RC349.R3B87   616.8′04757   80-24709
ISBN 0-443-08016-X

To our families
Anne, Emma, and Charlotte
Bette, Rick, and Patti

Preface

This book aims to provide the reader with an informed approach to the radiological investigation and interpretation of neurological disorders. It is based on the experiences of two neuroradiologists, one British and one American, whose careers span the complement of a number of different neuroradiological examinations and the significant changes which followed the introduction of computed tomography. During the years when this text was being prepared, this new technique had already altered neuroradiological practice and its impact upon existing contrast procedures had become clear. This is one of the first textbooks of neuroradiology to be written since the CT revolution. In addition to computed tomography, the appearances of lesions depicted by alternative investigative methods are described in detail, in order to provide radiologists with the answers they may require on plain skull and spine radiography, cerebral angiography, pneumography and scintigraphic imaging.

A second, scarcely less far-reaching change which this work records, is the successful introduction to neuroradiological practice of the water-soluble contrast agent, metrizamide. Realization of the need for whole-diameter myelography and radiculography and the combination of metrizamide with computed tomography have led the neuroradiologist into new and fertile fields. Such innovative studies of the spinal canal and its contents have enabled the neuroradiologist to reveal morphological abnormalities with an elegance and accuracy never before possible.

Volume 1 of this book provides a topic-oriented approach to neuroradiology which is mainly topographical. Each chapter is fully illustrated and augmented by references to the relevant recent literature in the English language. Volume 2 consists of 100 Exercises which further amplify and illustrate the text of Volume 1. These exercises are both didactic and for self-evaluation. When the reader has studied a particular chapter carefully, he should be able to answer the questions asked in each related exercise. These exercises may also be utilized alone as a test of acquired knowledge in neuroradiology, for example, in preparing for Board examinations.

About 20 of the illustrations in this book have appeared before in other publications. The authors gratefully acknowledge the generosity of others in permitting republication here. Credit to the original sources appears in the captions of those illustrations.

The authors wish to express their thanks to Dr. Ronald Murray of London and Alton, Hampshire for his encouragement and stimulation during the formative stages of this work. Robert Duncan, Carol Hoidra, Carole Baker, Lewis Reines, and the staff of Churchill Livingstone have our thanks for their much appreciated help. We would also like to express our thanks to Pamela Kimber, Ruth Chapman, Pat Hollingdale, David Whitcher and Peter Jack at Southampton General Hospital, and to Carole Wald, Eugene Bowers, Lascelles Ferguson and Myrna Weinberg at Montefiore Hospital and Medical Center, who were helpful in the preparation of the text and in providing photographic copies.

Contents

Volume 1

Volume 2

Part 1
Chapter-Related Exercises

Neuroradiology

Volume 1

1 The Skull

The neuroradiologist is concerned with diseases of the brain, its coverings and nerves, and this bias influences his interest in, and interpretation of, plain skull radiographs. He must be familiar with the patterns of involvement of the skull in intracranial diseases and be able to differentiate these patterns from other processes, some of which are local calvarial lesions and others cranial manifestations of systemic or generalized skeletal disease.

Plain skull radiographs retain a place in the intelligent management of intracranial disease processes, notwithstanding noninvasive brain scanning, as the following three cases illustrate: (1) head injury including fractured skull—only the skull radiographs reveal the fracture; (2) subdural hematoma with a pineal shift and ipsilateral clinical signs—if computed tomography is not available the direction of pineal shift indicates the appropriate carotid artery to inject; and (3) low-grade glioma with pressure sella, pineal shift and a false-negative scintigram—the patient might have been dismissed following the scintigram, if the skull changes had not indicated the need for further investigation.

EXAMINATION TECHNIQUE AND INTERPRETATION

Standard Projections

The traditional baseline for radiography of the skull is the tragocanthal or canthomeatal line (outer canthus of the eye to the midpoint of the external auditory meatus), to which the central ray of all projections is related. Five standard views of the skull are used in neuroradiology (Fig. 1–1):

   Lateral
   Anteroposterior 20° caudad tilt ("pineal view")
   Postero-anterior 25° caudad tilt (Caldwell's view)
   Anteroposterior 30° caudad tilt (Towne's view)
   Submentovertical (full axial, basal, Hirtz's view)

Some projections yield more diagnostic information than others. In intracranial lesions the lateral projection is the most useful: in this book 115 out of the 231 (50%) noncontrast radiographs of the skull are lateral views. However, a frontal view is necessary to make the most important observation in cranial neuroradiology, viz., the midline position of the calcified pineal gland. Thus two projections represent the minimum for an adequate examination: the lateral and the 20-degree anteroposterior. The posteroanterior 25° projection is also valuable because of the information present: the bony orbits, sphenoid ridge and the floor of the anterior midline.

About 50 structures can be identified in each view, but only about a dozen are unique for any given view (Potter, 1971). Those structures of greatest radiologic relevance will now be enumerated under each projection.

Lateral Projection: For this projection, a horizontal-ray beam is essential. No alternative radiographic technique is acceptable any longer, for three reasons: (1) Small fluid levels will not be overlooked, which are formed either by gas within the intracranial compartment or blood in the sphenoidal sinuses (see Ch. 4, Head Injuries). (2) The bones and joints of the craniovertebral angle are evaluated in the optimal functional and dynamic position, i.e., both skull and cervical spine are seen in true lateral

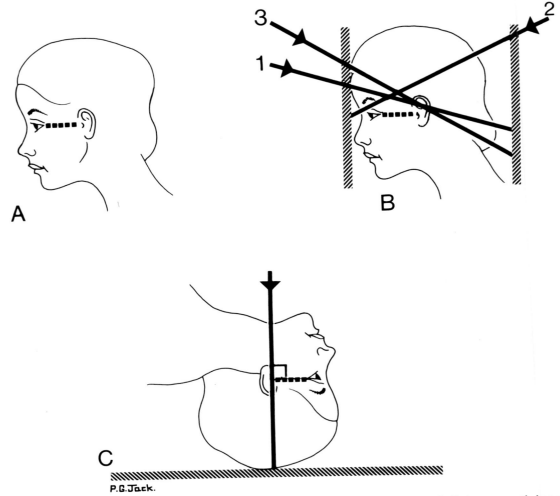

P.G.Jack.

Fig. 1–1 Radiographic projections of the skull. (A) The conventional radiographic baseline of the skull, the tragocanthal or canthomeatal line. (B) Three standard coronal views made with the baseline at a right angle to the radiograph. The arrow indicates the direction of the central beam of each projection and shows its point of entry, course of traverse and point of exit in relation to the skull. 1. Anteroposterior ("pineal view"), central ray 20° to the baseline. 2. Posteroanterior 25° (Caldwell's), central ray tilted 25° towards the feet. 3. Half-axial anteroposterior 30° (Towne's), central ray tilted 30° towards the feet. (C) Submentovertical (basal, Hirtz's), central ray at a right angle to the radiograph, but the head is thrown back to bring the baseline parallel to the radiograph.

view, and the patient's supine position during radiography maximizes any atlantoaxial subluxation or odontoid fracture which may be present. (3) Examination with the patient comfortable, and not carried out with his head forcibly rotated on his neck, is the best way of obtaining a lateral radiograph that will be neither tilted nor rotated.

The following areas and structures may be identified(Fig. 1–2):

(a) Pineal Calcification: Habenular commissure. Calcified glomus bodies.

(b) Pituitary Fossa (see Fig 5–1): Cortical floor. Posterior clinoid processes and dorsum sellae. Carotid sulcus. Anterior clinoid processes. Sphenoidal sinus.

(c) Cranial Vault: Vascular grooves—anterior and posterior for branches of both middle meningeal arteries, parietal "spider" and sphenobregmatic sulcus (Fig. 1–27). Pacchionian granulations. Inner and outer tables, and soft tissues of scalp (bright light!). Areas of physiological thinning (occipital squame above and below internal occipital protuberance and temporal squame) and thickening (parietal boss), sutures—coronal, lambdoid, sagittal and bregmatic.

(d) Floor of Skull: Midline of anterior cranial fossa (cribriform plate, sphenoid planum and chiasmatic sulcus) and the roofs of both bony orbits. Anterior limits of both temporal fossae, terminating above in the pterion on each side. Posterior cranial fossa. visible from the posterior rim of foramen magnum to the internal occipital protuberance.

(e) Craniovertebral Angle: Anatomical integrity of component bones (axis, atlas, and occiput with the foramen magnum), normal craniocervical funnel

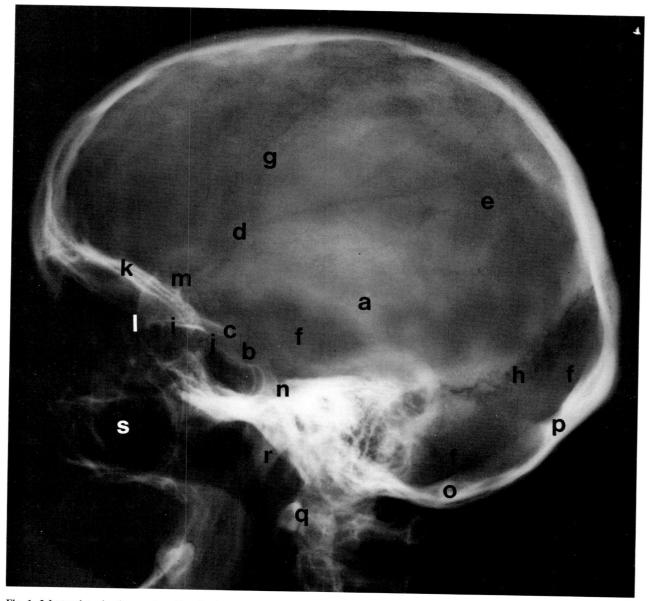

Fig. 1–2 Lateral projection made with a horizontal-ray beam—the most useful noncontrast radiograph for evaluating the skull. This case is also shown in Figures 1–3, 1–4 and 1–6. What is the diagnosis? The answer is given in the form of a captioned illustration elsewhere in Chapter 1. a. Pineal calcification. b. Pituitary fossa. c. Anterior clinoid process. d. Middle meningeal arteries. e. Parietal "spider" of veins. f. Physiological thinning of occipital and temporal squames. g. Coronal suture. h. Lambdoid suture. i. Sphenoid planum. j. Chiasmatic sulcus. k. Roofs of orbits. l. Anterior wall of temporal fossa (greater sphenoid wing). m. Pterion. n. Clivus. o. Posterior rim of foramen magnum. p. Torcular Herophili. q. Atlantoaxial joint. r. Soft tissues of nasopharynx. s. Maxillary antrum.

and clivocervical angle, absence of basilar impression or atlantoaxial instability (see Ch. 9).

(f) Nasopharynx: Width of soft tissues.

(g) Face: Fluid levels in the maxillary antra may be detected with the aid of a bright light. Underexposed views are useful to evaluate displacement of facial-bone fractures.

Anteroposterior 20° Projection: The following areas and structures may be identified (Fig. 1–3):

(a) Pineal Calcification: Of all the coronal projections, the pineal is best seen in this view, when not overlain by the external occipital protuberance or thickening of the occipital or frontal squames. In the normal patient, the calcified glomus bodies of the choroid plexus form a symmetrical triangle with the pineal gland.

(b) Cranial Vault (Middle Third): Examine and compare the two sides to study the integrity of inner and outer tables and the scalp tissues (bright light!). Lambdoid suture, external occipital protuberance, confluence of sinuses and grooves for lateral sinuses.

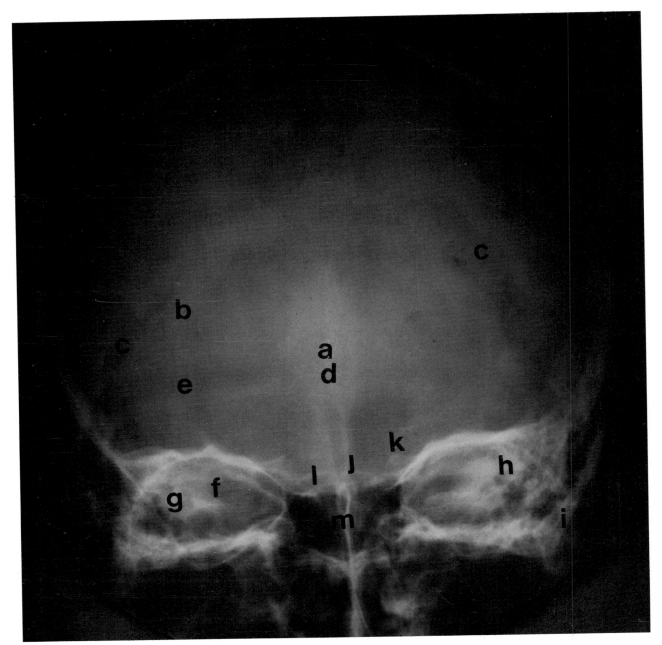

Fig. 1–3 Anteroposterior projection tilted 20° to the feet, a view favored by neurologists and otologists. It has three advantages over other coronal views, because it is more likely to demonstrate the position of the pineal calcification; it offers the best view of the middle and inner ear structures; and it shows the greatest volume of the supratentorial brain free of overlying facial bones, since the central ray passes roughly parallel to the inferior surface of the cerebral hemisphere. a. Pineal calcification. b. Glomus bodies of choroid plexus. c. Lambdoid suture. d. External occipital protuberance. e. Grooves for lateral sinus. f. Internal auditory canal, including posterior wall. g. Vestibule and cochlea. h. Semicircular canals. i. External auditory canal. j. Crista galli. k. Anterior clinoid process. l. Dorsum sellae. m. Ethmoidal and sphenoidal sinuses.

(c) *Ear:* Compare the width of the internal auditory canals and the porus acousticus on each side, note its well-defined posterior wall. Auditory structures visible within the petrous pyramid are the vestibule and cochlea, semicircular canals and sometimes the ossicles; also the external auditory canals.

For special examination: see Special Projections below.

(d) *Other Structures:* The crista galli, anterior clinoid processes, dorsum sellae and posterior clinoid processes may be dramatically highlighted. The ethmoidal and sphenoidal air cells are super-

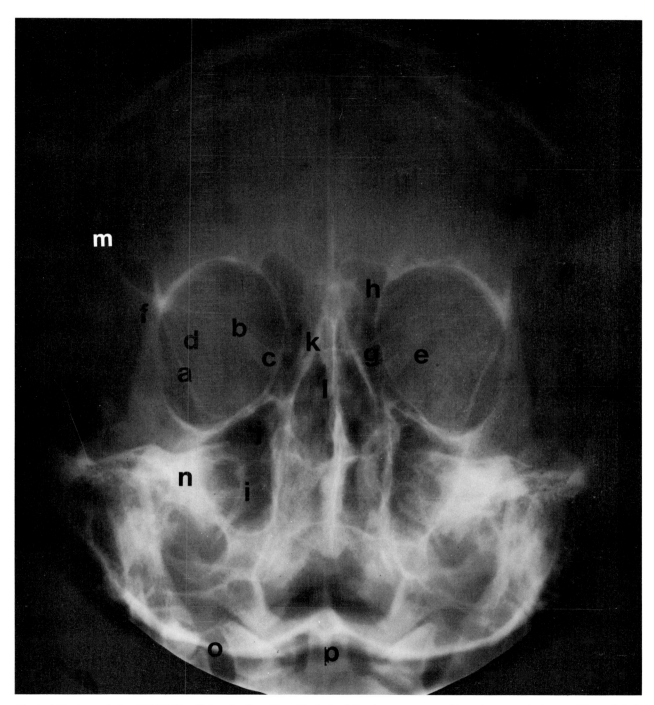

Fig. 1–4 Posteroanterior 20° (Caldwell's) projection. If omitted, the following structures will not be seen: the bony orbits and their walls, the sphenoid ridge and wings, and the various parts of the facial midline. Lesions such as sphenoid meningiomas may be missed. a. Innominate line. b. Sphenoid ridge. c. Lesser wing of sphenoid bone. d. Greater wing of sphenoid bone. e. Superior orbital fissure. f. Frontozygomatic synchondrosis. g. Ethmoidal sinuses. h. Frontal sinuses. i. Maxillary antrum. j. Foramen rotundum. k. Sphenoid planum. l. Floor of pituitary fossa. m. Pterion. n. Petrous pyramid. o. Floor of posterior fossa. p. Odontoid process.

imposed, but their roofs and lateral extent are clearly shown.

Posteroanterior 20° (Caldwell's) Projection: The following areas should be studied to identify the various structures listed (Fig. 1–4):

(a) Bony Orbits: Size, evaluated by measuring the vertical diameter of the margins, should not differ by more than 2 to 3 millimeters. The bony components should be carefully evaluated, including the following: oblique or innominate line, which represents the projected cross section of the squamozygomatic surface of the frontal bone; symmetry and integrity of the sphenoid ridge, the lesser and greater wings and the superior orbital fissure separating them; and following trauma the frontozygomatic suture and orbital walls forming the ethmoidal and maxillary sinuses (blow-out fracture).

(b) Paranasal Sinuses: The frontal and ethmoidal cells are best evaluated in this projection, also the roof of the maxillary sinus (blow-out fracture).

(c) Sphenoid Planum and Pituitary Floor: The sphenoid planum thickens in meningioma. The pituitary fossa is eroded and made asymmetrical by sellar masses (see Ch. 5).

(d) Cranial Vault (Anterior Third): The forehead and hairline part of the vault is seen in this projection, and the integrity and symmetry of its various features should be inspected, in the same way as the anteroposterior 20° projection is used to check those of the middle third. No sutures are visible, but the outer ends of the sphenoid ridge terminate in the pterion, which should be studied on each side. Linear vault fractures are often visible with the aid of a bright light.

(e) Floor of the Skull: This is a useful coronal view of the floor of the posterior fossa and the upper cervical vertebrae, which is particularly valuable in identifying occipital fractures and in basal craniometry involving the mastoid tips and odontoid processes (see Ch. 9).

Anteroposterior 30° (Towne's) Projection: The following areas and structures may be identified (Fig. 1–5):

(a) Pineal Calcification: Usually overlain by thick bone of the occipital protuberance, but it may be visible—especially if displaced from its normal midline position.

(b) Cranial Vault (Posterior Third): This is bisected horizontally by the attachment of the tentorium cerebelli along the margins of the grooves for the lateral sinuses. The parietal part of the cranial vault is highlighted. This is the most useful projection for evaluating asymmetry due to focal brain damage. The impression of the superior sagittal sinus appears as a notch in the inner table, and Pacchionian granulations may account for small lucencies in the parasagittal region (i.e., within 2 cm. on either side of the midline). The coronal suture projects as a semicircle across the vault but it is less well seen than the lambdoid suture, which bounds the supratentorial part of the occipital squame, and connects on each side with the occipitomastoid suture (not fracture!). A foramen for an emissary vein may lie at the head of the latter suture, but midline occipital emissary veins are probably more frequent.

(c) Petrous and Mastoid Temporal Bones: The contents of the petrous pyramid, particularly those not well seen in the anteroposterior 20° projection, can be adequately studied. From medial to lateral, these are: the apex, the internal auditory meatus and canal cochlea and vestibule lateral and superior semicircular canals and the lateral wall of the attic. The mastoid antrum is a well-defined lucency, projected lateral and superior to the middle ear structures. The mastoid air cells lie laterally.

(d) Foramen Magnum and Three Other Observations: A satisfactorily positioned Towne's projection includes the posterior half of the foramen magnum and, if slightly overtilted, the posterior arch of the atlas will be visible through it. Anatomical structures of great diagnostic importance are projected anteriorly in the foramen magnum; these are the components of the pituitary fossa, viz., the dorsum sellae, posterior clinoid processes and anterior clinoid processes. The second observation is the outline of the anterior part of the floor of the temporal fossa, which reflects the shape and volume of its contents. A dramatic asymmetry accompanies deforming lesions of the skull such as congenital subdural hygroma or orbital neurofibromatosis, and the normal cortical pattern will be altered in meningioma of the sphenoid wing. The third structure is the inferior orbital fissure that lies on the floor of the orbit, which is deformed by a depressed fracture (blow-out fracture into the maxillary antrum).

Submentovertical (Hirtz's) Projection: The following structures should be identified (Fig. 1–6):

(a) The Three Lines: On each side, three well-defined linear structures intersect. These are the lateral wall of the orbit, the anterior wall of the middle cranial fossa and the lateral wall of the maxillary antrum. Expanding processes of the middle fossa or bony orbit displace or deform these lines, and infiltrative lesions such as metastatic cancer or sphenoid meningioma alter their corticated appearance.

(b) Important Foramina: These are spinosum, ovale and magnum; the jugular foramen is not usually visible in the full axial view (see Special Projections below). In view of the wide range of normal asymmetry and individual variation in size of these foramina, only observations based on serial radiographic examinations showing progressive enlargement over a period of time possess value. Stenosis or off-center asymmetry of the foramen magnum is an important feature of achondroplasia or congenital anomalies of the craniovertebral angle. The foramen spinosum enlarges to accommo-

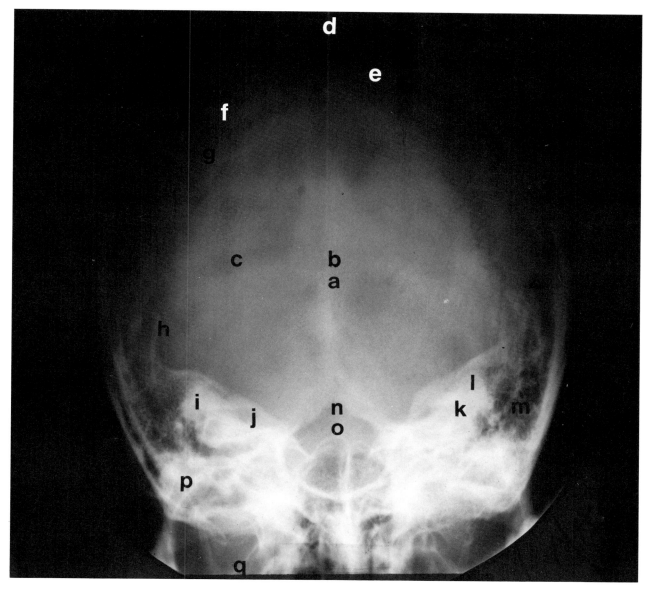

Fig. 1–5 The half-axial anteroposterior 30° (Towne's) projection. Alone of all the skull projections, Towne's projection provides an unencumbered view of the occipital squame and infratentorial compartment. If omitted, fractures and deposits of calcium in the posterior fossa will be missed, because in the lateral view the anterior half of the infratentorial compartment is obscured by the mastoid air cells. It is also useful to the otologist, providing the only view of the mastoid antra and air cells and permitting these structures to be compared with the opposite ones in the same radiograph. The middle ear structures are better seen than on the anteroposterior projection. a. Pineal calcification. b. Occipital protuberance c. Grooves for lateral sinus d. Notch for superior sagittal sinus. e. Pacchionian granulations. f. Coronal suture. g. Lambdoid suture. h. Occipitomastoid suture line. i. Petrous pyramid. j. Internal auditory canal. k. Vestibule and chochlea. l. Semicircular canals. m. Mastoid antrum. n. Foramen magnum, posterior half. o. Dorsum sellae. p. Floor of temporal fossa. q. Inferior orbital fissure.

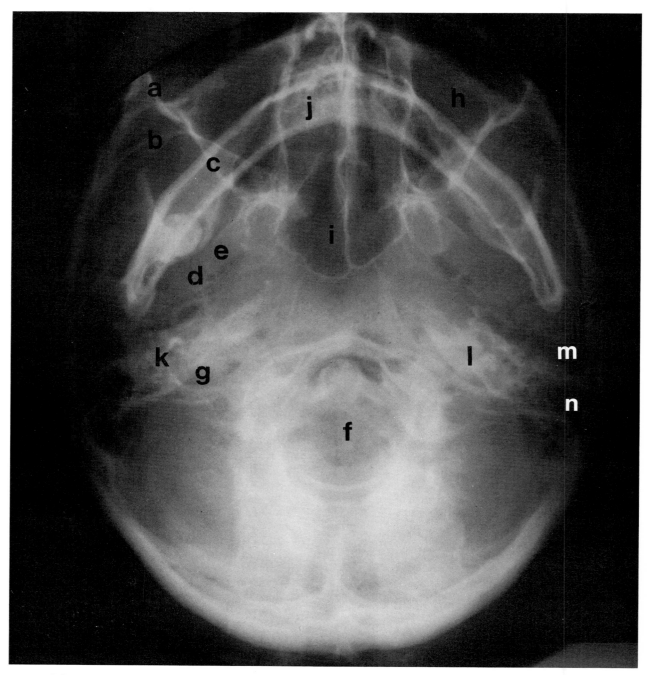

Fig. 1—6 Submentovertical, or full-axial or basal (Hirtz's) projection. Unique advantages of this projection are the detection of asymmetrical or destructive lesions of the skull base, congenital deformities of the craniovertebral angle and lesions of the paranasal sinuses. It is also useful for detecting early diastasis of the coronal suture in cases of raised intracranial pressure. a. Lateral wall of the orbit. b. Anterior wall of temporal fossa (greater sphenoid wing). c. Lateral wall of maxillary antrum. d. Foramen spinosum. e. Foramen ovale. f. Foramen magnum. g. Jugular foramen. h. Maxillary antrum. i. Sphenoidal sinus. j. Coronal suture. k. Petrous pyramid. l. Internal auditory canal. m. External auditory canal. n. Tip of mastoid process.

date a hypertrophied middle meningeal artery (meningioma or Paget's disease of the skull vault, or dural arteriovenous malformation). Destruction of the floor of the middle cranial fossa may be detectable only after the outlines of the foramen ovale or foramen spinosum have disappeared.

(c) *Paranasal Sinuses:* Only the submentovertical projection shows each sphenoidal sinus as a separate entity. Mucosal thickening in the maxillary antra is best evaluated, and sometimes diagnosable only in this view.

(d) *Coronal Suture:* The full axial view is the only projection which is made at right angles to the major part of the coronal suture. It reveals convincing suture separation at an earlier stage than lateral or frontal radiographs.

(e) *Petrous and mastoid temporal bone,* especially the petrous tip and middle ear structures: Only the submentovertical projection shows the malleus and incus as two separate structures.

Special Projections

The application of recent technical advances such as high-speed and fine focus tubes to neuroradiology has reduced the value of special-interest ("coned") views of specific structures. Provided only that these structures are visible in the sagittal or coronal planes, they are likely to be optimally seen in routine skull views.

Three paired structures are important exceptions: the optic canals, internal auditory canals and jugular foramina. These foramina lie at a tangent to both the coronal and sagittal planes, and specially angled projections are required to view them (Fig. 1–7).

Optic Canals: Each is a true canal 4 to 9 mm. long in adults, transmitting the optic nerve from the retina to the brain in a medial and upward direction. The central axis of each canal lies at an angle of 37° to the median sagittal plane, and of 20 to 30° to the canthomeatal line. Although geometric tomography can be used to demonstrate the profile of each optic canal in lateral or full-axial projection (Harwood-Nash, 1970; Lloyd, 1975), *en face* views remain the basis of clinical diagnosis. They are made by directing the beam along the central axis of each canal, in one of two techniques: (1) By fixing the position of the tube relative to the film, and then posturing the patient's head for each view—the "four-point landing," so called because four skin points of the face touch the cassette during the exposure, viz., forehead, cheek, chin and nose. Advantage: magnification no more than 15 per cent. Disadvantage: reproducibility is poor due to demands upon patient and technician (Rhese projection—see Goalwin, 1927). (2) By fixing the patient's head in the median-sagittal plane relative to the film, and then altering the angle of the tube to examine first the one canal and then the other. Using the Schönander

skull unit, Lysholm's original method (1931) was improved by Ruggiero (1960), but both possess the disadvantage of magnification. The only method that combines reproducibility with minimum magnification is that of Pfeiffer (1933), who devised a cassette tunnel for use with this technique (2). The optic canal is projected into the lower and outer quadrant of the orbit, lying between the sphenoid ridge and the anterior clinoid process.

Internal Auditory Canals: The neuroradiologist's major interest in the temporal region is the petrous part of the bone and notably the internal auditory canal. Lesions of the mastoid are of lesser neurological interest, and radiographic projections of the mastoid cells will not be discussed. Each internal auditory canal faces the other: in the dry skull, a matchstick inserted into both meatuses lies across the posterior fossa, to lie horizontally in the coronal plane. Diagnostic evaluation is concerned chiefly with the symmetry of the two meatuses and canals, rather than absolute measurements. The two canals, each measured from the vestibule to the well-defined posterior rim of the meatus, should not differ by more than 3 mm., and variations in the size of the meatuses are equally critical (Valvassori and Pierce, 1964; see Ch. 8, p. 387).

Adequate examination of the petrous temporal bones must include, in addition to views of the canals in the conventional radiographic planes, an *en face* projection of each meatus. Several projections have been described but none is superior for evaluating the size of the meatus to the original described by Stenvers (1917). Lysholm's modification, the famous Stockholm C view of the Schönander, makes Stenvers' projection more exact and reproducible. The patient is placed prone and his head lateral, with the temporal bone to be examined nearest the film, then the tube is angled 10° cephalad and positioned to make an angle of 28° to the vertical. The internal auditory canal is foreshortened but the meatus is projected 1 to 2 cm. above the ipsilateral temporomandibular joint. A better view of the middle ear is the modified Schüller projection (Runström, 1933) which shows the sinodural plate, the junction between the petrous bone and the lateral and sigmoid sinuses.

These views should be made routinely whenever a structural lesion of the adjacent soft tissue has to be ruled out—and especially in patients with unilateral sensorineural deafness, and tomography of the petrous bone is probably no substitute for them. The diagnostic yield from such practice is impressive. Osborn (1975), in reviewing the material of one of the present authors (E.H.B.) found that the proportion of patients with acoustic neuromas who show plain-film changes rises from 47 to 78.5 percent if the routine skull series is amplified by special views. The most valuable are the Stenvers and perorbital views. The additional yield

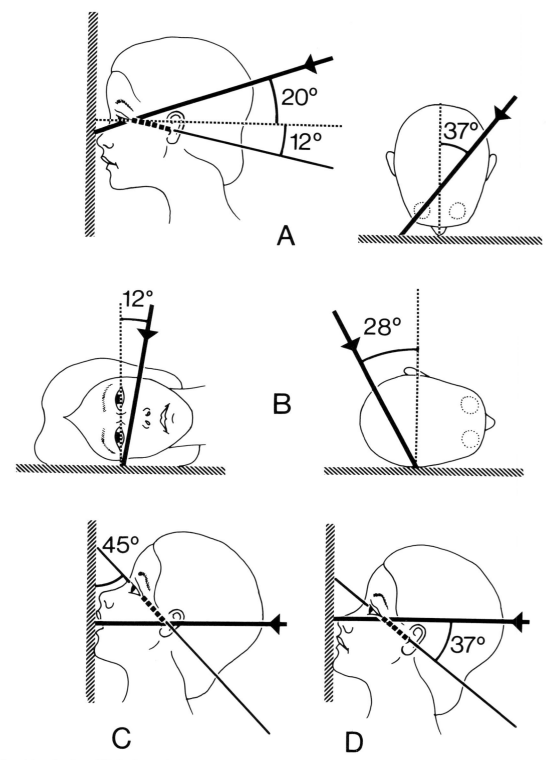

Fig. 1–7 Special projections. (A) Optic canals (Ruggiero's method): the head is fixed relative to the film, and the tube is angled so that the central beam subtends the angles shown in the diagrams. (B) Internal auditory canals (Stenvers' projection). (C) Jugular canals (Rovsing's projection): the tube is fixed at a right angle to the film, then the head is extended until the canthomeatal line lies at 45° to the central beam. Amplified by: (a) tomography, and/or (b) 45° rotation of the head away from the foramen under examination. (D) Facial skeleton—occipitomental (Waters') projection: the tube is fixed at a right angle to the film, then the head is extended until the cantho-meatal line lies at 37° to the central beam. This projection is useful for viewing paranasal sinuses and bony orbits and for lateralizing vault fractures.

from tomography, even pluridirectional sections, is less dramatic.

Jugular Canals: Neither of these paired foramina in the skull base is visible on any of the standard projections listed above. Each transmits an internal jugular vein (arising from the ipsilateral jugular bulb which molds the shape of the canal), three lower cranial nerves (glossopharyngeal, vagus and accessory) and meningeal branches of the terminal external carotid artery. The jugular foramina are not visible on any standard projection of the skull because their long axis is directed anteroinferiorly at 40 to 45° to the canthomeatal line, and also slightly laterally. Wide variations exist from subject to subject and from side to side in the same subject: one canal may be more than twice the diameter of the opposite one, without being abnormal. It is claimed that more than 20 different radiographic techniques have been devised to examine them. The simplest is Rovsing's projection, which is a modification of the occipitomental (Waters' projection) described below, amplified by tomography: the patient lies supine with his head extended so that the canthomeatal line is at 45° to the film. The central ray passes through the open mouth, and the tomographic cuts are made from the level of the external auditory meatus (Di Chiro, Fisher and Nelson, 1964; Hawkins, 1966). An *en face* view of one foramen may be obtained by additionally rotating the head 45° to the contralateral side. This view is especially useful during angiographic and venographic investigations.

Occipitomental (Waters') Projection: This projection was developed more than 50 years ago by an ear, nose and throat surgeon, as a modification of the original PA view of the skull, to examine the maxillary antra and other accessory sinuses (Waters, 1915). It provides the only unencumbered view of the antra, which are projected above the petrous pyramids (criterion of radiographic adequacy: entire floor of each antrum visible!). The view of the bony orbits is second only in value to that given by the PA 20° (Caldwell's) projection. Well shown above is the wall between the orbital roof and the frontal sinuses, which can be destroyed by mucocele, and this projection is particularly useful for evaluating frontal sinus opacity due to infection. Only in this projection are the ethmoidal cells separated: the anterior ones are projected above, the posterior ones below.

The importance of this projection in acute head trauma will be stressed in Chapter 4, where its advantages in lateralizing linear fractures of the skull vault and in detecting facial fractures justify its routine use. Thus, it reveals fractures of the mandible and zygomatic arch, traumatic diastasis of the frontozygomatic synchondrosis, as well as soft tissue damage to the orbit. In blow-out fractures into the maxillary antrum, the normal double floor is disrupted: the upper line on the radiograph corresponds to the palpable rim of the orbit; the lower one represents the orbital floor about 1 cm. behind the rim.

Other Special Projections: "Dedicated" projections are required for several other structures, areas and situations in neuroradiology, e.g., cranioverte-bral angle, head trauma. The chapters of this book have been written to reflect these areas of interest, and reference will be found in each to the appropriate radiographic techniques required.

How to Look at Skull Radiographs

The authors intend the first ten chapters of this book to be a comprehensive treatise of the radiological diagnosis of the skull, and this section is intended merely to provide guidelines for primary interpretation. The majority of the 50 structures which Potter (1971) claimed can be identified in each standard radiographic projection are, while anatomically interesting, not relevant clinically. The practicing neuroradiologist is concerned primarily with those observations that reflect the health of the brain, e.g., evidence of a spaceoccupying lesion or raised intracranial pressure. Therefore the following order is a logical scheme for viewing skull radiographs:

Midline position of the calcified pineal gland
Cortical floor of the pituitary fossa
Other features: focal calvarial changes, abnormal vascular grooves and fractures, opaque mastoids and sinuses, changes at the craniovertebral angle.

Pineal and Choroid Calcification: The position of the calcified pineal gland is the most important neuroradiological observation in plain skull radiographs.

It is so crucial to intracranial diagnosis, that requests to "x-ray skull" would be better phrased, "x-ray pineal," in order to encourage a more aggressive approach in technicians, radiologists and physicians towards identifying it. A displaced pineal gland is a neurosurgical emergency: if associated with a diminishing level of consciousness, the patient's life is probably at risk from imminent brain herniation. Then the duty of the neuroradiologist is clear: immediately to alert his clinical colleagues to the danger. Junior radiologists should be trained to adopt a positive approach, to assume that any laterally displaced pineal is caused by a potentially curable condition such as a subdural hematoma. Most pineal displacements are caused by incurable lesions, either supratentorial gliomas or neoplastic metastases.

Calcium salts are present in the pineal gland at birth and additional (physiological) deposition continues throughout life. Computed tomography invariably reveals calcium in the pineal gland and choroid glomus bodies (Fig. 1–8), but the x-ray photographic process is too insensitive always to demonstrate it. Pineal calcification is visible in the lateral radiographs of just over 50 percent of sub-

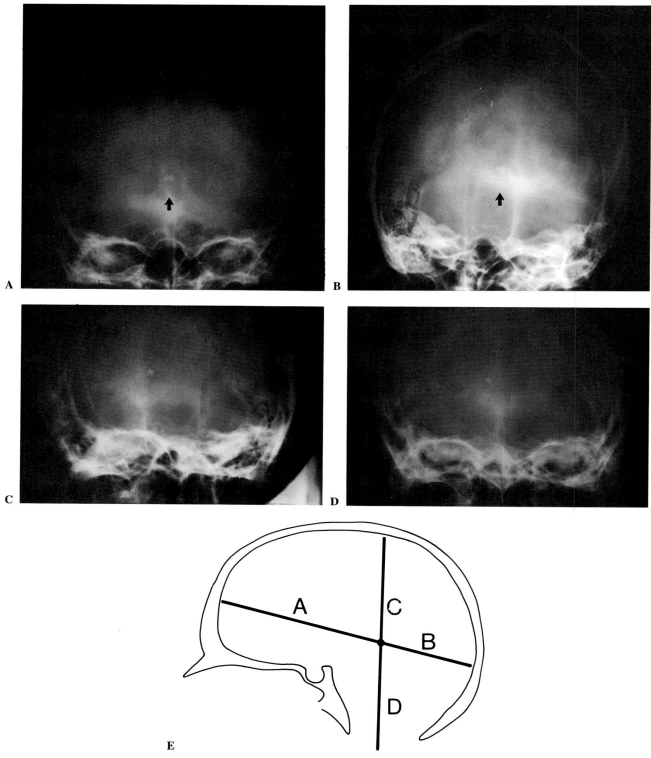

Fig. 1−8 The position of the pineal calcification. 1. *Sideways displacement:* Since the pineal lies in the same vertical plane as the odontoid process around which the skull rotates, a central pineal (*arrow,* A) will remain in the midline upon rotation of the head (B). For the same reason, pineal displacement to one side, when shown on a rotated film such as C, is usually a genuine sign, which may be confirmed by a straight coronal film (D, same patient). This patient had a left subdural hematoma. E. Measurements utilizing a lateral radiograph of the skull: AB = the longest anteroposterior internal diameter passing through the pineal, and CD = a vertical line drawn from the plane of the foramen magnum through the pineal to the inner table of the parietal bone. 2. *Anteroposterior displacement.* The formula of Powsner and Taveras (Taveras and Wood, 1964) gives the distance from the inner table of the frontal bone to the center of the pineal calcification ±5 mm. Thus, $\dfrac{A = 2(A + B) - 5 \text{ cm}}{3}$. 3. *Vertical displacement.* The measurements C and D may be read off in the charts of Vastine and Kinney (1927).

jects (Dyke, 1941). Fewer than 5 percent of children under the age of 10 years show it, and under 20 percent of teenagers, while it is present in more than 70 percent of people over 60 (Vastine and Kinney, 1927). Thus the percentage expectation of pineal calcification corresponds roughly to the chronological age of the patient.

Before measuring the position of the pineal in the coronal projections, a simple precaution is necessary: *verify that pineal calcification is visible on the lateral radiograph!* A solitary plaque of dural or tentorial calcification, a pedunculated external occipital protuberance or a similar density in the scalp of the forehead may mimic pineal calcification in the coronal projections. Calcification in the free edge of the tentorium cerebelli is usually linear, corresponding to its line of attachment. The midline of the brain is best determined by using a ruler and grease marking pencil, and bisecting the distance between both inner (or both outer) tables. The position of the pineal can then be related to the mark. Practically all pineal shifts from the midline are caused by supratentorial mass lesions: tumor, blood or pus within or over the contralateral cerebral hemisphere; the possibility of ipsilateral traction due to an atrophic process is remote. Traditionally a shift of 3 mm. or more is abnormal, but relevant clinical details such as a contralateral hemiplegia may make a lesser degree of displacement significant. Since the pineal gland lies in the same vertical plane as the odontoid process, rotation of the head does not displace it sideways. This observation is relevant to head injury patients, in whom satisfactory skull radiography is not always possible; the position of the pineal may be reliably determined from rotated frontal views, provided that the inner tables of the parietal bones can be identified. This remains possible until the head is rotated more than 20° (Fig. 1–8).

Assessment of pineal displacement from the lateral radiograph is less reliable or useful. A number of methods have been described. Vastine and Kinney (1927) produced tables of the normal range of position of the calcified pineal gland in the vertical plane. Displacement in the sagittal plane may be determined by using the formula of Powsner and Taveras (Fig. 1–8; Taveras and Wood, 1964).

Choroid plexus calcification is usually bilateral and has a stippled or cart-wheel appearance. Occasionally it may be strip-like, extending forward along the floor of the lateral ventricle and/or downward into the temporal horn (Fig. 1–9). Asymmetry is a less reliable sign of a supratentorial mass than pineal displacement, due to loose attachment of the calcified bodies within the ventricles, which permits them to slide forward when the head is prone. However, any significant disruption of the equilateral triangle formed by the glomera and pineal gland should be treated with suspicion, especially medial displacement of one body.

Pituitary Fossa: The neuroradiologist's first interest in the sella turcica is the state of its cortical lining, and not its size or shape. The cortex is a reliable morphological barometer of the intracranial compartment: when the pressure rises the cortex thins, and if the pressure is relieved the cortex will reform. See the next section, Generalized Raised Intracranial Pressure, and Chapter 5 (Fig. 5–3).

Other Features: Once the position of the pineal gland and the health of the sellar lining have been examined, the neuroradiologist should search for other clues of an intracranial lesion. Bone changes are usually found by comparing the two sides of the vault: the normal bone texture and vascular grooving has a symmetrical pattern, and any striking change on one side should prompt suspicion of a meningioma. Most brain abscesses in Western countries are complications of sinusitis or otitis media, therefore an opaque frontal sinus or mastoid may provide the vital diagnostic clue in an ill child. In an unconscious patient, skull radiography may reveal a fracture, intracranial gas or other evidence of head trauma. A small proportion of intracranial tumors and other lesions contain deposits of calcium, the site and pattern of which may enable an etiological diagnosis to be suggested.

THE SKULL IN INTRACRANIAL DISEASES

The nature of an intracranial disease process may be mirrored in the appearances of the plain skull radiographs—sometimes in a diagnostically specific way. In certain cerebral lesions, careful evaluation of the skull changes provides more information than contrast studies. Any or all of three effects may be visible:

1. **Calcium Deposits** within the intracranial lesion(s), which can be distinguished from physiological calcification or from calcium laid down in normal structures such as the basal nuclei.

2. **Generalized Raised Intracranial Pressure:** Recognizable radiological patterns accompany the various clinical hyperpressure syndromes such as the acute picture of papilledema, headache and vomiting and the chronic picture of low-grade hydrocephalus.

3. **Skull Abnormalities:** The response of the skull vault to intracranial processes involves four parameters. There may be changes from the normal in respect of one, two or all of the following:

Size: the head may be larger or smaller
Shape: the deformity may be generalized or focal
Width: the vault may be thicker or thinner (or absent)
Density: the vault may be sclerotic, rarefied or have a heterogeneous pattern.

The characteristic plain-film features of intra-

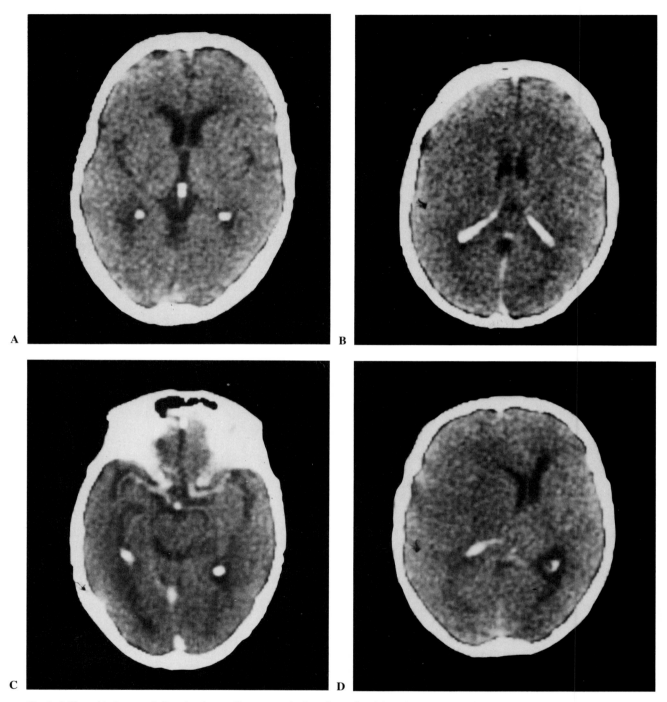

Fig. 1—9 Choroid plexus calcification is usually symmetrical, and may be either circular (A) or linear (B). The two glomus bodies form an equilateral triangle with the pineal calcification of the midline. Asymmetry, although occasionally a normal variant (C), should be viewed with suspicion. (D) A glomus body displaced medially and forwards by an extensive isodense subdural hematoma.

cranial tumors and certain other lestions will be described fully in succeeding chapters. These features include changes such as focal thinning or erosion of the pituitary fossa (chromphobe adenoma) or internal auditory canal (acoustic neuroma), bone destruction (nasopharangeal carcinoma) or reaction (meningioma). Special projections are required to detect erosion of the optic canal (glioma) or jugular foramen (chemodectoma).

The processes producing these changes cover a wide spectrum. They vary from lesions of early life, such as birth injury, to lesions that become

Table 1–1 Intracranial Lesions Deforming The Skull

1. *Generalized Deformity*
   a. Large head (macrocrania)
      Cerebral gigantism and other rare congenital syndromes
      Hydrocephalus
   b. Small head (microcrania): see text, Chapter 1
2. *Focal Deformity Including Asymmetry*
   Cranium bifidum, meningocele and encephalocele
   Craniovertebral-angle anomalies including basilar impression
      and the Chiari malformation: see Chapter 9
   Orbito-cranial dislocation syndromes: see Chapter 5
   Focal brain damage in early life, including hemiatrophy
   Meningioma
   Arteriovenous malformation: see Chapter 3
   Sundry intracranial neoplasms producing specific patterns of
      bone erosion, e.g., pituitary region tumors (Ch. 5), acoustic
      neuromas (Ch. 8)

manifest only in adulthood, such as meningiomas. A useful classification is difficult to devise: even the simplest, viz., lesions producing generalized deformities and lesions producing focal deformity (Table 1–1), does not escape radiological criticism, because of the overlap between entities and the similarity of appearances with the cranial lesions of certain non-neurological skeletal affections.

Pathological Intracranial Calcification
Radiologically visible intracranial deposits of calcium are the result of a variety of processes. In some there is a direct causal relationship, e.g., parasitic or other infection, hypercalcaemic metabolic state or trauma. In others the deposits represent dystrophic calcification in necrotic brain (abscess, neoplasms or tuberculoma) or organizing hematoma or exudate (tuberculous meningitis). In the majority of gliomas the nature of the calcified deposits is ill understood: they are rarely—if ever (Henschen, 1955)—merely a secondary degenerative change. No histological diagnosis can be made from the morphological appearances only, but useful conclusions are frequently possible by considering them in relation to their site and any adjacent bone changes (Kalan and Burrows, 1962).

Morphological Classification: Figure 1–10 illustrates several of the common types associated with unifocal lesions (see below); many deposits defy classification, being too amorphous or varied to describe. Computed tomography of the brain reveals far more intracranial calcification than conventional radiography, because of its greater sensitivity in detecting structures of different density (e.g., Fig. 1–16).

(a) Linear: "String of beads" or "tramline" calcification is traditionally associated with Sturge-Weber's disease or oligodendrogliomas, but this type occurs as frequently in astrocytomas, and also certain non-neoplastic lesions. Curvilinear calcification, i.e., calcium deposits in a ring or arc, possesses more specificity, because it denotes calcification in the wall of a cystic cavity. In calcified aneurysms and arteriovenous malformations, the

deposits are characteristically thin and delicate (see Fig. 5–6).

(b) Granular: Closely-packed nodules, often deposited within a well-defined outline, favors the diagnosis of meningioma, craniopharyngioma, ependymoma or choroid plexus papilloma. However, astrocytomas are commoner glial tumors than either ependymoma or choroid plexus papillomas, and about one-third of all calcified astrocytomas contain granular deposits.

(c) "Cotton-wool": Glioma, craniopharyngioma and non-neoplastic lesions, unlikely in meningiomas or vascular lesions.

(d) "Brain-stone": This term is applied to a dense focus of intracranial calcification, usually situated on the surface of the brain and denoting a meningioma or an organized hematoma. It should be distinguished from an osteoma, i.e., focal thickening of the inner or outer table of the skull, as well as from a "falx stone," which is a nonsignificant physiological phenomenon.

Diagnostic Approach: The neuroradiologist's evaluation of deposits of intracranial calcification should be a process of exclusion. Concerning the calcification, he should ask:

(a) Is it physiological?

(b) Is it abnormally deposited in normal structures?

(c) If pathological, is it a multifocal or unifocal process?

Dramatic artifacts may be produced on individual skull radiographs by scalp swellings such as a wen, greasy hair, poor hygiene or electroencephalogram paste and hair tied in ribbons. The wise neuroradiologist will always ensure that he can identify deposit(s) of calcium in at least two projections, preferably frontal and lateral, before embarking on a differential diagnosis.

(a) Physiological: Apart from pineal and choroid calcification mentioned in the previous section, the principal physiological type encountered is calcification in the dura mater. It occurs around the pituitary fossa (Ch. 5) and over the cortical edge of the cerebral hemispheres; a calcified V-shaped gutter for the superior sagittal sinus may be formed (Fig. 1–11). Dural calcification in the tentorium cerebelli may be mistaken for a deviated pineal gland.

(b) Abnormal Deposits in Normal Structures: These structures include:
   falx cerebri,
   carotid siphons,
   basal ganglia,
   hippocampus,
   dentate nuclei.
According to Dyke (1930), falcine calcification is present in 7 to 9 percent of adults and it may possess no significance, beyond being an aging phenomenon. The uncalcified falx is usually visible if seen end-on in frontal views, its fibrous texture

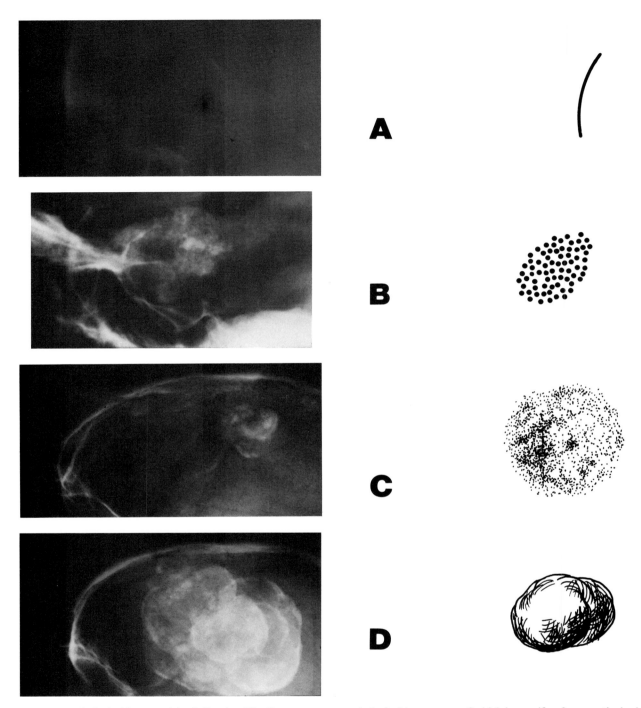

Fig. 1–10 Pathological intracranial calcification. The four common morphological types, none of which is specific of any particular lesion. (A) Linear or curvilinear (giant carotid aneurysm). (B) Granular or nodular (recurrent craniopharyngioma). (C) "Cotton-wool" (astrocytoma). (D) "Brain stone" (meningioma). A fifth type, rather inadequately described as amorphous calcification, represents deposits that are too varied in morphology or too light to reproduce.

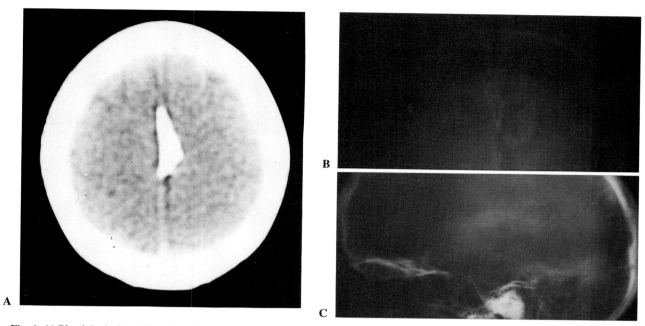

Fig. 1–11 Physiological calcification. (A) Deposits in the falx cerebri—usually ossification ("falx stone"). (B) Deposits in the dura on either side of the falx cerebri and superior sagittal sinus, but not laterally over the convexities of the hemispheres.

casting a linear density. Calcium or bone is deposited in plaques on the lateral side of its leaves. Excessive calcification occurs in hypercalcemic states such as chronic renal failure and hemodialysis (Ritchie and Davison, 1974; Batnitzky, Powers and Schechter, 1974) and hypervitaminosis D, the basal cell nevus syndrome (Amin, 1975) and lipoid proteinosis (Wiley, 1963; Gorlin and Pindborg, 1964).

Atheromatous plaques are frequently present in the internal carotid arteries, particularly at the origins and the siphons, but they are not seen distal to the superior limb. They are usually crescentic, taking the form and shape of one wall of the carotid artery. In coronal or full axial projections, they may project as complete or incomplete calcified ring shadows in the parasellar region (Cole and Davies, 1964).

Microscopic calcification in the basal ganglia and dentate nuclei is a common necropsy finding in the elderly, but deposits that are radiologically visible are infrequent. They are usually bilateral and present in the heads of the caudate nuclei, resembling the caput of the corpus callosum in lateral view and the upper halves of the limbs of a V in frontal views. Deposits in the caudate nuclei are comma-shaped, and obscured by the mastoid cells in lateral view. Two-thirds of patients with radiological evidence of basal ganglia calcification suffer from a disorder of calcium metabolism, usually hypoparathyroidism or pseudohypoparathyroidism (Fig. 1–12). About 50 percent of patients with these diseases show calcified basal ganglia (Bennett, Maffly and Steinbach,

1959). A cause only slightly less frequently seen is idiopathic basal ganglia calcification, and this condition may be familial (Palubinskas and Davies, 1959). Other rare associations are tuberose sclerosis and toxoplasmosis (Camp, 1947), anoxia (see Fig. 10–37), carbon monoxide poisoning and intracranial hemorrhage and arteriovenous malformations. Several ill-defined neurological syndromes with such deposits have been described, e.g., Fahr's disease, mental deficiency and epileptic states, but in all these the extrapyramidal system remains intact.

Calcification in the hippocampus and adjacent choroid plexus of each temporal horn may occur in generalized neurofibromatosis and lipoid proteinosis (Wiley, 1963; Zatz, 1968; Williams, Slimack and Fowler, 1972).

(c) Pathological Calcification: All other deposits are pathological, and often noncontrast radiology takes the diagnosis no further. When this stage of evaluation is reached in a specific case, three aspects should be considered, viz., (l) Multifocal or unifocal lesion? The term *multifocal* means that more than one lesion is present; almost always the deposits are bilateral and sometimes also infratentorial. Unifocal calcification may be a solitary deposit or satellite deposits scattered widely over a hemisphere (see calcified subdural hematoma, Fig. 1–13). A "butterfly" glioma of the corpus callosum may show calcified deposits in both hemispheres and yet it is a unifocal lesion. (2) Associated osseous changes, either in the skull, such as raised intracranial pressure, focal sclerosis or enlarged vas-

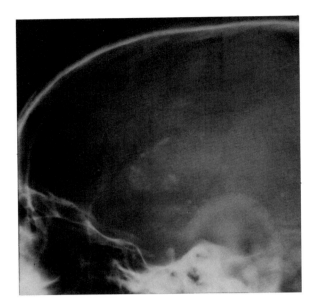

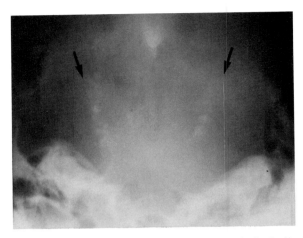

Fig. 1–12 Calcification in the basal ganglia. Deposits in the head of each caudate nucleus, in a 33-year-old woman with hypoparathyroidism due to a parathyroid adenoma. In frontal view the symmetrical deposits *(arrows)* make a V configuration.

cular channels, or elsewhere in the skeleton. (3) Site of calcification (suprasellar, basal ganglia or posterior cranial fossa). This approach narrows the diagnostic possibilities and may lead to recognition of a particular disease or lesion pattern. In this way, some specificity can be imparted to pathological deposits of intracranial calcification (Burrows, 1971).

Multifocal deposits usually denote an infective etiology, particularly in geographical regions where certain infestations are known to occur, such as toxoplasmosis or paragonimiasis. In Western countries tuberous sclerosis merits early exclusion as one of the few important causes of multiple deposits

of pathological calcification. For a comprehensive list of multiple intracranial calcifications, see Reeder (1976).

Unifocal intracranial calcification is the more frequent diagnostic situation, and the causes are legion (Table 1–2). In the authors' practice, astrocytomas and arteriovenous malformations account for the majority of calcified intracranial lesions; by comparison, inflammatory and other types of calcification that are solitary are rare.

Cytomegalic Inclusion Disease: Calcification is seen in about 25 percent of infants suffering from a congenital form of the disease; it does not occur in the adult cases. Calcium is deposited in the lining of the dilated lateral ventricles but, contrary to early descriptions, neonatal paraventricular calcification is not pathognomonic of the disease, since this pat-

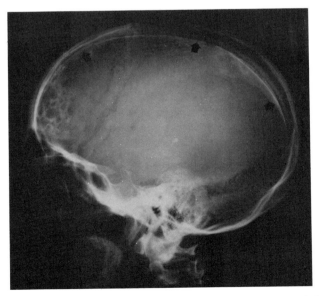

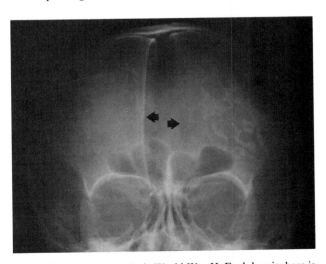

Fig. 1–13 Calcified bilateral subdural hematomas—the result of a head injury 20 years previously in World War II. Each hemisphere is enveloped in a calcified bag *(arrows)*. The subdural membrane over the left frontal lobe has appearances similar to those of calcified pleural deposits. (Reproduced by courtesy of Dr. Desmond Smith, Salisbury Infirmary, Salisbury.)

Table 1-2 Pathological Intracranial Calcification

See Mascherpa and Valentino, 1959; Burrows, 1971 and 1973; Ozonoff, 1971. For multiple foci, see Reeder, 1976.

Diseases Due to Pathogenic Microorganisms

Viruses   – Cytomegalic inclusion disease (25%)
                – Encephalitis (Williams and Fowler, 1972)
Bacteria   – Pyogenic
                – Tuberculosis – Tuberculoma
                                    – Postmeningitic treatment
Parasites   – Toxoplasmosis (59%)
                – Cysticercosis (57%)
                – Trichinosis, paragonimiasis (40%), echinococcosis
Fungi   – Torulosis, coccidiomycosis

Vascular Lesions

Arteriosclerosis
Arteriovenous malformation (20%)
Aneurysm (1%)
Hematoma   – Intracerebral
                – Subdural and extradural

Neoplasms

Glioma   – Astrocytoma (6%)
              – Oligodendroglioma (50%)
              – Medulloblastoma (–)
              – Ependymoma (15%)
              – Choroid plexus papilloma (25%)
              – Miscellaneous
Meningioma (6%)
Craniopharyngioma (75%)
Pearly tumor (epidermoid, dermoid, teratoma)
Pituitary adenoma (4%)
Solitary neurofibroma   – Acoustic (1%)
                              – Trigeminal
                              – Other
Chordoma (50%)
Chondroma, chondrosarcoma
Metastatic malignancy
Lipoma of the corpus callosum
Pinealoma

Miscellaneous

Lissencephaly
Basal cell nevus syndrome (Amin, 1975)
Phakomatoses   – Generalized neurofibromatosis
                      – Tuberous sclerosis
                      – Sturge-Weber's syndrome
Syndromes involving basal ganglia and dentate nucleus (hypoparathyroidism, Fahr's disease, ill-defined neurological syndromes: Bruyn et al., 1963)
Iatrogenic   – Antituberculous treatment
               – Methotrexate therapy
               – X-irradiation treatment
               – Hemodialysis (Ritchie and Dawson, 1974)
               – Ventriculoatrial shunts
               – Leukemia chemotherapy (Borns and Rancier, 1974)

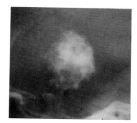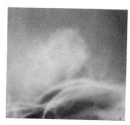

Fig. 1-14 Tuberculoma of the brain (histologically unproven). A 30-year-old man with established tuberculosis and right spasticity. The calcified lesion in the ganglionic region of the left hemisphere has a crenated edge.

percent of these lesions lie below the tentorium. The typical calcified tuberculoma is a solitary, dense brain stone with a crenated edge, but the diagnosis, resting merely on a strong history of infection, often remains unproved (Fig. 1–14).

Improved survival of patients with tuberculous meningitis following the discovery of tuberculostatic drugs has made healed meningeal tuberculous lesions the commonest form of iatrogenic intracranial calcification (Lorber, 1958). The suprasellar region and sylvian fissure are the most frequent sites (Fig. 5–6).

Toxoplasmosis: This is the commonest cause, both of multifocal deposits and of intracranial calcification in neonates. If the classical clinical features of chorioretinitis, psychomotor mental retardation and hydrocephalus are present, calcification is seen in over half of the patients. The deposits vary widely in appearance and are situated in the supratentorial compartment, affecting the meninges and parenchyma of both hemispheres (Fig. 1–15). The diagnosis is favored by identifying calcification in the heads of both caudate nuclei and the combination of parenchymal densities with involvement of the basal ganglia (Sutton, 1951; Müssbichler, 1968).

Other Parasites: In *cysticercosis,* encystment of the larvae in the brain may produce amorphous calcification (Santin and Vargas, 1966). The radiological diagnosis is most likely to be made by demonstrating calcified cysts in muscle masses, where they are uniformly bullet-shaped. Infestation with the oriental liver fluke *(paragonimiasis),* a common condition in parts of Asia, causes arachnoiditis, granulomas and cysts of the brain, and nearly half of these lesions calcify. The deposits are punctate or amorphous but clusters of calcified cysts may have a characteristic soap-bubble appearance (Oh, 1968). Calcification in hydatid cysts *(echinococcosis)* is rare.

Vascular Lesions: The calcification associated with intracranial arteriovenous malformation, aneurysm and atherosclerosis is discussed and illustrated in Chapter 3. Calcified subdural and extradural hematomas are mentioned in Chapter 4.

Gliomas: Any glial tumor may calcify at any age. Mathematical probability ensures that a glioma is

tern may also be seen in toxoplasmosis. Moreover, the ventricles continue to dilate after the calcium has been deposited, and the paraventricular pattern is lost (Molloy and Lowman, 1963).

Tuberculosis: Computed tomography has shown that brain tuberculomas occur more frequently than most Western neuroradiologists believed, because the proportion that calcify or exert space-occupying effects is very low. In Madras, India, tuberculomas account for 28 percent of all intracranial masses, of which only 1 to 8 percent calcify (Ramamurthi and Varadarajan, 1961; Varadarajan, 1965). About 50

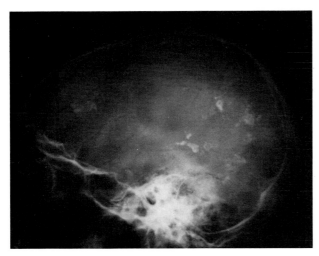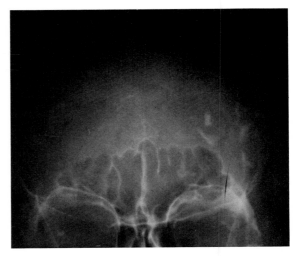

Fig. 1–15 Toxoplasmosis. Multifocal calcified lesions in both hemispheres, but there is no infratentorial calcification.

the most likely cause of any pathological calcification seen within the skull. In the largest group of cases ever collected, Kalan and Burrows (1962) found 149 calcified tumors in a total of 1608 histologically verified gliomas — an incidence of 9.3 percent. Classification according to the various tumor types revealed that while one-half of oligodendrogliomas and one-quarter of choroid plexus papillomas may be expected to calcify (Table 1–2), the most frequently encountered calcified glial tumor is the astrocytoma, because it is four times as prevalent as all the other glioma types combined. The incidence of calcification depends also on the histological grade of malignancy: one-quarter of grade I (Kernohan) astrocytomas calcify, but only 2 percent of grade IV astrocytomas.

The calcium salts indicate the approximate site of the tumor. However the morphological appearances of the deposits, considered by themselves, are valueless in differential diagnosis. All four morphological varieties shown in Figure 1–10 are represented in each glioma-type (exception: no ependymomas show linear deposits). Indeed, from the morphological appearances, the lesion need not be a glioma — or even a neoplasm. Occasionally additional radiological features endow the calcium salts with a glioma specificity: pressure thinning of the skull vault adjacent to calcium deposits almost invariably indicates glioma, not meningioma. Calcium salts in the posterior fossa of a child indicate benign cystic astrocytoma, not medulloblastoma. The incidence of glial calcification appears to be declining: Burrows (1973) in a comparable series of proven gliomas examined between 1966 and 1973, found only 4 percent calcified — a trend that may reflect earlier diagnosis.

Meningioma: Calcification in intracranial meningiomas is rare and overshadowed by an accompanying focal bone reaction which is common and often spectacular. A review of the world literature suggests that the incidence of meningioma calcification is well below 10 percent (Burrows 1971). Cushing and Eisenhardt (1938) observed that tumors lacking contact with the dura, e.g., intraventricular meningiomas, calcify more easily.

All four morphological types of calcification are encountered, but the cotton-wool and curvilinear varieties are rare. The differential diagnosis of well-defined granular deposits is ependymoma and, if suprasellar in situation, craniopharyngioma; that of a brain stone is a calcified intracerebral hematoma. The diagnosis of meningioma, if based on the presence of granular deposits or a brain stone, is greatly strengthened by two factors: (i) site of the calcification — parasagittal gutter, suprasellar region and posterior cranial fossa — and (ii) adjacent focal bone changes such as hyperostosis and/or enlarged middle meningeal artery channels. Calcified deposits near the surface of the brain combined with *thickening* of the adjacent vault or base is virtually pathognomonic of meningioma (Fig. 8–2). Tomography may be indispensable in identifying and elucidating the bone changes and the calcification, and in differentiating between the two.

Site-Dependent Calcification: The following chapters refer to calcified lesions in specific locations:

Chapter 3: aneurysm of the vein of Galen

Chapter 5: pituitary region (craniopharyngioma, pituitary tumors, chordoma, chondroma, trigeminal neuroma)

Chapters 6 and 7: supratentorial hemispheres (lipoma of corpus callosum, pinealoma)

Chapter 8: posterior cranial fossa (acoustic or hypoglossal neuroma, pearly tumor)

Tuberous Sclerosis: Sometimes the radiological appearance suggests the diagnosis in this protean neurocutaneous syndrome because of the particular scatter and multiplicity of lesions. In the brain, the

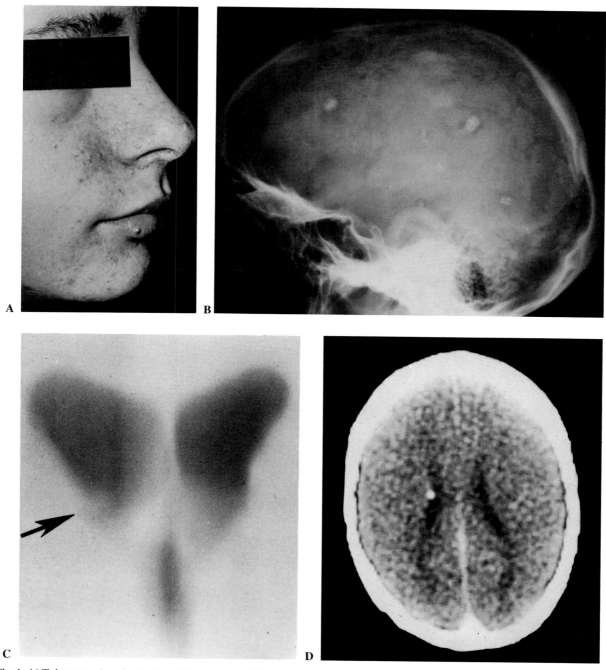

Fig. 1–16 Tuberous sclerosis. (A, B and C) A 9-year-old boy with the facial features of adenoma sebaceum and multifocal calcified intracranial deposits, in whom pneumoencephalography showed calcified tubers adjacent to both lateral ventricles *(arrow)*. (D) Unenhanced computed tomogram in another patient, showing a solitary calcified tuber in the roof of the left lateral ventricle — a pathognomonic picture. The patient was the 50-year-old father of a family of 3 mentally retarded children with epilepsy.

cortical and paraventricular nodules (called tubers by Bourneville in 1880) calcify and may project into the ventricles and/or obstruct the cerebrospinal-fluid pathway: focal calvarial sclerosis, multiple foci of intracranial calcification, hydrocephalus and "candle-guttering" are present in over 50 percent of cases. The nodules appear as ill-defined round de-

posits of amorphous calcification usually about 1 cm. in diameter; in fewer than one patient in four is the calcification solitary. Two features should prompt thought of the diagnosis: a basal ganglion or paraventricular distribution of the calcification and patchy sclerosis of the skull vault or base, which many cases show (Hawkins, 1959; Green, 1968).

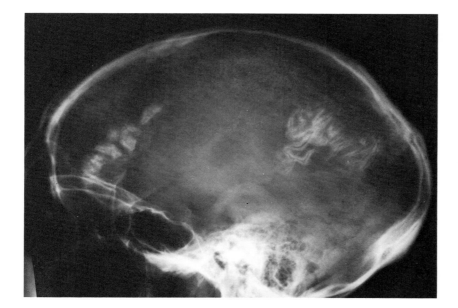

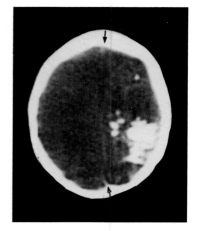

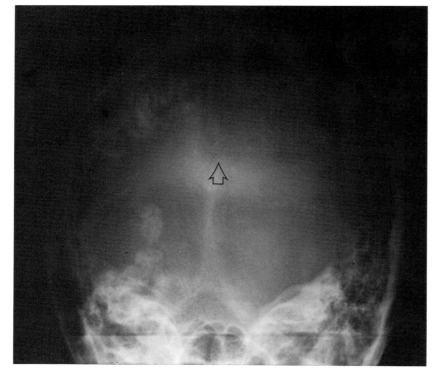

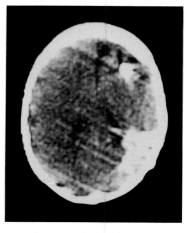

Fig. 1–17 Sturge-Weber's disease. Calcified venous angiomata of the frontal and occipital cortex of the right hemisphere, in a 25-year-old epileptic with a port-wine stain of the right cheek. The half-axial view shows a falx *(arrows)* central to the foramen magnum, but an underdeveloped thickened right side of the calvarium — thus the falx is in the midline, although it appears to be ipsilaterally displaced. Computed tomography confirms the cranial asymmetry midline falx *(arrows)* and thickened right side, and reveals severe focal cortical atrophy surrounding the calcification. Ventricular slices showed no enlargement or displacement of the right lateral ventricle. See Enzmann et al. (1977).

Tuberous calcification is unrelated to the presence of epilepsy or mental deficiency, or to the prognosis (Lagos, Holman and Gomez, 1968). The computed-tomographic appearances are pathognomonic in that all tubers, noncalcified as well as calcified, may be revealed, as well as "candle-guttering," dilated ventricles, associated glial tumors and retinal phakomas (Fig. 1–16). Remote alternative diagnoses to consider in certain cases are heterotopic transmigration of cortical gray matter and arteriovenous malformations of the midbrain (Bergeron, 1969; Medley, McLeod and Houser 1976).

Sturge-Weber's Syndrome (Encephalotrigeminal Angiomatosis): This syndrome which comprises a leptomeningeal venous angioma combined with a port-wine cutaneous stain in the distribution of the ipsilateral trigeminal nerve, is one of the hemisyndromes of early life. Calcification is present in 50 to 60 percent of patients (Coulam, Brown and Reese, 1976). Typically the calcium is deposited within the layers of the atrophic occipital or parietal cortex immediately beneath the angioma, in paired curvilinear lines that follow the cerebral convolutions (Fig. 1–17). Each pair of lines represents adjacent

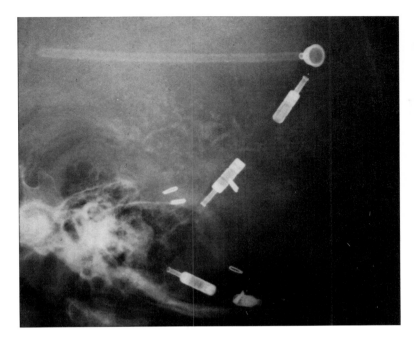

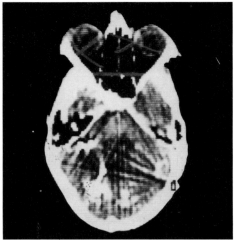

Fig. 1–18 Calcification after x-irradiation. Cystic astrocytoma of the cerebellum treated by excision and shunting. One year later calcified deposites were visible on skull radiography and computed tomography, but there was no evidence of recurrence. See also Figure 10–31.

calcified gyri. The deposits are rarely present before the age of 2 years, but subsequently they increase in density to adulthood. Poser and Taveras (1957) reviewed a large series of cases and found that cerebral angiography is more often abnormal in younger patients without calcified deposits than in older children, in whom calcification is more prevalent. An important diagnostic feature is the associated calvarial hemiatrophy which serves to differentiate the syndrome from other causes of linear calcification such as glioma or antileukemic chemotherapy (Fig. 1–18; Borns and Rancier, 1974; Flament-Durand et al. 1975). For cortical calcification following methotrexate therapy, see Figure 10–31.

Generalized Raised Intracranial Pressure

Intracranial hypertension covers a wide morphological spectrum, which is reflected in a variety of radiological patterns. These patterns are conditioned principally by two factors: (1) the age of the patient and (2) the rapidity of onset of the raised pressure. For example, the picture of acute pressure in a child with a medulloblastoma differs from that of a child with non-tumor chronic hydrocephalus, and both these skulls exhibit separate and different radiological patterns from those of two adults with raised intracranial pressure, in one acute and of recent onset, and in the other low-grade and present throughout life.

Confirmation of the presence of radiological signs of raised intracranial pressure is an important function of the neuroradiologist, a diagnosis in itself. Radiological signs may precede papilledema and other clinical evidence by weeks or even months, therefore they are directly relevant to management of the patient and to decisions about further investigation. The ingredients for a radiological diagnosis of generalized raised intracranial pressure are specific changes in the following structures:

cranial sutures

cortical lining of the pituitary fossa

skull vault: cranial capacity, normal brain impressions, thickness

other: sphenoid planum, optic canals, emissary veins.

Suture Diastasis: If raised intracranial pressure develops before the age of bony union, suture diastasis occurs (Fig. 1–19). There is no other cause of generalized sutural widening: traumatic diastasis is usually asymmetrical and other signs of hypothyroidism provide the diagnosis in untreated cretins with open sutures. Sutures may appear to be widened by regular destruction of bone along their margins due to neuroblastoma or leukemic deposits. Although not closed anatomically until adulthood, the coronal, sagittal and lambdoid sutures cease to spread readily in response to raised pressure after the age of 6 years. While some widening can still take place beyond this age, the possibility diminishes progressively. It should be assumed, for the purposes of practical diagnostic interpretation, that sutural union is complete by 16 years. However, long before this time, probably after the age of 10 years, suture diastasis is seldom seen until the intracranial pressure has been raised for many months. In these older children, it may be a useful confirmation that the lesion is a long-standing one. Du Boulay (1957) studied the relationship between the length of history and the presence of suture diastasis and sellar changes in a large group of children

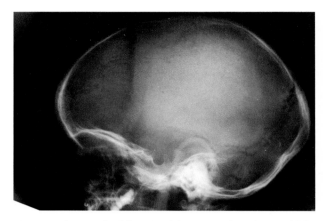 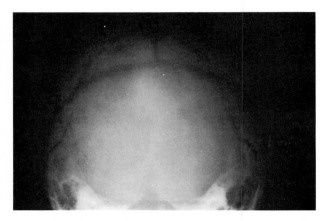

Fig. 1–19 Acute raised intracranial pressure in a 4-year-old boy, due to medulloblastoma. Selective suture diastasis is present, the coronal and sagittal sutures being more severely affected than the lambdoid sutures. The pituitary fossa is normal.

with raised intracranial pressure. He concluded that in children under 6 years suture diastasis may occur very rapidly (within 10 days) and that it may remain the only evidence of raised intracranial pressure for a long time—up to 4 years. In young children with slowly growing tumors, the onset of signs is probably delayed by suture diastasis, this process amounting to a partial decompression (Jupe, 1950).

The particular pattern of suture diastasis, i.e., all sutures equally spread or the coronal suture wider, probably depends on the speed of onset of the raised pressure, rather than its pathogenesis. Thus, most children with medulloblastoma show a preferentially widened coronal suture and, conversely, large-headed hydrocephalic children usually have intact sutures. The coronal suture may be studied in lateral projections that are slightly rotated, or rotated and tilted, but it is best evaluated in the submantovertical projection.

Sellar Changes: Prolonged acute raised intracranial pressure in adults will inevitably breach the cortical lining of the pituitary fossa and produce a "pressure sella" (Fig. 1–20). The early changes and the sequence of development and pathogenesis of this important radiological sign are fully dealt with in Chapter 5.

In younger children "pressure sella" is a less constant accompaniment of raised pressure: only 40 percent of Du Boulay's (1957) series of children under 6 years showed sellar changes, compared with 80 percent of those aged 6 to 16 years. He made two observations in respect of the pituitary fossa: (1) At least 6 weeks of high pressure usually precedes any sellar changes; after this duration of the illness the changes are found in children of any age. (2) In the absence of suture diastasis, erosion of the pituitary fossa in young children usually indicates a local pituitary tumor. An important negative finding: 1 in 4 of the children studied by Du Boulay exhibited no plain-film evidence of the intracranial lesion or of the hyperpressure state it had produced.

Prominent Digital Impressions: Du Boulay (1956) confirmed that a rise in intracranial tension increases the digital impressions of the child's skull ("copper-beating," "increased convolutional markings"). In a careful comparative study he showed that after 10 weeks of raised pressure the impressions in the frontal and parietal regions are significantly more prominent than in health. However, he was forced to the conclusion that this feature is of secondary importance as a radiological sign of raised pressure because: (1) too many normal children have prominent markings and, conversely, a significant number of children with increased pressure never show them; and (2) suture diastasis and sellar changes are likely to have developed before the impressions become striking. "Deep impressions which alone are of no importance may, in the presence of other signs, point towards a long-standing condition."

In adults, accentuated digital markings may be the most dramatic feature of chronic, low-grade raised intracranial pressure, as in a non-tumorous condition such as aqueduct obstruction (Fig. 1–21). An increased cranial capacity and usually a deformed pituitary fossa are integral features of this radiological syndrome. Very occasionally, intracranial neoplasms accentuate the digital markings before producing a "pressure sella," and here correct interpretation requires the caution of experience.

Increased Cranial Capacity and Generalized Calvarial Thickening: Hydrocephalus which starts in infancy or childhood and remains unrelieved will enlarge the vault and thicken it (Fig. 1–22). This situation represents the end of the spectrum of generalized raised intracranial pressure, and will be considered in the next section, Generalized Deformity, Macrocrania.

Other Features: Other secondary radiological features of raised intracranial pressure are: (1) thinning of the floor of the anterior cranial fossa and the

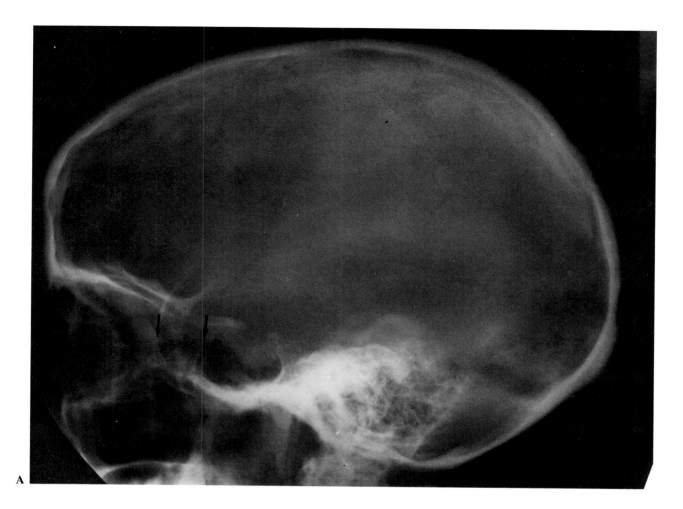

A

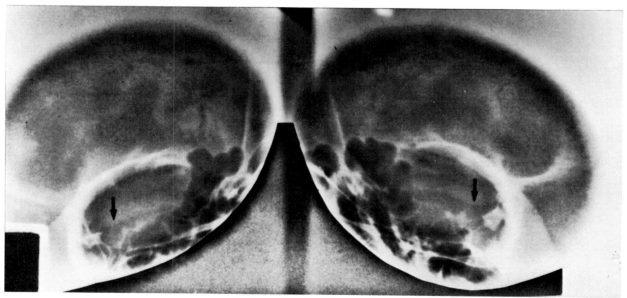

B

Fig. 1–20 Acute raised intracranial pressure in a young adult, caused by a malignant parietal glioma. (A) Lateral view, showing loss of the cortical lining of the pituitary fossa, the sphenoid planum and the cribriform plate *(arrows)*. (B) Special views of the optic canals. The cortical lining of each canal has virtually disappeared, and the position of each *(arrow)* is best identified by the prominent landmarks on its lateral side, the anterior clinoid process. The canals are not abnormally enlarged, although some magnification is present.

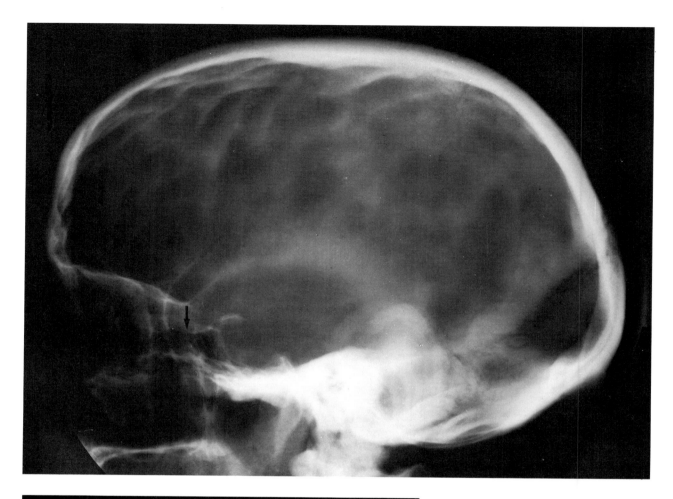

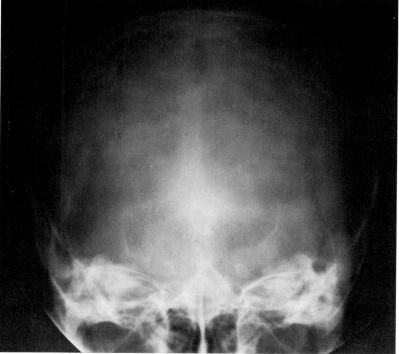

Fig. 1—21 Chronic raised intracranial pressure in an adult due to nontumor aqueduct stenosis. The head is enlarged and the vault shows accentuated digital markings but the sutures are not abnormally wide. The pituitary fossa shows a characteristic deformity, the effects of long-standing compression by a dilated third ventricle. The floor of the anterior cranial fossa is deepened *(arrow)*.

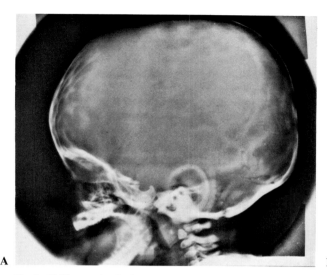 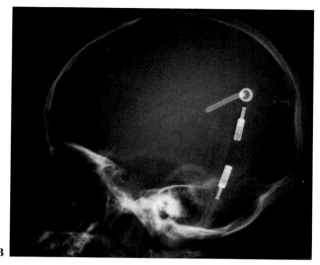

A   B

Fig. 1–22 Obstructive hydrocephalus in a child caused by basal adhesions. (A) Infant, before treatment: the vault is enlarged and paper-thin, the sutures are not properly visible. Cronqvist index = 65. (B) Five years later, after successful ventricular-atrial drainage: the vault has thickened, digital markings are absent, and the sutures have united. Despite normal growth of the skull over five years, the cranial capacity is smaller than before treatment. Cronqvist's index = 53.

planum sphenoidale, and (2) loss of the cortical lining of the optic canals (Fig. 1–19). (3) Enlargement of calvarial emissary veins, particularly that in the occipital midline near the torcular Herophili.

Raised Pressure Patterns: Abnormally raised pressure is a continuous process but the child's skull behaves differently from the adult's skull, thus there are two continuous processes to consider. In either child or adult, the picture of acute pressure will change into one of chronic pressure, if the patient survives. For practical purposes, there are at least four radiological pressure patterns.

(a) Acute in Children (Fig. 1–19): The best example is a rapidly-growing malignant tumor such as medulloblastoma. Diastasis of the sutures may be the only sign, with the coronal suture more widely spread than the lambdoid. Discrepant sutural spread reflects the acuteness of onset of the raised pressure rather than merely the presence of obstructive hydrocephalus. The pituitary fossa may be abnormal but in such instances in older children without striking suture diastasis, the possibility of erosion from an adjacent tumor should always be considered.

(b) Chronic in Children (Fig. 1–22): In non-tumor lesions, the child's head is large to clinical and radiological measurements. The sutures are usually normal and a "pressure sella" is never present. The pituitary fossa, if abnormal, shows the curious deformity of chronic hydrocephalus (see Fig. 5–3). The vault may be thinner than normal, but tends with time and molding to become thicker: bossing is a feature of chronic hydrocephalics. Slowly growing neoplasms may present a more dramatic picture: very prominent digital impressions and thinning of the vault, with inconstant in-

volvement of sutures and sella. In such cases, a search should be made for infratentorial deposits of calcium, indicating a cystic cerebellar astrocytoma.

(c) Acute in Adults (Fig. 1–20): The primary sign is the "pressure sella" and it may be the only one present. Other signs such as accentuated digital impressions or erosion of the sphenoid planum or optic canals, are of secondary significance. See Chapter 5 and Figure 5–3.

(d) Chronic in Adults (Fig. 1–21): See the next section, Generalized Deformity, Macrocrania.

Generalized Deformity
This section is confined to a review of those intracranial conditions which make the skull larger (macrocrania) or smaller (microcrania) than normal. All partial or asymmetrical deformities are discussed in the next section, Focal Changes.

Before discussing the changes in the size of the skull it is necessary to define the range of normal variation. The cranial vault is molded by the brain, and its shape and size are largely controlled by the size and rate of growth of the brain. Unfortunately the range of normal provided by absolute measurements of the skull, based on its length, height and width, is too wide to be useful, and the cranium is better evaluated by relating its volume to the size of the face. Craniofacial proportions alter with age: at birth the cranial volume is eight times as great as the facial volume, but at 6 years the index is 3:1; and by 18, 2:1. Cronqvist (1968) utilized these facts to construct an index of cranial size which requires only lateral and anteroposterior radiographs of the skull (Fig. 1–23). It is easy to use, and American authors have confirmed its reliability, although they found that the index falls through Cronqvist's

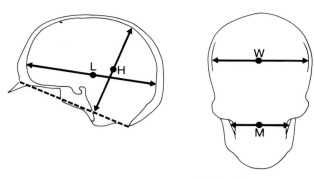

Fig. 1–23 Cronqvist's cranial index $= \dfrac{H + L + W}{M} \times 10$. Using standard lateral and anteroposterior views, the greatest distance between the inner tables is measured in cm. in three directions: H = height, being the maximum perpendicular distance between the vault and a line joining the nasion to the posterior rim of the foramen magnum, W = width, and L = length. The sum of the 3 measurements is divided by the distance between the inner margins of the necks of the mandible (M), and this quotient is then multiplied by 10. Normal range: 51–57, ± 2 standard deviations.

range, from 57 to 53, in the first 5 years of life (Austin and Gooding, 1971).

Large Head (Macrocrania): A symmetrically enlarged head indicates hydrocephalus in the majority of cases (Kingsley and Kendall, 1978). But before this diagnosis can be made, two other groups of conditions must be discussed, which enlarge the head symmetrically. These are (1) diseases that thicken the bones of the skull without significantly altering the intracranial volume, e.g., Paget's disease, acromegaly and chronic severe anemias such as thalassemia (Cooley's Mediterranean anemia), sickle-cell disease and congenital spherocytosis. (2) Diseases associated with hypertrophy of cerebral substance such as cerebral gigantism (Sotos' disease), a very rare entity caused by hypothalamic hypersecretion, or infantile hydranencephaly, an equally rare disturbance analogous to hydrocephalus which converts the neonatal brain into a bag of fluid (see Fig. 10–35). Combined macrocrania and macroencephaly has been reported in generalized neurofibromatosis (Holt and Kuhns, 1976) and acromegaly (Rådberg, 1974).

Certain radiological patterns of hydrocephalus may be defined, which depend predominantly on the interrelationship between the enlarged brain and growth of the skull vault. The picture varies with its speed of development, and whether the process is "active" or arrested.

(a) In the acute hydrocephalus of childhood caused by neoplasm, lymphoma or leukemia, the outstanding feature is suture diastasis (Fig. 1–19).

(b) In the commoner variety, non-neoplastic hydrocephalus, the characteristic feature of the enlarged head is the thinned vault indicating that while brain volume is outstripping calvarial ossification

(Fig. 1–22), the pace of expansion of the brain is so slight that it is totally compensated by the new bone deposited along the suture margins. Consequently the sutures do not separate, although the interdigitations may lengthen. The appearances do not vary with different causes, which are those of non-neoplastic obstruction of the cerebrospinal fluid pathway in early life, viz., meningitis or subarachnoid bleeding (see Ch. 10).

(c) Spontaneous or therapeutically-induced arrest of hydrocephalus causes the head to cease enlarging further (although it may remain abnormally large), and then excess bone is deposited on the inner table along suture lines (Fig. 1–22).

Premature closure of the sutures and excessive thickening of the skull may follow the insertion of a ventriculoatrial valve and other surgical shunting maneuvers (Fig. 1–50; Anderson, Kieffer and Wolfson, 1970).

(d) Dysostosis Multiplex (Gargoylism, Hurler-Hunter's Syndrome): Children with this type of mucopolysaccharidosis are mentally retarded dwarfs with large heads and faces. The diagnosis is usually made from the grotesque and repulsive facies which is characteristic. The hydrocephalus is thought to be caused by basal obstruction of the cerebrospinal fluid pathway by the mucopolysaccharide, heparitin sulfate (Russell, 1949). The radiological appearances of the enlarged head are striking: thick vault, especially the frontal squame, which has a geometric curve in lateral projection, thickened supraorbital plates, complete absence of sagittal markings and a J sella in about two-thirds of cases (Horrigan and Baker, 1961). Neuhauser and his colleagues (1968) suggested that the pituitary changes are the result of suprasellar arachnoid cysts.

(e) Non-tumor Aqueduct Stenosis: Infants with this condition may sometimes be recognized by the disproportionate enlargement of the supratentorial part of the vault, compared with the face, craniovertebral angle and squamous part of the occipital bone. The condition may present for the first time in young adults who are mentally normal, and the skull shows characteristic radiological features of chronic low-grade hydrocephalus described above (Fig. 1–21).

(f) Non-tumor Outlet Obstruction (Including Dandy-Walker's Syndrome): See Chapter 10.

Small Head (Microcrania): A small head is far more likely to be the result of a damaged brain that has failed to stimulate a normal skull to grow, than the result of a normal brain being restricted by a skull that cannot expand (generalized craniostenosis). Thus a microcrania usually reflects a microcephaly. The etiology of microcephaly is a subject of pediatric neurology, but the neuroradiologist should be aware of the importance of fetal injury as a cause of failure of normal growth. Total-brain

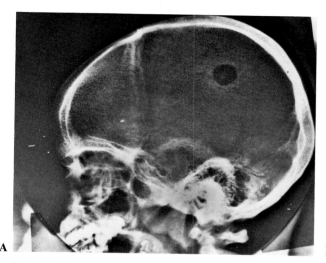
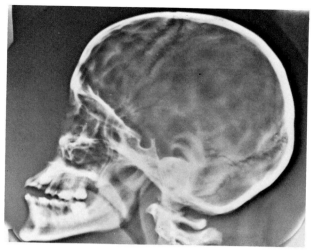

A   B

Fig. 1–24 Microcrania in brain-damaged children. (A) A high-grade mental defective with a history of perinatal trauma and subsequent burrhole evacuation of a subdural hematoma. The thick vault shows no digital markings and possesses a uniform "gritty" texture. The sutures have sclerotic margins. The striking feature is the small cranial capacity, Cronqvist's cranial index = 46. (B) Mongol, aged 8 years. The craniofacial disproportion is caused by the microcephaly. Sutures remain patent, but the vault is not abnormally thin and digital markings are present. Cronqvist's cranial index = 47.

growth may be retarded by genetic deficits such as phenylketonuria or abnormal lesions such as trisomy 13–15 or mongolism; by x-irradiation or German measles; and by infections such as toxoplasmosis and cytomegalic inclusion disease (Farmer, 1964).

Specific radiological features other than microcrania may be associated with microcephaly (Gordon, 1970). The most severe retardation of brain growth produces a cranium that compensates for the reduced intracranial content. Severe craniofacial disproportion is present, and radiologically the face looks as large as the brain, the forehead slopes backwards, the vault is thickened and digital impressions are absent—a "gritty" skull (Fig. 1–24). Mongols and other children whose mental deficit is compatible with a long lifespan, show less dramatic changes: the vault may not be thick, digital impressions may be present, and the sutures are patent or abnormally wide (Fig. 1–24B). In most, the cranial capacity is markedly reduced (Ingalls, 1947; Burwood, Gordon and Taft, 1973).

Focal Changes Including Asymmetry

Intracranial lesions may produce five types of localized change of the skull bones, viz.:

sclerosis: increased density
hyperostosis: increased thickness
erosion: thinning from pressure resorption
destruction: from infiltration
deformity: a misshapen skull, both tables being involved.

All the intracranial pathological processes responsible for such changes will be mentioned in this section and the neuroradiologist should be familiar with them, in order to be able to identify "non-neu-

rological" diseases that may produce similar focal changes of the skull.

Meningioma and Its Differential Diagnosis: The bone reaction evoked by this tumor is so variable that the presence of any focal abnormality of the skull, not necessarily only in adults, should prompt consideration of this diagnosis (Fig. 1–25). Although meningiomas account for less than one-quarter of intracranial tumors, their potentially benign nature enhances their neurosurgical importance.

Two epidemiological features are relevant in radiological diagnosis: (1) site: about 50 percent of intracranial meningiomas occur on the vertex of the brain, over the convexity or in the parasagittal gutter of a hemisphere. Most of the remainder lie on the floor of the skull, involving especially the sphenoid bone (pterion, wings and planum) cribriform plate, suprasellar and parasellar region, also on the clivus and in the posterior fossa. (2) Age of the patient: traditionally, meningiomas are tumors of middle age, but they are sufficiently prevalent in children and adolescents to reduce the value of the age factor in differential diagnosis.

Four groups of changes may be present in the skull radiographs of patients with meningiomas. They are:

nonspecific signs of an intracranial mass: one-third of cases
calcification: under 10 percent
focal bone changes: about 50 percent
abnormal vascular grooves: about 10 percent.

Focal bone changes, if present, most often take the form of bone production. Thickening, or hyperostosis, cannot be separated from an increase in density, or sclerosis—an element of both is usually present.

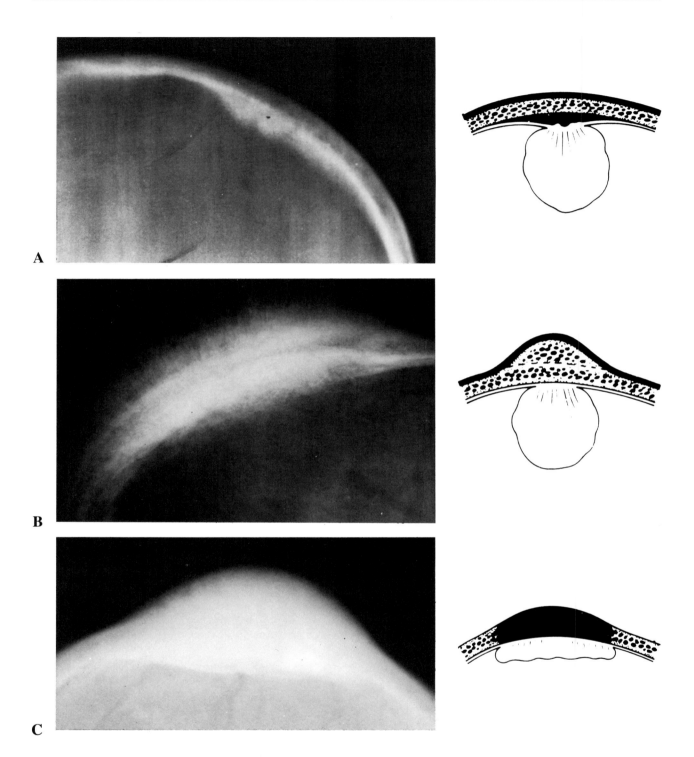

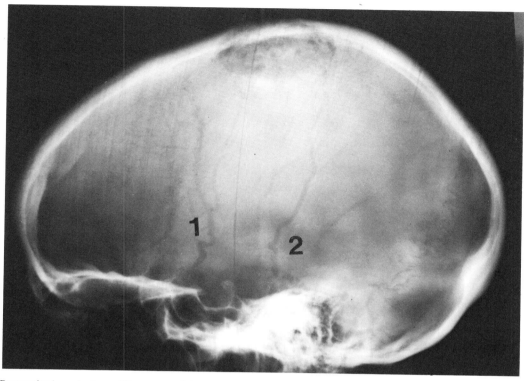

B

Fig. 1–28B Parasagittal meningioma. The nature of the lytic lesion on the parietal vault is obvious from the hypertrophied blood vessels that supply it. 1. Middle meningeal groove (inner table). 2. Groove in outer table for hypertrophied superficial temporal artery.

the distal parts of either the anterior or posterior branches are unusually prominent; normally these vessels taper and do not reach the inner table on the lateral radiographs. These changes are often bilateral, and hypertrophied dural branches of the vertebrobasilar circulation that feed the lesion also may groove the skull. Thus, meningiomas with a dural attachment can show a similar abnormal vascular pattern to dural arteriovenous malformations (see Fig. 3–29).

Prominent vascular grooves including enlargement of a foramen spinosum are often difficult to diagnose with certainty as abnormal, especially if bilateral, due to the wide range of normal variation (Fig. 1–27). However, unilateral increased vascularity may be present to indicate the site of an underlying meningioma: this is the pepper-pot appearance of the skull, a cluster of discrete translucencies produced by enlarged branches of the superficial temporal artery perforating the skull to supply the lesion (Schunk, Davies and Drake, 1964; Fig. 1–28).

The differential diagnosis of meningioma depends on the particular bone reaction manifested by the tumor. Fibrous dysplasia of bone and osteosclerotic metastases invading the skull base may be indistinguishable from an *en plaque* meningioma, and meningiomatous bone production on the skull

vault can resemble a variety of diverse conditions (see Table 1–3).

The neuroradiological relevance of the conditions

Table 1–3 Sclerosis and /or Hyperostosis of the Skull

Generalized
Arrested hydrocephalus
Severe chronic anemias, e.g., Cooley's Mediterranean anemia
Microcephalic and brain damage states
Paget's disease
Acromegaly
Hyperparathyroidism
Fluorine intoxication
High vitamin D levels
Hyperphosphatasemia (Van Buchem's disease)
Progressive diaphyseal dysplasia (Engelmann's disease)
Osteopetrosis (Albers-Schönberg's disease)
Myotonia congenita (Thomsen's disease)
Craniometaphyseal dysplasia (Pyle's disease)
Pycnodysostosis
Focal
Metastases
Meningioma
Fibrous dysplasia of bone
Hyperostosis frontalis interna
Osteoma
Hemangioma
Osteogenic sarcoma
Cerebral hemiatrophy (Davidoff-Masson-Dyke's syndrome)
Cephalhematoma
Chronic osteomyelitis
Tuberous sclerosis

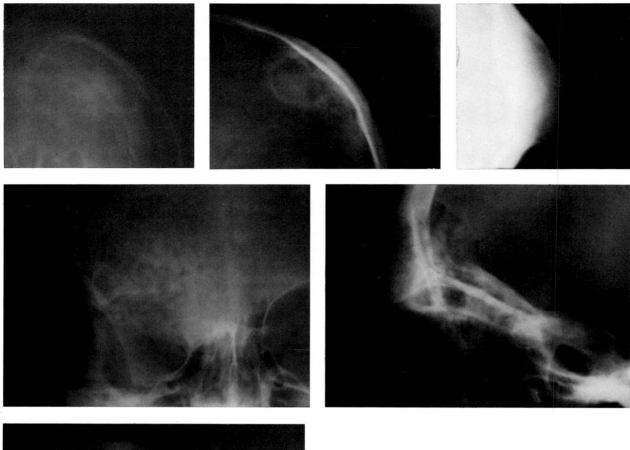

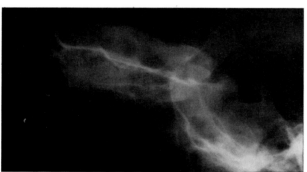

Fig. 1–29 Fibrous dysplasia of bone, three types. *(Top)* Cystic lesion of the vault. The inner table is not involved, the extent of deformity of the outer table is shown by the tangential projection. *(Middle)* Mixed type ("pips in a jelly")—cystic lesion of the frontal squame deforming the orbit, combined with sclerotic deformity of the right sphenoid wings including the anterior clinoid process. *(Bottom)* Homogeneous sclerotic lesion of the body and left sphenoid wings.

discussed below lies chiefly in differentiating the bone lesions they produce from those of meningioma.

(a) Fibrous Dysplasia: Two types of lesion are found in the skull, and there are also mixed lesions (Fig. 1–29). The radiolucent (cystic) type affects the vault, especially the parietal and the supraorbital regions. The edge of the lesion is well defined; often there is a peripheral border of sclerosis. The inner table is normal and the diploic widening causes a bulging outer table: tangential views reveal the outward bulge and the absence of intracranial extension (Leeds and Seaman, 1962). The sclerotic type has a predilection for the body of the sphenoid bone and adjacent facial bones. The deformed bone usually has a ground-glass appear-

ance which is lacking in *en plaque* meningiomas. The mixed type contains features of both: thickened bone, well-defined border, bulging outer table and a homogeneous cystic content occupied by osseous foci ("pips in a jelly"). Fibrous dysplasia occurs in young subjects and progression, when it occurs, takes place only during the years of growth. Other useful differential-diagnostic points from meningioma are the distinctive appearances and distribution of the skull lesions and the different clinical picture: fibrous dysplasia deforms but it only rarely causes neurological signs such as blindness, deafness and raised intracranial pressure.

(b) Hyperostosis Frontalis Interna: Bilateral, symmetrical bone deposition on the frontal squame is seen in many older women. The condition is re-

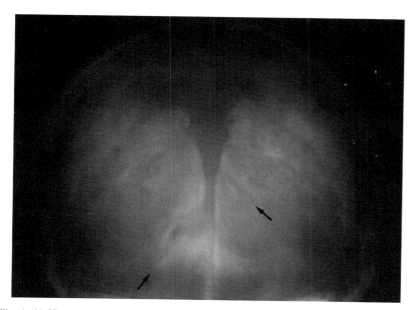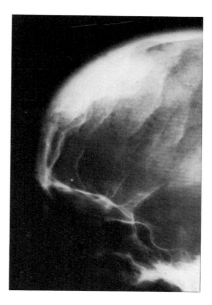

Fig. 1–30 Hyperostosis frontalis interna. Bilateral thickening of the inner table of the frontal squame, with sparing of the midline (falcine attachment) and the channels for the cortical veins (arrows).

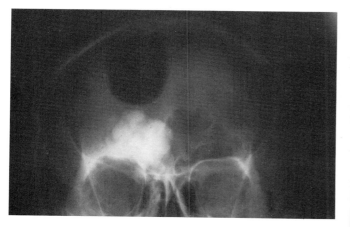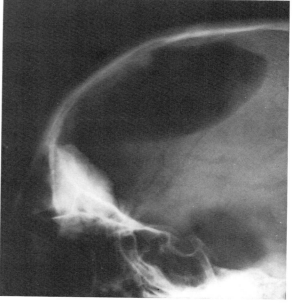

Fig. 1–31 Osteoma of the right frontal sinus producing intracranial complications, viz., space-occupying effects on the contents of the anterior cranial fossa and pneumatocele following perforation of the intracranial dura. Clinical presentation: acute pyogenic meningitis.

garded as harmless and symptomless but its almost exclusive occurrence in postmenopausal females has led to postulation of an endocrine, i.e., estrogen-linked, association; many of the women are very fat. However, identical changes are occasionally encountered in males and young females. The association of bone change, obesity and virilism has been called Morgagni's syndrome; that of the bone change, obesity and mental abnormality, the Stuart-Morel syndrome (Moore, 1955). The radiological diagnosis depends on the site and distribution of the new bone (Fig. 1–30). It is usually confined to the inner table of the squamous part of the frontal bone, and it projects into the cavity of the cranium with a nodular or smooth surface to which the dura mater is tightly adherent. The hyperostosis extends to and across the diploe, but does not transgress the outer table, and characteristically it spares the frontal air sinuses, the median groove of the superior sagittal sinus and the channels for its tributary cortical veins (Burrows, 1950).

(c) Osteoma: Osteomas are probably the com-

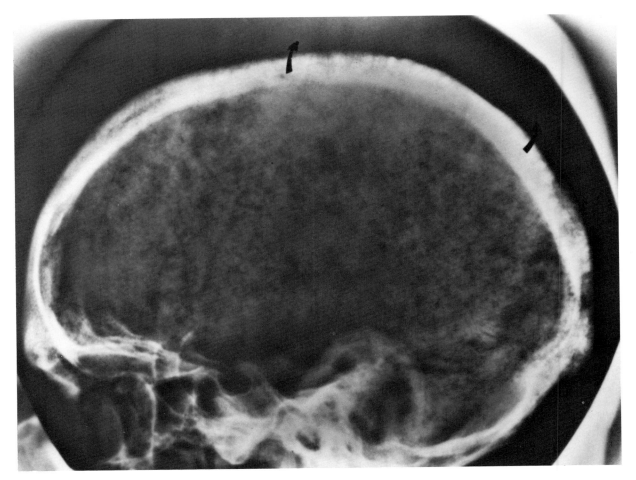

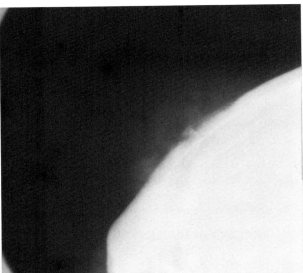

Fig. 1−32 Osteogenic sarcoma. *(Top)* Secondary to Paget's disease. A 60-year-old man with bone changes of the vault and a large soft-tissue mass *(arrows)*. Pagetoid changes were present in the pelvis and a tibia. *(Bottom)* Primary in a 30-year-old man with a large soft-tissue swelling of forehead. The soft tissue lateral view shows destruction of the outer table with irregular new bone formation.

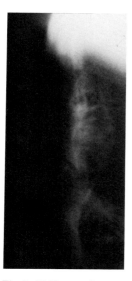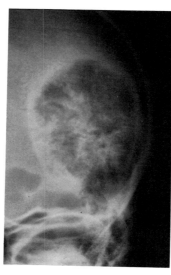

Fig. 1–33 Hemangioma of bone. A radiolucent lesion with well-defined margins and a characteristic honeycomb appearance. The profile view permits the differential diagnosis from osteogenic sarcoma: in hemangioma the spicules are coarser and the spiculation is carried into the depth of the bone; usually there is no soft-tissue mass.

Table 1–4 Lytic Skull Lesions

Congenital
  Cranium bifidum
  Craniolacunia
  Parietal foramina
  Cleidocranial dysostosis
  Generalized neurofibromatosis (sphenoid and lambdoid defects)
Traumatic
  Operative and traumatic defects
  Leptomeningeal cyst
Inflammatory
  Acute osteomyelitis (pyogenic, tuberculous, etc.)
Neoplastic and Infiltrative
  Epidermoid and dermoid
  Meningioma
  Neuroblastoma
  Leukemia
  Fibrosarcoma
  Osteogenic sarcoma
  Metastasis
  Lymphoma
  Myeloma
  Histiocytosis-X (eosinophil granuloma, Hand-Schüller-Christian's, Letterer-Siwe's syndromes)
  Sarcoidosis
  Osteoclastoma (base and mandible)
Miscellaneous
  Radiation necrosis
  Fibrous dysplasia of bone
  Symmetrical parietal thinness
  Paget's disease (osteoporosis circumscripta)

monest benign tumors of the skull. They grow from the outer table (exostosis), or the inner table (enostosis) or the wall of a paranasal sinus. Although osteomas do not invade the diploe or the other skull table, a solitary benign cortical enostosis may be indistinguishable from a bone-producing meningioma. When osteomas occur in the paranasal sinuses they may grow to a giant size and pressure-erode adjacent structures. Modes of clinical presentation then include meningitis or rhinnorhea (dural perforation, Fig. 1–31) and pneumocephalus, proptosis (orbital spread) or mental changes (frontal lobe displacement) (Hudolin et al., 1961).

(d) Osteogenic Sarcoma: This malignant tumor of bone may be encountered in the skull vault, albeit only very rarely: in Southampton over the past decade, 8 cases have been seen, compared to 255 intracranial meningiomas. Two were secondary to Paget's disease, and the other 6 were primary lesions in young men (Fig. 1–32). A specific diagnosis may be impossible, although the combination of a disproportionately large soft-tissue swelling and underlying calvarial changes should always prompt consideration of a malignant bone tumor. Radiating marginal spiculation does occur, but it is more frequently seen in osteosarcomas of the long bones.

(e) Hemangioma of the Vault: This well-defined focal abnormality of the diploe and outer table may be confused both with meningioma and sarcoma. It consists of a honeycomb of large vascular spaces arranged vertically which expands the outer table into a palpable lump. The profile of the honeycomb may have a sunray appearance due to the bony spicules, but unlike osteogenic sarcoma the spiculation

is coarser and carried into the depth of the lesion and the lump has no soft-tissue elements. *En face* a cart-wheel arrangement of the bony diploe may be present (Fig. 1–33). If diagnostic doubt exists, selective external carotid angiography may be helpful (Rosenbaum et al., 1969).

Meningiomas infiltrating the diploe and destroying bone are so rare that more frequent causes of calvarial destruction should take priority in the differential diagnosis of a solitary lytic lesion (Table 1–4). It is narrowed by factors favoring meningioma, viz., adult age of the patient (only in respect of differentiating non-Pagetoid sarcoma), preferential locations such as the parasagittal gutter, and a palpable bony lump. The most likely diagnoses to be considered are: lytic or mixed metastatic deposits from a primary renal, thyroid or bronchial carcinoma, osteomyelitis, histiocytosis-x, hemangioma of bone and, very rarely, fibrosarcoma (Fig. 1–34). If the meningiomatous infiltration extends over a sufficiently large area of the skull, it may resemble osteoporosis circumscripta (see Paget's disease, below).

Arteriovenous Malformation: See Chapter 3, pages 140–142.

Focal Brain Damage in Early Life: Brain damage or trauma of a generalized type in early life produces microcrania (see previous section). Less extensive lesions cause asymmetrical focal deformities of the skull, and there may be other evidence of disturbed brain growth such as a reduced

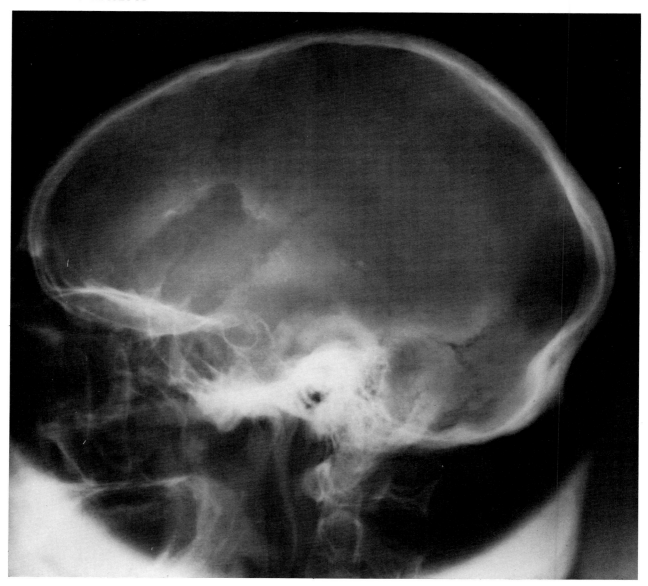

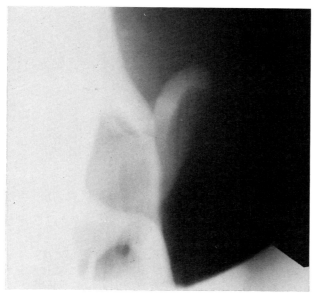

Fig. 1–34 Fibrosarcoma. Destruction of the outer table of the vault only, with a tangential arrangement of newly-formed trabeculae. No specific diagnosis is possible from the radiological appearances, although the large soft-tissue swelling *(tangential view)* indicates the likelihood of a primary malignant neoplasm.

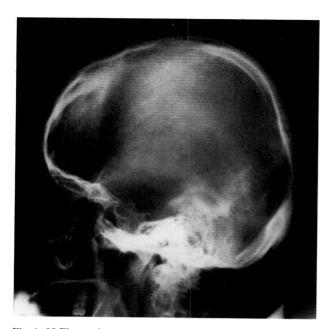

Fig. 1–35 Flat occiput associated with brain damage of early life. The vault molds in this fashion because the infant's head lies motionless on the pillows. The patient was a 54-year-old mental defective who had spent his whole life in an institution. Cronqvist's cranial index = 48.

cranial capacity and a thickened skull vault.

(a) Postural Asymmetry: Neuroradiologists sometimes see minor degrees of asymmetry of the vault or base which they tend to dismiss as insignificant. There is some evidence that such changes are more frequent in epileptics and others with evidence of brain damage in early life (McRae, 1948). The simplest significant deformity is a flattening of the parieto-occipital vault, a deformity of the skull caused by inability of the backward infant to lift his head from the pillows (Fig. 1–35).

(b) Cerebral Hemiatrophy (Dyke-Davidoff-Masson Syndrome): The most severe focal brain damage is an arrest of development of one cerebral hemisphere which then atrophies. Normal growth of the opposite hemisphere produces a striking asymmetry of the skull which involves the base as well as the vault. On the affected side, the skull appears to expand inwards by thickening, literally to compensate for the atrophic hemisphere (Dyke, Davidoff and Masson, 1933). Thus, some or all of the following features may be present: elevated petrous pyramid, enlarged frontal sinuses and mastoid cells, thickening and flattening of the ipsilateral half of the vault, absent digital markings, ipsilateral displacement of the sagittal suture and/or angulation of the falx (Fig. 1–36). Cases of the Sturge-Weber syndrome may show a similar picture (Fig. 1–17; Poser and Taveras, 1957).

The cranial asymmetry of cerebral hemiatrophy must be differentiated from plagiocephalic craniostenosis, in which one half of the coronal suture fuses prematurely, and also from the cranial hemihypertrophy syndromes (temporal arachnoid cyst, orbital neurofibromatosis). The most useful points of differentiation are the appearances of the ipsilateral sphenoid ridge and bony orbit, which are invariably deformed in plagiocephaly and orbital neurofibromatosis (see Table 5–1).

(c) Infantile Extracerebral Collection (Arachnoid Cyst): An extracerebral space-occupying lesion, if present for a long time in infancy and childhood, will cause local bulging and thinning of the vault. The commonest site of the so-called chronic juvenile subdural hygroma is the middle cranial fossa (Fig. 1–37) but superficially situated pools of cerebrospinal fluid associated with focal expansion of the vault are also found over the frontal and parietal lobes (Fig. 1–38). The radiological features of temporal subdural hygromas of childhood have been well documented (Davidoff and Dyke, 1938; Bull, 1949; and Cronqvist and Efsing, 1970). They are: expansion of an entire middle fossa, i.e., forward displacement of its anterior margin as shown on the lateral view, outward displacement of its lateral wall (full axial view) and elevation of the lesser wing of the sphenoid bone and distortion of the innominate line (PA 20° view). These changes may be mimicked by other growing temporal fossa lesions: temporal lobe agenesis syndrome (Robinson, 1964), neurofibromatosis (Burrows, 1963, 1978), and very rarely glioma (Childe, 1953).

Porencephalic cysts, the cystic formations that develop from contusions, hemorrhages and probably other lesions of the cerebral parenchyma, are not usually space occupying—they *re*place and do not *dis*place brain substance (see Ch. 10). Thus skull radiographs give no clue to their presence.

Intracranial Neoplasms Deforming the Skull: An area of thinning of the vault is occasionally caused by an intracranial tumor, but the thinning is often more obvious to the surgeon than the neuroradiologist, and it is easily missed (Fig. 1–39). The vault may be reduced to eggshell thickness in the affected area, which may appear in *en face* views as a translucency. Any such area of diminished density, or any superficially situated focus of pathological calcification, should prompt a search for focal thinning of the inner table: the combination of focal thinning and calcification indicates a low-grade glioma (Burrows, 1971).

Local bulging of the vault is a very rare manifestation of an intracranial tumor (except neurofibromatosis), although well-documented instances in young children are recorded (Childe, 1953; Du Boulay, 1965). The presence of a bulging asymmetry, particularly if enlarging the middle cranial fossa, points to an alternative diagnosis: either subdural hygroma or generalized neurofibromatosis.

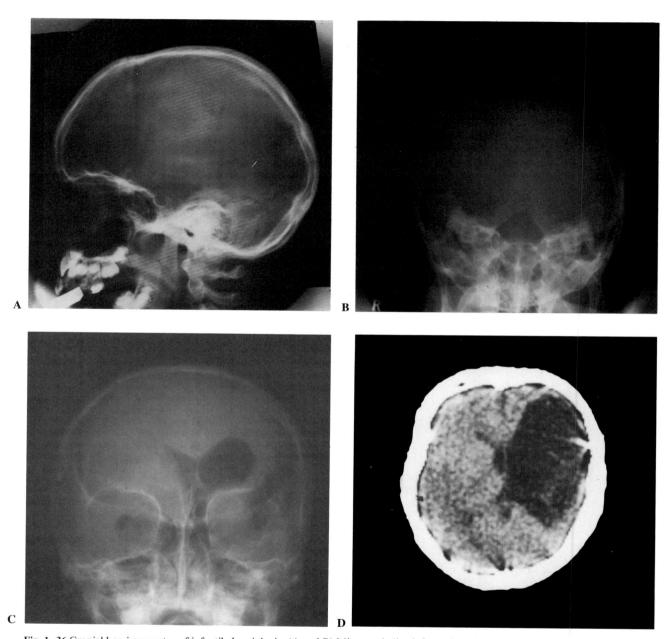

Fig. 1–36 Cranial hemisymmetry of infantile hemiplegia. (A and B) Microcephalic, deformed vault showing an off-center position of the sagittal suture, thickening and other signs of arrested growth of the left side of the vault. No other features of the classical Davidoff-Dyke-Masson syndrome are present. (C) Pneumoencephalogram: the left lateral ventricle including its temporal horn is grossly dilated due to the atrophic left hemisphere. In this patient, the midline shift is not caused by a mass of the right hemisphere (which is normal), but by failure of the left side of the vault to grow. Thus the word "traction" is incorrect in describing the mechanism of the shift. (D) Computed tomogram of a 20-year-old mental defective, with spastic hemiplegia caused by a damaged right cerebral hemisphere. Note the diffusely thickened vault, which may reflect generalized brain damage.

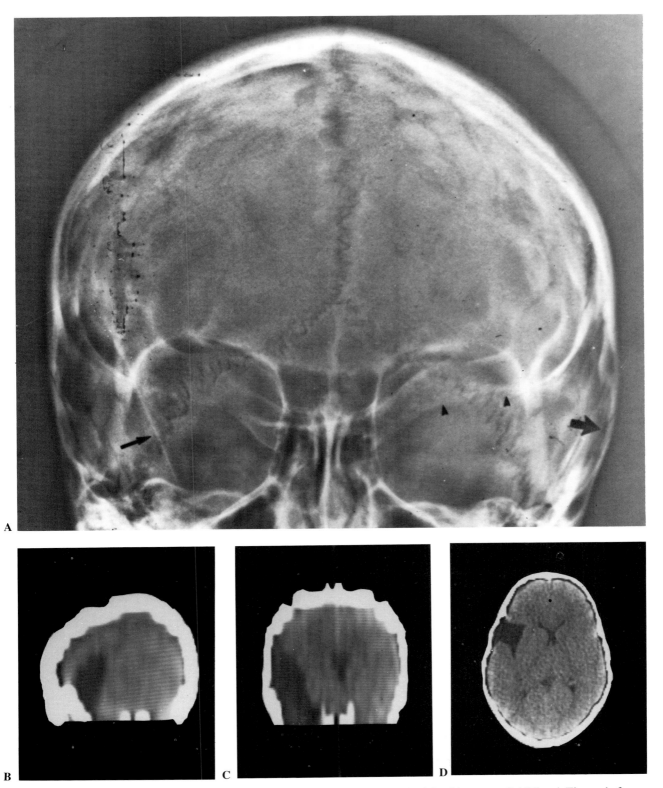

Fig. 1–37 Cranial asymmetry due to infantile extracerebral collection: 1. Temporal subdural hygroma of childhood. The pool of cerebrospinal fluid around the tip of the small temporal lobe acts as a mass which deforms the skull. (A) The "bare orbit": the sphenoid ridge is elevated *(arrowheads)*, the temporal squame is displaced outwards and open *(arrow)*, carrying the innominate line with it *(arrow on normal opposite line)*; the bony orbit is not enlarged. (B, C and D) Computed tomogram, showing the extent of the extracerebral collection which extends over the convexity of the hemisphere, producing displacement of the ventricular system in three projections.

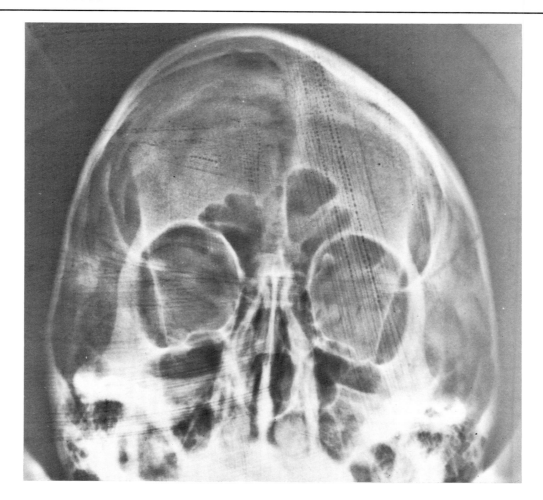

A

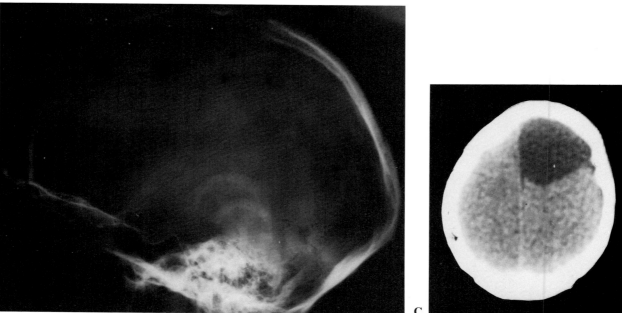

B

C

Fig. 1−38 Cranial asymmetry due to infantile extracerebral collection (continued): (1) Frontal subdural hygroma of childhood in a 14-year-old boy with a history of birth trauma. (A) Frontal view shows asymmetry of the frontal squame due to a bulging and thinned right side. (B) Lateral view shows thinning of the frontal squame and asymmetrical deformity of the anterior half of the vault. (C) Computed tomography reveals the extent of the hygroma. The apparently thicker vault is a technical artifact — for explanation, see Paxton and Ambrose (1974).

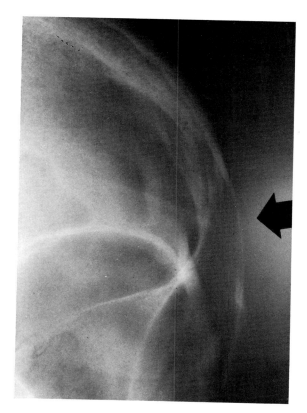

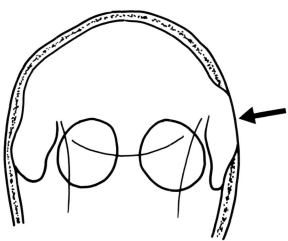

Fig. 1–39 Vault thinning due to a slow-growing glioma. A 51-year-old woman with a long history of epilepsy caused by an astrocytoma of the left temporal lobe. The frontal radiograph shows the left temporal squame reduced to eggshell thickness, due to pressure resorption of the inner table and diploe.

Focal thinning of the skull due to intracranial pressure erosion is an important element of neuroradiological interpretation, which will be discussed fully in succeeding chapters. For example, the inner table of the vault is eroded in distinctive patterns by arteriovenous malformations (Ch. 3); the pituitary fossa is excavated by adjacent masses according to

recognizable patterns (Ch. 5); the acoustic porus and internal auditory canal are widened by auditory nerve tumors in the cerebellopontine angle (Ch. 8); and the foramen magnum and upper cervical canal may be funnelled by congenital malformations of the hindbrain (Ch. 9). Pressure erosion of an optic canal or jugular foramen will be identified only with the use of special radiographic projections.

Meningoencephalocele and Its Differential Diagnosis: The brain and/or its coverings may herniate through any defect in the skull. Usually the defect lies in the midline of the vault between the foramen magnum and the root of the nose, and the lesion is a congenital defect involving the full thickness of the bone. Secondary encephaloceles may develop through linear fractures or surgical defects in which the dura remains ununited (leptomeningeal cyst, "expanding fracture of childhood"; Taveras and Ransohoff, 1953), and also through the sphenoid defect of generalized neurofibromatosis (Burrows, 1963). Depending on the extent of herniation, different terms are used: *cranium bifidum* describes the isolated bone defect, if no intracranial contents have herniated; a *meningocele* is present if a fluid-filled meningeal diverticulum is palpable on the scalp; and a *meningoencephalocele* refers to herniation of cerebral tissue. In the latter entity, the mass may have a volume greater than the infant's cranial capacity which is proportionately reduced, and the skull defect is much larger.

The essence of meningoencephalocele is the midline position of the bone defect and its presence from birth. The size may vary from an occipital emissary foramen to an extensive trough-shaped defect of the occipital squame confluent with the foramen magnum. According to Lodge (1975), the size of the encephalocele can be deduced from the diameter of the defect. The edges may be ill-defined in cranium bifidum but herniated intracranial contents render them smooth, and in *en face* views they may appear to be sclerotic due to elevation of the inner table (Fig. 1–40). Most encephaloceles are found in the occipital squame. The next commonest site is the root of the nose, where the intracranial contents herniate through the cavity of a paranasal sinus or into the nasopharynx, and may give rise to symptoms of respiratory obstruction. Small lesions may be impossible to demonstrate radiologically; larger defects may be revealed only by tomography or pneumoencephalography. Hyperteleorism is a common finding (Pollock, Newton and Hoyt, 1968). Parietal cranium bifidum is associated with craniofacial dysostosis (Crouzon's disease) and may be mistaken for the early vault defects of cleidocranial dysostosis (see Fig. 1–62).

Several developmental defects of the vault will be conveniently considered in the differential diagnosis

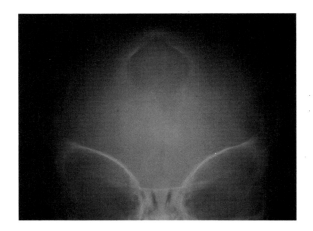
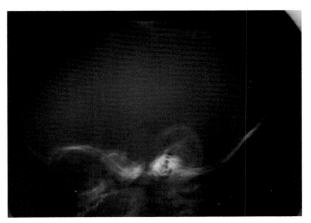
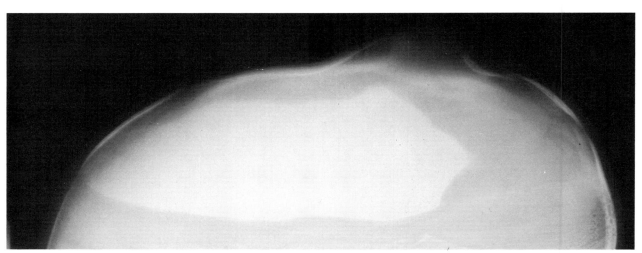
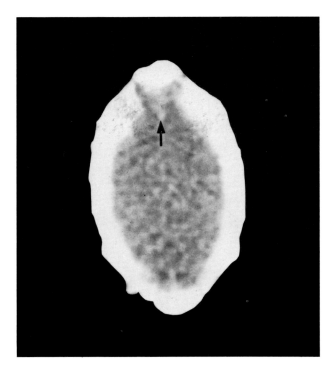

Fig. 1−40 Encephalocele in a patient with Crouzon's disease (craniofacial dysostosis). The boat-shaped vault points to premature synostosis of the sagittal suture. The "harlequin" face is caused by bilateral tethering of both lesser sphenoid wings, which are elevated due to premature coronal synostosis. The parietal midline defect has well-defined and everted edges, and computed tomography showed it to contain cerebral tissue (*arrow*), thus a true encephalocele.

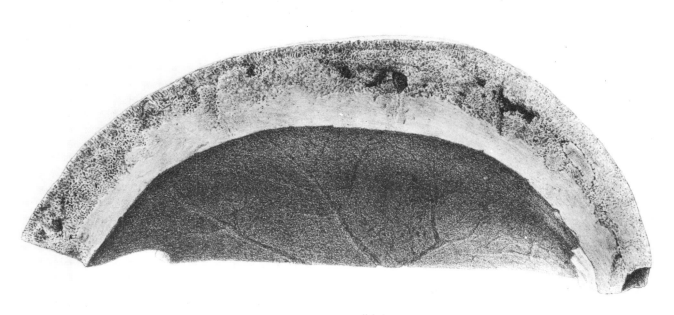

Fig. 1–45 Paget's disease. Skull cap of Sir James Paget's original case, showing the salient features of cranial involvement: grossly thickened vault, loss of differentiation between inner table, diploë and outer table, and widened vascular grooves. Well shown is the fact that the inner table is replaced by compact bone and the outer table by cancellous bone. (From *Medico-Chirurgical Transactions, London, 1877.*)

increases with age, and it has a remarkable geographical distribution, being relatively more frequently seen in the British Isles and in Australians of British stock than in North America or Continental Europe; it is rare in indigenous Africans and Asiatics (Barry, 1969). The skull is affected in only slightly more than half of the patients with the disease—it may be the solitary site, or it may escape completely in the presence of florid involvement of other bones.

(a) Radiological Appearances: Three radiological patterns are found, which are probably stages of the same process. (1) Osteoporosis circumscripta: Sosman, the Boston radiologist, was the first to associate this destructive lesion with Paget's disease of the skull (1927). Osteoporosis circumscripta is an integral part of the disease process and not a precursor of the more florid, classical forms. It may be present up to 8 years before Pagetoid lesions appear elsewhere in the skeleton and, if followed up for a sufficiently long time, can be observed to alter to mixed and sclerotic forms. The osteoporotic process itself is progressive, starting in either the occipital or the frontal squame and usually extending equally to both sides and crossing suture lines, over the course of 5 years or more (Steinbach and Dodds, 1968). The affected areas, which stand out clearly at autopsy or biopsy as purplish or reddish in contrast to the normal bone (Collins and Winn, 1955), consist of thinned skull tables and diploe.

The normal diploic venous channels disappear but the grooves for the meningeal arteries remain visible and may hypertrophy (see below). The characteristic radiological features are the sharply demarcated interface between diseased and normal bone, and the extensive area of the vault usually involved (Fig. 1 – 46). (2) Mixed lesions: These are commonest (Fig. 1 – 47). The radiolucent osteoporotic bone slowly thickens and becomes denser. The process of fibrous thickening affects both tables and the diploe but its extent is not initially visible: carotid angiography may show the superior sagittal sinus to be displaced from the inner table, and a bright light is necessary to outline the outer table. The process of sclerosis commences in a patchy fashion, through the appearance of sclerotic bone islands of oval or irregular outline within the radiolucent diploë. This patchy sclerosis imparts the "cotton-wool" radiographic appearance so characteristic of the thickened Pagetoid skull. (3) Eventually the sclerotic areas coalesce into a uniformly thickened, dense vault, in which the inner and outer tables, vascular markings and suture lines are no longer identifiable. The inner table is always very thick and dense, eventually new bone is also formed in the outer table and no further radiological changes occur: the disease is considered quiescent. Before this stage, the vault tends to collapse over the facial skeleton and the cervical spine giving rise to constriction of neural foramina and cavities, and basilar

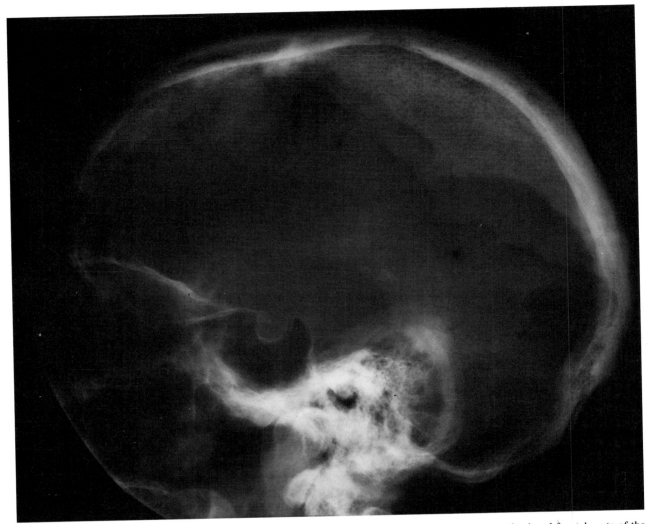

Fig. 1–46 Paget's disease – osteoporosis circumscripta. Both sides of the skull are rarefied, only the parietal and frontal parts of the vault remain intact. Diagnostic features are the extensive area of destruction and its sharp edge.

impression (see Ch. 9). Now the skull base also is involved and becomes uniformly dense (Fig. 1–48).

The high vascularity of the Pagetoid skull lesion evokes an increased abnormal blood supply which is reflected in hypertrophy of the meningeal vascular markings. The increased diameter of the middle meningeal arteries can be confirmed not only by bilateral carotid angiography, but widened and tortuous vascular grooves are visible in about 50 percent of mixed and early sclerotic lesions (Bull et al., 1959): the grooves are not hypertrophied in the early destructive (osteoporotic) stage, and they become invisible when the vault becomes sclerotic.

(b) Associated Neoplasms: Two neoplasms of adolescence or young persons occur in the skulls of patients with Paget's disease. One, the benign giant cell tumor (osteoclastoma) of long bones, is exceedingly rare (Barry, 1969), and radiological diagnosis

is impossible. The other neoplastic tendency, viz., sarcomatous transformation, is the feature that distinguishes Paget's disease from metastatic bone diseases. The incidence is impressive: one-quarter of all primary malignant bone tumors occurring in subjects over the age of 40 years are sarcomas associated with Paget's disease, and this proportion rises steeply with increasing age. Of the series of 287 patients with Paget's disease collected by Barry, 44 (15%) died of sarcomatous degeneration.

The skull vault is a preferential site for sarcomatous change. Usually sarcoma develops in a Pagetoid skull but it may occur in a "normal" skull in a subject with Paget's disease elsewhere in the skeleton. The clue to the diagnosis lies in the advanced age of the patient: in an old person, any hard scalp swelling overlying a lytic area is ominous, and especially if accompanied by intractable pain. A skeletal survey may reveal evidence of Paget's disease in

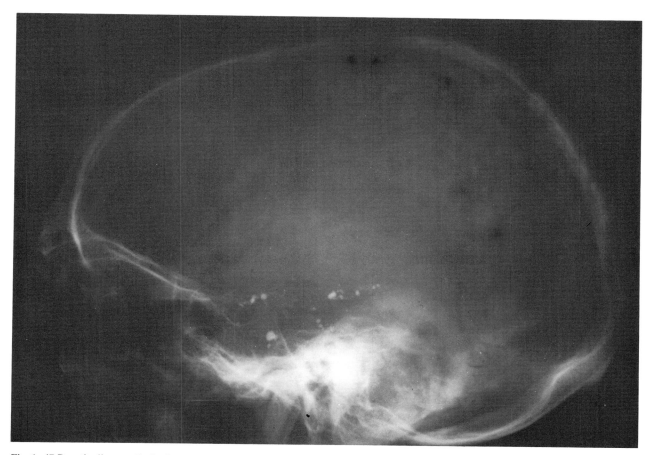

Fig. 1–47 Paget's disease. Early "cotton-wool" changes in the parietal vault. The diploë and the outer table are no longer identifiable (oil residues from a previous myelogram).

other bones. For radiological features of sarcoma, see Figure 1–32.

(c) Differential Diagnosis: The appearance of extensive osteoporosis circumscripta is specific and no other condition mimics it. If the lesion is less widespread and unilateral, the destroyed area of the vault with its well-defined edge might be mistaken, in an elderly subject, for meningiomatous change or a lytic metastatic deposit.

Once focal cotton-wool lesions appear, sclerosing metastatic deposits become difficult or impossible to differentiate, since the skull may show patchy but generalized involvement. When prostatic cancer is the primary tumor, the raised serum acid phosphatase level may be more useful in diagnosis than the radiological appearances.

Diseases producing generalized sclerosis and/or hyperostosis of the skull are listed in Table 1–3. Very few conditions *thicken* the vault as greatly or as diffusely as Paget's disease. One of these is thalassemia and other severe chronic anemias which both thicken and sclerose the vault: the radiating spiculated pattern, if florid, is unmistakable (Fig. 1–49). The only other condition that shows com-

parable degrees of generalized thickness to advanced Paget's disease is arrested intracranial growth—either diffuse brain damage of early life or arrested hydrocephalus; in both, other radiological signs make the correct diagnosis obvious (Fig. 1–50). In hyperparathyroidism both tables and the diploe are altered into a homogeneous, thickened fibrous mass, but sclerosis is absent (Fig. 1–51). Bone cysts ("brown tumors"), which are a feature of this disease in the long bones, occur relatively rarely in the skull. Diseases that produce generalized cranial sclerosteosis do not as a rule thicken the vault as much as Paget's disease, and the hyperostosis is more uniform (Beighton, Cremin and Hamersma, 1976).

Endocrine Diseases

Acromegaly: The pituitary growth hormone stimulates skeletal growth and the formation of endochondral and membranous bone, without affecting skeletal maturation. Tumors of the eosinophilic cells of the anterior lobe cause a peculiar overgrowth of the skeleton and soft tissues called acromegaly. Skeletal hypertrophy is manifest by en-

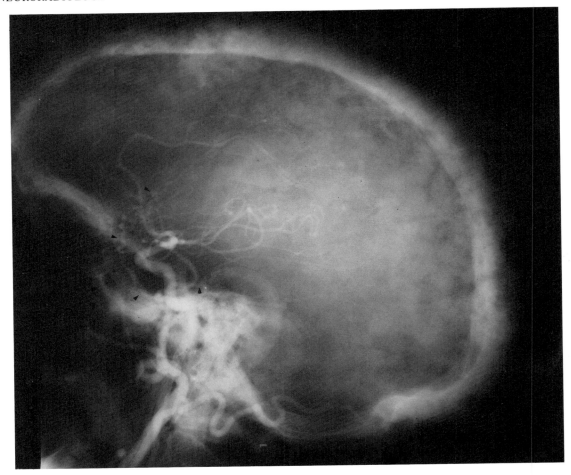

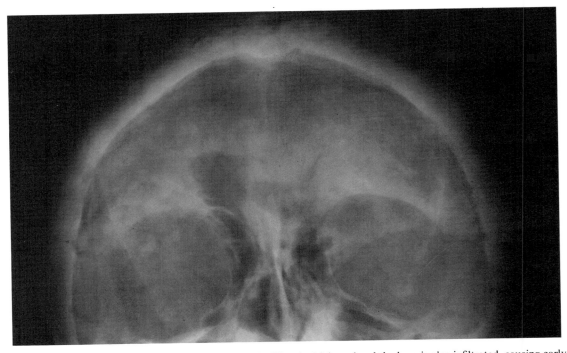

Fig. 1–48 Paget's disease, a more advanced stage. The vault is diffusely thickened and the base is also infiltrated, causing early basilar impression. The frontal view shows the dense, well-demarcated surface of the inner table, with grooves for the hypertrophied middle meningeal arteries—compare Figure 1–45. The carotid angiogram reveals hypertrophied middle meningeal *(arrowheads)* and occipital arteries, supplying respectively the inner and outer tables of the vault which has a greatly increased vascularity.

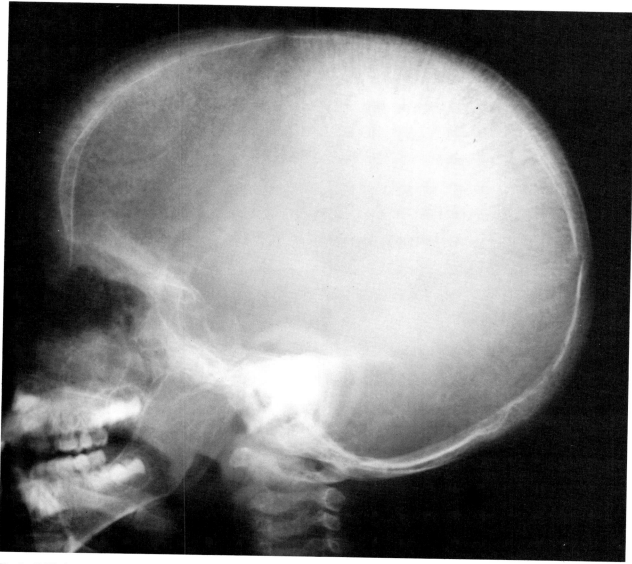

Fig. 1–49 Thalassemia. Excessive marrow hyperplasia is reflected by thickening of the diploe and inner table, especially the frontal squame, with a pattern of vertical striations. The characteristic "rodent facies" is the result of maxillary overgrowth which obliterates the antra; however, the ethmoidal sinuses are usually spared. Cortical atrophy of the mandible and medullary expansion results in loss of the mandibular angle.

chondral and periosteal new bone formation, and both the skull and the vertebral column show characteristic changes.

The lateral skull shows more of the typical features than any other view: an abnormally enlarged pituitary fossa (Ch. 5), expanded frontal sinus and mastoid air cells, a diffusely thickened calvarium and especially the external occipital protuberance, and a prognathic mandible (Fig. 1–52). Mandibular elongation and widening of its angle are a good example of the deforming effect of the exaggerated apposition of bone in one part and resorption of bone in another part. The prognathism is the result of accelerated endochondral ossification of the con-

dyles. An element of macrocrania also is present, according to Rådberg (1974), who found a significantly increased brain volume by measurement in 30 acromegalics submitted to pneumoencephalography. These typical changes are not invariably present: Lang and Bessler (1961) found that only one out of four acromegalics in a series of patients they examined exhibited expanded frontal or mastoid air cells, a thickened vault or an enlarged external occipital protuberance. The abnormal pituitary fossa is commonly identified and was absent in only 1 out of 19 consecutive cases of acromegaly seen in the Wessex Neurological Centre in recent years.

Radiological confirmation of acromegaly may be

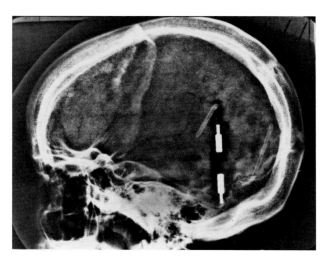

Fig. 1–50 Arrested hydrocephalus. The enormously thickened vault, due to the deposition of layered bone on the inner table, marginal sclerosis of the sutures and the absence of convolutional markings or a "pressure sella" confirm that the Spitz-Holter valve is functioning satisfactorily.

obtained from studying the appearances of other parts of the skeleton and soft tissues. The terminal digits of the toes, fingers and thumbs are tufted and their soft tissues show a homogeneity through loss of the normal fascial planes. Cartilaginous hyperplasia at the costochondral joints causes an acromegalic rosary with lengthening of the ribs and an expanded chest. An increase in the sesamoid index may be present.

Hyperparathyroidism: Hypersecretion of parathyroid hormone reduces the reabsorption of inorganic phosphate by the renal tubules and mobilizes calcium from the skeleton. Bone changes ("fibrocystic disease of bone") are present in about one-third of cases and in half of these the skull is involved (Steinbach et al., 1961). The most frequent finding is a generalized granular or mottled calvarial demineralization. As the process advances, the mottling disappears and the calvarium assumes a homogeneous, ground-glass appearance. It becomes impossible to identify the outer table, diploic markings or vascular grooves (Fig. 1–53). Cysts, although rare in the skull, do occur. The vault may be greatly thickened (Fig. 1–51). Successful treatment leads to a return to normal.

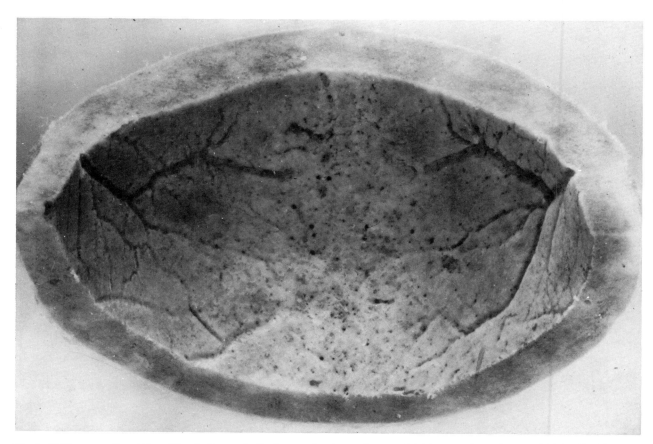

Fig. 1–51 Hyperparathyroidism. The skull cap of a fatal case, showing an increased thickness, a loss of anatomical detail of the vault and enlarged middle meningeal vessels comparable to Paget's disease. (This case was described and illustrated by H. J. Burrows in Modern Trends in Orthopaedics, 1950.)

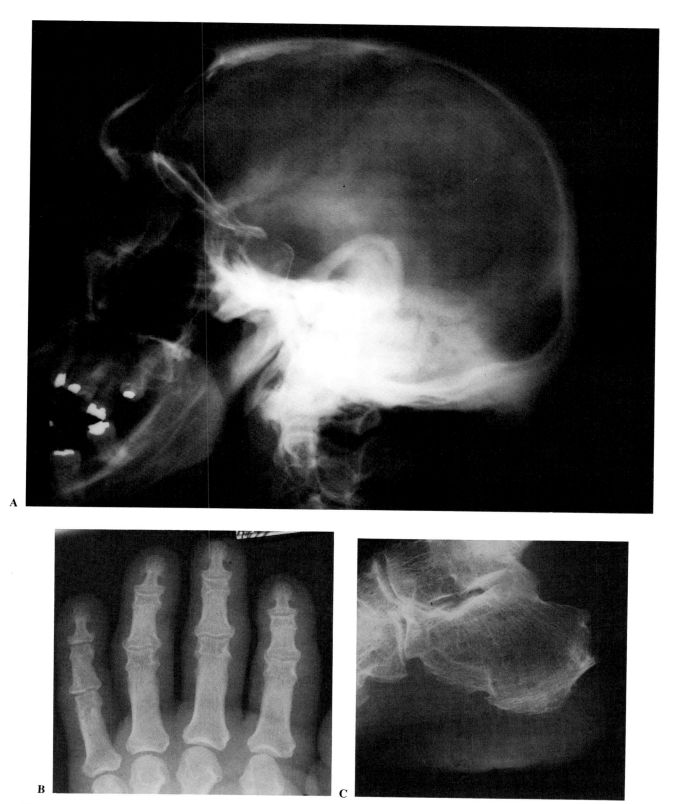

Fig. 1–52 Acromegaly due to eosinophilic pituitary adenoma. (A) Lateral view of the skull, showing enlarged pituitary fossa, large par-anasal sinuses, prognatic jaw and prominent external occipital protuberance. All the classical features are not invariably present in ac-romegaly, but a normal pituitary fossa is rare. (B) Digits of the hand, showing tufted terminal phalanges and a loss of the tissue planes and thickening of the soft tissues. (C) Thickened heel pads. Heel pads thicker than 22 mm. are likely to indicate acromegaly.

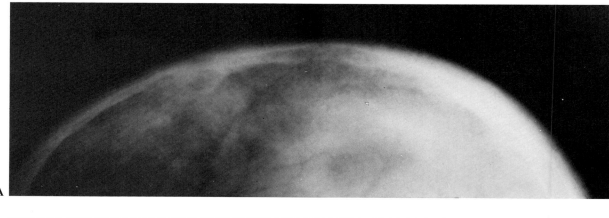

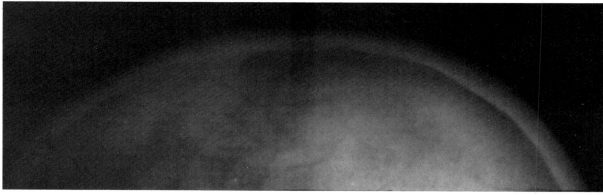

Fig. 1—53 Hyperparathyroidism. A 52-year-old woman in whom adenomas of the parathyroid gland were resected. (A) Before operation: the vault has a fuzzy appearance, and the inner and outer tables are poorly defined but no thickening is present. (B) Six months after successful operation: a return to normal appearances, sharp outlines of inner and outer tables.

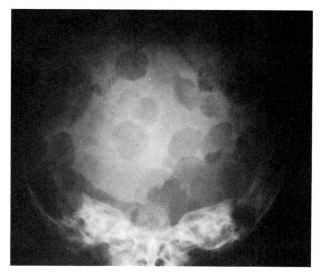

Fig. 1—54 Histiocytosis-X. Hand-Schüller-Christian's disease in a 6-year-old boy. Suture diastasis caused by meningeal deposits.

In the skull the changes of secondary hypoparathyroidism due to renal failure (renal osteodystrophy) are indistinguishable radiologically from those of the primary disease caused by hyperplasia or neoplasia of the parathyroid gland. However, the combined high-calcium-, high-phosphate-state of renal failure predisposes to renal calculi and the deposition of calcium in the soft tissues, which is uncommon in the primary disease. According to Steinbach et al. (1961), a combination of mottled granularity of the skull and falcine or tentorial calcification is probably specific for secondary hyperparathyroidism. Skull radiographs also may be useful in the differential diagnosis of fibrocystic lesions elsewhere in the skeleton: if these lesions are caused by hyperparathyroidism, the process is diffuse and involves the entire vault, while the calvarial lesions of fibrous dysplasia of bone are always focal in nature.

Hypoparathyroidism: See Pathological Intracranial Calcification.

Hypothyroidism (Cretinism): Adequate thyroid hormone is necessary for normal growth of bone and cartilage and skeletal maturation, and the skulls of cretins display retardation of these parameters.

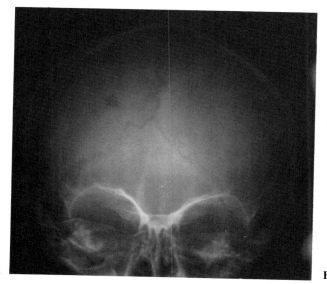

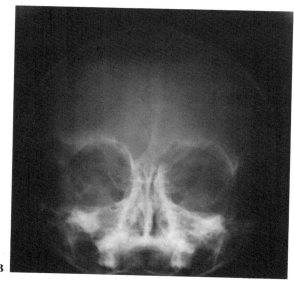

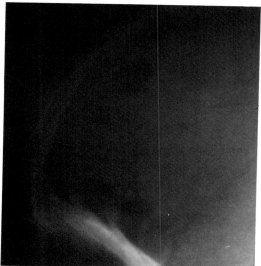

Fig. 1–55 Histiocytosis-X. Eosinophil granuloma in a 8-year-old girl. (A) Two irregular lucencies are visible on the vault. (B) One year later: both lucencies had disappeared, but a fresh destructive lesion of the margin of the left bony orbit is now present, causing proptosis. The maxillary antra and ethmoidal cells are opaque due to histiocytic infiltration. (C) Three months later still: the proptotic lesion remains but an additional deposit has appeared in the frontal squame.

Underdevelopment of the skull base prevents forward growth of the face and the frontonasal angle is unusually acute (see Achondroplasia, below). The retarded ossification of the membranous skeleton is reflected in patent sutures, wormian bones and a poorly developed diploic space.

Hypogonadism: Various workers (Keats and Burns, 1964; Kosowicz and Rzymski, 1975; Rzymski and Kosowicz, 1975) have associated a specific pattern of radiological features—each of which is a normal variant of the skull rather than an abnormal sign—with male hypogonadism (Klinefelter's syndrome) and eunochoidism and gonadal dysgensis (Turner's syndrome). They include, in male hypogonadism: flattening of the normal temporal squame, thinning of the vault bones and defective ossification in the vicinity of the anterior fontanelle, excessive marginal ossification of the coronal suture and shortening of the mandibular ramus. In Turner's syndrome, small facial bones, and hyperpneumatized paranasal sinuses have been demonstrated.

Bone Marrow and Neoplastic Diseases

These two etiological groups of diseases will be discussed together for the sake of convenience. Some appear as lytic or lucent focal, or multifocal areas of the skull, and they thus present similar problems of differential diagnosis.

Histiocytosis-X: Lichtenstein in 1953 suggested this name for a group of conditions, of which the histological lesion is an inflammatory histiocytosis. At the mildest end of the spectrum are the lesions of eosinophil granuloma that remain confined to the skeleton and carry a good prognosis. The diffuse syndrome, Hand-Schüller-Christian's disease, is less benign and the infantile form, Letterer-Siwe disease, is a malignant condition. The majority of cases of histiocytosis-X occur in children or adolescents. The skull is the commonest skeletal site, being affected in about two-thirds of cases, but the classical triad of proptosis, diabetes insipidus and skull lesions is rare (the original cases described by Hand in 1893, Schüller in 1915 and Christian in 1918, all by chance showed this triad!).

The characteristic lesion of the eosinophil granuloma is a punched-out area of destruction of well-defined, regular margins which, because of rapid growth, shows no bone reaction. Unequal destruction of the inner and outer tables may produce a

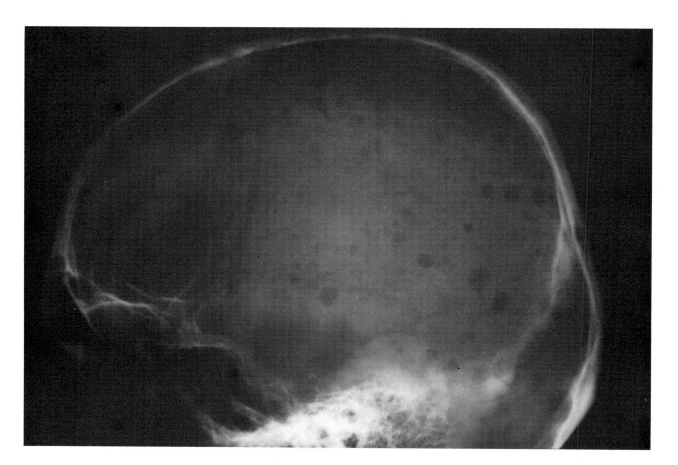

Fig. 1—56 Myelomatosis. Discrete, "punched-out" lesions with well-defined and nonsclerotic margins involve the whole vault. Their relatively uniform size and round shape are important features in differentiating myelomatosis from malignant metastases. The serum alkaline phosphatase level is always very high.

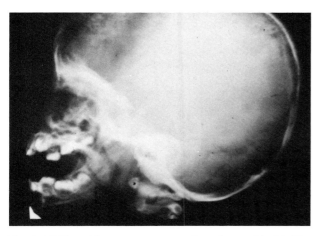

Fig. 1–57 Neuroblastoma metastases in a 4-year-old girl. The vault shows patchy destruction due to tumor infiltration, the orbital roofs characteristically being preserved ("spectacles"). At autopsy examination one week later, the appearances of the coronal sutures were shown to have been caused by a combination of sutural diastasis due to intracranial deposits and perisutural destruction of the vault.

bevelled margin. Multiple lesions, with coalesence of several, produces the typical "geographical skull" of Hand-Schüller-Christian's disease (Fig. 1–54). Sequestra may occasionally be present within the defects, mimicking the appearances of tuberculous osteomyelitis (Wells, 1956). Large lesions may be expansive, presenting as a scalp swelling, or even growing intracranially as proved by carotid angiography (Ennis, Ross and Middlemiss, 1973). Two preferential sites of involvement in the skull are the petrous and mastoid parts of the temporal bones and the superior orbital margin (Fig. 1–55); otitis media and proptosis are well-known clinical signs. The paranasal sinuses, if developed, may be opaque due to secondary involvement in the histiocytic process.

A tendency to spontaneous regression in histiocytosis-X makes the disease one of three conditions in which lytic calvarial lesions may vanish and the bone return to normal: the others being osteomyelitis (Fig. 1–61) and hyperparathyroidism (Fig. 1–53). However, dense sclerosis of previously lytic lesions of the orbital roofs following spontaneous healing or radiotherapy may occur (Nesbit et al., 1970).

Myeloma: Malignant proliferation of plasma cells in the bone marrow produces a profound anemia, and it usually destroys the bone. The generalized osteoporosis that affects the skeleton is uncommon in the skull, which is customarily involved in the process and exhibits either a solitary lytic, palpable lesion (*plasmacytoma*) or numerous punched-out areas (*myelomatosis, multiple myeloma*). The solitary variety tends to involve the skull base: large areas of destruction of the petrous temporal bone, clivus or sella may result. The trabecular pattern is completely effaced from the center of these lesions, and the margins show no bone reaction. Radiological diagnosis is based on the punched-out appearance and on the fact that the lesions vary less in size than those of metastatic cancer (Fig. 1–56). Very rarely myelomatosis may manifest itself as a patchy sclerosis of the vault: no radiological diagnosis is possible, but it is important always to consider this condition in the differential diagnosis of cranial sclerosteosis (Moseley, 1971).

Lymphoma Including Hodgkin's Disease: Cranial involvement is rare in Hodgkin's disease: only about 50 percent of cases show skeletal lesions and only 15 percent of these involve the skull. The vault changes may be both proliferative and destructive, and the affected areas have ragged margins. The radiological appearances are not specific. Lesions of the more malignant lymphomas such as reticulum cell sarcoma are almost entirely lytic.

Leukemia: About two-thirds of children with leukemia show skeletal lesions, frequently in the skull. The diploic spaces become infiltrated with leukemic cells, and the most frequent radiological findings according to Caffey (1973), are poorly defined areas of rarefaction of the vault; they are so widespread that the impression may be gained of a generalized osteoporosis. In addition, lytic areas are encountered with ragged nonreactive margins. Intracranial involvement in the form of a leukemic meningitis often produces diastasis of the cranial sutures. The diagnosis of leukemia may be ventured in a child in whom the skull shows a combination of suture diastasis and focal lysis of the vault. See Neuroblastoma Metastases, below.

Neuroblastoma Metastases: All children with neuroblastomas eventually develop cranial deposits. They produce a moth-eaten appearance of the vault but tend preferentially to involve the margins of the bony orbits and the sutures, as well as the meningeal spaces, resulting in the familiar picture of an emaciated child with large ecchymoses and palpable soft-tissue lumps of the scalp. The deposits are in three locations: (1) intracranial: usually extradural (subendocranial), causing suture diastasis; (2) intradiploic, often along the suture lines, partly destroying the serrated edge; and (3) scalp (subpericranial) causing the palpable lumps and sometimes sunray spiculation. Although local erosion of the suture margins by extradural deposits is an established pattern (Fig. 1–57; Carter et al., 1968; Pascaul-Castroviejo et al., 1975), neuroradiologists consider that most cases of suture diastasis result directly from raised intracranial pressure.

Sarcoma: See Meningioma, Paget's Disease.

Neoplastic Metastases: Blood-borne metastases are common in the vault. They may be multiple or solitary, osteolytic or osteoblastic. The pattern most frequently seen in breast and lung cancer is that of multiple lesions which are ill-defined, incom-

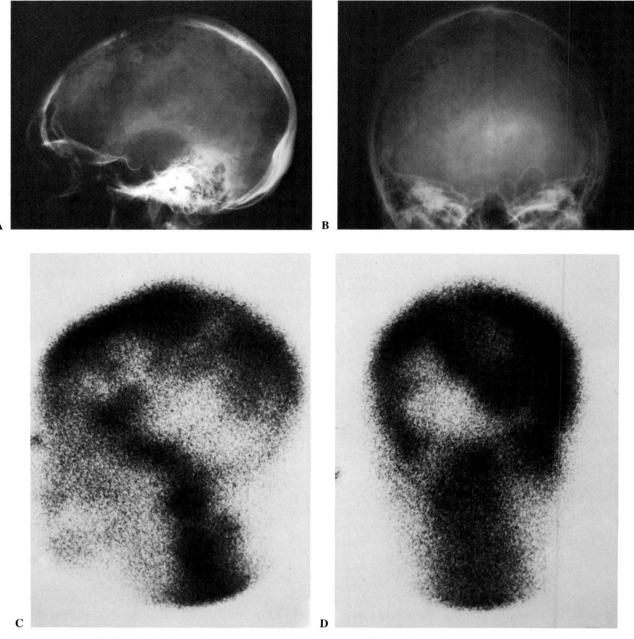

Fig. 1–58 Metastatic deposits of primary breast cancer. (A and B) Lateral and frontal views, showing patchy and ill-defined lytic lesions of the diploë, spreading to destroy both tables of the vault. (C and D) Radiopolyphosphate scintigram of the same patient, revealing more extensive neoplastic infiltration of the vault bones. The accuracy of detecting neoplastic metastases by conventional radiography is enhanced by combining it with scintigraphic imaging.

plete translucencies when visible (Fig. 1–58), or frankly osteolytic (Fig. 1–59). The two appearances are probably different stages of the same process: intradiploic deposits are ill-defined until they break through the outer table, and they may then be palpable as small soft tissue swellings. There is no marginal sclerosis. As a rule, the lesions are irregular and vary greatly in diameter. If they are rounded

and diffuse and of more uniform size, differentiation from multiple myeloma may be impossible.

Solitary osteolytic metastases usually arise from primary thyroid, renal or bowel cancer. The entire thickness of the vault is destroyed, usually over a wide area, and a large scalp swelling is visible and palpable. Sometimes, satellite erosions are present along the margin, and the metastasis resembles an

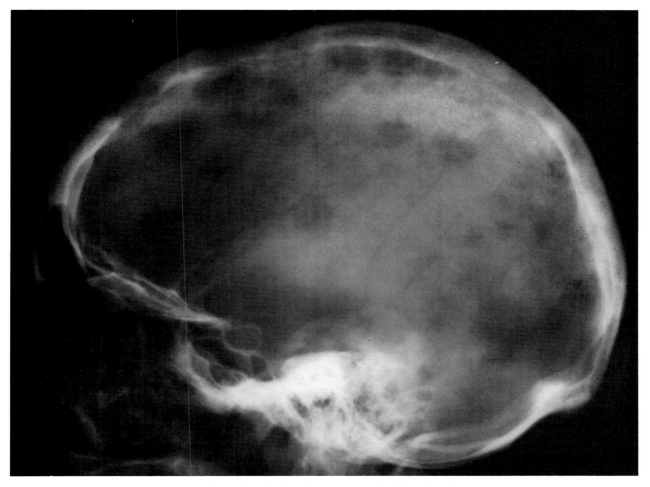

Fig. 1−59 Metastatic deposits of primary breast cancer. Multiple, ill-defined lytic lesions.

acute osteomyelitis. It is not surprising that the lesions of neoplastic metastases and osteomyelitis should appear identical, due to the similar mode of spread of both processes through the vault bones (Du Boulay, 1965).

Prostatic cancer produces sclerotic deposits which may mimic the hyperostosis of a meningioma (Fig. 1−60). A sclerotic element also may be present in breast metastases ("mixed deposits") and if generalized the appearances may be similar to those of advanced Paget's disease, except that the skull is not thickened and both tables remain well preserved. Basal osteosclerosis may be a manifestation of tumor invasion (Tsai et al., 1975).

Carcinomas of the nasopharynx and paranasal sinuses, which are rare, not infrequently spread onto adjacent portions of the skull. By contrast, giant-cell tumors of bone of the base and chordoma of the clivus (see Ch. 9) do not involve the vault.

Osteomyelitis

Acute calvarial osteomyelitis differs from the appearances of this lesion in other bones, in that subperiostial new bone forms less readily and that sequestra are uncommon in the skull. Diploic continuity is assured by its system of veins (Breschet's canals) — the paranasal sinus and mastoid cells may be regarded for this purpose as eroded diploë — and there is no resistance to the spread of pus, involvement of the inner and outer tables (osteomyelitis) and invasion of the venous system (septic thrombophlebitis). Prior to antibiotics, skull osteomyelitis was a distinct and dreaded entity which carried a high mortality. Nowadays it is viewed with less alarm, more as part of the presenting features that bring a patient to hospital and the main concern is for its intracranial complications, viz., abscess (extra- or sub-dural, intra-cerebral or -cerebellar), meningitis, and venous sinus thrombosis. In an unconscious patient, focal rarefaction of the vault, especially if combined with an opaque frontal sinus or mastoid, should alert the neuroradiologist to the correct diagnosis. These signs give specificity to any intracranial mass that might be demonstrated by scanning or contrast studies.

Acute osteomyelitis of the vault is commonly a

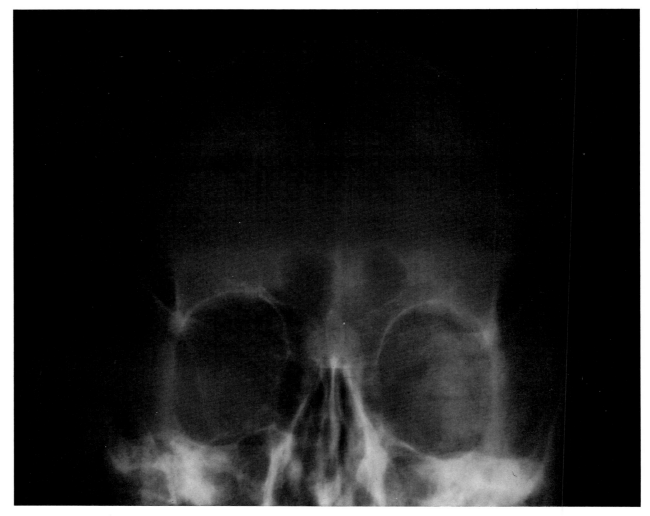

Fig. 1–60 Metastatic deposits of primary prostatic cancer. Bone-producing skull deposits are rare in malignant disease. The deposit in the left sphenoid wing is similar in appearance to a sphenoid-wing meningioma (see Fig. 1–67), but there are also patchy deposits in the vault of this elderly male with a high serum acid phosphatase level.

secondary infection, arising from the frontal sinus or the mastoid cells, or from sepsis in scalp tumors or wounds such as compound fractures, craniotomy flaps and traction tongs. Acute hematogenous osteomyelitis of the vault is extremely rare. The earliest radiological evidence of suppurative osteomyelitis is multiple small areas of rarefaction making perpendicular streaks through the bone: these are produced by the infection spreading along the diploic channels. However, it must be stressed that these changes lag behind the clinical evidence of a lesion by several weeks: not only will the scalp swelling ("Pott's puffy tumor") be present before the bone changes appear, but the bone changes will remain long after the swelling disappears. If untreated, the small rarefied areas coalesce to form a single focus of bone destruction with irregular margins (Fig. 1–61). After some weeks, a marginal

sclerosis may develop, giving the lesion a "moth-eaten" appearance.

The radiologist's duty, whenever osteomyelitis is suspected as the cause of a lytic lesion, is to search for evidence of sinus infection—fluid levels, an eroded sinus wall or a primarily obstructive cause such as fibrous dysplasia or mucocele—and for pineal displacement, indicating a serious intracranial complication.

Infection of a craniotomy wound is usually confined to the flap: its edges become blurred and a patchy mottling develops. The process may go on to complete resorption of the flap. An identical appearance may follow avascular necrosis of a bone flap without infection (Du Boulay, 1965).

Clinical low-grade skull infections, such as those caused by tuberculosis, syphilis, coccidiomycosis, actinomycosis or coccal infections complicating

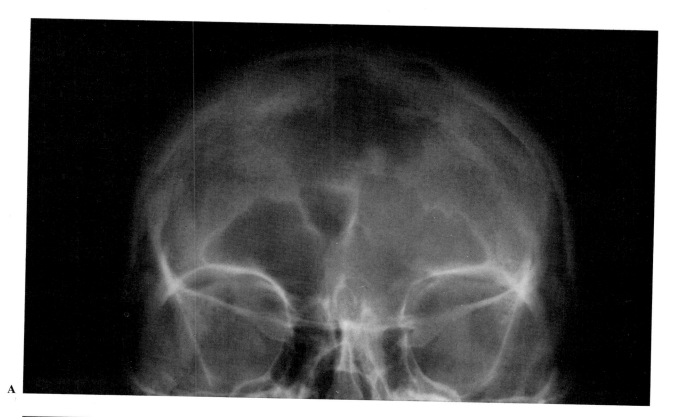

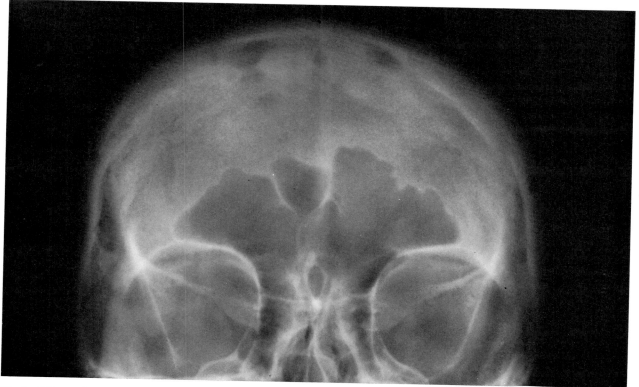

Fig. 1–61 Pyogenic osteomyelitis of the vault secondary to frontal sinusitis. The patient was an unconscious adolescent with a brain abscess. (A) Examination on admission: solitary "moth-eaten" lesion of the vault, adjacent to an opaque left frontal sinus that lacks part of the cortical lining of its roof. Intracranial contrast studies revealed a large frontal abscess. (B) Two years later: the bone lesion had completely healed (burrholes visible); normal frontal sinus.

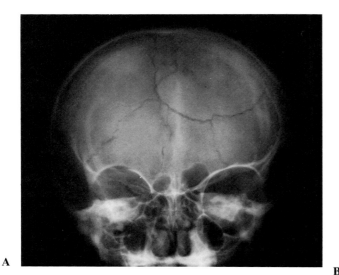

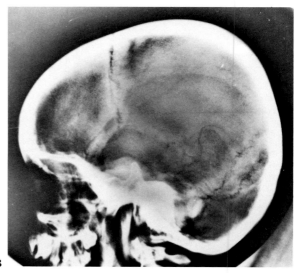

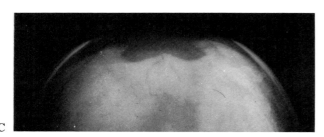

A

B

C

Fig. 1-62 Cleidocranial dysostosis in a 26-year-old woman. (A and B) Wormian bones are present and the sutures are unusually prominent, but there is no other evidence of defective membrane ossification. The stunted growth of the base (basal angle = 90°) and face (deformed mandible and small maxilla, delayed dentition) indicates a gross disturbance of endochondral ossification. (C) Another case, a 2-year-old girl with absent clavicles, in whom symmetrical defects in the closing stages resembled parietal foramina, but a mosaic of wormian bones was visible. (This case was reported and illustrated by Sir Thomas Lodge in the British Journal of Radiology, 48, 421–434, 1975.)

scalp neoplasms, usually produce a sclerotic bone reaction of nonspecific type, and a laboratory diagnosis is required. Tuberculous osteomyelitis of the skull may be purely osteolytic and resemble the lesions of histiocytosis-X in children; later they may harbor sequestrum-like material.

Fractures and Other Traumatic Sequelae
See Chapter 4.

Dysplasias, Dysostoses and Other Affections of Bone
This section is disproportionately brief since the entities discussed within it belong to the realms of skeletal and pediatric radiology. They concern the neuroradiologist, apart from differential diagnosis, only in that in some the clinical pictures may include mental deficiency or retardation or be complicated by neurological deficits due to foraminal constriction or basilar invagination.

Defective ossification is the fundamental fault in a number of generalized conditions that alter the skull (Gorlin and Pindborg, 1964). The fault may lie in defective synthesis of either the cartilaginous skeleton (skull base) or the membranous skeleton (vault), or both. Defective development of membrane bone is seen in cleidocranial dysostosis, osteogenesis imperfecta, pycnodysostosis, hypophosphatasia, mongolism and hypogonadism. The cartilaginous base fails to develop completely

in achondroplasia, and less completely in mongolism and hypogonadism. The appearances of the skull in each of these conditions is described below.

Cleidocranial Dysostosis: The membranous calvarium shows various degrees of imperfect ossification. The base ossifies normally. The sutures often fail to close, and large Wormian bones are present in the parietal and occipital vault (Fig. 1–62). The anterior fontanelle is large and may never close, although usually the midline defect—sometimes confused with large congenital parietal foramina (Lodge, 1975)—disappears in adolescence. The lateral ends of the clavicles are defective, and other symmetrical bones meeting at the midline may not ossify, such as the pubis, mandible and vertical neural rami. The face is underdeveloped and the malar bones and maxilla including its sinuses are hypoplastic. Dentition is faulty. The permanent teeth often fail to erupt due to impaction, and deciduous teeth may be present into adulthood.

Osteogenesis Imperfecta: This condition is a defect which involves bone, teeth, sclerae and certain other connective tissues. The most severe form occurs in the infant who may show multiple fractures, blue sclerae and otosclerosis, and in whom the calvarium remains a membranous container covered with patches of thin bone forming a mosaic of Wormian bones. More attenuated forms of skele-

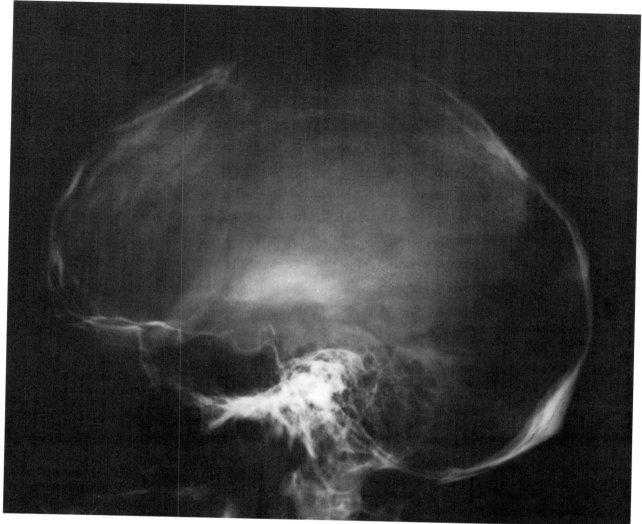

Fig. 1—63 Osteogenesis imperfecta. Skull of adult man with a mild form of the disease, showing evidence of poor skeletal mineralization—a thin vault and numerous Wormian bones along the lambdoid suture. No basilar impression is present.

tal fragility are compatible with a long life ("fragilitas ossium tarda"). The skulls of adults with the disease are thin and poorly mineralized, and the diagnosis is made by the recognition of Wormian bones and basilar impression (Fig. 1–63).

Pycnodysostosis: This autosomal recessive dysplasia of bone first described as a separate entity in 1962 (see Dusenberry and Kane in 1967, Grünebaum and Landau in 1968), is characterized by short stature, increased density of bones and hypoplastic terminal phalanges. The radiological appearances of the skull combine the findings of cleidocranial dysostosis with those of osteopetrosis, viz., patent sutures and fontanelles and poorly developed but dense facial bones (hypoplastic paranasal sinuses), absent mandibular angle and defective dentition.

Hypophosphatasia: The low level of alkaline phosphatase activity hampers normal bone forma-

tion in this condition, but the range of severity of the skeletal manifestations varies from a nearly complete absence of skeletal ossification in the neonate to normal bones in adults (Currarino et al., 1957). The skull of adults with the disorder contain plaque-like areas of ossified bone, wide sutures and a bulging anterior fontanelle. Survivors commonly have craniostenosis, but the microcephaly is unaccompanied by mental retardation. The extremities show the features of severe rickets.

Achondroplasia: This is the circus dwarf suffering from partial failure of endochondral ossification which stunts the growth of his limbs and the base of his skull. The chondrocranium, consisting of the ethmoid and parts of the sphenoid and the occipital bones, is foreshortened by defective growth, as well as by premature synostosis of the spheno-occipital synchondrosis. As a result, the foramen magnum is small and the basal angle reduced to a right angle

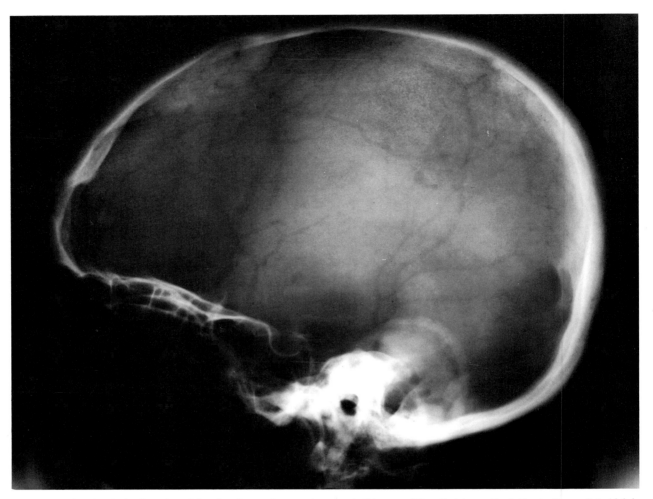

Fig. 1—64 Achondroplasia. Stunting of the chondrocranium produces a skull base and face that is small relative to the vault (which is normal, although it may appear hydrocephalic). The basal angle is reduced to nearly 90° and there is stenosis of the foramen magnum — see Chapter 9.

(see Ch. 9). Ossification of membranous bone proceeds normally, and the discrepancy between the normal vault and underdeveloped base of the skull is reflected in the clinical and radiological features (Fig. 1–64), viz., prominent forehead and occiput, flattened bridge of the nose and sometimes maloccluded jaws. The ethmoid bone, being of cartilaginous origin, remains abnormally small and fails to deliver the maxilla into normal apposition to the mandible. The vault, although prominent and apparently hydrocephalic, shows a normal growth pattern: the brain is often normal. Hydrocephalus is distinctly rare: when present, it is associated with an outlet obstruction caused by the basal deformity (Du Boulay, 1965; see also Chs. 9 and 11).

Generalized cranial sclerosteosis accompanies some, but not all, skeletal affections in which the bones are thicker or denser than normal (Beighton, Cremin, and Hamersma, 1976). They are osteopetrosis, progressive diaphyseal dysplasia, craniometaphyseal dysplasia, pycnodysostosis and hyper-

phosphatasemia. Myotonia congenita, and fluorine and vitamin D intoxication and tuberous sclerosis may also cause sclerosis of the skull base.

Osteopetrosis (Albers-Schönberg's Disease): This rare skeletal dysplasia which results in a generalized increase in bone density and thickness, consistently involves the base and frequently the vault and face. Ossification in cartilaginous bone proceeds normally but no resorption occurs. Thus, no medullary cavity forms and the bones assume a chalklike appearance which obscures all normal markings ("marble bones"). The optic canals and other cranial nerve foramina may be obliterated. Sufferers from the disease may present with a fatal anemia, an osteomyelitis of the jaw due to periodontal infection, fractures of long bones or cranial nerve lesions (blindness, facial palsy or deafness). The condition most likely to be confused with osteopetrosis is progressive diaphyseal dysplasia.

Progressive Diaphyseal Dysplasia (Engelmann's Disease): The shafts of long bones are thickened in-

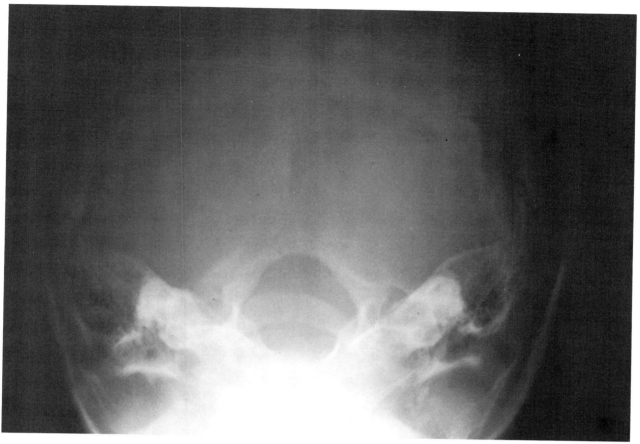

Fig. 1–65 Generalized neurofibromatosis. Characteristic defect of the lambdoid suture on the left side, associated with underdevelopment of the ipsilateral mastoid process.

ternally as well as externally, and the metaphyses and epiphyses are normal. The skull base is nearly always sclerotic while the bones of the membranous *anlage* may be normal. No foraminal impingement occurs. Therefore the appearance of the skull is similar to that of osteopetrosis, but a skeletal survey always provides the correct diagnosis.

Hyperphosphatasemia ("Juvenile Paget's Disease") and Hyperphosphatasemia Tarda (Van Buchem's Disease): A high alkaline phosphatase level is common to these two conditions which occur respectively in children and young adults. In the childhood type, the skull shows typical Pagetoid features, and the shafts of long bones are thickened. In the adult type, only the shafts of long bones are involved and there is extreme thickening of the vault, facial bones and the base of the skull; foraminal impingement may produce cranial nerve palsies (Van Buchem et al., 1962; Scott and Gautby, 1974; Owen, 1976).

Myotonia Congenita (Thomsen's Disease): Patients with this rare, multisystem abnormality possess a typical facial appearance: frontal baldness, hollow cheeks and drooping eyelids; the head hangs for-

ward due to the muscular weakness. Skull radiographs show all or some of the following features in a large proportion of cases: small pituitary fossa, hyperostosis frontalis interna or more extensive thickening of the vault, large frontal sinuses and a wide mandibular angle (Caughey, 1952; Gleeson et al., 1967).

Generalized Neurofibromatosis (Von Recklinghausen's Disease): This hereditary disease resulting from dysplasia of neuroectodermal and mesodermal tissues may affect any organ or system of the body. It is the commonest neurocutaneous syndrome found, and the skin manifestations, pigmented (café au lait) patches and the characteristic nipple-like tumors (fibrosum molluscum) are present in 80 to 90 percent of patients. The brain is frequently—and inevitably—involved, either through an undefined genetic aberration during embryonic life or secondarily due to tumor or hydrocephalus. It is said that about 50 percent of patients with generalized neurofibromatosis have brain tumors (Klatte, Franken and Smith, 1976). These are gliomas, frequently of the optic, facial or auditory nerves, or meningiomas; often they are multiple. A multiplicity of intra-

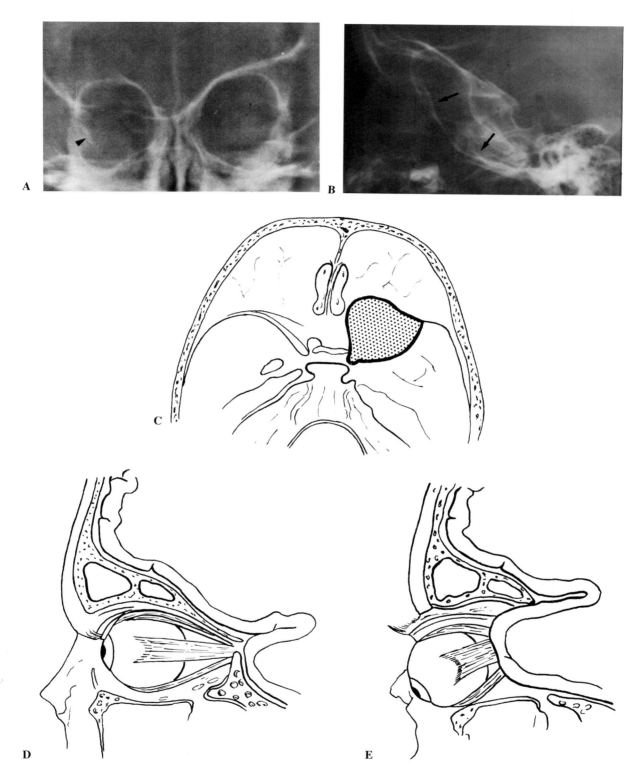

Fig. 1–66 Generalized neurofibromatosis. Orbital encephalocele produced by defective development of the sphenoid wings on one side. (A and B) A 3-year-old child with right proptosis. Radiographs show an enlarged bony orbit which is "bare" due to congenital absence of the greater and lesser wings, elevation of the sphenoid ridge, and lateral displacement of the innominate line (arrowhead in frontal view points to the normal opposite line). The arrows in lateral view indicate the anterior margins of the right temporal fossa. Unlike temporal subdural hygroma, the bony orbit of generalized neurofibromatosis is usually enlarged (Seaman and Furlow, 1954; Burrows, 1963). (C, D and E) Diagram of a typical defect of the sphenoid ridge and wing involving the posterior wall of the orbit, as viewed (C) from above and (E) from the side. Anterior herniation of the temporal lobe through the bony defect with consequent displacement of the eyeball is well demonstrated in lateral view, by comparing the normal arrangement (D) with (E). (This diagram illustrated the paper of E. H. Burrows in the British Journal of Radiology, *36*, 549–561, 1963.)

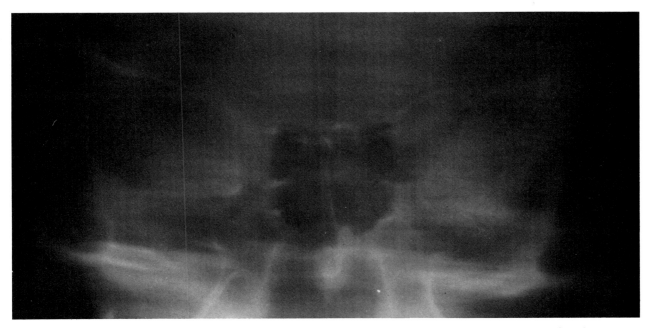

Fig. 1–67 The answer to Figs. 1–2, 1–3 and 1–4: meningioma of the left sphenoidal wings. Sphenoid zonogram confirms involvement of both lesser and greater wings and thickening of the adjacent part of the sphenoid ridge.

cranial lesions, or a combination of tumors and unrelated skull or other skeletal abnormalities, always suggests this diagnosis.

Two mesodermal defects of the skull are characteristic of the disease, and several associated abnormalities have been reported:

(a) Periosteal defect of the lambdoid suture, usually on the left side (Fig. 1–65). It may be associated with underdevelopment of the ipsilateral mastoid (Joffe, 1965):

(b) Sphenoid wing defect producing an orbital encephalocele and pulsating unilateral exophthalmos (Fig. 1–66). Cases are described in which the defect is unassociated with any neurofibromatous tissue, and no asymmetry of the orbital margin is present (Burrows, 1963). More usually a plexiform neuroma is found in the soft tissues above the eyeball, which deforms the bony orbit (see cranial hemihypertrophy syndromes, above; also Table 1–5). Another form of presentation of orbital neurofibromatosis is glioma of the optic nerve. Various combinations of the three forms are found (Burrows, 1978).

(c) Isolated skull defects, including cranium bifidum, have been described (Hunt and Pugh, 1961). Macrocrania, reported by Holt and Kuhns (1976), is presumably caused by a macroencephaly.

Craniofacial Anomalies: Brief reference is made below, for the sake of completeness, to the diagnostic maze that comprises this particular aspect of pediatric radiology, which is the subject of a masterly review by Campbell (1971).

(a) Anomalies related to cranial or generalized skeletal growth affections. These comprise the deformities associated with various types of craniostenosis, particularly Crouzon's and Apert's syndromes, and hyperteleorism (Greig's syndrome); and second, the generalized anomalies of gargoylism, achondroplasia, cleidocranial dysostosis and osteogenesis imperfecta.

(b) Anomalies related to embryonic midline defects, viz., arhinencephaly (holoprosencephaly, see Fig. 10–34) and the medial cleft face syndrome. This latter title covers a variety of effects of failure of midline fusion, such as forehead lipoma, orbital hyperteleorism, occult frontonasal encephalocele, cleft nose and cleft palate.

(c) Anomalies related to defects of the first and second branchial arches. These include rare syndromes of defective development of more than one of the following parts: facial bones, mandible, dentition, orbits, lens, digits. The best known are the chinless wonders: the Treacher-Collins and Pierre-Robin syndromes.

REFERENCES

Amin, R.: Basal cell naevus syndrome. British Journal of Radiology, *48*, 402–407, 1975.

Anderson, R., Kieffer, S. A. and Wolfson, J. J.: Thickening of the skull in surgically treated hydrocephalus. American Journal of Roentgenology, *110*, 96–101, 1970.

Austin, J. H. M. and Gooding, C. A.: Roentgenographic measurement of skull size in children. Radiology, *99*, 641–646, 1971.

Banna, M. and Appleby, A.: Some observations on the angiography of supratentorial meningiomas. Clinical Radiology, *20*, 375–386, 1969.

Barry, H. C.: Paget's Disease of Bone. Edinburgh: E. and S. Livingstone, 1969.

Batnitzky, S., Powers, J. M. and Schechter, M. M.: Falx "calcification" – does this exist? Neuroradiology, 7, 255–260, 1974.

Beighton, P., Cremin, B. J. and Hamersma, H.: The radiology of sclerosteosis. British Journal of Radiology, 49, 934–939, 1976.

Bennett, J. C., Maffly, R. H. and Steinbach, H. L.: The significance of bilateral basal ganglia calcification. Radiology, 72, 368–378, 1959.

Bergeron, R. T.: Radiographic demonstration of cortical heterotopia. Acta Radiologica Diagnosis, 14, 561–568, 1973.

Borns, P. F. and Rancier, L. F.: Cerebral calcification in childhood leukemia mimicking Sturge-Weber syndrome. American Journal of Roentgenology, 122, 52–55, 1974.

Bruyn, G. W., Bots, G. T. and Staal, A.: Familial bilateral vascular calcification in the central nervous system. Psychiatria, Neurologia, Neurochirurgia, 66, 98–119, 1963.

Bull, J. W. D.: The diagnosis of chronic subdural haematoma in children and adolescents. British Journal of Radiology, 22, 68–80, 1949.

Bull, J. W. D., Nixon, W. L. B., Pratt, R. T. C. and Robinson, P. K.: Paget's disease of the skull and secondary basilar impression. Brain, 82, 10–22, 1959.

Burrows, E. H.: Bone changes in orbital neurofibromatosis. British Journal of Radiology, 36, 549–561, 1963.

Burrows, E. H.: Intracranial calcification. In Newton, T. H. and Potts, D. G., Eds.: Radiology of the Skull and Brain. Vol. 1, book 2. St. Louis: C. V. Mosby, 1971.

Burrows, E. H.: Calcification in intracranial gliomas. Journal Belge de Radiologie, 56, 359–362, 1973.

Burrows, E. H.: Orbitocranial asymmetry. British Journal of Radiology, 51, 771–781, 1978.

Burrows, H. J.: The bone dystrophies. In Platt, H. Ed.: Modern Trends in Orthopaedics. London: Butterworth and Company, 1950.

Burwood, R. J., Gordon, I. J. S. and Taft, R. D.: The skull in mongolism. Clinical Radiology, 24, 475–480, 1973.

Caffey, J.: Pediatric X-ray Diagnosis. 6th Ed. Chicago: Year Book Medical Publishers, 1973.

Camp, J. D.: Symmetrical calcification of cerebral basal ganglia; its roentgenographic significance in diagnosis of parathyroid insufficiency. Radiology, 49, 568–577, 1947.

Campbell, J. A.: Craniofacial anomalies. In Newton, T. H. and Potts, D. G., Eds.: Radiology of the Skull and Brain. Vol. 1, book 2. St. Louis: C. V. Mosby, 1971.

Carter, T. L., Gabrielsen, T. O. and Abell, M. R.: Mechanism of split sutures in metastatic neuroblastoma. Radiology, 91, 467–470, 1968.

Caughey, J. E.: Radiological changes in the skull in dystrophia myotonica. British Medical Journal, 1, 137–139, 1952.

Childe, A. E.: Localized thinning and enlargement of the cranium, with special reference to the middle fossa. American Journal of Roentgenology, 70, 1–22, 1953.

Cole, M. and Davies, H.: Carotid siphon calcification. British Journal of Radiology, 36, 289–293, 1964.

Collins, D. H. and Winn, J. M.: Focal Paget's disease of the skull (osteitis deformans). Journal of Pathology and Bacteriology, 69, 1–9, 1955.

Cooper, R.: Acrocephalysyndactyly: with report of a case. British Journal of Radiology, 26, 533–538, 1953.

Coulam, C. M., Brown, L. R. and Reese, D. F.: Sturge-Weber syndrome. Seminars in Roentgenology, 11, 55–60, 1976.

Cronqvist, S.: Roentgenologic evaluation of cranial size in children. A new index. Acta Radiologica Diagnosis, 7, 97–111, 1968.

Cronqvist, S. and Efsing, H. O.: Skull size and ventricular dilatation in subdural hygroma in infants. Acta Radiologica Diagnosis, 10, 11–16, 1970.

Currarino, G., Neuhauser, E. B. D., Reyersbach, G. and Sobel, E.: Hypophosphatasia. American Journal of Roentgenology, 78, 392–419, 1957.

Cushing, H. and Eisenhardt, L.: Meningiomas; their classification, regional behavior, life history and surgical results. Springfield: Charles C Thomas, 1938.

Davidoff, L. M. and Dyke, C. G.: Relapsing juvenile chronic subdural hematoma: a clinical and roentgenographic study. Bulletin of the Neurological Institute of New York, 7, 95–111, 1938.

Di Chiro, G., Fisher, R. L. and Nelson, K. B.: The jugular foramen. Journal of Neurosurgery, 21, 447–460, 1964.

Du Boulay, G.: The significance of digital impressions in children's skulls. Acta Radiologica, 46, 112–122, 1956.

Du Boulay, G.: The radiological evidence of raised intracranial pressure in children. British Journal of Radiology, 30, 375–377, 1957.

Du Boulay, G. H.: Principles of X-ray Diagnosis of the Skull. London: Butterworths, 1965.

Dusenberry, J. F. and Kane, J. J.: Pyknodysostosis. American Journal of Roentgenology, 99, 717–723, 1967.

Dyke, C. G.: Indirect signs of brain tumor as noted in roentgen examinations; displacement of pineal shadow; survey of 3000 consecutive skull examinations. American Journal of Roentgenology, 23, 598–606, 1930.

Dyke C. G.: The roentgen-ray diagnosis of diseases of the skull and intracranial contents. In Golden, R.: Diagnostic Roentgenology New York: Thomas Nelson Sons, 1941.

Dyke, C. G. Davidoff, L. M. and Masson, C. G.: Cerebral hemiatrophy with homolateral hypertrophy of the skull and sinuses. Surgery, Gynecology and Obstetrics, 57, 588–600, 1933.

Ennis, J. T., Ross, F. G. M. and Middlemiss, J. H.: The radiology of the bone changes in histiocytosis X. Clinical Radiology, 24, 212–220, 1973.

Enzmann, D. R., Hayward, R. W., Norman, D. and Dunn, R. P.: Cranial computed tomographic scan appearance of Sturge-Weber disease: unusual presentation. Radiology, 122, 721–724, 1977.

Farmer, T. W.: Pediatric Neurology. New York: Harper and Row, 1964.

Flament-Durand, J., Ketelbant-Balasse, P., Maurus, R., Regnier, R. and Spehl, M.: Intracerebral calcifications appearing during the course of acute lymphocytic leukaemia treated with methotrexate and x-rays. Cancer, 35, 319–325, 1975.

Gleeson, J. A., Swann, J. C., Hughes, D. T. D. and Lee, F. I.: Dystrophia myotonica—a radiological survey. British Journal of Radiology, 40, 96–100, 1967.

Goalwin, H. A.: One thousand optic canals: clinical, anatomic and roentgenologic study. Journal of the American Medical Association, 89, 1745–1748, 1927.

Gold, L. H. A., Kieffer, S. A. and Peterson, H. O.: Intracranial meningiomas. A retrospective analysis of the diagnostic value of plain skull films. Neurology, 19, 873–878, 1969.

Goldsmith, W. M.: Catlin mark: inheritance of unusual opening in parietal bones. Journal of Heredity, 13, 69–71, 1922.

Gordon, I. R. S.: Microcephaly and craniostenosis. Clinical Radiology, 21, 19–31, 1970.

Gorlin, R. J. and Pindborg, J. J.: Syndromes of the head and neck. New York: McGraw-Hill Book Company, 1964.

Green, G. J.: The radiology of tuberose sclerosis. Clinical Radiology, 19, 135–147, 1968.

Greig, D. M.: On symmetrical thinness of the parietal bones. Edinburgh Medical Journal, 33, 546–671, 1926.

Grünebaum, M. and Landau, B.: Pycnodysostosis. British Journal of Radiology, 41, 359–361, 1968.

Harwood-Nash, D. C.: Axial tomography of the optic canals in children. Radiology, 96, 367–374, 1970.

Hawkins, T. D.: Radiological bone changes in tuberose sclerosis. British Journal of Radiology, 32, 157–161, 1959.

Hawkins, T. D.: Radiological investigation of glomus jugulare tumors. Acta Radiologica Diagnosis, 5, 201–210, 1966.

Henschen, F.: Intrakranielle Verkalkungen. In Lubarsch, O., Kenke, F. and Roessle, R., Eds.: Handbuch der speziellen pathologischen Anatomie und Histologie. Vol. 13, part 3. Berlin: Springer, 1955.

Hirtz, E. J.: La radiographie de la base du crâne. Journal de Radiologie, d'Électrologie et Archives d'Électricité Médicale, 6, 253–263, 1922.

Holt, J. F. and Kuhns, L. R.: Macrocrania and macroencephaly in neurofibromatosis. Skeletal Radiology, 1, 25–28, 1976.

Horrigan, W. D. and Baker, D. H.: Gargoylism: a review of the roentgen skull changes with a description of a new finding. American Journal of Roentgenology, 86, 473–477, 1961.

Hunt, J. C. and Pugh, D. G.: Skeletal defects in neurofibromatosis. Radiology, 76, 1–20, 1961.

Hudolin, V., Riessner, D., Kadrnka, S. and Knezevic, M.: A huge osteoma in the anterior cranial fossa. Journal of Neurology, Neurosurgery and Psychiatry, 24, 80–83, 1961.

Ingalls, T. H.: Etiology of mongolism; epidemiologic and teratologic implications. American Journal of Diseases of Childhood, 74, 147–165, 1947.

Joffe, N.: Calvarial bone defects involving the lambdoid suture in neurofibromatosis. British Journal of Radiology, 38, 23–27, 1965.

Jupe, M. H.: Central nervous system. In A Text Book of X-Ray Diagnosis by British Authors. Vol. 1. London: H. K. Lewis, 1950.

Kalan, C. and Burrows, E. H.: Calcification in intracranial gliomata. British Journal of Radiology, 35, 589–602, 1962.

Keats, T. E. and Burns, T. W.: The radiographic manifestations of gonadal dysgenesis. Radiologic Clinics of North America, 2, 297–313, 1964.

Kingsley, D. and Kendall, B. E.: The value of computed tomography in the evaluation of the enlarged head. Neuroradiology, 15, 59–71, 1978.

Klatte, E. C., Franken, E. A. and Smith, J. A.: The radiographic spectrum in neurofibromatosis. Seminars in Roentgenology, 11, 17–33, 1976.

Kosowicz, J. and Rzymski, K.: Radiological features of the skull in Klinefelter's syndrome and male hypogonadism. Clinical Radiology, 26, 371–378, 1975.

Lagos, J. C., Holman, C. B. and Gomez, M. R.: Tuberous sclerosis: neuroroentgenologic observations. American Journal of Roentgenology, 104, 171–176, 1968.

Lang, E. K. and Bessler, W. T.: The roentgenologic features of acromegaly. American Journal of Roentgenology, 86, 321–328, 1961.

Lee, K. F.: The diagnostic value of hyperostosis in midline subfrontal meningioma. An analysis of 66 cases. Radiology, 119, 121–130, 1976.

Leeds, N. E. and Seaman, W. B.: Fibrous dysplasia of the skull and its differential diagnosis. Radiology, 78, 570–582, 1962.

Lichtenstein, L.: Histiocytosis X: integration of eosinophilic granuloma of bone, Letterer-Siwe disease and Schüller-Christian disease as related manifestations of single nosologic entity. Archives of Pathology, 56, 84–102, 1953.

Lorber, J.: Intracranial calcifications following tuberculous meningitis in children. Acta Radiologica, 50, 204–210, 1958.

Lloyd, G. A. S.: Axial hypocycloidal tomography of the orbits. British Journal of Radiology, 48, 460–464, 1975.

Lodge, T.: Developmental defects in the cranial vault. British Journal of Radiology, 48, 421–434, 1975.

Lysholm, E.: Apparatus and technique for roentgen examination of the skull. Acta Radiologica Supplementum, 12, 1931.

McRae, D. L.: Focal epilepsy. Correlation of the pathological and radiological findings. Radiology, 50, 439–457, 1948.

Mascherpa, F. and Valentino, V.: Intracranial Calcification. Springfield: Charles C Thomas, 1959.

Medley, B. E., McLeod, R. A. and Houser, O. W.: Tuberous sclerosis. Seminars in Roentgenology, 11, 35–54, 1976.

Molloy, P. M. and Lowman, R. M.: The lack of specificity of neonatal intracranial paraventricular calcifications. Radiology, 80, 98–102, 1963.

Moore, S.: Hyperostosis Cranii. Springfield: Charles C Thomas, 1955.

Moseley, J. E.: Hematologic disorders. In Newton, T. H. and Potts, D. G., Eds.: Radiology of the Skull and Brain. St. Louis: C. V. Mosby, 1971.

Moss, M. L.: The pathogenesis of premature cranial synostosis in man. Acta Anatomica, 37, 351–370, 1959.

Müssbichler, H.: Radiologic study of intracranial calcifications in congenital toxoplasmosis. Acta Radiologica Diagnosis, 7, 369–379, 1968.

Nesbit, M. E., Wolfson, J. J., Kieffer, S. A. and Peterson, H. O.: Orbital sclerosis in histiocytosis X. American Journal of Roentgenology, 110, 123–128, 1970.

Neuhauser, E. B. D., Griscom, N. T., Gilles, F. H. and Crocker, A. C.: Arachnoid cysts in the Hurler-Hunter syndrome. Annales de Radiologie, 11, 453–469, 1968.

Oh, S. J.: Roentgen findings in cerebral paragonimiasis. Radiology, 90, 292–299, 1968.

Osborn, J. D.: A comparative study of special petrous views and tomography in the diagnosis of acoustic neuromas. British Journal of Radiology, 48, 996–999, 1975.

Owen, R. H.: Van Buchem's disease (hyperostosis corticalis generalisata). British Journal of Radiology, 49, 126–132, 1976.

Ozonoff, M. B.: Intracranial calcification. In Newton, T. H. and Potts, D. G., Eds.: Radiology of the Skull and Brain. Vol. 1, book 2. St. Louis: C. V. Mosby, 1971.

Paget, J.: On a form of chronic inflammation of bones. Medico-Chirurgical Transactions (London), 60, 38–63, 1877.

Palubinskas, A. J. and Davies, H.: Calcification of the basal ganglia of the brain. American Journal of Roentgenology, 82, 806–822, 1959.

Pascaul-Castroviejo, I., Lopez-Martin, V., Rodriguez-Costa, T. and Pascaul-Pascaul, J. I.: Radiological and anatomical aspects of the cranial metastases of neuroblastomas. Neuroradiology, 9, 33–38, 1975.

Paxton, R. and Ambrose, J.: The EMI scanner. A brief review of the first 650 patients. British Journal of Radiology, 47, 530–565, 1974.

Pfeiffer, R. L.: A new technique for roentgenography of the optic canals. American Journal of Roentgenology, 29, 410–415, 1933.

Pollock, J. A., Newton, T. H. and Hoyt, W. F.: Transsphenoidal and transethmoidal encephaloceles; a review of clinical and roentgen features in eight cases. Radiology, 90, 442–453, 1968.

Poser, C. M. and Taveras, J. M.: Cerebral angiography in encephalo-trigeminal angiomatosis. Radiology, 68, 327–336, 1957.

Potter, G. D.: Sectional anatomy and tomography of the head. An atlas of the normal sectional anatomy of the head. New York: Grune and Stratton, 1971.

Rådberg, C.: Brain volume in acromegaly. An encephalographic investigation. Acta Radiologica Diagnosis, 15, 113–133, 1974.

Ramamurthi, B. and Varadarajan, M. G.: Diagnosis of tuberculomas of the brain; clinical and radiological correlation. Journal of Neurosurgery, 18, 1–7, 1961.

Reeder, M. M.: Multiple intracranial calcification. Seminars in Roentgenology, 11, 13–14, 1976.

Ritchie, W. G. M. and Davison, A. M.: Dural calcification: A complication of prolonged periodic haemodialysis. Clinical Radiology, 25, 249–353, 1974.

Robinson, R. G.: The temporal lobe agenesis syndrome. Brain, 87, 87–106, 1964.

Rosenbaum, A. E., Rossi, P., Schechter, M. M. and Sheehan, J. P.: Angiography of haemangiomata of the calvarium. British Journal of Radiology, 42, 682–687, 1969.

Ruggiero, G.: A technique for the examination of the optic foramina, Acta Radiologica, *53*, 120–124, 1960.

Runström, G.: Roentgenological study of acute and chronic otitis media. Acta Radiologica Supplementum, 17, 1933.

Russell, D. S.: Observations of the pathology of hydrocephalus. Medical Research Council Special Report Series No. 265. London: H. M. Stationery Office, 1949.

Rzymski, K. and Kosowicz, J.: The skull in gonadal dysgenesis, a roentgenometric study. Clinical Radiology, *26*, 379–384, 1975.

Santin, G. and Vargas, J.: Roentgen study of cysticercosis of the central nervous system. Radiology, *86*, 520–528, 1966.

Schunk, H., Davies, H. and Drake, M.: A study of meningiomas with correlation of hyperostosis and tumor vascularity. American Journal of Roentgenology, *91*, 431–433, 1964.

Schunk, H. and Maruyama, Y.: Two vascular grooves of the external table of the skull which simulate fractures. Acta Radiologica, *54*, 186–194, 1960.

Scott, W. C. and Gautby, T. H. T.: Hyperostosis corticalis generalisata familiaris. British Journal of Radiology, *47*, 500–503, 1974.

Seaman, W. and Furlow, L. T.: Anomalies of the bony orbit. American Journal of Roentgenology, *71*, 51–59, 1954.

Shillito, J. and Matson, D. D.: Craniosynostosis, a review of 519 surgical patients. Pediatrics, *41*, 829–853, 1968.

Sosman, M. C.: Radiology as an aid in the diagnosis of skull and intercranial lesions. Radiology, *9*, 396–404, 1927.

Steinbach, H. L. and Dodds, W. J.: Clinical radiology of Paget's disease. Clinical Orthopedics, *57*, 277–297, 1968.

Steinbach, H. L., Gordon, G. S., Eisenberg, E., Crane, J. T., Silverman, S. and Goldman, L.: Primary hyperparathyroidism: a correlation of roentgen, clinical and pathologic features. American Journal of Roentgenology, *86*, 329–343, 1961.

Stenvers, H. W.: Roentgenology of the os petrosum. Archives of Radiology and Electrotherapy, *22*, 97–112, 1917.

Sutton, D.: Intracranial calcification in toxoplasmosis. British Journal of Radiology, *24*, 31–37, 1951.

Taveras, J. M. and Ransohoff, J.: Leptomeningeal cysts of the brain following trauma, with erosion of the skull. Journal of Neurosurgery, *10*, 233–241, 1953.

Taveras, J. M. and Wood, E. H.: Diagnostic Neuroradiology. Baltimore: Williams and Wilkins, 1964.

Tod, P. A. and Yelland, J. D. N.: Craniostenosis. Clinical Radiology, *22*, 472–486, 1971.

Tsai, F. Y., Lisella, R. S., Lee, K. F. and Roach, J. F.: Osteosclerosis of base of skull as a manifestation of tumor invasion. American Journal of Roentgenology, *124*, 256–264, 1975.

Tytus, J. S. and Pennybacker, J.: Pearly tumours in relation to the central nervous system. Journal of Neurology, Neurosurgery and Psychiatry, *19*, 241–259, 1956.

Valvassori, G. E. and Pierce, R. H.: The normal internal auditory canal. American Journal of Roentgenology, *92*, 1232–1241, 1964.

Van Buchem, F. S. P., Hadders, H. N., Hansen, J. and Woldring, J.: Hyperostosis corticalis generalisata. American Journal of Medicine, *33*, 387–397, 1962.

Varadarajan, M. G.: Statistics of the Department of Neurosurgery, General Hospital, Madras, India. Personal communication, 1965.

Vastine, J. H. and Kinney, K. K.: Pineal shadow as an aid in localization of brain tumors. American Journal of Roentgenology, *17*, 320–324, 1927.

Walker, J. C., Koenig, J. A., Irwin, L. and Meijer, R.: Congenital absence of skin (aplasia cutis congenita). Plastic and Reconstructive Surgery, *26*, 209–218, 1960.

Waters, C. A.: A modification of the occipitofrontal position in the roentgen examination of the accessory nasal sinuses. Archives of Radiology and Electrotherapy, *20*, 15–17, 1915.

Wells, P.: The button sequestrum of eosinophilic granuloma of the skull. Radiology, *67*, 746–747, 1956.

Wiley, C. J.: Lipoid proteinosis—a new roentgenologic entity. American Journal of Roentgenology, *89*, 1220–1221, 1963.

Williams, J. P. and Fowler, G. W.: Gyriform calcifications following encephalitis. Neuroradiology, *4*, 57–59, 1972.

Williams, J. P., Slimack, N. M. and Fowler, G. W.: Radiographic hippocampal calcifications. Neuroradiology, *4*, 159–161, 1972.

Zatz, L. M.: Atypical choroid plexus calcifications associated with neurofibromatosis. Radiology, *91*, 1135–1139, 1968.

2 Vascular Abnormalities

Table 2–1 Abnormalities of the Arterial Wall

1. Infective arteritis (bacterial including pyogenic, tuberculous and fungal meningitis), in:
   a. Meningitis
   b. Meningoencephalitis
   c. Encephalitis
   d. Abscess (cerebral, subdural and epidural empyema)
   e. Cavernous sinus thrombophlebitis
   f. Osteomyelitis
   g. Embolism
2. Atherosclerotic vascular disease
3. Cranial arteritis
4. Collagen vascular disease
5. Necrotizing angiitis
6. Granulomatous disease (including sarcoidosis, see Lawrence et al., 1974)
7. Hypertension
8. Neoplastic disease (glioma, metastasis, lymphoma, leukemia, carcinomatous meningitis)
9. Fibromuscular dysplasia
10. Takayasu's disease
11. Drug abuse (including oral contraceptives)
12. Radiation damage
13. Trauma (stenosis and occlusion associated with hematoma, thrombosis, infarction, and aneurysm formation)
14. Phakomatosis (neurocutaneous syndromes)
15. Miscellaneous
    a. Acute hemorrhagic leucoencephalopathy
    b. Sickle cell anemia (Stockman et al., 1972; Russell et al., 1976)
    c. Chemical arteritis
    d. Migraine

DISEASES OF CEREBRAL ARTERIES

Numerous disease processes produce morphological changes in the walls of the blood vessels which can be seen in cerebral angiograms. Table 2–1, adapted from Ferris and Levine (1973), lists some of these conditions. The luminal changes identifiable by angiography include narrowing, irregularity, occlusion and aneurysm formation, and these morphological changes may be focal, multifocal or disseminated.

An artery can respond to a pathological process in only a limited number of ways. The various conditions that may affect the intracranial and extracranial cerebral vessels can therefore produce similar angiographic patterns. Certain morphological changes or combinations of changes may be more characteristic of one condition than of another, but frequently differential diagnosis is impossible without pertinent clinical and laboratory information.

Narrowing of the lumen of a vessel may be focal or segmental, smooth or irregular. The constriction may be the result of involvement by a meningeal process; external compression by tumor, pus, blood or edema (entrapment, encasement); infiltration of the wall of the blood vessel by tumor, edema or emboli. Other complications of damage to the wall include occlusion or aneurysm formation. Occlusion may also result from thrombosis or embolism.

Dilatation can be observed as a result of the opening up of collateral channels associated with occlusion and/or as a consequence of increased flow of blood to an area of shunting; an upset of cerebral autoregulation with hyperperfusion or inflammatory hyperemia; or as a result of increased metabolism (Lassen, 1966; Davis et al., 1970; Leeds and Goldberg, 1971). In many of these abnormalities, particularly inflammatory processes, the arterial changes are accompanied by venous thrombosis.

A hypervascular pattern or vascular staining may be caused by the accumulation of acid metabolites

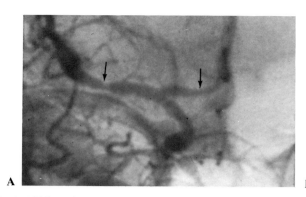
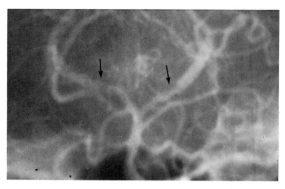

Fig. 2–1 Tuberculous meningitis affecting arteries at the base of the brain. (A) Irregularities are present in the proximal segments of the anterior and middle cerebral arteries *(arrows)*. (B) Another proven case affecting the posterior cerebral arteries *(arrows)*.

and carbon dioxide, with resulting dilatation of the capillary bed and shunting of blood into the veins (early filling dense veins). This is referred to as "luxury perfusion" (Lassen, 1966) or hyperperfusion (Leeds and Goldberg, 1973). These abnormal zones of hyperemia, with or without early filling veins, have to be distinguished from neoplasms and other mass lesions (see p. 275; Ferris et al., 1968). If angiography reveals that such a lesion is space-occupying, the following conditions should be considered as the possible cause of the mass: hemorrhage, infarction, or edema.

The vascular changes of the disease process may be nonspecific, yet their location and distribution — whether they are focal, multifocal or disseminated — frequently offer clues to its etiological nature. Usually the differential diagnosis is further narrowed by the history and appropriate laboratory information.

Inflammatory Arteritis — Meningitis, Encephalitis, "Cerebritis", Abscess

Meningitis: The arteries at the base of the brain are most commonly affected by pneumococcal, staphylococcal, tuberculous and fungal agents, meningeal or meningovascular syphilis, and occasionally *Hemophilus influenzae.* This is because pus accumulates on the floor of the skull, with consequent irritation, edema or actual inflammatory infiltration of the arterial wall. These changes may produce a shaggy angiographic configuration. Such stenotic areas have a variable distribution: short or long segments are involved circumferentially, with occasionally shaggy or irregular margins. Less common are thrombosis or aneurysmal dilatation, due to weakening of the vessel wall (Adams et al., 1948; Dodge and Swartz, 1965; Davis and Taveras, 1967; Ferris et al., 1968; Leeds and Goldberg, 1971; Ferris and Levine, 1973).

If the process is confined to the arteries at the base of the brain in a patient with meningitis, the differential diagnosis should include tuberculous, pneumococcal, fungal and luetic meningitis (Fig. 2–1). If the process is disseminated, i.e., involving

sylvian and convexity branches as well as the basal arteries, all these conditions as well as staphylococcal and *Hemophilus influenzae* meningitis must be considered. An inflammatory lesion affecting exclusively the peripheral vessels may be *Hemophilus influenzae,* pneumococcal or viral meningitis. Involvement of the convexity vessels usually produces a multifocal pattern (Fig. 2–2). The abnormalities observed in the peripheral cerebral arteries appear to be confined to the brain, not having been reported elsewhere in the body (Dodge and Swartz, 1965), and this pattern may point to an anatomical peculiarity of the leptomeningeal arteries.

Tuberculosis has never been observed to involve only the convexity vessels (Fig. 2–3; Lehrer, 1966; Leeds and Goldberg, 1971). *Hemophilus influenzae* meningitis has been reported to be disseminated or to involve the convexity vessels alone (Adams et al., 1948; Lyons and Leeds, 1967) and is com-

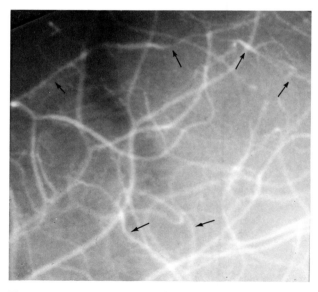

Fig. 2–2 Pneumococcal meningitis. Luminal constrictions, irregularities and dilated segments of many convexity branches are present *(arrows)*. The basal vessels were spared.

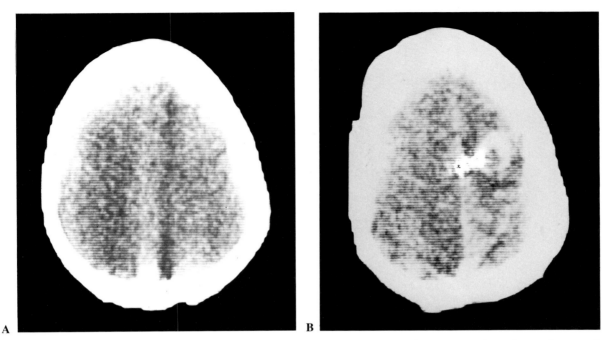

A   B

Fig. 2–7 Cerebral abscess revealed by computed tomography and not shown by angiography. (A) Nonenhanced scan shows no abnormality. (B) Enhanced scan made at the same level shows a thick-walled "doughnut" lesion in the right parietal region. Angiographic study failed to demonstrate a ring lesion.

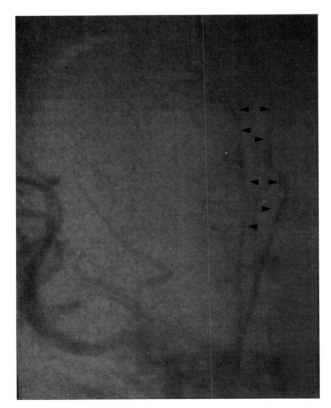

Fig. 2–8 Interhemispheric subdural empyema. Ipsilateral displacement of each pericallosal artery with midline separation *(arrowheads)* indicates an interhemispheric collection—in this case, an empyema.

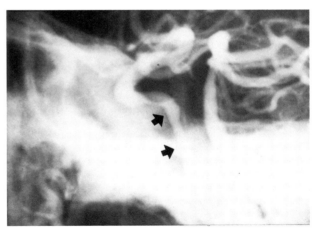

Fig. 2–9 Actinomycosis of the sphenoidal sinus. The extradural and cavernous portions of the internal carotid artery are displaced, with luminal stenosis and irregularity due to the involvement of the arterial wall *(arrows)*. Clouding of the sphenoidal sinus and sclerosis of the sphenoid bone were caused by osteomyelitis affecting the skull base secondary to actinomycosis.

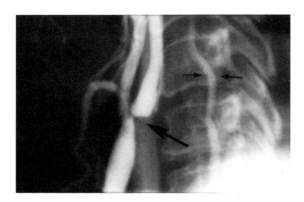

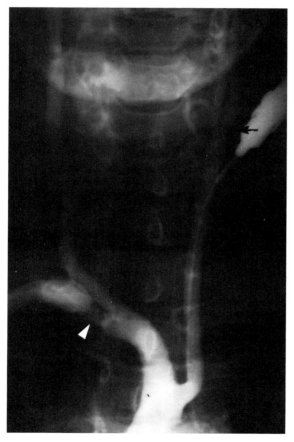

Fig. 2–10 Circumferential stenosis of the cervical portion of the left internal carotid artery due to arteriosclerosis. The stenotic cuff at the mouth of the artery *(large arrow)* reduces its lumen to thread-like dimensions. Retrograde catheterization revealed that the left common carotid arises from the innominate artery. A second atheromatous plaque narrows the right subclavian artery *(arrowhead)*. Filling is observed at the *right* vertebral artery, which is hypoplastic *(small arrows)*.

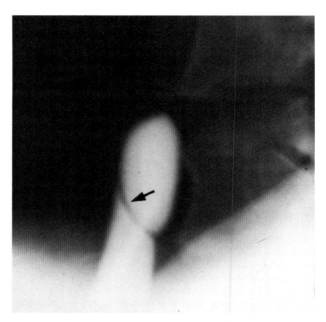

Fig. 2–11 Subintimal injection. The apparent obstruction to flow is not an occlusion but results from subintimal injection of the contrast medium. The raised intimal flap can be identified *(arrow)*.

Couch, 1960). In the latter, the intima is elevated and contrast medium is retained in the subintimal layer. When a stenosis is hemodynamically significant, the slow perfusion time after contrast injection may result in prolonged contact of the contrast medium with the cerebral vasculature which gives rise to complications (Broman and Olsson, 1956). Downstream (retrograde) carotid injection reduces this potential complication by diluting the contrast medium and thus promoting more physiological intracranial filling (see Figs. 2–10 and 2–12). Stenosing plaques may have smooth or rough surfaces. Plaques with irregular surfaces are often difficult to distinguish from atheromatous ulceration (Kishore et al., 1971).

Ulceration of the endothelium most frequently involves the common carotid bifurcation and the proximal 1 cm. of the internal carotid artery, but it also occurs at other sites. The angiographic diagnosis of ulceration depends upon observations of contrast material entering, and being retained, in the atheromatous plaques (Figs. 2–12, 2–13 and 2–14; Maddison and Moore, 1969; Hugh and Fox, 1970; Kilgore and Fields, 1974). A rough or ulcerated plaque may form the bed of an intraluminal thrombus or act as a source of intracranial emboli (see Fig. 2–12). Kishore and his colleagues demonstrated brain emboli in 20 out of 61 patients with ulcerated or irregular plaques in the brachiocephalic arteries. Stenosis or occlusion may occur suddenly as a result of bleeding into the wall of the artery beneath a plaque. An intraluminal thrombus may be

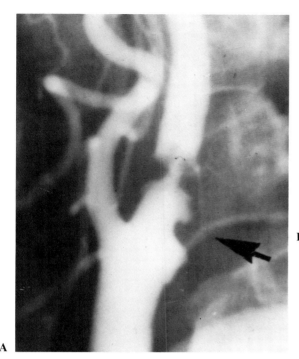

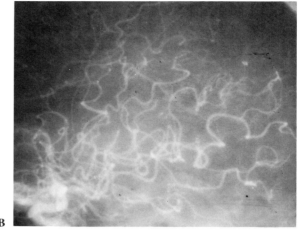

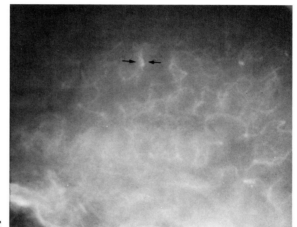

Fig. 2–12 Patient with ulcerated plaque and stenosis of the internal carotid artery, with delayed emptying of the peripheral middle cerebral vessels, possibly due to embolism. (A) A tight stenosis of the lumen is present, with an irregular outpouching of the contrast column, indicating an ulcerated plaque *(arrow)*. (B) Reduced flow occurs through the anterior and middle cerebral arteries as a consequence of the severe carotid stenosis. (C) Contrast retention in a peripheral sylvian branch *(arrows)*, after draining of almost all the contrast medium from the arteries. The possibility of an embolus from the ulcerated plaque was suspected, but there were no confirmatory clinical signs.

recognized in patients with an ulcerated or an irregular plaque: only rarely is a thrombus found without either (Fig. 2–15). Roberson et al. (1973) were able to demonstrate luminal thrombi at the site of carotid stenosis in 7 out of 80 patients with severe stenosis. Since intraluminal thrombi serve as a source of emboli and since propagation of the clot inevitably results in carotid occlusion, it is important to demonstrate and recognize them. Immediate remedial treatment is indicated.

The commonest sites of arterial ectasia secondary to weakening of the elastic tissue in the arterial wall are the extracranial and extradural intracranial parts of the internal carotid artery and the trunk of the basilar artery (Fig. 2–16). Other diffuse abnormalities of the wall include elongation, looping and kinking, producing fusiform aneurysms (Wallace and Jaffe, 1967). Calcification may occur in association with plaques or ulceration. The atherosclerotic process may also involve the small arteries of the brain: it is usually disseminated although it may appear to be focal or multifocal. The distinguishing feature of each arteriosclerotic plaque is that it is

discrete and focal, a notch-like defect involving only one wall (Fig. 2–17). However, the picture may be complicated by coalescence of plaques or thrombus formation. Emboli arising from ulcerated plaques or thrombi from the extracranial carotid artery may give rise to arterial occlusion or stenosis within the skull (Fig. 2–12).

Cerebral infarction occurs as a result of vascular occlusion or reduced perfusion of an area of the brain. Luxury perfusion may be encountered in some patients—that is, a zone of increased vascularity with early filling veins at the periphery of the lesion (Fig. 2–18; Ferris et al., 1966, 1968). These hypervascular areas may cause diagnostic errors if the criteria for diagnosing the luxury perfusion are not carefully understood (Leeds and Goldberg, 1973).

The acute infarct may provoke an appreciable amount of swelling, which results in midline displacement. Careful scrutiny may reveal an arterial occlusion (Taveras et al., 1969). Hemispheric swelling in the presence of an identifiable arterial occlusion must always be assumed to be caused by

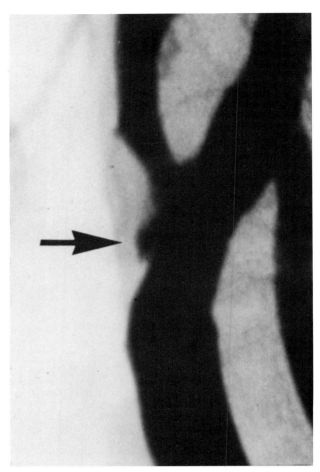

Fig. 2–14 Atheromatous ulcer of the anterior wall of the carotid bifurcation. A saucer-like defect is present in the anterior wall of the common and external carotid arteries with an ulcer crater (arrow).

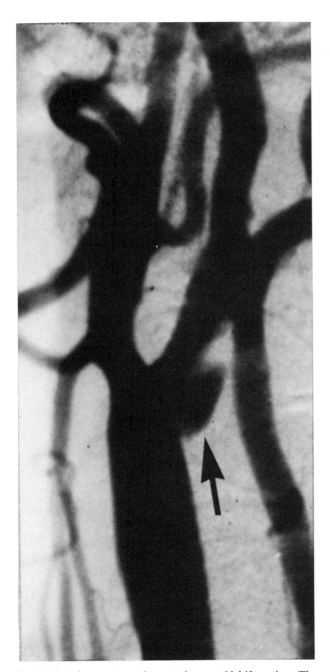

Fig. 2–13 Atheromatous ulcer at the carotid bifurcation. The large extraluminal collection of contrast medium (arrow) was shown at operation to represent an ulcerated plaque. Only minimal stenosis or irregularity of the internal carotid artery is present.

infarction, and not a tumor (Burrows and Lascelles, 1965).

Computed tomography demonstrates infarction as a lesion of low density (Fig. 2–19) or isodensity, compared to normal brain, but associated bleeding (hemorrhagic infarction) may cause a heterogeneous density. Early on, the computed tomogram may reveal no abnormality. According to Davis et al. (1975), the optimal time for examination is 10 days after the ictus. If the parenchyma is damaged, hyperperfusion may occur in the area of damage, which usually shows a gyral or wedge-shaped configuration and exhibits vivid enhancement upon injection of contrast medium (Fig. 2–20; Yock and Marshall, 1975). The hyperemia may sometimes be confirmed angiographically by the presence of dilated vessels (Figs. 2–21 and 2–22). Midline displacement or ventricular compression may occur, but it is usually disproportionately small compared to the infarcted area—an important feature in the differential diagnosis of an enhancing lesion (see

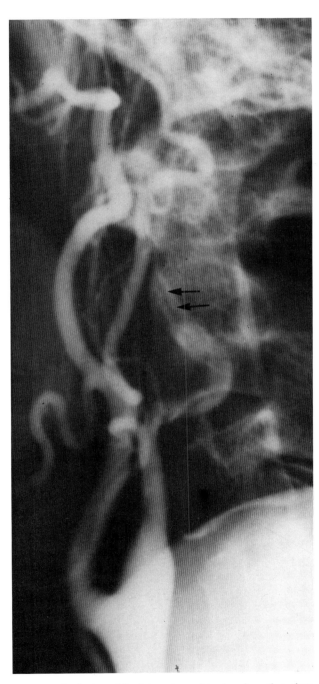

Fig. 2–15 Occlusion of the internal carotid artery by a thrombus. The internal carotid artery is occluded at a distance beyond its mouth, and the linear filling defect within the lumen *(arrows)* represents a thrombus. Note the narrow lumen of the artery as a result of reduced flow.

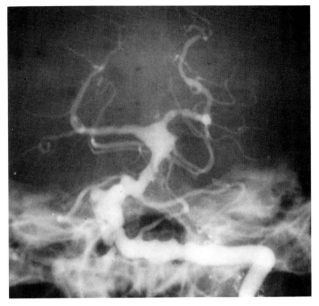

Fig. 2–16 Ectasia of the basilar artery. Irregularity and dilatation of the arterial lumen are present, in addition to ectasia of the artery. This appearance is sometimes called an atherosclerotic aneurysm.

Fig. 2–19). Differentiation may be difficult, but examination after an interval demonstrates a situation that is resolving, while a neoplastic lesion will be static or show progression.

For the radionuclide appearances and the value of serial scanning in cerebral infarction, see Chapter 6, page 256.

Cranial Arteritis

This curious entity, which affects young subjects, is an occlusive disease process of the extracranial and intracranial parts of the carotid arteries. There is preferential involvement of the internal carotid artery in the neck just above the bifurcation and the supraclinoid segment of the internal carotid artery (Wisoff and Rothballer, 1961; Bickerstaff, 1964; Shillito, 1964; Taveras, 1969). Several cases affecting the extracranial part of the internal carotid artery have been attributed to an infective process in contiguous structures such as the nasopharynx or inner ear (Banker, 1961; Shillito, 1964), but no consistent laboratory evidence of an inflammatory etiology has been produced. The possibility of the lesion's being a true arteritis has often been suspected, but it is rarely proved (Hilal et al., 1971). Hilal and his colleagues have proposed a classification into five groups based upon the morphological changes demonstrated by cerebral angiography, viz., basal arterial occlusion without telangiectasia, basal occlusion with telangiectasia, nontraumatic stenosis of the cervical internal carotid artery in children, primary distal-branch occlusion, and small-artery disease.

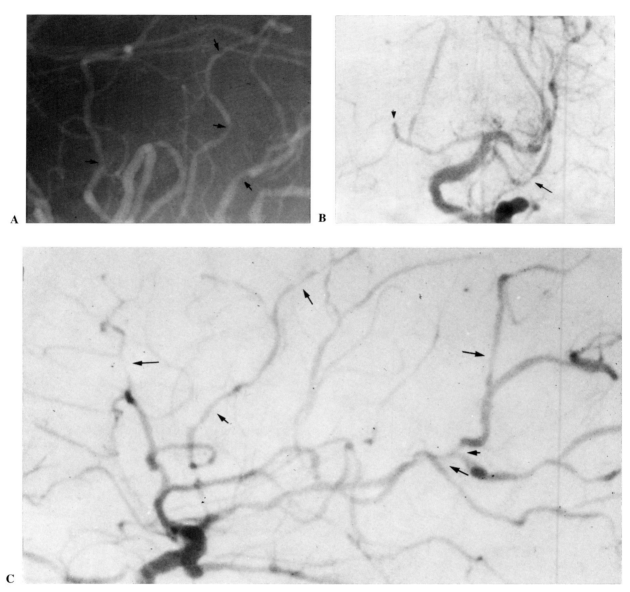

Fig. 2–17 Diffuse arteriosclerotic intracranial disease. (A) Atherosclerotic plaques *(arrows)* produce numerous notch-like defects, usually lying along one wall of the affected intracranial branches. (B and C) Another case illustrates notch-like defects as well as long and short stenotic segments affecting the middle cerebral artery *(arrows)* and superior cerebellar artery *(arrow)*. The right posterior cerebral artery is occluded *(arrowhead)*.

Patients in whom a stenotic segment in the internal carotid artery in the neck is observed 1 to 2 cm. above the bifurcation often have no known cause for the lesion. The arterial segment involved may be long or short and it has smooth margins, and the carotid may be dilated beyond it. No abnormality of soft tissues is apparent clinically or radiographically, and no evidence of associated trauma or infection has been demonstrated, despite the morphological similarity with arterial changes observed secondary to inflammation and trauma (Banker, 1961; Shillito, 1964; Walker et al., 1973). The dif-

ferential diagnosis includes trauma from angiography (needles, guide wires and catheters), inflammatory lesions, trauma (Shillito, 1964; Hilal et al., 1971), fibromuscular dysplasia (Houser et al., 1971) and dissecting aneurysm (Brice and Crompton, 1964; Brown and Armitage, 1973). Hilal et al. make the observation that in their cases as well as others, an arteritis is suspected but rarely proved.

Stenosis of the supraclinoid part of the internal carotid artery may occur without complicating branch occlusion of the middle cerebral artery, and if major pathways are preserved telangiectasia does not occur. As in the neck, the stenosis is smooth and the segment may be long or short. Without an associated clinical history or pertinent laboratory findings, these changes are indistinguishable from the arterial lesions associated with subarachnoid hemorrhage, anemia, or inflammatory or neoplastic disease involving the meningeal envelope.

Telangiectasia develops on account of the profusion of collateral channels that may develop in basal occlusion (Fig. 2–23; Leeds and Abbott, 1965). This rich collateral network arising from the supraclinoid part of the internal carotid artery, and from the anterior choroidal, posterior communicating and lenticulostriate arteries, is required to nourish the basal ganglia and to act as collateral channels in the re-formation of other intracranial branches. This picture should not be confused with a tumor stain, and Japanese workers have named it Moya-Moya (a Japanese term meaning "little cloud or puff of smoke"; see Suzuki and Takaku, 1969). It does not represent a disease entity but rather a nonspecific response of the cerebral vasculature to an occlusion at the base of the brain. Recently it has been described in patients with arteriosclerotic occlusive lesions (Hinshaw et al., 1976) and secondary to tumor encasement (Rosengren, 1974). Radionuclide imaging reveals nonspecific increased activity which demands carotid angiography for correct interpretation (Mori et al., 1970).

Another rich basal network is the "rete mirabile" or transdural supply from the external carotid artery, which in the presence of occlusive disease penetrates the dura and serves as collateral channels to re-establish the leptomeningeal branches of the three major cerebral arteries (Fig. 2–23; Leeds and Abbott, 1965; Taveras 1969).

Patients with the Moya-Moya picture may present as cases of subarachnoid hemorrhage because the rich network of thin-walled capillaries acting as collateral channels can easily rupture when subjected to systemic blood pressure levels. Six out of seven patients showing the Moya-Moya picture who were examined by one of the authors (N. E. L.) exhibited blood-stained cerebrospinal fluid; one patient had a fatal hemorrhage.

Stenosis or occlusion of major branches of the internal carotid artery should always prompt a search for a source of emboli: an inflammatory focus, collagen vascular disease or necrotizing angiitis (see the next section). Occasionally patients with neurocutaneous syndromes or phakomatoses may present with occlusion of a cerebral artery (Hilal et al., 1971).

Collagen Vascular Disease and Necrotizing Angiitis
A variety of collagen vascular diseases and necrotizing angiitis may affect the internal carotid and intracranial arteries (Table 2–2). The clinical signs and symptoms will depend on the particular vessel affected. Both leptomeningeal branches and the larger basal arteries may be involved (Fig. 2–24; Trevor et al., 1972; Ferris and Levine, 1973). Luminal involvement is usually focal but may be disseminated.

In lupus erythematosus, vegetations on the cardiac valves serve as a source of emboli and they may be identified as the cause of embolic intracranial lesions (Fig. 2–25). The luminal changes accompanying this disease are often nonspecific and indistinguishable angiographically from other diseases of arteries. An additional finding that may distinguish these conditions is the occurrence, in addition to luminal irregularities, of peripheral aneurysms. These aneurysms, which may be multiple, have been observed in patients with lupus erythematosis, periarteritis nodosa and temporal (giant-cell) arteritis (Ferris and Levine, 1973). None of the shaggy vessels identified with inflammatory lesions is found. Beading of arteries, due to short segments of constriction alternating with dilatation, may occur (Fig. 2–24). Arterial ectasia dilatation and aneurysm formation may occur as a result of intimal disease. Occlusion may be the only detectable abnormality (George et al., 1971). Venous occlusion may occur concomitantly or alone.

Complications include hemorrhage due to rupture of the thin-walled aneurysm or cerebral infarction secondary to the vascular occlusion. Occlusion or hemorrhage produces a mass, in addition to the arterial lesions. The external carotid artery may also be involved, particularly in temporal arteritis (Stanson et al., 1976).

Radionuclide imaging (Fig. 2–24) and computed tomography (Fig. 2–26) demonstrate the parenchymal damage complicating arterial stenosis or occlusion.

Hypertension
The hypertensive patient frequently has a normal cerebral angiogram. Compared to other patients, the cerebral circulation time may be reduced, because the brain responds to autoregulation to maintain the steady state (Lassen, 1966; Leeds and Taveras, 1969). If the hypertension is complicated by hypertensive encephalopathy, cerebral vasoconstriction and swelling may develop (manifested as hyperperfusion), and also cerebral hemorrhage (Fig. 2–27). This vasoconstriction is nonspecific and is usually secondary to cerebral edema or the vasospasm observed after subarachnoid hemorrhage: the hemispheric vessels show a smooth decrease in caliber (Yamaguchi et al., 1973).

The vessels most selectively affected in hypertension are the lenticulostriate arteries. The significance of abnormalities in these arteries in hyper-

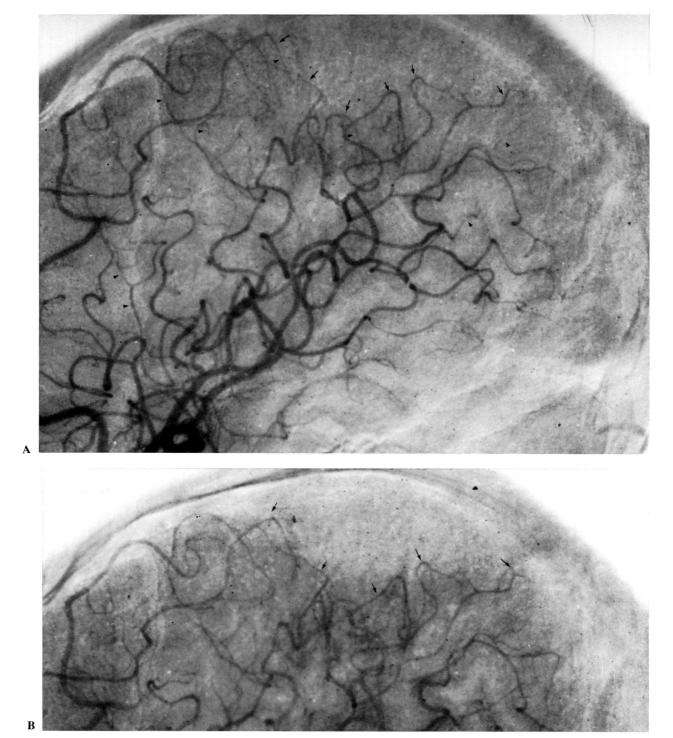

Fig. 2–18 Infarct of the right parietal region with hyperperfusion, which dates the insult to 2 – 3 weeks previously. (A) Diffuse atherosclerotic disease is observed affecting many peripheral branches of the middle cerebral artery *(arrowheads)*. In addition, an avascular zone is observed on the parietal convexity *(arrows)*. (B) Late arterial phase (1.5 seconds later), the avascular zone is better defined *(arrows)*. (C) Intermediate phase: early filling of a cortical vein and the vein of Labbé are observed, both arising from the inferior margin of the avascular zone *(arrows)*. The arrowheads point to opacified branches of the external carotid artery. (D) Early venous phase (one second later): the early filling veins are denser *(arrows)* than neighboring veins. The late appearance of the early filling veins and the fact that they are visualized just prior to normal venous filling indicates that the insult is approximately 3 weeks old.

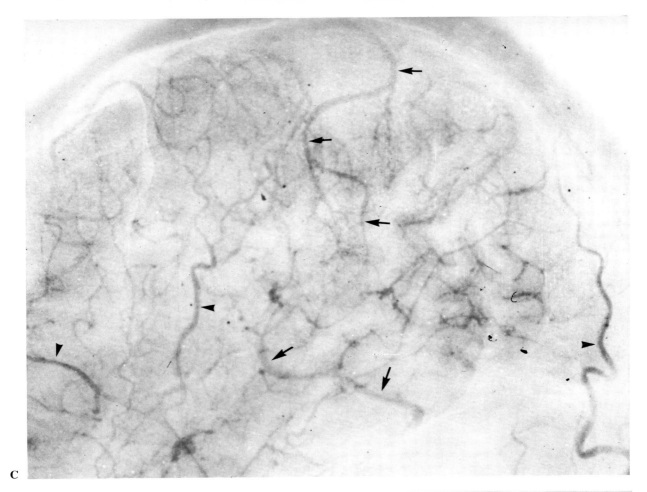

C

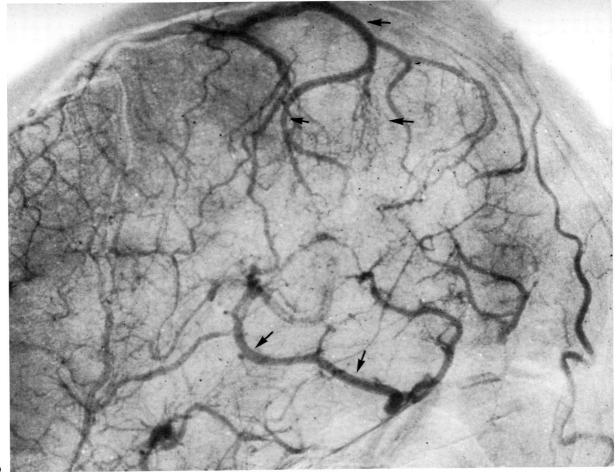

D

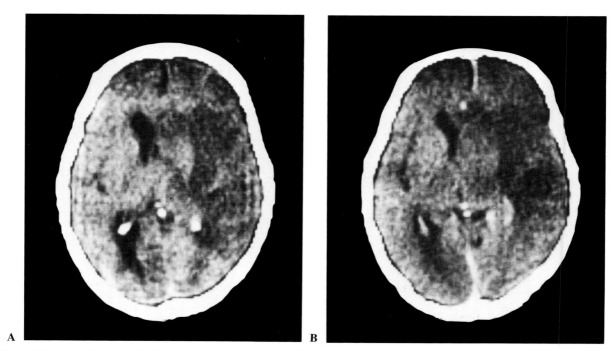

Fig. 2–19 Acute infarction. (A) Noncontrast slice shows an irregular lesion, predominantly of low density, in the ganglionic and temperoparietal region of the right hemisphere. Ventricular compression and moderate displacement of the midline structures to the left side are present, due to edema. The faint density observed within the low-density area is thought to represent normal brain. (B) Enhanced slice made at the same level shows no change, apart from the physiological blanching effect of the contrast medium on the entire brain.

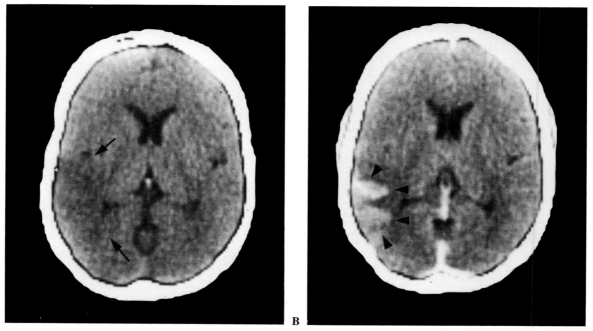

Fig. 2–20 Acute infarction. (A) Noncontrast slice shows a faintly perceptible low-density lesion in the posterior temporal part of the left hemisphere *(arrows)*. (B) Enhanced slice at the same level reveals a wedge-shaped image of increased attenuation in the region of the lesion — so-called gyral blushes *(arrowhead)*.

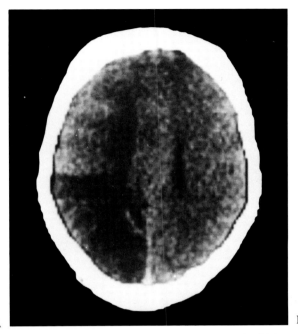 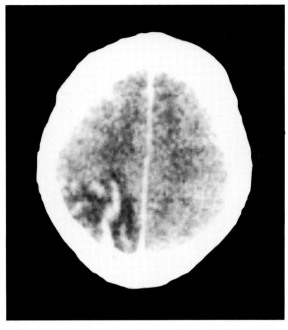

A   B

Fig. 2–21 A 12-day-old infarct in the territory of the left middle cerebral artery. A wedge-shaped low-density lesion is observed in the posterior half of the left hemisphere. (B) Enhanced slice at a slightly higher level shows serpiginous and linear densities, probably dilated draining veins or gyral blushes.

tensive patients was first emphasized in microangiographic examinations performed by Ross Russell (1963) and Cole and Yates (1972). Cole and Yates demonstrated that microaneurysms are more often present and at an early stage of the illness in these patients (46 out of 100 brains studied), than in the elderly normotensive subject (7 out of 100 brains studied). This high frequency of aneurysms and severe disease of the lenticulostriate arteries probably accounts for the increased incidence of capsular hemorrhage in these patients. The abnormalities of the lenticulostriate arteries that can be demonstrated by good quality magnification/subtraction angiography include: elongation, luminal irregularity, reduction in number of branches, occlusion, dilatation, tortuosity and microaneurysms (Fig. 2–28; Gargano et al., 1968; Leeds and Goldberg, 1970; Wollschlaeger et al., 1970). Occlusion may occur but this will often be identified only with angiotomography (Fig. 2–29).

Neoplastic and Radiation Vasculopathy
All types of morphological abnormality may be found in the cerebral arteries of patients with brain neoplasms—constriction, irregularity, dilatation, stenosis, occlusion and aneurysms (Lin and Siew, 1971; Leeds et al., 1971; Leeds and Rosenblatt, 1972; Launay et al., 1977; Solé-Llenas et al., 1977). These abnormalities are not well known as a manifestation of intracranial neoplasia. Changes in the contour of arteries within neoplastic lesions

may be an important clue to the site of the mass, but they provide no information about its histology because diverse entities may cause similar abnormalities (Table 2–1). They are the result of actual involvement of the arterial wall by one or more of the following processes: the neoplasm itself, perivascular edema with cerebral compression, tumor emboli, involvement of the Virchow-Robin spaces, and lymphocytic infiltration of the brain parenchyma with perivascular cuffing. The shaggy or constricted vessel demonstrated within the confines of a mass is caused by tumor encasement. Neoplastic involvement may also dilate or smoothly constrict blood vessels, and these appearances may be mistaken for atheromatous stenosis or occlusion (Figs. 2–30 and 2–31).

Luminal changes in lymphomas are due to involvement of the Virchow-Robin spaces resulting in arterial entrapment. Contiguous and noncontiguous lesions may occur in patients with malignant neoplasms, notably lymphomas, a breakdown in the immune mechanism of the host is considered responsible for the arterial changes, the microscopic lesion being lymphocytic infiltration of brain parenchyma with perivascular cuffing (Ridley and Cavanagh, 1971). Another mechanism of arterial constriction in lymphoma is direct involvement or secondary spread of the process from the dura to the meninges. Consequently patients with lymphoma may exhibit focal, multifocal or disseminated arterial changes.

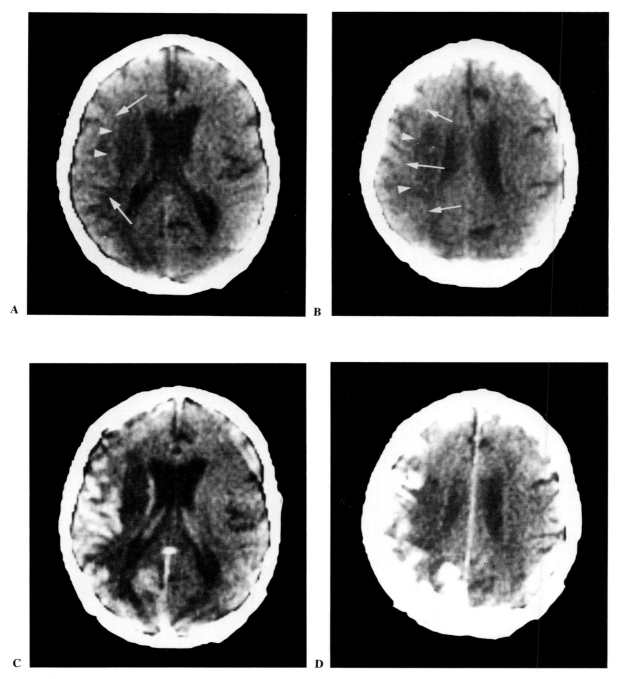

Fig. 2–22 Occlusion of the left internal carotid artery with massive infarction. (A and B) Noncontrast slices show increased density of the cortex of the left hemisphere *(arrows)* with a low-density lesion in the left paraventricular region beneath it *(arrowheads)*. (C and D) Enhanced cuts reveal intense blushing of the area of increased density. The blushing lesion has the configuration of sulci. Note that the midline is virtually undisplaced, despite the large size of the lesion (differential diagnosis of neoplasm!).

Leukemia may infiltrate the meninges diffusely and affect the brain, resulting in similar changes to those identified in patients with pyogenic meningitis. The basal and convexity arteries may be involved exclusively or together.

Meningeal carcinomatosis (Fig. 2–32) produces constrictive or shaggy arteries at the base of the brain or over the hemispheres (Latchaw et al., 1974). These changes are identical to those observed in patients with meningitis and leukemic meningeal infiltration. They are not invariably present, and in some cases the only angiographic abnormality present is a symmetrical hydrocephalus due to obstruction of the cerebrospinal fluid pathways. The entities most often implicated are metastases from melanoma or from primary tumors of the lung, breast or gastrointestinal tract, and subarachnoid seeding from medulloblastoma and pinealoma.

Radiation treatment may result in arterial constriction or occlusion. This process may be focal or diffuse and a mass may occasionally be present due to swelling or hemorrhage (Darmody et al., 1967; Kagan et al., 1971; Painter et al., 1975).

Fibromuscular Carotid Dysplasia

Fibromuscular disease has been observed in both the extracranial and intracranial segments of the cerebral arteries. The cervical part of the internal carotid is the artery most frequently affected. The lesion is found well above the bifurcation, characteristically in the segment of the vessel lying adjacent to the axis vertebra (Houser et al., 1971). The lesions may be bilateral. The characteristic arteriographic appearance is a corrugated or plicated segment of the internal carotid artery which resembles a string of beads (Fig. 2–33). Only a few cases have been examined microscopically and these have revealed only medial fibroplasia in the carotid arteries — in contrast to the various types of fibroplasia demonstrated in the renal arteries.

The diagnosis is usually established by radiological examination. As a rule, only 1 cm. of the artery is affected but occasionally longer lesions are seen. The characteristic "string-of-beads" appearance is such that the dilated segments are wider than the normal lumen and the constricted segments about 40 percent narrower. The stenosis is rarely of hemodynamic significance but the turbulence resulting from the changes in caliber may produce emboli.

According to Houser and his colleagues, carotid involvement is frequently seen in women, and often discovered incidentally — it can be expected in about 1 percent of cerebral angiograms. Less commonly, the intracranial segment of the internal carotid or the vertebral arteries may be involved (Zimmerman et al., 1977). The arterial wall abnormalities account for the complications that may occur which include aneurysm formation, caroticocavernous fistula and branch occlusion.

Takayasu's Disease

Takayasu's arteritis is an occlusive arterial process encountered in adolescents and young adult women. The abnormalities affect the mouth of one or more vessels arising from the aortic arch and may extend for variable lengths. Skip areas are common. The common carotid and proximal internal carotid arteries may be affected but the intracranial vessels are spared.

Drug Abuse

The increase in drug addiction in recent years, and particularly the self-administration of a variety of drugs intravenously, has given rise to various neurological complications. Abnormal vascular patterns may be demonstrated by cerebral angiography (Fig. 2–34; Rumbaugh et al., 1971). Despite the fact that on the whole these are unreliable patients, a picture is emerging in the literature of a vasculopathy consisting of arterial changes resembling inflammatory lesions. The vascular abnormalities, inflammatory lesions and intracranial hemorrhage are sufficient to account for the neurological deficits.

The injected solutions containing the drug or a combination of drugs may be incompletely dissolved in a vehicle of alcohol, tap water, milk or some other unsterile material. It may also include other particulate matter and contaminants. Consequently the angiographic lesions may be secondary to the drug, emboli, an autoimmune response, a hyperergic phenomenon or local or systemic infection due to the injection of infected material. Other factors to be considered are starvation, hypoglycemia, trauma, the effects of repeated injections and the question of sensitization. Rumbaugh and colleagues demonstrated the effect of methamphetamines on intracranial vessels in monkeys. The drug resulted in vasoconstriction and microaneurysms.

While the precise etiology may therefore be difficult to identify, there is no longer any doubt about the abnormal vascular pattern of drug abuse. Citron and his colleagues (1970) demonstrated changes similar to a necrotizing angiitis in drug addicts, particularly those taking methamphetamines. This finding suggests the possibility of an autoimmune or hyperimmune response to the drug or the vehicles used. In addition to arterial changes, Margolis and Newton (1971) claimed that individuals taking methamphetamines are more likely to suffer intracranial hemorrhage.

Lesions Related to the Use of Oral Contraceptives

The introduction of the oral contraceptive agents heralded an increase in the incidence of unexplained strokes in healthy young women. Bickerstaff (1975), in a study of strokes in women of childbearing age in a region of England, found an incidence of 2 to 3 strokes per year prior to the era of contraceptive medication. This incidence in-

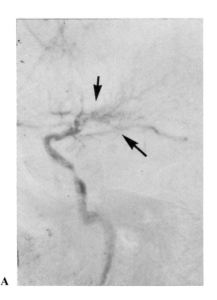

A

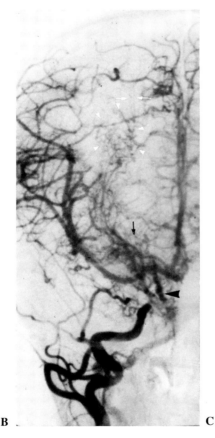

B

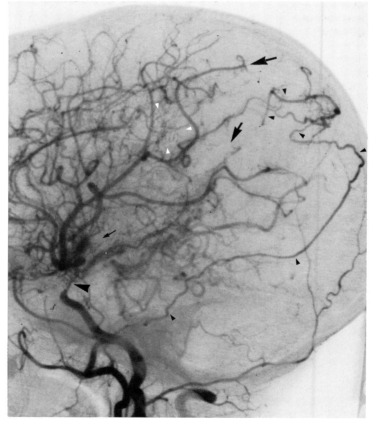

C

Fig. 2–23 The Moya-Moya pattern. (A) A middle-aged adult with diabetes and arteriosclerosis, in whom the right carotid angiogram shows a supraclinoid occlusion with a teleangiectatic flare *(arrows)*. This pattern is seen in Moya-Moya disease. (B and C) A 4-year-old child with cranial arteritis. The right carotid angiogram shows marked stenosis of the supraclinoid part of the siphon *(large arrowhead)*, peripheral vascular occlusions *(large black arrows)*, a teleangiectatic collateral pattern at the base of the brain *(small black arrow)* and in the white matter *(small white arrowheads)*, a transdural meningeal collateral circulation *(small black arrowheads)*.

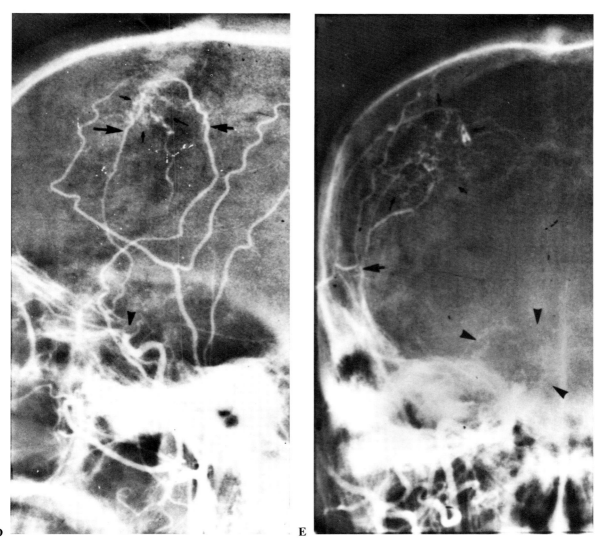

D   E

Fig. 2–23 continued (D and E) A 58-year-old man with severe arterial hypertension. The internal carotid artery is occluded in its su-praclinoid part *(arrowhead, lateral projection)*, and the cervical part is narrow due to reduced flow. There is an adjacent teleangiectatic blush *(frontal arrowheads)*. A prominent middle meningeal artery is present *(large arrows)*, which penetrates the dura to supply intra-cranial structures. There is a teleangiectatic blush in the distribution of the anterior and middle cerebral arteries *(small arrows)*. The patient died suddenly, and autopsy revealed an intracerebral hematoma in the region of the teleangiectatic blush.

Table 2–2 Collagen Vascular Disease and Necrotizing Angiitis

1. Collagen vascular disease
   a. Lupus erythematosus
   b. Scleroderma
   c. Dermatomyositis
   d. Thrombotic thrombocytopenic purpura
   e. Rheumatoid arthritis
2. Necrotizing angitis (Adams and Jennett, 1967)
   a. Periarteritis nodosa
   b. Hypersensitivity angiitis
   c. Rheumatic arteritis
   d. Allergic granulomatous angiitis
   e. Temporal (giant-cell) arteritis
   f. Wegener's syndrome
   g. Carotid and cranial arteritis

creased significantly following the introduction of the "pill," to 8 to 9 a year. Bickerstaff concluded that this increase was related to the use of contraceptives, because all the women beyond the expected incidence were taking the pill. An increased risk of stroke is present in all women on contraceptive medication, but nulliparous women do not appear to be at greater risk than young women in general.

The possible etiological factors include the following (Bickerstaff, 1975): (1) increased blood coagulability; (2) metabolic changes that predispose to the development of thrombosis; (3) hypertension

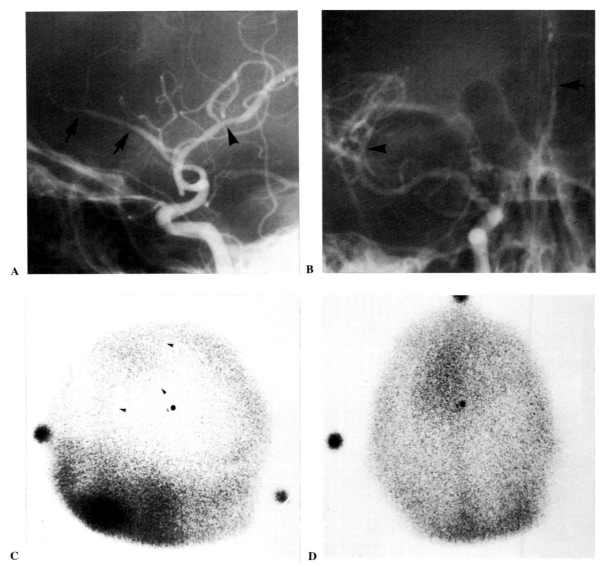

Fig. 2–24 Arterial lesions in a patient with lupus erythematosus. (A and B) Right carotid angiography demonstrates luminal irregularity and beading of the anterior cerebral artery (arrows) and middle cerebral artery (arrowhead) due to involvement of the arterial walls. (C and D) Radionuclide scan demonstrates an area of increased uptake in the distribution of the right anterior cerebral artery, which is consistent with cerebral infarction (arrowheads). Central dot on these views is a camera artifact.

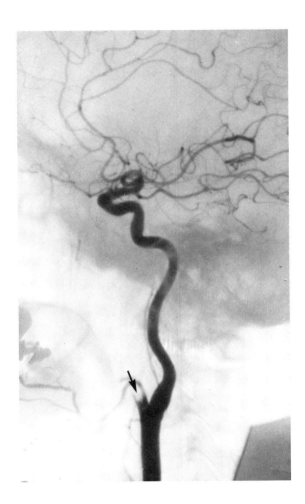

Fig. 2–25 Intracranial emboli of cardiac origin in a patient with lupus erythematosus. Carotid angiography demonstrates a cup-shaped defect in the proximal external carotid artery (arrow) from an embolus. There is also an avascular zone in the distribution of the middle cerebral artery caused by branch occlusion due to emboli.

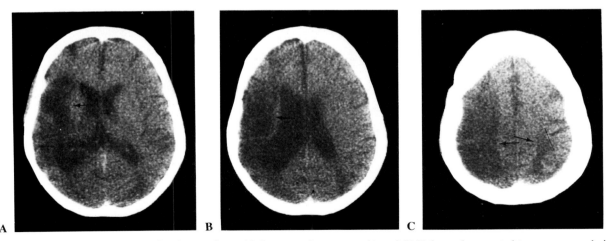

Fig. 2–26 Bilateral cerebral infarction in a patient with lupus erythematosus. (A and B) Enhanced computed tomograms made in a cephalad direction reveal a low-density lesion occupying the *left* temporal lobe, part of the ganglionic region and the parietal lobe *(arrow)*, accompanied by ipsilateral ventricular enlargement but not midline displacement. (C) Enhanced slice made at a higher level shows a low-density lesion in the *right* parietal lobe *(arrow)* in addition to the large left hemispheric lesion *(arrow)*. These findings imply vascular insults in the distribution of both internal carotid arteries.

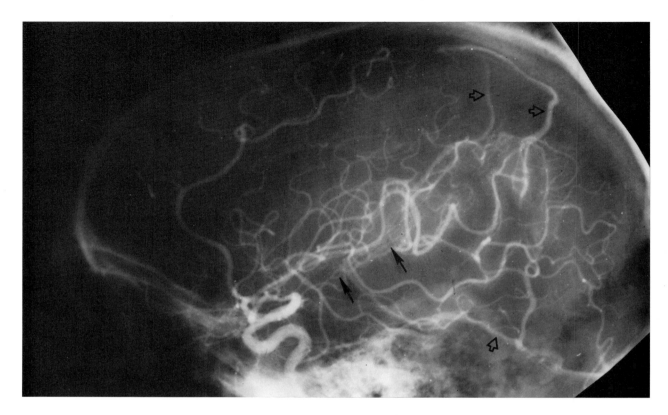

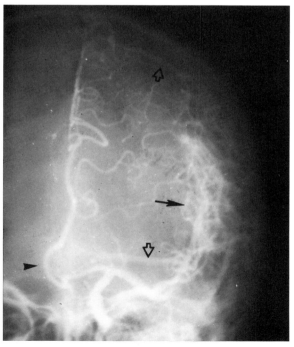

Fig. 2–27 Basal ganglionic hemorrhage in a patient with hypertensive encephalopathy. The middle cerebral artery is slightly elevated and compressed laterally *(black arrows)* by the hematoma. A low round shift of the anterior cerebral artery *(black arrowhead, frontal view)* is present. A disturbance of cerebral autoregulation due to the hemorrhage and hypertensive encephalopathy produces a hyperperfusion with dense and early filling of cortical veins during the arterial phase *(open arrows)*.

and increased incidence of cerebrovascular accidents; (4) mural blood vessel changes favoring thrombus formation; (5) luminal changes within blood vessels predisposing to the development of ischemic episodes; and (6) embolization to healthy cerebral vessels from other parts of the body.

The arterial lesions include occlusions and luminal changes in peripheral arteries (Fig. 2–35) and occlusion of larger arteries (Fig. 2–36; Bergeron and Wood, 1969; Okawara and Calkens, 1973).

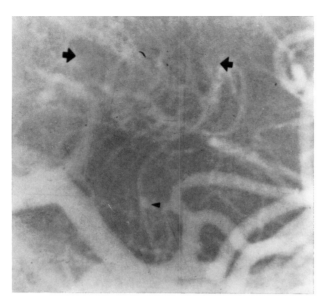

Fig. 2-28 A case of hypertensive hemiparesis. The lenticulo-striate arteries are elongated, tortuous and dilated *(arrows)*. In addition, a microaneurysm *(arrowhead)* is visible, producing localized dilatation of one artery. No midline shift or mass is evident. The patient was a middle-aged hypertensive man who complained suddenly of headache and a right hemiparesis.

INTRACRANIAL VENOUS THROMBOSIS

Venous thrombosis of the brain is a process that is easily overlooked, clinically and radiologically (Scotti et al., 1974). Careful scrutiny of the venous phase of the cerebral angiogram is necessary to examine the appearances of the superficial cortical veins, deep-vein complex and anastomotic veins to avoid this error. The venous discharge varies greatly in normal subjects, and a difference in appearance between the two hemispheres is more common than an identical configuration (Di Chiro, 1962). Numerous pathological lesions causing venous thrombosis have been documented in the literature (Yasargil and Damur, 1974). The most frequent causes are: infection, both distant and local; post-traumatic; neoplastic, particularly meningioma or metastasis; arteritis (Gabrielsen and Heinz, 1969); pregnancy; dehydration; hypercoagulation states and primary or aseptic meningitis.

Patients with venous thrombosis may present with bloodstained cerebrospinal fluid, and cerebral hemorrhage or swelling. Papilledema may be present due to raised intracranial pressure. Venous thrombosis is one of the entities grouped together under the term "pseudotumor cerebri."

The angiographic changes include thrombosis of the superior sagittal sinus (Fig. 2-37), less often of the straight sinus (Fig. 2-38) or the lateral sinus (Fig. 2-39). Occlusion of the superior sagittal sinus is commonly seen in meningiomas arising in the parasagittal gutter (see Ch. 6). In addition to thrombosis of the sinus, which is manifested angiographically by a demonstrable obstructive lesion or absence of the sinus, the direction of flow of the venous blood may be reversed—as shown by the presence of collateral vessels or abnormal or unusual cortical veins (Fig. 2-37). It may be possible to identify numerous corkscrew surface veins (Figs. 2-5 and 2-40; Gettelfinger and Kokmen, 1977).

Cavernous sinus thrombosis may be a difficult diagnosis to make by means of cerebral angiography. It is necessary to identify collateral channels

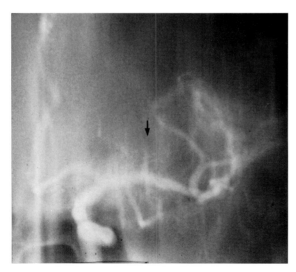

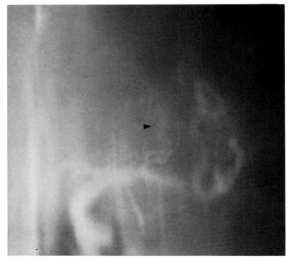

Fig. 2-29 Atherosclerotic disease, branch occlusion of the lenticulostriate arteries. Angiotomography reveals an occluded branch of a lenticulostriate artery *(arrow)*. A slice made 2 cm. posteriorly demonstrates that the other lenticulostriate arteries *(arrowhead)* are tortuous, elongated and dilated. (Reproduced by courtesy of Dr. Herbert I. Goldberg, Hospital of the University of Pennsylvania, Philadelphia, Pennsylvania.)

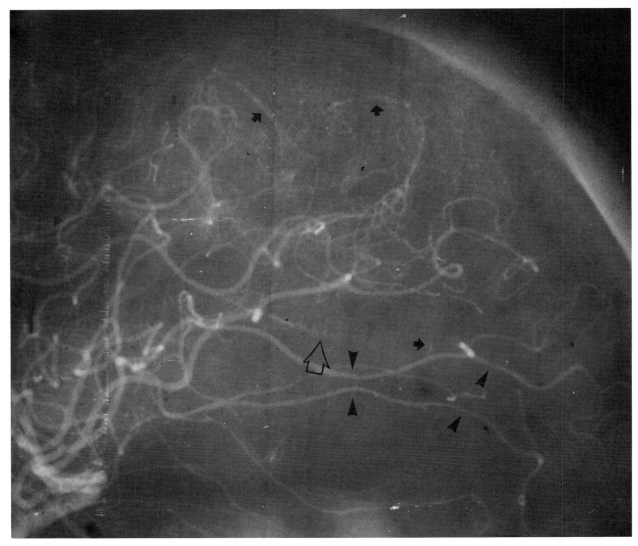

Fig. 2–30 Glioblastoma multiforme simulating small-artery occlusion. Several occluded branches are present in the posterior parietal and temporal regions. Stretched, irregular and occluded arteries suggesting vascular disease and swelling can be identified in the parietal and posterior temporal regions *(small arrows)*. In addition there is an occluded artery plugged with a thrombus *(open arrow)*. Stretching of the distal middle cerebral arteries suggests cerebral edema *(arrowheads)*. These diffuse changes were interpreted as evidence of atherosclerotic disease rather than neoplasm, in view of the multifocal pattern and the absence of midline displacement. However, the patient became clinically worse and a second angiogram 10 days later revealed midline displacement. A glioblastoma multiforme involving both the parietal and temporal lobes in contiguity was found at operation.

such as the superior ophthalmic vein, basilar venous plexus or pterygopalatine veins. The cavernous sinus may be occluded by inflammatory lesions (Fig. 2–41), fungal disease and pituitary and parapituitary neoplasms.

A variety of technical factors may result in overdiagnosis of venous thrombosis. These include: (1) poor technique; (2) normal variations in vessel filling, particularly of the superior sagittal sinus; (3) arterial occlusion with resultant poor perfusion; and (4) vascular spasm or marked prolongation of the circulation time (Yasagil and Damur, 1974).

COLLATERAL CHANNELS

The vascular supply of the brain if interrupted may be restored through collateral vascular channels.

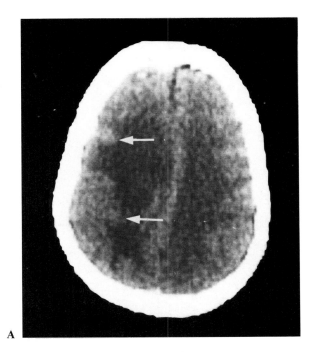

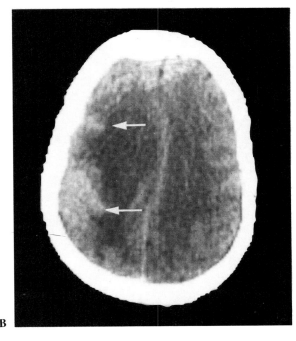

Fig. 2–31 Glioblastoma multiforme infiltrating the frontal and parietal lobes. (A) Noncontrast computed tomogram of the vertex showing two separate zones of increased density with surrounding edema *(arrows)*. (B) Both lesions enhance *(arrows)*. (C) In frontal view a distal shift of the anterior cerebral artery is present with subfalceal herniation *(small arrowhead)*. The sylvian point is depressed and displaced medially by a suprasylvian mass *(large arrowhead)*. A faint blush can be seen in the parietal region (arrows). (Fig. continues on next page.)

These are numerous pathways that are immediately available if the primary anatomical source of supply becomes reduced or is abolished. Additional collateral channels may open up in an attempt to maintain a satisfactory perfusion. Children are as likely to show the collateral pattern as adults (Wisoff and Rothballer, 1961; Savage et al., 1977).

Collateral channels may form to supply the carotid siphon and branches after occlusion of the proximal internal carotid artery. These channels link the external carotid artery with the intracranial circulation, usually running between the internal maxillary branch to the nasal and ethmoidal branches that communicate with the ophthalmic artery in which flow is reversed, so that blood passes into the carotid siphon (Fig. 2–42). Similar collateral channels from the middle meningeal artery supply the cavernous part of the internal carotid artery by means of communication with the artery of the inferior cavernous sinus (Fig. 2–43).

Intracranially, an intact circle of Willis provides the best collateral circulation. However, an intact

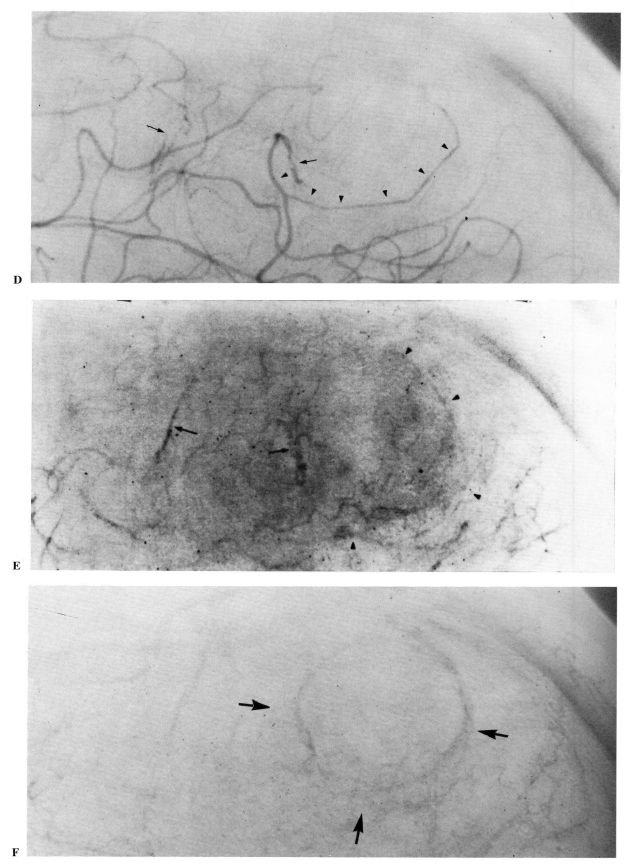

Fig. 2−31 continued (D, E and F) Left carotid angiogram: shaggy vessels due to encasement are seen in the posterior frontal and parietal regions (D, *arrows*). A parietal convexity branch is bowed (D, *arrowheads*). The intermediate phase shows residual contrast medium remaining in the encased arteries (E, *arrows*) and a ring blush is present in the area defined by the stretched artery (E, *arrowheads*). In the venous phase the ring blush persists (F, *arrows*). An infiltrating glioblastoma was found at operation.

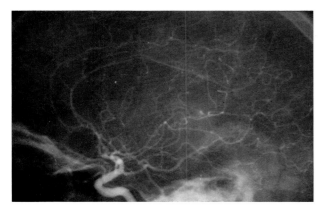

Fig. 2–32 Carcinomatous meningitis in a patient with breast cancer. The branches of the anterior and middle cerebral arteries are reduced in caliber, particularly the insular segment and convexity branches of the middle cerebral artery.

circle is present in only about one-quarter of humans, (Riggs and Rupp, 1963). An intact circle enables compensatory circulation to flow from an anterior cerebral artery via the anterior communicating artery to supply the opposite hemisphere, or from the posterior circulation via the posterior communicating artery to irrigate the carotid circulation (Fig. 2 – 44).

After the circle of Willis, the leptomeningeal anastomoses provide the most important intracranial collateral circulation (Vander Eecken and Adams,

1953). These potential communications link the peripheral branches of the three major intracranial arteries, the anterior cerebral, middle cerebral and posterior cerebral. They are physiologically dormant communications that are pressure-related: if a major branch occludes, the resultant fall in blood pressure stimulates them immediately to open and to supply the deprived territory in retrograde fashion (Fig. 2 – 45).

An occlusion of the internal carotid artery proximal to the origins of its anterior and middle cerebral branches opens collateral channels arising from the carotid siphon and the posterior communicating and anterior choroidal arteries. This proliferation of collateral channels causes a telangiectatic blush, which has been called Moya-Moya (see Fig. 2 – 23).

Occlusion of peripheral arterial branches intracranially may provoke distal medullary arterial branches and capillaries to open up in an attempt to supply the deprived region. Again, a telangiectatic blush may be observed but it is distally situated rather than central (Fig. 2 – 46; Zülch et al., 1974).

Collateral channels may also develop through the skull, from the external carotid to the internal carotid artery by branches that penetrate the dura and connect with peripheral branches of the internal carotid artery (see Fig. 2 – 23). An external carotid-vertebral anastomosis is also known (Schechter, 1964).

The lenticulostriate arteries, although originally

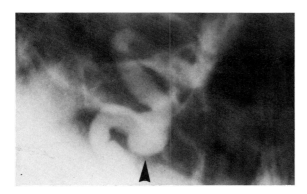

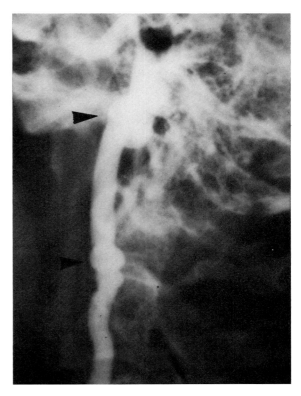

Fig. 2–33 Fibromuscular dysplasia of the internal carotid artery. The internal carotid artery at and above the level of the axis vertebra has a corrugated appearance, including some areas of localized dilatation *(arrowheads)*.

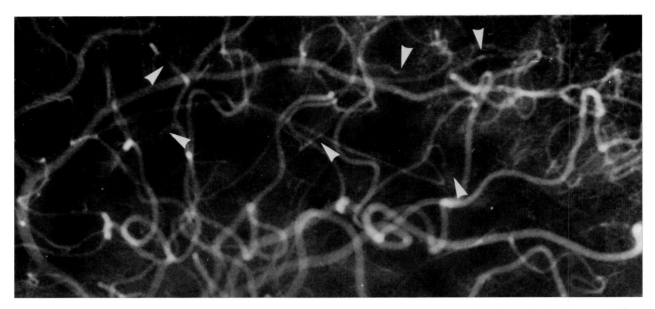

Fig. 2–34 Arterial lesion in a drug-abuse patient with sudden stupor and right hemiparesis. Carotid angiography demonstrates diffuse arterial disease affecting the peripheral branches of the middle cerebral artery. The arrowheads point to luminal irregularity and occlusions. (Reproduced by courtesy of Dr. Calvin Rumbaugh, Peter Bent Brigham Hospital, Boston, Massachusetts.)

considered to be end arteries, can be observed to act as collateral channels if the middle cerebral artery is occluded (see Fig. 2–47; Leeds and Goldberg, 1970). In the event of occlusion of the basilar artery, reconstitution may occur from the posterior inferior cerebellar artery via the superior cerebellar artery, and from the middle and anterior cerebral arteries via the posterior cerebral artery (Latchaw et al., 1974). Rarely, the spinal arteries may be the source of supply (Fig. 2–48).

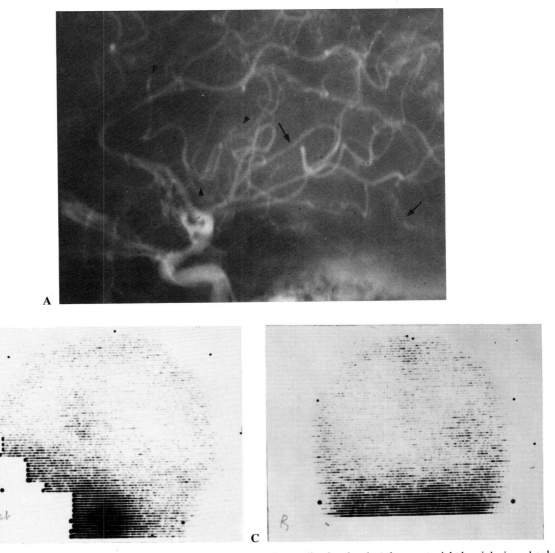

Fig. 2–35 "Contraceptive infarct." A 30-year-old woman on contraceptive medication developed an acute right hemiplegia and aphasia which resolved in 10 days. (A) Several convexity branches of the middle cerebral artery are occluded *(arrowheads)*. Luminal irregularity is also present *(arrows)*. (B) Radionuclide scan demonstrates a focal area of increased activity in the proximal distribution of the middle cerebral artery characteristic of cortical infarction.

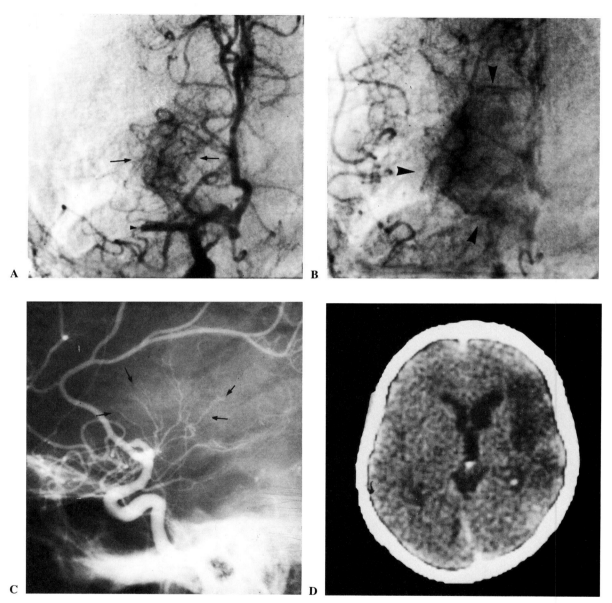

Fig. 2–36 "Contraceptive infarct." A 26-year-old woman on antiovulatory medication suddenly developed a left hemiparesis. (A, B and C) Right carotid angiogram shows nonfilling of the middle cerebral artery beyond the lenticulostriate arteries as a result of occlusion. The frontal view shows the impacted embolus in the trunk of the artery (A, *arrowhead*). A more diffuse and intense blush occurs in the ganglionic region (B, *arrowheads*), as a result of hyperperfusion, at the margin of the infarcted zone. Note the homogeneity of the blush and its relation to the dilated lenticulostriate arteries (A, *arrows*), and the absence of a mass. In the lateral view, the fan-shaped configuration of the lenticulostriate arteries is well shown, in the absence of the overlying middle cerebral artery (C, *arrows*). (D) Enhanced computed tomogram made 2 months later demonstrates the end-result of occlusion of the middle cerebral artery. A rectangular low-density lesion affecting the ganglionic region and part of the frontal and temporal lobes is present. The ipsilateral lateral ventricle and third ventricle are enlarged by focal atrophy.

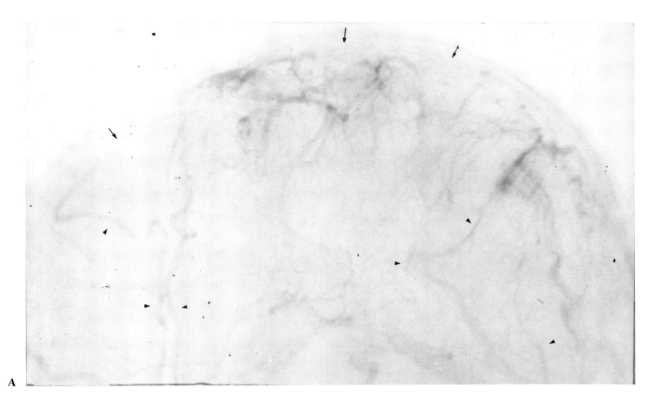

A

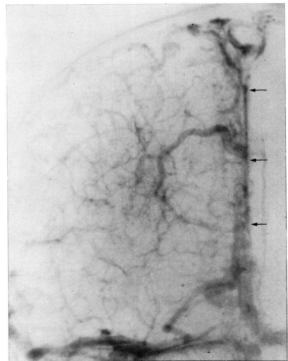

B

Fig. 2–37 Inflammatory thrombosis of the superior sagittal sinus in a child. (A) The superior sagittal sinus is not visualized on the lateral venogram *(arrows)* and the superficial cortical veins are engorged, indicating a redirection of flow inferiorly *(arrowheads)*. (B) Frontal venogram. The mosaic of engorged cortical veins is well shown. Extensive thrombus produces a filling defect in the superior sagittal sinus *(arrows)*.

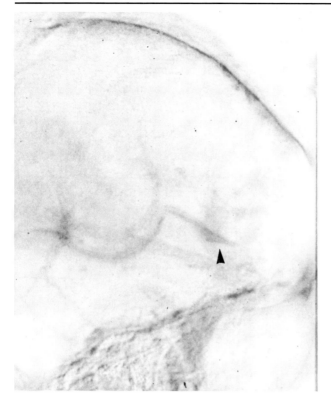

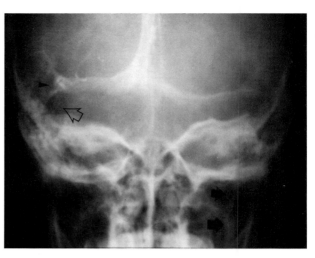

Fig. 2–39 Occlusion of a lateral sinus due to mastoid disease in a young patient with raised intracranial pressure ("pseudotumor cerebri"). The right lateral sinus is occluded *(arrowhead)* and collateral venous channels are present *(open arrow)*. There is no jugular opacification on the right but the left jugular vein is visible *(large arrows)*.

Fig. 2–38 Occlusion of the straight sinus in a patient with sarcoma arising from the superior surface of the tentorium. The occlusion *(arrowhead)* results from tumor invasion of the tentorium and encasement of the straight sinus.

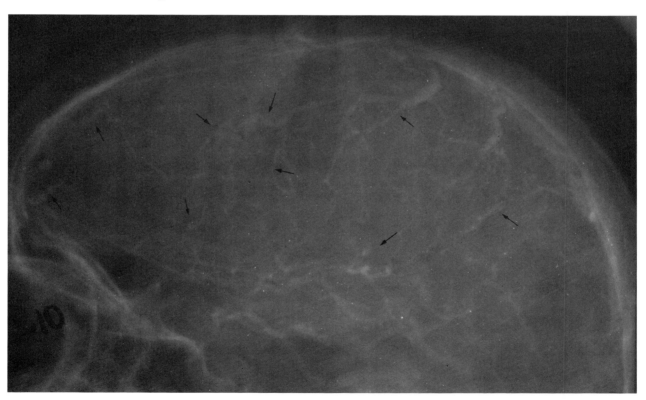

Fig. 2–40 Cortical venous thrombosis in a patient with meningitis. An abundance of irregular and corkscrew veins *(arrows)* is shown, because occlusion of the sinus leads to engorgement and dilatation of the cortical venous channels that remain patent.

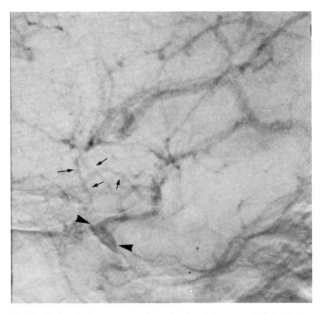

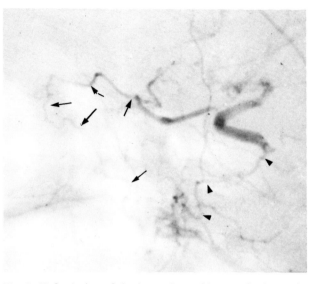

Fig. 2–41 Postinflammatory thrombosis of the superficial sylvian vein and cavernous sinus. The superficial sylvian vein is usually identifiable as a prominent venous channel running in the sylvian fissure and discharging into the cavernous sinus. In this patient, the superficial sylvian vein fails to fill and is replaced by several small collateral channels *(arrows)*. The cavernous sinus is partly occluded, its contrast outline being sharp *(arrowheads)* rather than its usual irregular configuration.

Fig. 2–43 Occlusion of the internal carotid artery in the neck, with compensatory opacification of the cavernous carotid via middle meningeal branches to the artery of the inferior cavernous sinus and ethmoidal twigs to the ophthalmic artery. Branches of the middle meningeal artery anastomose with the artery of the inferior cavernous sinus and reform the internal carotid artery *(arrowheads)*. Collateral channels are also present from the internal maxillary artery to the ethmoidal branches *(arrows)* which opacify the ophthalmic artery with retrograde filling of the carotid siphon.

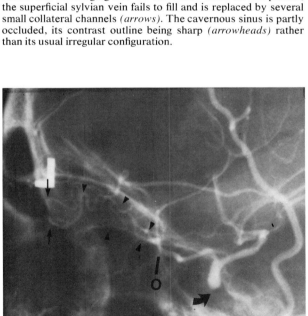

Fig. 2–42 Atherosclerotic occlusion of the internal carotid artery in the neck, with collateral flow to the ophthalmic artery from nasal and ethmoidal branches of the external maxillary artery. Nasal and ethmoidal channels *(arrows)* carry the contrast blood in retrograde direction *(arrowheads)* to fill the ophthalmic artery (big O), which then opacifies the internal carotid artery *(curved arrow)* and its branches. Profuse filling of external carotid branches is noted.

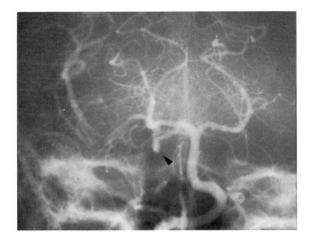

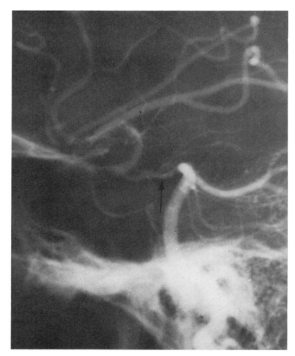

Fig. 2–44 Occlusion of the right internal carotid artery with collateral circulation from the vertebrobasilar circulation. Injection of the right vertebral artery opacifies the supraclinoid part of the right internal carotid artery *(arrowhead)* via an intact circle of Willis through the right posterior communicating artery *(arrow)*.

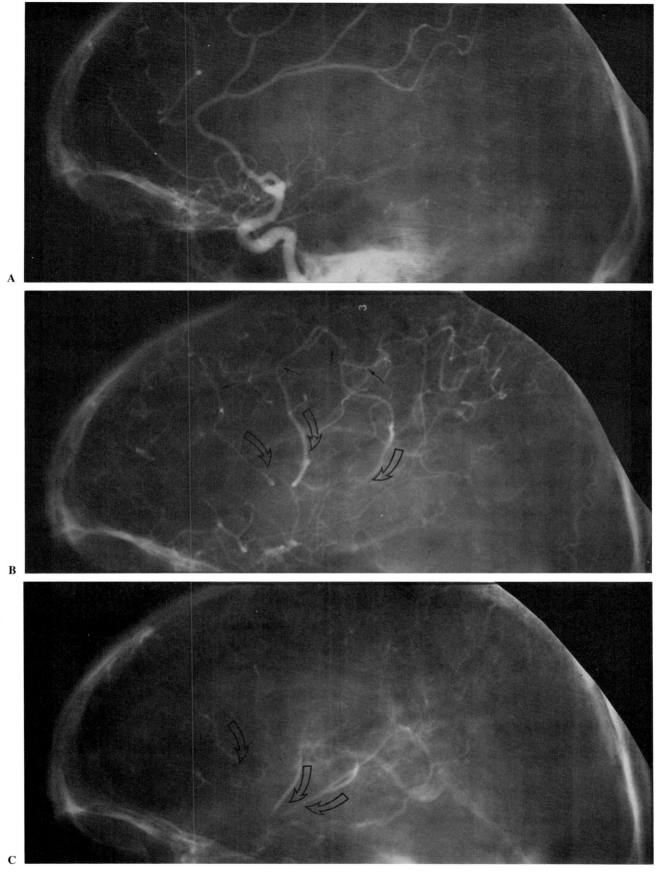

Fig. 2–45 The leptomeningeal anastomosis. (A–C) Case 1. The middle cerebral artery is occluded. The curved open arrows (B and C) point to the sylvian branches filling in retrograde direction from cortical branches of the anterior cerebral artery (B, *arrows*). (Fig. continues on next page.)

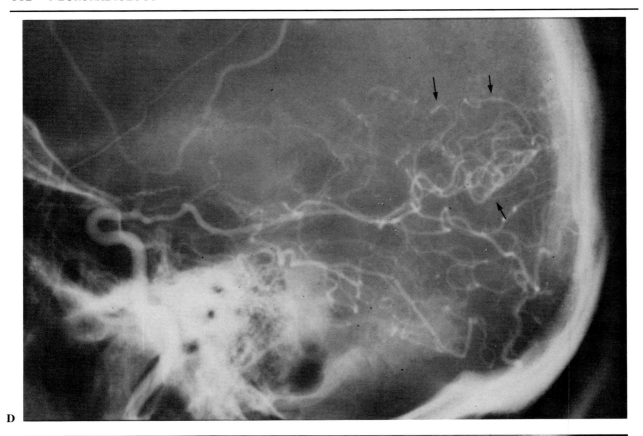

D

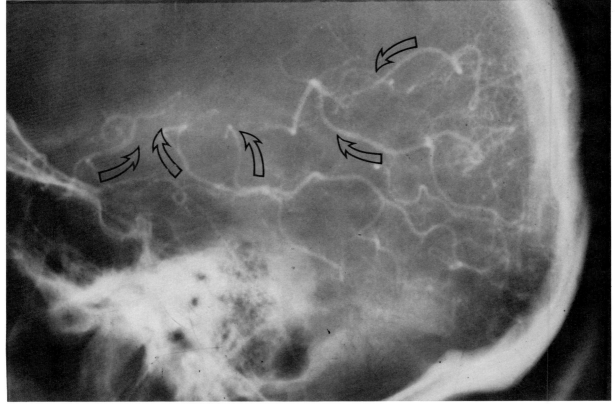

E

Fig. 2–45 continued (D and E) Case 2. The internal carotid artery is occluded just beyond the origin of the posterior communicating artery, and the anterior and middle cerebral arteries fail to fill. However, there is delayed retrograde opacification of temporal branches of the middle cerebral artery (E, *open arrows*) from the supratentorial branches of the posterior cerebral artery (D, *arrows*).

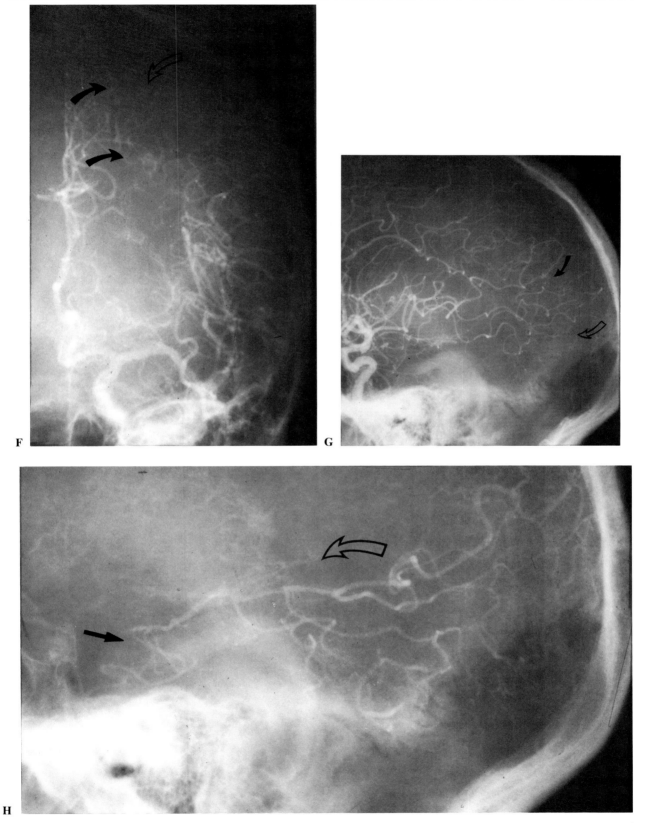

Fig. 2–45 continued (F, G and H) Case 3. A patient with occlusion of the basilar artery. Left carotid angiography reveals retrograde filling of the posterior cerebral artery via leptomeningeal collateral channels from both the anterior cerebral artery *(black curved arrow)* and the middle cerebral artery *(open curved arrow)*. The intermediate-phase lateral view shows filling of the posterior cerebral territory almost to the occluded basilar artery (H, *black arrow*).

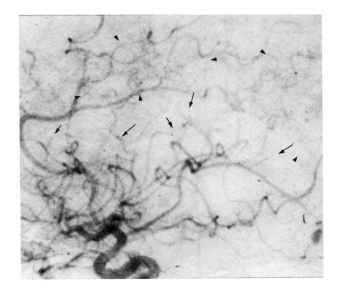

Fig. 2–46 Diffuse vasculopathy of unknown cause with multiple peripheral arterial occlusions and irregularity, and dilated medullary collateral channels. Angiography in a middle-aged patient with a sudden-onset hemiparesis revealed diffuse disease in the middle cerebral territory. Occluded small vessels and luminal irregularities are visible *(arrows)*. There are also clusters of dilated medullary vessels which have the appearance of a telangiectatic blush *(arrowheads)*, representing 3rd-order penetrating collateral channels. Individual medullary arteries can be identified within the blush.

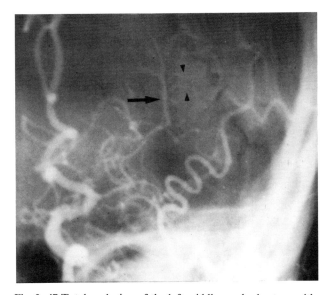

Fig. 2–47 Total occlusion of the left middle cerebral artery with collateral vessels penetrating from the lenticulostriate arteries. The trunk of the middle cerebral artery is occluded beyond the origin of the lenticulostriate arteries. The lenticulostriate arteries are prominent *(arrow)* and penetrating collateral channels are shown to extend laterally *(arrowheads)*, supplying the territory of the middle cerebral artery.

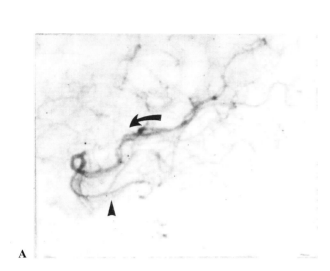

A

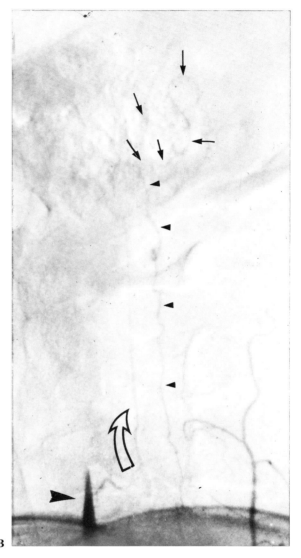

B

Fig. 2–48 Occlusion of the basilar artery with filling of the posterior cerebral artery via leptomeningeal collateral channels from the anterior and middle cerebral arteries, and filling of the posterior inferior cerebellar artery from the posterior spinal artery. (A) The intermediate phase of the vertebral angiogram demonstrates retrograde filling of the posterior cerebral artery *(curved black arrow)* via leptomeningeal collateral channels from the anterior and middle cerebral arteries. The terminal basilar artery also fills, to opacify a superior cerebellar artery *(arrowhead)*. (B) The vertebral artery is occluded in the neck *(arrowhead)*, and the anterior spinal artery fills from the proximal vertebral *(open curved arrow)*. The posterior spinal artery fills from the ascending cervical trunk *(small arrowheads)* and provides collateral channels for opacification of the posterior inferior cerebellar artery *(arrows)*. The gap separating the anterior and posterior spinal arteries is occupied by the spinal cord.

REFERENCES

Adams, J. H. and Jennett, W. B.: Acute necrotizing encephalitis: a problem in diagnosis. Journal of Neurology, Neurosurgery and Psychiatry, *30*, 248–260, 1967.

Adams, R. D., Kubik, C. S. and Bonner, F. J.: Clinical and pathological aspects of influenzal meningitis. Archives of Pediatrics, *65*, 354–376; 408–441, 1948.

Amin, P. H.: Radiological findings in herpes simplex encephalitis. British Journal of Radiology, *45*, 652–658, 1972.

Banker, B. Q.: Cerebral vascular disease in infancy and childhood. 1. Occlusive vascular diseases. Journal of Neuropathology and Experimental Neurology, *20*, 127–140, 1961.

Beller, A. J., Sahar, A. and Praiss, I.: Brain abscess. Review of 89 cases of a period of 30 years. Journal of Neurology, Neurosurgery and Psychiatry, *36*, 757–768, 1973.

Bergeron, R. T. and Wood, E. H.: Oral contraceptives and cerebrovascular complications. Radiology, *92*, 231–238, 1969.

Bickerstaff, E. R.: Aetiology of acute hemiplegia in childhood. British Medical Journal, *2*, 82–87, 1964.

Bickerstaff, E. R.: Neurological complication of oral contraceptives. Oxford: Clarendon Press, 1975.

Brice, J. G. and Crompton, M. R.: Spontaneous dissecting aneurysms of the cervical internal carotid. British Medical Journal, *2*, 790–792, 1964.

Broman, T. and Olsson, O.: Technique for the pharmaco-dynamic investigation of contrast medium for cerebral angiography. Acta Radiologica, *45*, 96–100, 1956.

Brown, O. L. and Armitage, J. L.: Spontaneous dissecting aneurysms of the cervical internal carotid artery. Two case reports and a survey of the literature. American Journal of Roentgenology, *118*, 648–653, 1973.

Burrows, E. H. and Lascelles, R. G.: The contribution of radiology to the diagnosis and prognosis of occlusions of the middle cerebral artery and its branches. British Journal of Radiology, *38*, 481–493, 1965.

Citron, B. P., Halpern, M., McCarron, M., Lundberg, G. D., McCormick, R., Pincus, I. J., Totter D., and Haverback, B. J.: Necrotizing angiitis associated with drug abuse. New England Journal of Medicine, *283*, 1003–1011, 1970.

Cole, F. M. and Yates, P.: Intracerebral microaneurysms and small cerebrovascular lesions. Brain, *90*, 759–768, 1967.

Cole, F. M. and Yates, P. O.: The occurrence and significance of intracerebral micro-aneurysms. Journal of Pathology and Bacteriology, *93*, 392–411, 1967.

Cope, V. and Howieson, J.: Radiological findings in acute necrotising encephalitis due to herpes simplex virus. Clinical Radiology, *18*, 109–111, 1967.

Courey, W. R., New, P. F. J. and Price, D. L.: Angiographic manifestations of craniofacial phycomycosis. Radiology, *103*, 329–334, 1972.

Crawford, E. S., Wukasch, D. W. and Debakey, M. E.: Hemodynamic changes associated with carotid artery occlusion: an experimental and clinical study. Cardiovascular Research, *1*, 3–10, 1962.

Darmody, W. R., Thomas, L. M., and Gurdjian, E. S.: Postirradiation vascular insufficiency syndrome. Neurology, *17*, 1190–1192, 1967.

Davis, D. O., Dilenge, D. and Schlaepfer, W.: Arterial dilatation in purulent meningitis. Journal of Neurosurgery, *32*, 112–115, 1970.

Davis, D. O. and Taveras, J. M.: Radiologic aspect of inflammatory conditions affecting the central nervous system. Clinical Neurosurgery, *14*, 172–210, 1967.

Davis, K. R., Taveras, J. W., New, P. F. J., Schnur, J. A. and Roberson, G. H.: Cerebral infarction diagnosis by computerized tomography. American Journal of Roentgenology, *124*, 643–660, 1975.

Di Chiro, G.: Angiographic patterns of cerebral convexity veins and superficial dural sinuses. American Journal of Roentgenology, *87*, 308–321, 1962.

Dodge, P. R. and Swartz, M. N.: Bacterial meningitis – a review of selected aspects. II. Special neurologic problems, post-meningitis complications and clinicopathological correlations. New England Journal of Medicine, *272*, 954–960, 1965.

Ferris, E. J. and Ciembroniewicz, J.: Subdural empyema: Report of a case demonstrating the unusual angiographic triad. American Journal of Roentgenology, *92*, 838–843, 1964.

Ferris, E. J., Gabriele, O. F., Hipona, F. A. and Shapiro, J. H.: Early venous filling in cranial angiography. Radiology, *90*, 553–567, 1968b.

Ferris, E. J. and Levine, H. L.: Cerebral arteritis: Classification. Radiology, *109*, 327–341, 1973.

Ferris, E. J., Rudikoff, F. C. and Shapiro, J. H.: Cerebral angiography of bacterial infection. Radiology, *90*, 727–734, 1968a.

Ferris, E. J., Shapiro, J. H. and Simeone, F. A.: Arteriovenous shunting in cerebrovascular occlusive disease. American Journal of Roentgenology, *98*, 631–636, 1966.

Gabrielsen, T. O. and Heinz, E. R.: Spontaneous aseptic thrombosis of the superior sagittal sinus and cerebral veins. American Journal of Roentgenology, *107*, 579–588, 1969.

Gado, M., Axley, J., Appleton, D. B. and Prensky, A. L.: Angiography in the acute and post-treatment phases of Hemophilus influenzae meningitis. Radiology, *110*, 439–444, 1974.

Gargano, F. P., Flaten, P. A. and Meringoff, B. N.: The angiographic criteria for the diagnosis of basal ganglionic hemorrhages and their extensions. Radiology, *91*, 1119–1123, 1968.

George, A. E., Kishore, P. R. S. and Chase, N. E.: Primary diseases of the cerebral blood vessels. Seminars in Roentgenology, *6*, 34–47, 1971.

Gettelfinger, D. M. and Kokmen, E.: Superior sagittal sinus thrombosis. Archives of Neurology, *34*, 2–6, 1977.

Handa, J., Hanakita, J., Koyama, T. and Handa, H.: Interhemispheric subdural empyema with an enlarged tentorial artery and vein. Neuroradiology, *9*, 167–170, 1975.

Handel, S. F., Klein, W. C. and Kim, Y. W.: Intracranial epidural abscess. Radiology, *111*, 117–120, 1974.

Harwood-Nash, D. C. and Fitz, C. R.: Neuroradiology in infants and children. St. Louis: C. V. Mosby, 1976.

Hilal, S. K., Solomon, G. E., Gold, A. P., and Carter, S.: Primary cerebral arterial occlusive disease in children; Part I. Acute acquired hemiplegia. Radiology, *99*, 71–86, 1971.

Hilal, S. K., Solomon, G. E., Gold, A. P. and Carter, S.: Primary cerebral arterial occlusive disease in children. Part II. Neurocutaneous syndromes. Radiology, *99*, 87–94, 1971.

Hinshaw, D. B., Thompson, J. R. and Hasso, A. N.: Adult arteriosclerotic Moya-Moya. Radiology, *118*, 633–636, 1976.

Houser, O. W., Baker, H. L., Jr., Sandok, B. A. and Holley, K. E.: Cephalic arterial fibromuscular dysplasia. Radiology, *101*, 605–611, 1971.

Huckman, M. S., Weinberg, P. E., Kim, K. S. and Davis, D. O.: Angiographic and clinio-pathologic correlates in basal ganglionic hemorrhage. Radiology, *95*, 79–92, 1970.

Hugh, A. E. and Fox, J. A.: The precise localization of atheroma and its association with stasis at the origin of the internal carotid artery – a radiographic investigation. British Journal of Radiology, *43*, 277–283, 1970.

Jordan, E. E., James, A. E. and Hodges, III, F. J.: Comparison of the cerebral angiogram and the brain radionuclide image in brain abscess. Radiology, *104*, 327–331, 1972.

Kagan, A. R., Bruce, D. W. and Di Chiro, G.: Fatal foam cell arteritis of the brain after irradiation for Hodgkin's disease: angiography and pathology. Stroke, *2*, 232–238, 1971.

Kaufman, D. M. and Leeds, N. E.: Focal abnormalities with subdural empyema. Neuroradiology, *11*, 169–173, 1976.

Kaufman, D. M. and Leeds, N. E.: Computed tomography (CT) in the diagnosis of intracranial abscess, subdural empyema and epidural empyema. Neurology, *27*, 1069–1073, 1977.

Kilgore, B. B. and Fields, W. S.: Occlusive disease in adults. In Newton, T. H. and Potts, D. G., Eds.: Radiology of the skull and brain. Vol. 2, book 4. St. Louis: C. V. Mosby, 1974.

Kishore, P. R. S., Chase, N. E. and Kricheff, I. I.: Carotid stenosis and intracranial emboli. Radiology, *100*, 351–356, 1971.

Lassen, N. A.: The luxury-perfusion syndrome and its possible relation to acute metabolic acidosis localised within the brain. The Lancet, *2*, 1113–1115, 1966.

Latchaw, R. E., Gabrielsen, T. O. and Seeger, J. F.: Cerebral angiography in meningeal sarcomatosis and carcinomatosis. Neuroradiology, *8*, 131–139, 1974a.

Latchaw, R. E., Seeger, J. E. and Gabrielsen, T. O.: Vertebrobasilar arterial occlusions in children. Neuroradiology, *8*, 141–147, 1974b.

Launay, M., Fredy, P., Merland, J. J. and Bories, J.: Narrowing and occlusion of arteries by intracranial tumors. Review of literature and report of 25 cases. Neuroradiology, *14*, 117–126, 1977.

Lawrence, W. F., El Gammal, T., Pool, W. H. Jr., and Apter, L.: Radiological manifestations of neurosarcoidosis: Report of three cases and a review of the literature. Clinical Radiology, *25*, 343–348, 1974.

Leeds, N. E. and Abbott, K. H.: Collateral circulation in cerebrovascular disease in childhood via rete mirabile and perforating branches of anterior choroidal and posterior cerebral arteries. Radiology, *85*, 628–634, 1965.

Leeds, N. E. and Goldberg, H. I.: Lenticulostriate artery abnormalities: value of direct serial magnification. Radiology, *97*, 377–383, 1970.

Leeds, N. E. and Goldberg, H. I.: Angiographic manifestations in cerebral inflammatory disease. Radiology, *98*, 595–604, 1971.

Leeds, N. E., and Goldberg, H. I.: Abnormal vascular patterns in benign intracranial lesions: pseudo tumors of the brain. American Journal of Roentgenology, *118*, 576–585, 1973.

Leeds, N. E. and Rosenblatt, R.: Arterial wall irregularities in intracranial neoplasms: the shaggy vessel brought into focus. Radiology: *103*, 121–124, 1972.

Leeds, N. E., Rosenblatt, R. and Zimmerman, H. M.: Focal angiographic changes of cerebral lymphoma with pathologic correlation. Radiology, *99*, 595–599, 1971.

Leeds, N. E., and Taveras, J. M.: Dynamic Factors in Diagnosis of Supratentorial Brain Tumors by Cerebroangiography. Philadelphia: W. B. Saunders, 1969.

Lehrer, H.: The angiographic triad in tuberculous meningitis. Radiology, 87, 829–835, 1966.

Liebeskind, A. L., Cohen, S., Anderson, R., Schechter, M. M. and Zingesser, L. H.: Unusual segmental cerebrovascular changes. Radiology, 106, 119–122, 1973.

Lin, J. P. and Siew, F. P.: Glioblastoma multiforme presenting angiographically as intracranial atherosclerotic vascular disease. Radiology, 101, 353–354, 1971.

Lyons, E. L. and Leeds, N. E.: The angiographic demonstration of arterial vascular disease in purulent meningitis. Report of a case. Radiology, 88, 935–938, 1967.

Maddison, F. E. and Moore, W. S.: Ulcerated atheroma of the carotid artery: arteriographic appearance. American Journal of Roentgenology, 107, 530–534, 1969.

Margolis, M. T. and Newton, T. H.: Methamphetamine ("speed") arteritis. Neuroradiology, 2, 179–182, 1971.

Mori, H., Maeda, T., Suzuki, Y., Hisada, K. and Kadoya, S.: Brain scan in cerebrovascular Moya-Moya disease. American Journal of Roentgenology, 124, 583–589, 1975.

Newton, T. H. and Couch, R. S. C.: Possible errors in the arteriographic diagnosis of internal carotid artery occlusions. Radiology, 75, 766–773, 1960.

Nielsen, H. and Halaburt, H.: Cerebral abscess with special reference to the angiographic changes. Neuroradiology, 12, 73–78, 1976.

Okawara, S. and Calkens, R.: Cerebral arterial occlusive disease with telangiectasia associated with oral contraceptives. Archives of Neurology, 29, 60–62, 1973.

Olmstead, W. W. and McGee, T. P.: The pathogenesis of peripheral aneurysms of the central nervous system: A subject review from the AFIP. Radiology, 123, 661–666, 1977.

Painter, M. J., Chutorian, A. M. and Hilal, S. K.: Cerebrovasculopathy following irradiation in childhood. Neurology, 25, 189–194, 1975.

Patton, J. T. and Hitchcock, E.: Angiographic features of falcine subdural empyema. Clinical Radiology, 19, 229–232, 1968.

Pexman, J. H. W.: The angiographic and brain scan features of acute herpes simplex encephalitis. British Journal of Radiology, 47, 179–184, 1974.

Raimondi, A. J.: Pediatric Neuroradiology, p. 665. Philadelphia: W. B. Saunders, 1972.

Ridley, A. and Cavanagh, J. B.: Lymphocytic infiltration in gliomas: Evidence of possible host resistance. Brain, 94, 117–124, 1971.

Riggs, H. E. and Rupp, C.: Variations in form of circle of Willis. Archives of Neurology, 8, 8–14, 1963.

Roberson, G. H., Scott, W. R. and Rosenbaum, A. E.: Thrombi at the site of carotid stenosis. Radiology, 109, 353–356, 1973.

Rosengren, K.: Moya-Moya vessels—collateral arteries of the basal ganglia. Malignant occlusion of the anterior cerebral arteries. Acta Radiologica Diagnosis, 15, 145–151, 1974.

Ross Russell, R. W.: Observations on intracerebral aneurysms. Brain, 86, 425–442, 1963.

Rumbaugh, C. L., Bergeron, R. T., Fang, H. C. H. and McCormick, R.: Cerebral angiographic changes in the drug abuse patient. Radiology, 101, 335–344, 1971.

Russell, M. O., Goldberg, H. I., Reis, L., Friedman, S., Slater, R., Reivich, M. and Schwartz, E.: Transfusion therapy for cerebrovascular abnormalities in sickle cell disease. Journal of Pediatrics, 88, 382–387, 1976.

Savage, J. P., Gilday, D. L. and Ash, J. M.: Cerebrovascular disease in childhood. Radiology, 123, 385–391, 1977.

Schechter, M. M.: The occipital vertebral anastomosis. Journal of Neurosurgery, 21, 758–762, 1964.

Scotti, L. N., Goldman, R. L., Hardman, D. R. and Heinz, E. R.: Venous thrombosis in infants and children. Radiology, 112, 393–399, 1974.

Shaw, M. D. M. and Russell, J. A.: Cerebellar abscess: a review of 47 cases. Journal of Neurology, Neurosurgery and Psychiatry, 38, 429–435, 1975.

Shillito, J. Jr.: Carotid arteritis: a cause of hemiplegia in childhood. Journal of Neurosurgery, 21, 540–551, 1964.

Solé-Llenas, J., Mercader, J. M. and Pons-Tortella, E.: Morphological aspects of the vessels of the brain tumors. Neuroradiology, 13, 51–54, 1975.

Stanson, A. W., Klein, R. G. and Hunder, G. G.: Extracranial angiographic findings in giant cell (temporal) arteritis. American Journal of Roentgenology, 127, 957–963, 1976.

Stockman, J. A., Nigro, M. A., Mishkin, M. M. and Oski, F. A.: Occlusion of large cerebral vessels in sickle-cell anemia. New England Journal of Medicine, 287, 846–849, 1972.

Suzuki, J. and Takaku, A.: Cerebrovascular "moyamoya" disease. Archives of Neurology, 20, 288–299, 1969.

Taveras, J. M.: Multiple progressive intracranial arterial occlusions: A syndrome of children and young adults. American Journal of Roentgenology, 106, 235–268, 1969.

Taveras, J. M., Gilson, J. M., Davis, D. O., Kilgore, B. and Rumbaugh, C. L.: Angiography in cerebral infarction. Radiology, 93, 549–558, 1969.

Thomson, J. L. G.: The computed axial tomograph in acute herpes simplex encephalitis. British Journal of Radiology, 49, 86–87, 1976.

Trevor, R. P., Sondheimer, W. J., Fessel, W. J. and Wolpert, S. M.: Angiographic demonstration of major cerebral vessel occlusion in systemic lupus erythematosus. Neuroradiology, 4, 202–207, 1972.

Vander Eecken, H. and Adams, R. D.: The anatomy and functional significance of the meningeal arterial anastomoses of the human brain. Journal of Neuropathology and Experimental Neurology, 12, 132–157, 1953.

Walker, R. J., El Gammal, T. and Allen, M. B.: Cranial arteritis associated with herpes zoster. Radiology, 107, 109–110, 1973.

Wallace, S. and Jaffe, M. E.: Cerebral arterial ectasia with saccular aneurysms. Radiology, 88, 90–93, 1967.

Wisoff, H. S. and Rothballer, A. B.: Cerebral arterial thrombosis in children. Archives of Neurology, 4, 213, 1961.

Wollschlaeger, P. B., Wollschlaeger, G., Lopez, V. F. and Krautmann, J. J.: Tortuosity of the perforating arteries. Neuroradiology, 1, 195–199, 1970.

Yamaguchi, K., Takahashi, H., Uemeura, K., Kowada, M. and Kawakami, H.: Venous filling abnormalities observed in hypertensive intracerebral hemorrhage. Neuroradiology, 5, 102–106, 1973a.

Yamaguchi, K., Uemura, K. and Takahashi, H.: An angiographic study of sequential changes in hypertensive intracranial haemorrhage, British Journal of Radiology, 46, 125–130, 1973b.

Yasargil, M. G. and Damiur, M.: Thrombosis of the cerebral veins and dural sinuses. In Newton, T. H. and Potts, D. G., Eds.: Radiology of the skull and brain. Vol. 2, book 4. St. Louis: C. V. Mosby, 1974.

Yock, D. H. and Marshall, W. H.: Recent ischaemic brain infarcts at computed tomography: appearance pre- and post-contrast infusion. Radiology, 117, 599–608, 1975.

Zimmerman, R. D., Leeds, N. E. and Naidich, T. P.: Carotid-cavernous fistula associated with intracranial fibromuscular dysplasia. Radiology, 122, 725–726, 1977.

Zulch, K. R., Dreesbach, H. A. and Eschbach, O.: Occlusion of the middle cerebral artery with the formation of an abnormal arterial collateral system—moya moya type—23 months later. Neuroradiology, 7, 19–24, 1974.

3 Subarachnoid Hemorrhage

A case of subarachnoid hemorrhage may be defined as a patient with frank blood in the cerebrospinal fluid, although lumbar puncture is not essential for a presumptive clinical diagnosis. The picture of sudden severe headache, associated with stiff neck and photophobia and other signs of cerebral irritability, often in a young and previously healthy subject, is sufficiently familiar and adequate to dispense with confirmatory lumbar puncture, which may be dangerous. In both primary diagnosis and in the day-to-day management of such patients, the radiological investigations are crucially important, and in no other field of intracranial diagnosis is the aid of an experienced neuroradiologist more valuable.

INTRODUCTION

Etiology
During the 11-year period ending in December 1976, 1588 patients with subarachnoid hemorrhage were admitted to the neurosurgical service of the Wessex Neurological Centre, Southampton. The following causes were demonstrated by radiological investigation, operation and/or autopsy:

Aneurysm	931 (58.6%)
Arteriovenous malformation	160 (9.9%)
Intracerebral hemorrhage	152 (9.5%)
Not determined	345 (21.7%)

These figures may be distorted in two respects by local practice: (1) angiography was undertaken to fulfill surgical requirements and the vertebrobasilar circulation was examined in less than one-third, therefore some aneurysms may have been missed; and (2) very few cases of traumatic subarachnoid hemorrhage are included.

A finding in this series which should be pointed out is the absence of neoplasms—stressing the infrequency with which brain tumors present as subarachnoid hemorrhage. Odom and his colleagues (1966) in their series of 151 intracranial hematomas included only 3 which complicated neoplasms, and experience of computed tomography since this date has confirmed this observation. Oldberg (1933) in his morbid-anatomical study of 832 patients with gliomas, was the first to emphasize this fact: he recorded that signs of spontaneous hemorrhage were present in only 31 (3.7%) and there was clinical evidence of intracranial hemorrhage in only 7 (0.8%).

Investigative Policy
The timing and scope of cerebral angiography in subarachnoid hemorrhage depends largely on the local approach to the surgery of ruptured aneurysms. If early operation is favored, then subarachnoid hemorrhage is an indication for emergency angiography. The completeness with which it is carried out, i.e., single-, two-, three- or four-vessel injection, is controlled by two factors: (1) the absence of clinical contraindications to angiography, e.g., advanced age or poor clinical status which may contraindicate craniotomy absolutely, irrespective of the lesion demonstrated; and (2) availability of emergency computed tomography which, by demonstrating clotted blood, indicates the primary

affected area. If the hematoma lies within the territory of one cerebral artery, injection of that territory may provide the surgeon with all the preoperative information he requires to deal with the causative lesion. Some surgeons take the view that, while additional angiography may reveal further lesions, such procedure does not contribute to the immediate clinical management of the patient. The practice of routine four-vessel angiography must be challenged wherever a conservative neurosurgical approach exists to the treatment of subarachnoid hemorrhage, e.g., posterior-fossa aneurysms. Unless contraindications exist, complete angiography is indicated because of the frequency of multiple aneurysms.

Radiological Tactics
The radiological investigation of subarachnoid hemorrhage is dominated by the likelihood of a ruptured aneurysm being the causative lesion (Fig. 3–1). The particular investigative routine for such cases should be modified only in those patients in whom the clinical circumstances indicate another cause, such as acute head injury (or in an unconscious patient, the suspicion of recent trauma),

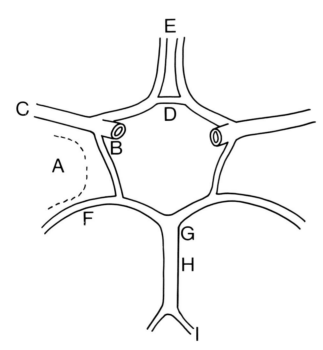

Fig. 3–1 Sites of 1000 consecutive cases of ruptured aneurysm seen in the Wessex Neurological Centre, Southampton, between 1965 and 1977. (A) Cavernous (extradural): 9. (B) Posterior communicating/internal carotid: 296. (C) Middle cerebral (sylvian): 286. (D) Anterior communicating: 355. (E) Distal anterior cerebral (callosomarginal): 13. (F) Distal posterior cerebral: 4. (G) Terminal basilar: 15. (H) Basilar trunk: 3. (I) Vertebral (posterior inferior cerebellar): 9. Note: Multiple: 130; space-occupying, i.e., lumen over 2 cm diameter: 16; calcified: 11.

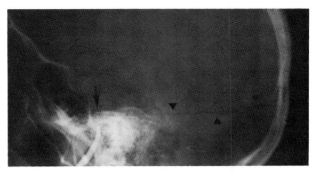

Fig. 3–2 Unconscious patient with bloodstained cerebrospinal fluid. Common carotid angiogram shows "pseudo-occlusion" of the internal carotid artery caused by terminal raised intracranial pressure *(arrow)*. The skull fracture *(arrowheads)* indicated the traumatic nature of the lesion, and autopsy revealed extensive cerebral contusion and hemorrhage.

the patient's youth—ruptured arteriovenous malformation is a commoner cause of hemorrhage in children and adolescents—or severe arterial hypertension, when subarachnoid bleeding is likely to be secondary to an intracerebral hematoma.

(1) **Skull radiographs** remain an essential preliminary of any definitive study. An unsuspected finding can materially influence the diagnosis and alter the sequence of contrast investigations particularly in an unconscious patient, e.g., fracture, intracranial foreign body such as a bullet, pineal shift, pathological calcification or raised intracranial pressure (Fig. 3–2).

(2) **Computed tomography** is the investigation of choice for locating the primary affected area, as a preliminary to "dedicated" angiography which is required to demonstrate the cause of the hemorrhage. Kendall and his colleagues have shown that computed tomography provides, apart from localization, vital information for clinical management which angiography may not offer as completely. This information includes the nature and extent of any process present, such as hemorrhage, infarction or edema, and the reason for any clinical deterioration, such as hemorrhage/infarction or hydrocephalus. In lesions which the computed scan shows to be inoperable, angiography can be avoided altogether (Kendall and Claveria, 1976; Kendall et al., 1976; Scotti et al., 1977; Liliequist et al., 1977).

(3) **Cerebral Angiography:** Most intracranial aneurysms and arteriovenous malformations will be demonstrated by adequate studies, therefore angiography in the majority of cases of subarachnoid hemorrhage will provide an etiological diagnosis. It fails to do so in the presence of arterial spasm or occlusion by thrombosis or in terminal raised intracranial pressure. Basal ganglionic hemorrhage, which gives rise to a devastating clinical picture, may present as a case of subarachnoid hemorrhage

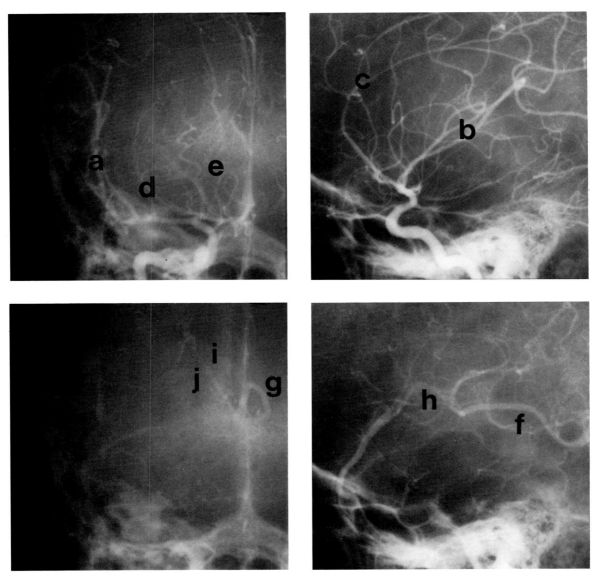

Fig. 3–3 Intracerebral hematoma (right basal ganglion). Right carotid angiogram shows "the mass without a shift" and reveals a wealth of diagnostic detail. Signs of a dilated lateral ventricle are present: the sylvian arteries are stretched and displaced outward (a) and upward (b); and the pericallosal artery is stretched and arched outward (c). Signs of the basal ganglionic mass are: the lenticulostriate arteries are stretched and bowed outward (d); and the thalamostriate arteries are displaced medially (e); the internal cerebral vein has lost its smooth curve (f) due to contralateral midline shift (g); the venous angle is widened (h); and the thalamostriate veins are displaced medially (i) and upward (j).

with surprisingly few angiographic abnormalities (Fig. 3–3).

A neurosurgical requirement in the diagnosis of small lesions such as aneurysms, is that they should be visible in at least two radiographic planes of the circulation, e.g., frontal and lateral (Table 3–1). The number of additional views necessary will become obvious in the course of the procedure as the diagnosis unfolds. If a direct puncture technique is used, failed or inadequate angiography is usually the result of inappropriate anesthesia. It may be impossible to inject the carotid arteries of a patient who is tense with apprehension or whose systolic blood pressure is below 90 mm. Hg. The commonest cause of poor intracranial contrast visualization is a low pCO_2 level of the arterial blood (Du Boulay et al., 1968).

(4) Scintigraphy: Static brain imaging fails to detect about one-third of extracerebral hematomas and an even greater proportion of intracerebral hematomas. The appearance of large arteriovenous malformations may be diagnostic (Fig. 3–4), but

Table 3–1 Optimal Views for Demonstrating Intracranial Aneurysms

Projection	Site of Aneurysm						
	Cavernous carotid	Anterior communicating	Posterior communicating	Middle cerebral	Posterior cerebral	Basilar	Vertebral, including posterior inferior cerebellar
AP–15°, straight		1	2	3			
AP–15°, contralateral oblique 30°		3					
AP–15°, ipsilateral oblique 30°		4					
AP–35°, straight					1	1	
AP–35°, contralateral oblique 30°							1
AP–35°, ipsilateral oblique 30°							2
AP–perorbital, straight	1				1	4	4
AP–perorbital, contralateral oblique 30°			3				
Lateral, straight	2	2	1	2	2	2	
Lateral, tilted or oblique		5	4				
Submentovertical	3			4	3	3	3

smaller ones and most aneurysms will not be seen (Fig. 3 – 25; Waltino et al., 1973). Radioisotope cisternography is useful to confirm obstruction of the cerebrospinal fluid pathways following subarachnoid hemorrhage.

(5) Pneumography: Lumbar pneumoencephalography serves no diagnostic purpose and is contraindicated in acute cases but it may be useful at a later stage in revealing cerebral atrophy, tentorial-block hydrocephalus and other chronic complications (Fig. 3 – 5). Air ventriculography may be required (in the absence of computed tomography) in postoperative management. According to Cronqvist

(1967), about 10 percent of the patients who survive a subarachnoid hemorrhage develop hydrocephalus. This complication, which is frequently associated with dementia, is caused by basal arachnoiditis.

ANEURYSMS

An aneurysm is a localized bulging of the lumen of an artery caused by weakness of its wall. The cause of the so-called berry, or congenital aneurysm which is the commonest variety to affect the cere-

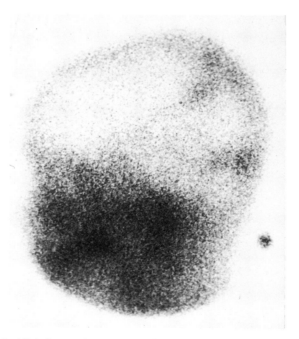
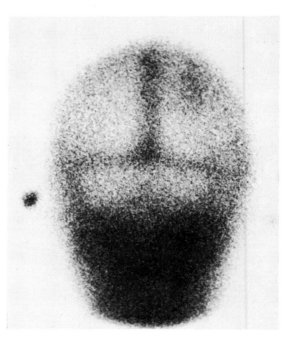

Fig. 3–4 Scintigram of an 8-year-old boy with subarachnoid hemorrhage. The wedge-shaped convexity activity is typical of a large arteriovenous malformation.

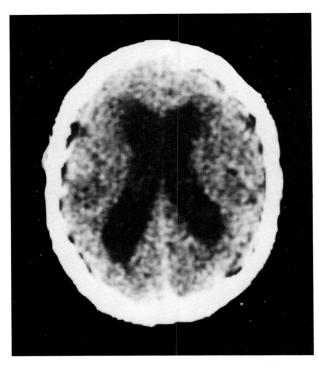

Fig. 3–5 Hydrocephalus due to convexity and tentorial blockage in a 32-year-old man. Computed tomogram performed 15 months after an attack of subarachnoid hemorrhage from an inoperable anterior communicating aneurysm.

bral vessels, is not clear. Forbus (1930) noted the presence of a medial defect at the points of bifurcation of the larger cerebral vessels, but failed to explain why aneurysms develop only at 6 or 7 such points (Fig. 3–1). Others have stressed the prevalence of arteriosclerosis and arterial hypertension in patients dying from ruptured aneurysms, and it seems likely that a multiplicity of factors is involved in their pathogenesis (Hassler, 1965; Crompton, 1966a). In Padget's (1944) celebrated embryological study, aneurysms occurred twice as commonly in congenitally anomalous cerebral arterial trees as in normal ones.

Classification
Bull's (1962) etiological classification incorporated most intracranial aneurysms: (1) congenital—probably 98 percent; (2) atherosclerotic; (3) infective (mycotic, monilial, syphilitic, Pseudomonas etc.); (4) traumatic; (5) aneurysm associated with specific conditions, e.g., intracranial arteriovenous malformation or other vascular anomaly and systemic hypertension.

A more practical radiological classification depends upon the morphology of the aneurysm—the size of its sac and whether it is fusiform or saccular in shape. Thus, there are two types:

1. "Berry" aneurysm—these are usually congenital and only occasionally associated with head trauma, intracranial vascular anomalies, and systemic disease or infection.

2. Giant aneurysm—most are arteriosclerotic in origin and some situated in the extradural space (infraclinoid cavernous aneurysm).

As a rule, these two types are well-defined and separate entities, clinically and radiologically, although space-occupying aneurysms can rupture and produce bloodstained cerebrospinal fluid, and berry aneurysms may exert a mass effect.

Clinical Presentation
The sac of the aneurysm acts as a space-occupying lesion if sufficiently large, and the following focal neurological deficits merit angiography to exclude aneurysm:

- unilateral oculomotor palsy, especially if accompanied by retro-orbital pain (ipsilateral posterior communicating aneurysm). About one-third of the patients with an isolated ocular palsy have an aneurysm; not all posterior communicating aneurysms affect the nerve (Soni, 1974);
- unilateral external ophthalmoplegia (3rd to 6th cranial nerves) suggesting a parasellar lesion (infraclinoid cavernous carotid aneurysm);
- chiasmal syndrome (anterior communicating aneurysm). Any unexplained bitemporal hemianopia requires *bilateral* carotid angiography to exclude aneurysm;
- raised intracranial pressure/obstructive hydrocephalus syndrome (terminal basilar or other large posterior fossa aneurysm.

The vast majority of intracranial aneurysms remain clinically silent until rupture. The signs and symptoms they then produce depend on the size of the hematoma and the direction in which it tracks. The extreme end of the spectrum is a devastating hematoma that destroys the patient through raised intracranial pressure—the arterial "pseudo-occlusion" syndrome (Fig. 3–2; Davies and Sutton, 1967). Nonfatal cases exhibit coma and other nonlateralizing signs such as a stiff neck, photophobia and severe headache. It is important to search for focal neurological deficits both in the history and physical examination of the patient, to pinpoint the source of the hemorrhage.

Angiographic Considerations
Preliminary noninvasive imaging methods such as plain skull radiographs and computed tomography should not be omitted (see Investigative Policy, above). "The angiographic examination should be designed to show whether an aneurysm is present; if so, its size and shape and the width of its neck should be demonstrated. Its relation to the parent vessel and other vessels in the region and evidence of hematoma or spasm should also be determined" (Allcock, 1974). In fulfilling this double task, name-

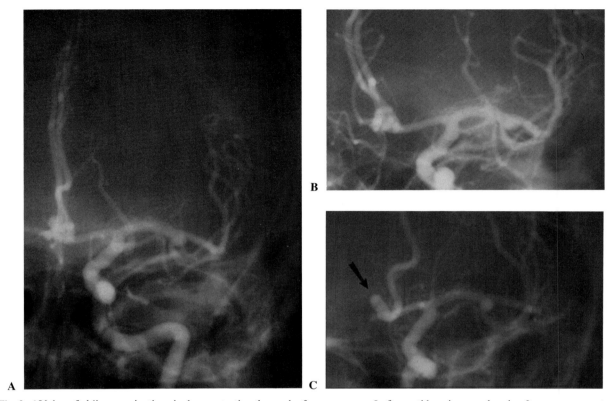

Fig. 3–6 Value of oblique projections in demonstrating the neck of an aneurysm. Left carotid angiogram showing 2 aneurysms: anterior communicating and middle cerebral trifurcation. Both anterior cerebral arteries fill spontaneously from the left carotid, and in the frontal projection, the neck of the anterior communicating aneurysm is hidden. Rotation of the head to the right side (B) gives no help, but rotation towards the side of injection (C) clears the aneurysm *(arrow)* of overlying vessels and reveals its neck.

ly reaching a primary diagnosis of aneurysm and providing aid to the surgeon, the neuroradiologist should be guided by three important facts. They are: (1) Over 95 percent of intracranial aneurysms arise within one inch (2.5 cm.) of the carotid bifurcation (Fig. 3–1). (2) A minimum of two views (preferably at a right angle) is necessary of any aneurysm that is likely to be treated by a torsion bar across its neck. (3) Multiplicity of lesions is a common finding, and the diagnosis of an aneurysm should always prompt a careful search for an alternate source of bleeding (see Figs. 3-8 and 3-10).

Technique: Subarachnoid hemorrhage demands high-quality imaging of the intracranial vascular tree, and aneurysms will be missed if technical standards are low. Selective injection of the particular cerebral artery under study is essential, because nonselective techniques such as aortic-arch, brachial or subclavian angiography result in unpredictable intracranial contrast opacification. Selective entry of the internal carotid artery offers an advantage over common carotid injection by eliminating confusion with overlying external vessels in lateral view, and by ensuring a higher rate of filling of the posterior cerebral artery. Sufficient serial films in frontal and lateral planes are necessary to view the

sac of the aneurysm and to evaluate arterial spasm and displacements. Single-film additional views can be made in other planes to define the neck of the aneurysm. An oblique view (the patient's nose turned away from the side of injection is always useful. However, the other oblique view (nose *towards* the injection) may be required to demonstrate the neck of an aneurysm (Fig. 3–6). Oblique views made with the following projectional tilts are appropriate (Lin and Kricheff, 1972):

Anterior communicating artery: AP–15°–35°

Middle cerebral artery: straight or ipsi- or contralateral perorbital–15°–20°

Posterior communicating artery: perorbital, paraorbital–55°

Posterior inferior cerebellar artery: AP–35°. The submentovertical view is invaluable and may be essential for viewing aneurysms of the anterior middle and posterior cerebral arteries and the basilar bifurcation (Fig. 3–7). Table 3–1 lists a personal choice of radiographic projections for aneurysm angiography.

Cross Compression: Digital occlusion of the contralateral common carotid artery during injection provides a useful view of the arteries supplying both hemispheres (Fig. 3–8). The total filling of the anterior communicating artery territory achieved by this

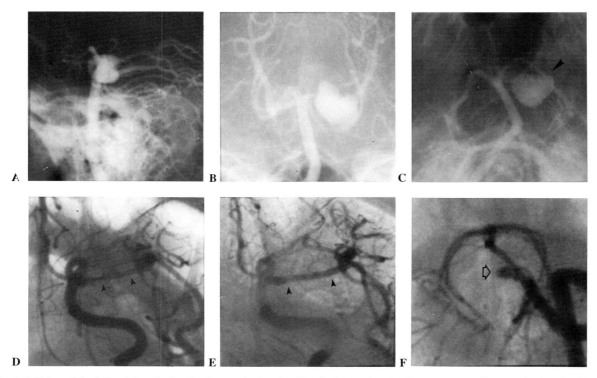

Fig. 3–7 Value of the full-axial projection for demonstrating the site of origin and neck of an aneurysm when standard projections fail, particularly on the vertebrobasilar tree. (A, B and C) Posterior cerebral aneurysm. The vertebral angiogram was repeated to obtain (C) at the surgeon's request, since (A) and (B) failed to show the precise point of origin of the aneurysm *(arrow)*. (D and E) Middle cerebral aneurysm, serial angiograms made 16 days apart, showing the relief of arterial spasm (arrowheads). (F) Posterior inferior cerebellar aneurysm *(open arrow);* same patient as Figure 3 – 9.

maneuver may reveal an aneurysm or hemispherical displacement due to hematoma. Apart from diagnosis, cross-compression angiography may be invaluable in surgical management, e.g., in evaluating the patient's suitability for carotid ligation.

Additional Aids: The techniques of stereoscopy, magnification and subtraction are useful adjuncts, but all are less valuable than an appropriate additional view which shows the neck of the aneurysm in profile. Routine subtraction in the course of ver-

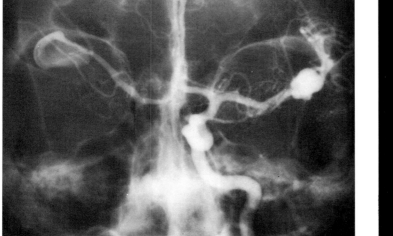

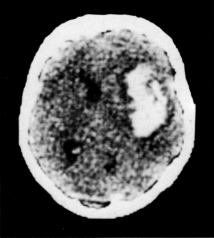

Fig. 3–8 Value of the perorbital projection in demonstrating bilateral middle cerebral artery aneurysms, also of the cross-compression technique in aneurysm angiography. The right middle cerebral trunk is elevated, suggesting a hematoma around the aneurysm. Computed tomography reveals a right sylvian hematoma, confirming that the right aneurysm had ruptured.

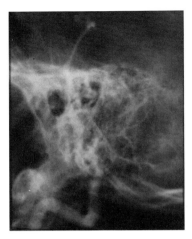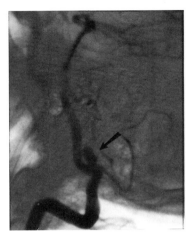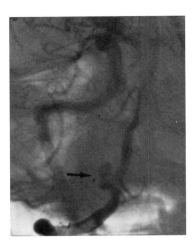

Fig. 3–9 Value of the subtraction technique for revealing aneurysms, especially of the vertebrobasilar tree. Aneurysm of the posterior inferior cerebellar artery, shown only after subtraction *(arrow)*. For full axial projection of same aneurysm, see Figure 3–7F.

tebral angiography occasionally permits the appropriate view to be made before the procedure is terminated (Fig. 3–9).

Accuracy of Detection: The only type of aneurysm likely to come to clinical notice before rupture is the space-occupying variety (see below). The detection rate of ruptured "berry" aneurysms varies greatly in the reports in the literature of series of patients with subarachnoid hemorrhage. In the Comparative Study, which included a total of nearly 6000 patients with blood-stained cerebrospinal fluid, the findings were (Locksley et al., 1966):

Ruptured aneurysm   50%
Arteriovenous malformation   36%.

The detection rate also depends on the completeness of the angiography: if more arteries are injected, more aneurysms are found. The highest positive findings are reported in patients in whom all four vessels were routinely studied: 75 percent showed aneurysms (Björkesten and Halonen, 1965; Donaldson, 1966).

An aneurysm may be missed for several reasons, other than the failure to inject all four arteries: (1) arterial spasm in the acute stage, which seals off its neck and prevents contrast filling of the sac—often a transient phenomenon; (2) thrombosis of the sac may occur, providing a spontaneous cure; (3) inadequate technique: in experienced hands, poor contrast filling is most often caused by inappropriate anesthesia and only rarely by an incorrectly placed catheter or needle. Subtraction and/or magnification is essential for viewing arterial segments overlain by dense bone such the vertebrobasilar tree (Fig. 3–9). (4) Observer error, which is particularly liable to occur with multiple lesions, e.g., multiple aneurysms or arteriovenous malformation associated with aneurysm. In such situations, the most obvious lesion is identified, but the arterial tree is often not carefully scrutinized for a second or even third source of bleeding (Figs. 3–10 and 3–11).

Aneurysms may appear subsequent to a hemorrhage—within weeks, in locations that may initially have been well demonstrated and shown to be free both of spasm and aneurysm. In the Comparative Study, repeat carotid angiography revealed aneurysms in 207 of 1251 patients (16.5%) in whom the first angiogram had been normal (Perret and Nishioka, 1966).

"Berry" Aneurysms
Through usage this term is applied to the congenital variety of aneurysm within the subarachnoid compartment. Morphologically, however, mycotic, post-traumatic and other "secondary" aneurysms possess no intrinsic features that enable radiologists to distinguish them from congenital aneurysms. The angiographic differential diagnosis depends on the presence of associated features—see below.

Incidence:
(1) Age, Sex and Familial Factors: "Berry" aneurysms tend to rupture later in life than arteriovenous malformations—in the 3rd and 4th decades, but any adult with subarachnoid hemorrhage may harbor an aneurysm. The disease is very uncommon before the age of 18 years, and aneurysms in children and adolescents are usually associated with systemic disease. Matson (1966) described 14 young patients with aneurysms, 3 of whom had coarctation of the aorta, one a subacute bacterial endocarditis and two "segmental atherosclerosis." The youngest patient in the Southampton series was a 14-year-old boy with arterial hypertension due to polycystic kidneys (Fig. 3–12). There is no sex predominance. The literature contains reports of aneurysms occurring in several members of the same family.
(2) Sites: Table 3–1 shows the distribution of 1000 consecutive aneurysms seen in Southampton in 12 years. All of these were "berry" aneurysms

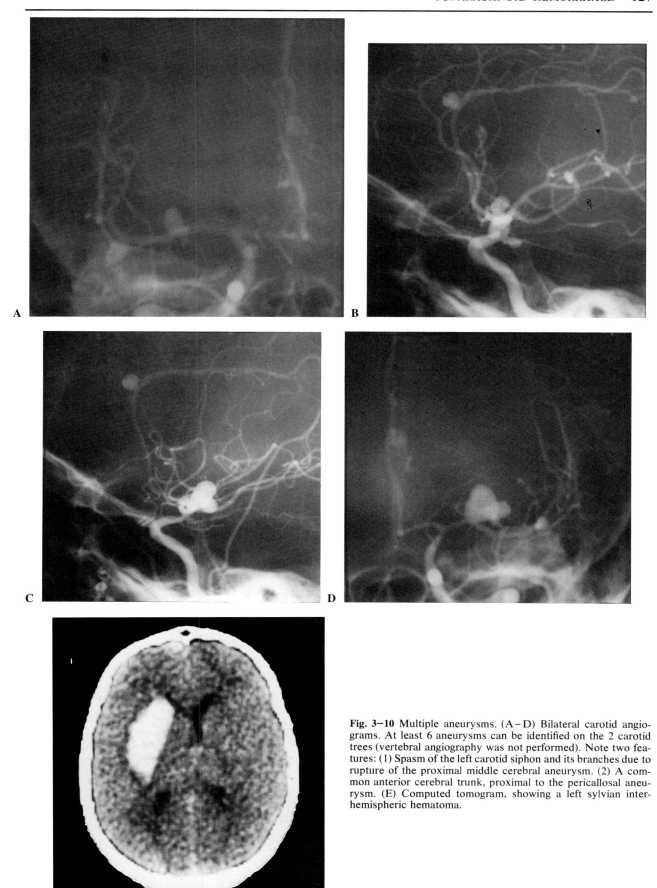

Fig. 3–10 Multiple aneurysms. (A–D) Bilateral carotid angiograms. At least 6 aneurysms can be identified on the 2 carotid trees (vertebral angiography was not performed). Note two features: (1) Spasm of the left carotid siphon and its branches due to rupture of the proximal middle cerebral aneurysm. (2) A common anterior cerebral trunk, proximal to the pericallosal aneurysm. (E) Computed tomogram, showing a left sylvian interhemispheric hematoma.

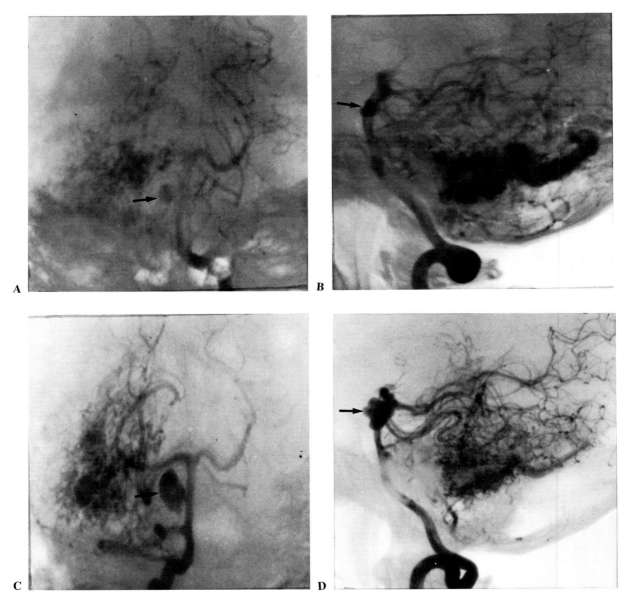

Fig. 3-11 A 25-year-old woman with subarachnoid hemorrhage. Combined infratentorial arteriovenous malformation and aneurysm of basilar artery *(arrow)*. (A and B) Left vertebral angiogram, initial examination. (C and D) Right vertebral angiogram made 34 months later, after second and fatal attack of hemorrhage. The striking feature is enlargement of the basilar aneurysm *(arrow)*, which was shown at autopsy to have ruptured. Same patient, see Figure 3-32.

except 16, of which 9 were cavernous (i.e., extradural) and 7 were space-occupying aneurysms in the subarachnoid compartment. The majority were revealed when they ruptured. The apparent low incidence of vertebrobasilar aneurysms (3.1%) is probably distorted by the local neurosurgical practice of confining the investigation of supratentorial aneurysms to bilateral carotid angiography. Björkesten and Halonen (1965) estimated that vertebrobasilar aneurysms account for about 10 percent of all intracranial aneurysms. Sharr and Kelvin (1973), in a review of the Southampton series, con-

firmed the findings of Sutton and Trickey (1962). Thus, in about 12 percent of patients with subarachnoid hemorrhage in whom bilateral carotid angiography is negative, unilateral vertebral angiography may be expected to reveal an aneurysm. If such three-vessel angiography also is negative, injection of the opposite vertebral artery may show an aneurysm in another 5 percent.

(3) Associated Features: The most frequent intracranial association is a second aneurysm. Autopsy studies show that the incidence of microaneurysms (diameter less than 2 mm.) is unusually high, there-

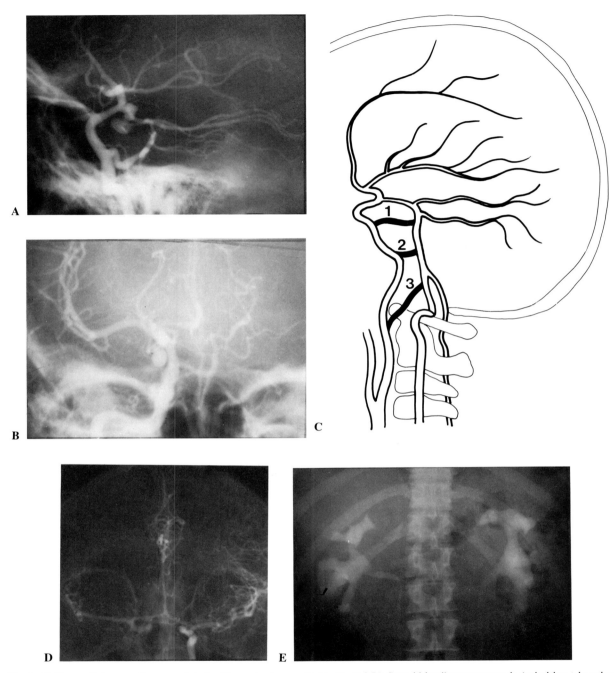

Fig. 3–12 Congenital anomalies associated with cerebral aneurysms. (A and B) Carotid-basilar anastomosis (primitive trigeminal artery), associated with aneurysm of the ipsilateral posterior communicating artery (Bingham & Hayes, 1961; Handa et al., 1971). (C) Persistent primitive connections between the carotid and basilar arteries. 1. Trigeminal artery. 2. Acoustic artery. 3. Hypoglossal artery. (D) Single proximal anterior cerebral trunk associated with a distal anterior cerebral aneurysm (aneurysm not visible in this view, due to spasm). (E) Polycystic kidneys in a 14-year-old boy with arterial hypertension who suffered an attack of subarachnoid hemorrhage from a ruptured posterior communicating aneurysm.

fore the presence of multiple aneurysms should not surprise. McKissock et al. (1964) reviewed 1686 patients with intracranial aneurysms, and 251 (14.9%) of these had more than one aneurysm. Aneurysms of the middle cerebral and posterior cerebral arteries tend to be symmetrical on the two

sides—so-called mirror aneurysms (Fig. 3–8). For the problem of deciding from the angiographic appearances which aneurysm has ruptured when more than one is present, see below.

About one case of cerebral aneurysm in every 100 is associated with an arteriovenous malforma-

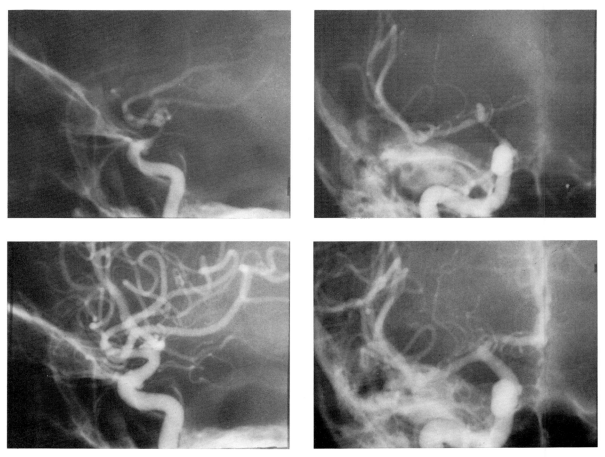

Fig. 3-13 Arterial spasm accompanying a small aneurysm of the terminal internal carotid artery *(top)*. Operation deferred and repeated angiography 20 days later *(bottom)* showed that the arteries had regained their normal caliber and that the aneurysm was no longer visible — presumably thrombosed.

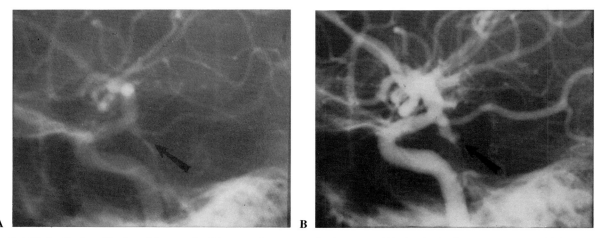

Fig. 3-14 Infundibular widening of the mouth of the posterior communicating artery (A), developing into an aneurysm which ruptured 8 years later (B). Infundibula are found at this site in about one per cent of subjects, and are sometimes viewed as "pre-aneurysms." The infundibulum is an enlarged part of the artery, whereas an aneurysm usually lies alongside the posterior commmunicating artery (Hassler and Saltzman, 1959; Fox et al., 1964). (Reproduced by courtesy of Dr. D. C. Bernstein, Whittington Hospital, London.)

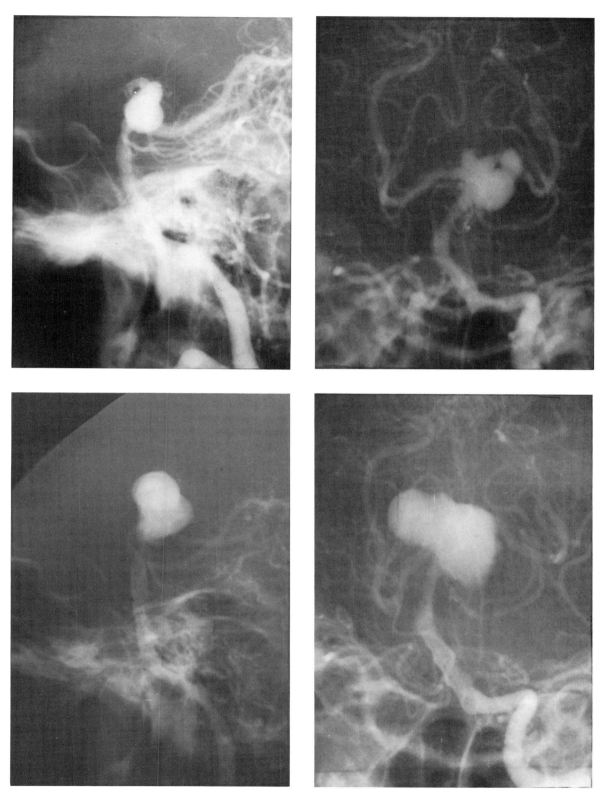

Fig. 3–15 Terminal basilar aneurysm *(top)* which had doubled in size 6 years later *(bottom)*.

Table 3–2 Rare Arterial Syndromes

Encephalofacial angiomatosis (Sturge-Weber)
Intracranial arteriovenous malformation with extracranial and retinal malformation (Wyburn-Mason)
Hereditary hemorrhagic telangiectasis (Rendu-Osler)
Arteriovenous anomaly of the Galenic system (aneurysm of vein of Galen)
Carotid-cavernous fistula
Orbital vascular malformations
Traumatic cervical arteriovenous malformations

tion, and the spectacular angiographic appearances of the latter may result in the aneurysm being overlooked. Such aneurysms have two features: they may be multiple, and often they are located on the major feeding artery of the malformation (Fig. 3–11). Autopsy evidence suggests that in such cases of subarachnoid hemorrhage, the aneurysm is the lesion more likely to rupture (Anderson and Blackwood, 1959; Perret and Nishioka, 1966).

Associated systemic lesions should be suspected whenever the picture contains discrepant features, e.g., a patient under 18 years of age, aneurysms peripherally situated and especially if multiple. Such lesions include bacterial endocarditis and other infective sources and certain diseases producing arterial hypertension (coarctation of the aorta, fibromuscular hyperplasia of the renal arteries, polycystic kidneys, Fig. 3–12).

(4) Natural History: Serial angiographic observations show that aneurysms are rarely static; their changing morphology reflects the various pathogenetic factors responsible for producing them. Thus, an aneurysm may disappear spontaneously—presumably sealed off and cured by mural thrombus (Lyall, 1966; Fig. 3–13). If this does not occur, the aneurysm continues to grow, and subsequent angiography shows a larger sac, often with an altered shape and new loculus (Figs. 3–14 and 3–15). Altered appearances are usually interpreted as evidence of further bleeding, and this may occur silently. The risk of re-rupture remains as long as any part of the lumen is patent, but very large "berry" aneurysms may exert mass effects on the brain (see Space-Occupying Aneurysms, below).

Radiology of Ruptured Aneurysm: If a ruptured aneurysm continues to bleed, eventually the intracranial pressure will exceed the arterial blood pressure, and flow into the head will cease. For the angiographic diagnosis of arterial "pseudo-occlusion" and cerebral death, see Fig. 3–2 and Chapter 7, page 318.

Aneurysmal Sac: Most aneurysms burst through the apices of their sacs and the point of rupture seals off promptly. Angiograms made before and after the incident usually reveal an alteration in the shape of the sac (Figs. 3–15 and 3–16). Only extraordinary coincidence will ordain that angiography takes place actually during the course of rup-

ture, therefore contrast extravasation from the aneurysmal sac is only very rarely observed. There are no features from which the age of an aneurysm can be predicted. Adjacent arterial spasm also alters the appearances of the sac.

Hematoma: The track followed by the hematoma, and the clinical features it produces, depend on the primary location of the aneurysms. Those lying on or close to the circle of Willis rupture first into the subarachnoid space then into the brain substance, ventricular system or both. Peripherally situated aneurysms such as those on the distal anterior cerebral artery may produce an interhemispheric hematoma (Fein and Rovit, 1970, Fig. 3–10), and deeply situated aneurysms may rupture direct into the ventricles or midbrain. Computed tomography is the most accurate method of demonstrating the extent and direction of the hematoma and it may also indicate the source of hemorrhage (Figs. 3–17 and 3–18; Hayward and O'Reilly, 1976). In cerebral angiography, the displacements caused by intracerebral hematomas must be distinguished from the other hemispherical effects of ruptured aneurysm; see below. Especially liable to misinterpretation are the pneumographic appearances of intracerebral hematoma and intraventricular blood (Fig. 3–38).

Arterial Spasm: Next to fatal hemorrhage, spasm of the adjacent arteries is the most dreaded complication of ruptured aneurysm and it is the commonest cause of death. Probably 30 to 50 percent of patients with ruptured aneurysms show spasm at some time during the first month. No specific pattern has been shown in regard to the extent, time of onset or duration of spasm. Successive studies have failed to demonstrate any association with either angiography or operative measures (Steven, 1966; Griffith et al., 1972; Du Boulay and Gado, 1974). If spasm around an aneurysm persists beyond three weeks, it is safe to assume that the aneurysm has ruptured again.

Which Aneurysm Has Ruptured? In patients with subarachnoid hemorrhage in whom more than one aneurysm is demonstrated by angiography, the problem arises: Which one has bled? Computed tomography in about half of the cases shows a hematoma or other localizing feature (Turnbull, 1979), and angiograms may contain useful diagnostic pointers. The aneurysm that is larger and has the more irregular shape, i.e., with an irregular pattern of contrast opacification of its loculi, is usually the source of hemorrhage. Wood (1964) in his study of 105 patients with multiple aneurysms, considered arterial spasm to be the least valuable of the localizing angiographic signs, since it may be present at a distance from the ruptured aneurysm.

The angiographic appearance of spasm may be similar to that of the irregular arteries seen in arte-

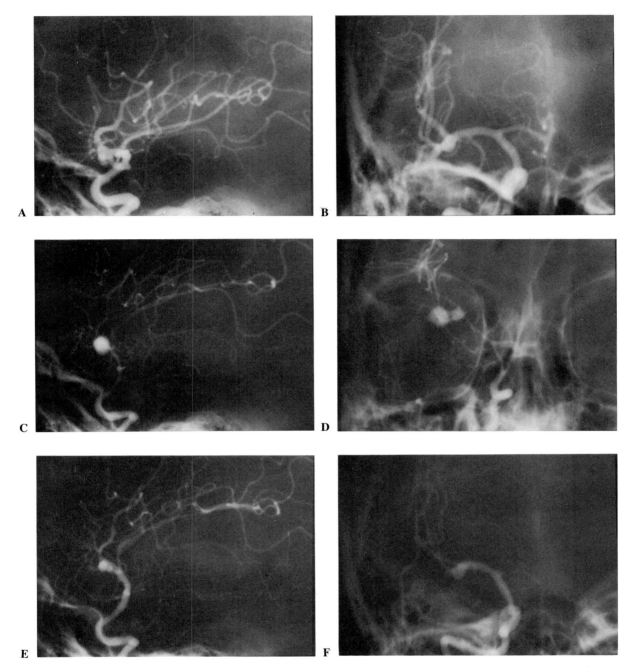

Fig. 3–16 Arterial spasm and hemorrhage from a right middle cerebral aneurysm. (A) Initial angiogram, 3 days after the first hemorrhage. Unilobular trifurcation aneurysm is present, but there is no evidence of arterial displacement or spasm. (B) Second angiogram, performed 3 weeks after the first angiogram and 9 days after a second hemorrhage. The proximal vessels are reduced in caliber—the internal carotid from its point of entry through the dura and the middle cerebral trunk. The aneurysm is now bilobed and larger, and the sylvian vessels are elevated by hematoma. (C) Third angiogram 14 days after the second. Spasm is receding and the aneurysmal sac is smaller. At subsequent craniotomy the hematoma was evacuated and the aneurysm successfully clipped.

riosclerosis and in some normal subjects around the carotid siphon. A feature of spasm is that, although the actual lumina may be reduced to thread-like dimensions, points of bifurcation retain a triangular appearance, because the arterial walls there cannot be constricted further. Beyond the affected region,

the distal arterial branches assume their normal dimensions (Fig. 3–16).

The hemispherical effects of spasm are the result of partial (transient) occlusion of the adjacent arteries. In the patient illustrated in Figure 3–19, a second hemorrhage from an anterior communicating

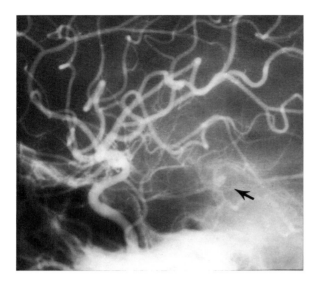

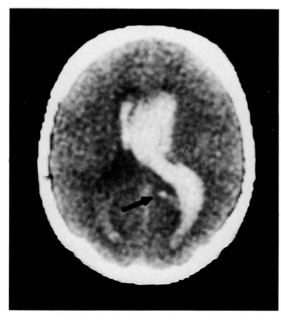

Fig. 3–17 Peripheral posterior cerebral aneurysm *(arrow)*, with rupture into the ventricular system. Computed tomography shows the dilated, blood-filled lateral ventricles, as well as the aneurysm *(arrow)*, and the track of rupture. The patient, a 27-year-old man, survived the hemorrhage, and the aneurysm was successfully ligated.

aneurysm produced a hemodynamic disturbance in the anterior cerebral territory, sufficient to evoke a compensatory collateral circulation. Cerebral edema (and infarction) provoked by the ischemia is best revealed by computed tomography (Fig. 3 – 19). Angiographically, a swollen hemisphere accompanying an aneurysm represents either diffuse edema or an intracerebral hematoma, and the differential diagnosis in life may be impossible without computed tomography.

Surgical Angiography: Allcock and Drake (1963) were the first to insist that the success of surgical ligation of an aneurysm can be claimed only if postoperative angiography confirms that the aneurysmal sac has been obliterated. In separate reviews totalling over 1,000 postoperative angiograms of patients operated upon in Glasgow and London, Ontario, the incidence of aneurysmal sacs continuing to opacify was 15 percent (Steven, 1966; Drake and Allcock, 1973). Another complication of surgical ligation shown by these workers is occlusion of a major artery or branch, present in 15 to 20 percent. Thus, postoperative angiography may reveal a situation that requires immediate reoperation. The fate of partially ligated aneurysms is uncertain: sometimes angiography at a subsequent date shows that the aneurysm is small or no longer present – presumably a "thrombotic cure" (Crompton, 1966b; Cummins et al., 1974). Figures 3 – 20 and 3 – 21 illustrate the angiographic features of these complications.

Ligation of a carotid artery in the neck is a form of treatment practiced for certain inaccessible aneurysms. It is aimed at provoking a thrombosis or reducing the blood pressure directly. Angiography in such patients reveals a profuse compensatory collateral circulation from the vertebrobasilar and contralateral carotid trees. The aneurysmal sac may be expected, in the course of time, to shrink or to disappear (Tindall et al., 1966). Occasionally it enlarges, and the patient illustrated in Figure 3 – 22 presented with visual failure due to a suprasellar aneurysm which had grown to space-occupying proportions. In the immediate postoperative period after craniotomy for aneurysm surgery, deterioration in the patient's level of consciousness may herald a fatal complication. Emergency computed tomography provides a ready answer because it will reveal blood clot, infarction due to spasm or hydrocephalus. Carotid angiography is less helpful in this situation, and it may be valueless in distinguishing between postoperative edema and hemorrhage.

Late Complications: The adhesive arachnoiditis following repeated attacks of subarachnoid hemorrhage obliterates the basal cisterns and the tentorial opening, leading to failed absorption of cerebrospinal fluid. The incidence of tentorial or convexity-block hydrocephalus in ruptured aneurysms may be as high as 30 percent (Galera and Greitz, 1970). Focal atrophy of the white matter is the end result of severe arterial spasm or occlusion. Both generalized and focal atrophy is a feature of computed tomograms or pneumoencephalograms performed on aneurysm survivors.

Space-occupying Aneurysms
Figure 3 – 1 shows that less than 2 percent of intracranial aneurysms are space-occupying, i.e., they possess an internal diameter exceeding 2.5 cm.

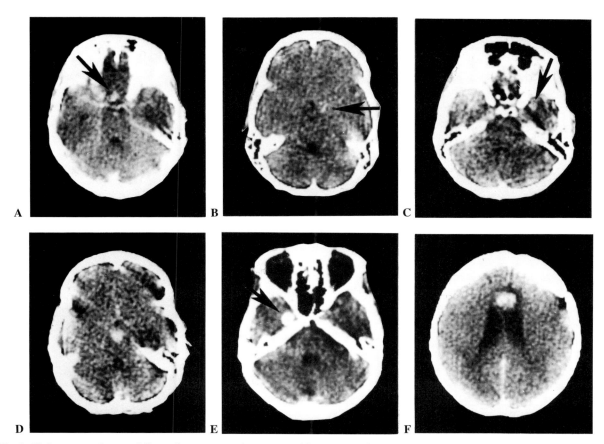

Fig. 3–18 Aneurysmal sacs of "berry" aneurysms demonstrated by computed tomography. (A) Anterior communicating artery. (B) Posterior communicating artery. (C) Middle cerebral artery. (D) Terminal basilar artery. (E) Cavernous part of internal carotid artery. (F) Callosomarginal artery, aneurysm wrapped (same case as Fig. 3–12D).

Such aneurysms seldom rupture nonfatally, more usually they present clinically as intracranial masses. Of the 16 giant aneurysms in the Southampton series, 9 were extradural, arising from the cavernous (infraclinoid) portion of the internal carotid artery (Fig. 3–23). Several arose from the basilar artery, deforming it into an S-shaped, elongated tube, reaching above the level of the pituitary fossa and indenting the floor of the third ventricle (Pribram et al., 1969; Bull, 1969; Sutton, 1971; Sarwar et al., 1976). The remainder were suprasellar or temporal-fossa masses—being aneurysms on the anterior communicating or middle cerebral arteries that had grown by repeated leakage to extraordinary dimensions (Fig. 3–24).

Radiological Features

Calcification: These are segments of delicate, curvilinear deposits called Albl's rings, after the German physician who first described them. These rings, which outline the outer surface of the aneurysm, were visible in 11 of the 16 giant aneurysms—representing calcification in 1.1 percent of all intracranial aneurysms. Schunk (1964) in a study of thrombosis in aneurysms, observed that calcifi-

cation does not take place without thrombosis. However, in most patients the thrombotic process remains incomplete, and the presence of calcified deposits does not necessarily indicate that an aneurysm has been rendered innocuous by total thrombosis of its lumen.

Bone Erosion: The petrous apex or one side of the superior surface of the sphenoid bone may be eroded by giant suprasellar aneurysms. The characteristic pattern of bone erosion in infraclinoid aneurysms is described in Chapter 5, Fig. 5–8.

Thick Aneurysmal Wall: The thickness of the thrombosed wall of the aneurysm can be shown by computed tomography or by comparison between its calcified outer rim and its contrast-filled lumen (Figs. 3–23 and 3–24). If the thrombosis is complete, angiography will be negative (Burrows, 1971).

Arterial Occlusion: The thrombotic mural thickening of the aneurysm may involve the peripheral artery and occlude its lumen (Fig. 3–26).

Mass Effect: Intracranial imaging shows that giant aneurysms exert clinical effects appropriate to their space-occupying characteristics, e.g., temporal-lobe epilepsy (Fig. 3–24), visual failure (Fig. 5–24) or unilateral sensorineural deafness (Fig. 8–81).

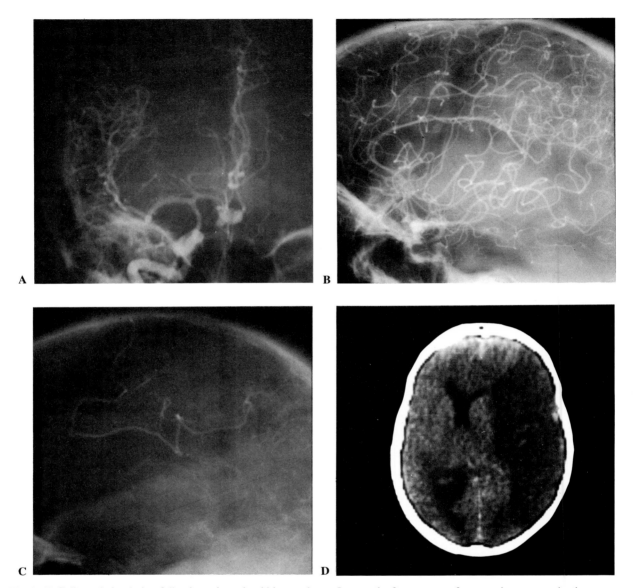

Fig. 3–19 Collateral circulation following subarachnoid hemorrhage. One week after rupture of an anterior communicating aneurysm the patient experienced a second hemorrhage. (A and B) Repeat carotid angiography showed arterial spasm around the aneurysm and some filling of the distal anterior cerebral system, ruling out thrombosis. (C) Late-phase vertebral angiography revealed retrograde filling of the pericallosal and other distal branches of the anterior cerebral artery. (D) Another case of 52 y.o. Patient with posterior communicating artery aneurysm, who presented with subarachnoid hemorrhage. An infarct in the right middle cerebral artery distribution is visualized.

Giant aneurysms of the posterior fossa may mimic brain tumors (Pribram et al., 1969; Michael, 1974; Danziger and Bloch, 1975).

Rupture: Only one of the seven intradural giant aneurysms of the Southampton series presented as a case of subarachnoid hemorrhage, stressing the relative infrequency of this mode of presentation.

Aneurysm of the Vein of Galen
Aneurysmal enlargement of the Galenic vein is a rare entity which is more likely to present clinically as a space-occupying lesion or a "steal" phenome-

non than as subarachnoid hemorrhage. It is appropriate to consider Galenic aneurysms between aneurysm and arteriovenous malformations in this chapter, since they may be of two types:

(1) True or primary aneurysms, in which the blood passes directly into the sac from normal albeit hypertrophied feeding arteries (Fig. 3–27); and

(2) Secondary dilatation of the Galenic system of venous drainage, which is part and parcel of an arteriovenous malformation (Fig. 3–27).

Both types compress the midbrain and produce profound supratentorial obstructive hydrocephalus due to aqueduct stenosis which may not be relieved

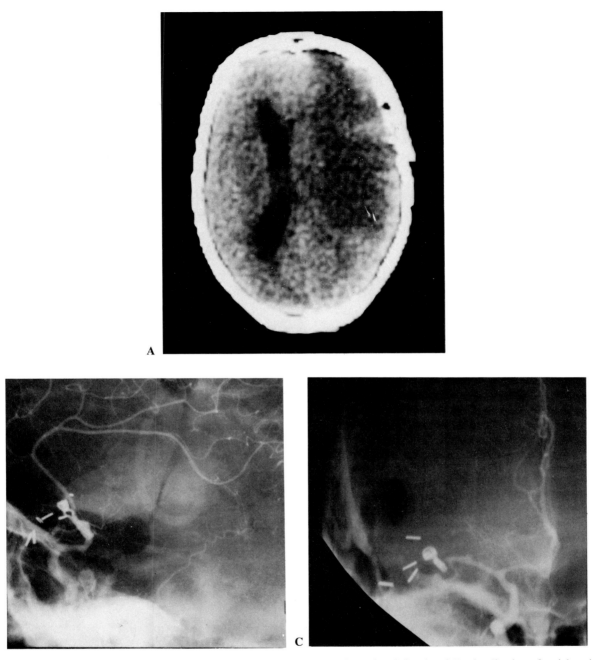

Fig. 3–20 Operative complications. (A) Computed tomogram showing hemispherical infarction following ligation of a right middle cerebral aneurysm. (B and C) Right carotid angiogram shows that the torsion bar while totally excluding the sac, also occludes the trunk of the middle cerebral artery.

without shunting after successful aneurysm surgery (Amacher and Shillito, 1973). In neonates the presenting features may be severe cardiac failure accompanied by a cranial bruit and increasing head size. If the patient survives early life, the aneurysm may appear in the teens or even later, with nonspecific signs such as headache or syncope (due to a "steal" phenomenon). Skull radiographs may provide the diagnosis, because most cases of Galenic aneurysm observed in subjects over the age of 15 years exhibit ring or curvilinear calcification, which is unmistakable (Russell and Newton, 1964). In the absence of this calcification, the computed-tomographic appearances of the lesion are not less specific. Angiography including opacification of the vertebrobasilar tree is necessary to evaluate the type of the lesion and the origins of its arterial supply.

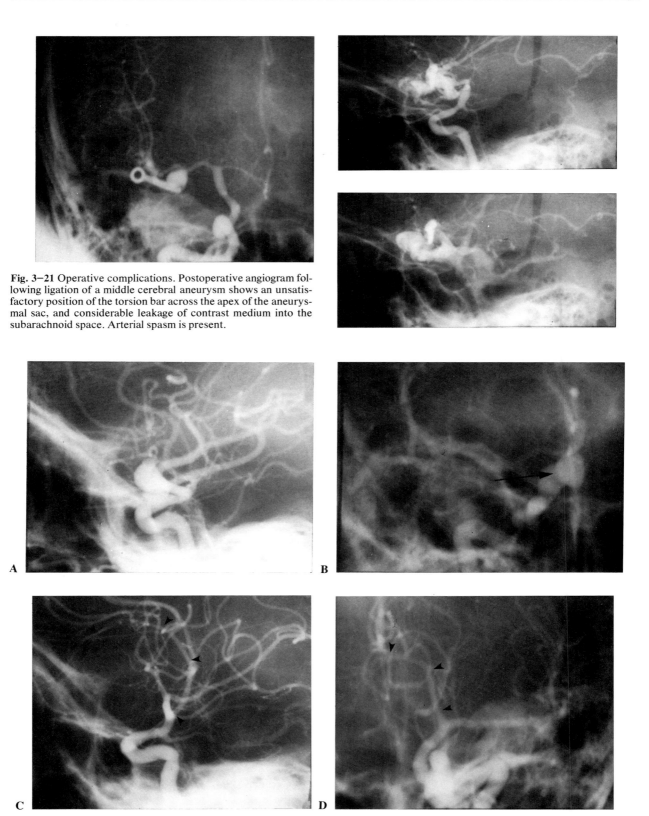

Fig. 3–21 Operative complications. Postoperative angiogram following ligation of a middle cerebral aneurysm shows an unsatisfactory position of the torsion bar across the apex of the aneurysmal sac, and considerable leakage of contrast medium into the subarachnoid space. Arterial spasm is present.

A

B

C

D

Fig. 3–22 Effects of carotid ligation. (A and B) A 25-year-old woman with a ruptured internal carotid (suprasellar) aneurysm was treated by right carotid ligation, because the aneurysm was inaccessible to direct surgical attack. Six years later the patient presented with visual deterioration and a chiasmal syndrome. (C and D) Left carotid angiography revealed an increase in the overall dimensions of the mass *(arrowheads)*. *(Fig. continues on next page.)*

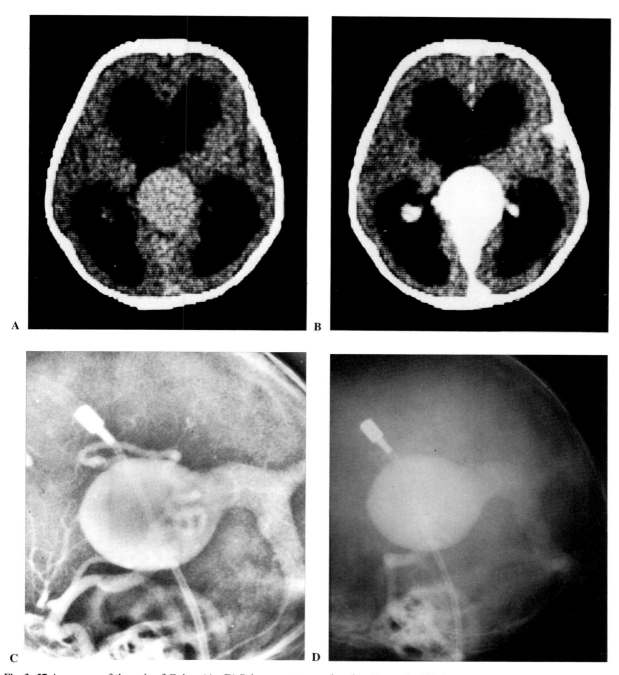

Fig. 3–27 Aneurysm of the vein of Galen. (A – D) Primary or true variety in a 7-month-old baby presenting with increasing head size. Computed tomograms made before and after contrast enhancement, showing gross symmetrical supertentorial hydrocephalus produced by aqueductal obstruction. The left carotid and vertebral angiograms show the midline aneurysm to be supplied by hypertrophied posterior cerebral and anterior choroidal arteries, and to drain mainly into the straight sinus. (Reproduced by courtesy of Dr. R. M. Paxton, Plymouth General Hospital, Plymouth.) *(Fig. continues on next page.)*

raphy. Diagnostic accuracy and yield is high: over 90 percent (Pressman et al., 1975; Kendall and Claveria, 1976). Computed tomography frequently reveals details of the extent of the lesions and associated complications such as hemorrhage, edema or obstructive hydrocephalus better than angiography, and it may answer crucial surgical decisions, e.g.,

whether a lesion involving a lateral ventricle is confined to the choroid plexus or also involves the basal nuclei (Fig. 3 – 29).

(3) **Angiography:** For cerebral angiography to be adequate, it must be both selective and comprehensive in order to visualize the flow pattern (including drainage) from each feeding vessel separately.

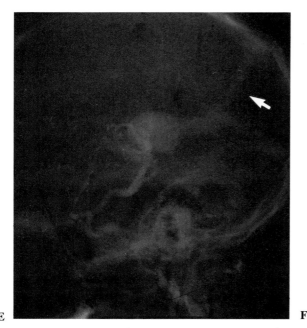
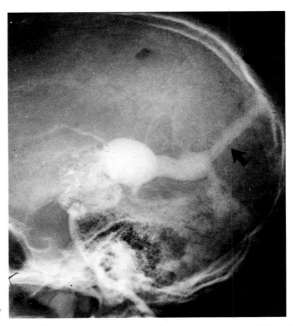

E   F

Fig. 3–27 continued. (E and F) Secondary variety, representing part of the dilated venous drainage of an arteriovenous malformation. Right carotid and vertebral angiograms show that the malformation is supplied mainly by terminal branches of the vertebrobasilar tree and also the posterior cerebral arteries. An anomalous vein *(arrow)* is identified that is often seen with this malformation.

Transfemoral catheterization is therefore desirable, so that each internal carotid, external carotid and vertebral artery may be injected separately. Super-selective studies, e.g., occipital angiography, may be necessary. Rapid serial films and multiprojectional imaging, supplemented by subtraction and perhaps magnification techniques, are particularly important.

The appearances of the various types of arteriovenous malformation are shown as follows:

Dural malformation: Fig. 3 – 28.

Pial malformation: arterial (arteriovenous) type – Figs. 3 – 31 and 3 – 32; venous type – Fig 3 – 35.

Mixed malformation: Fig. 3 – 29.

The angiographic differential diagnosis between small arteriovenous malformations and malignant brain neoplasms may be difficult (see Ch. 6). Two reliable differentiating points are the enlarged feeding vessels carrying the blood to and from the malformation, and the regular "ball of string" appearance of its constituent blood vessels. Early venous filling is a nonspecific sign.

Angiographic demonstration of an arteriovenous malformation should always prompt a search for associated features:

(1) An aneurysm will be present in every tenth case of arteriovenous malformation – usually located on a feeding artery. The importance of identifying an associated aneurysm in patients with subarachnoid hemorrhage is underlined by the experience of the Comparative Study, namely that, if the two lesions coexist, the hemorrhage usually arises

from the aneurysm (Perret and Nishioka, 1966; Cronqvist and Troupp, 1966).

(2) Other associated lesions: occasionally silent angiomas are found in patients with other lesions, e.g., trigeminal artery (Fig. 3 – 12), stroke, or meningioma.

(3) Signs of hemorrhage: rupture of the angioma itself produces vessel displacement characteristic of an intracerebral hematoma (see below). Lesions with mixed or dural feeding arteries may rupture into the subdural space. Arterial spasm may follow acute rupture and – similar to the situation with ruptured aneurysms – it may hide important diagnostic features (Nishimura and Hawkins, 1975). Serial angiography in arteriovenous malformations may be completely normal under two conditions: in the so-called cryptic angiomas, the abnormal vessels may seal off during rupture as described above; and spontaneous cure may follow total thrombosis of the vessels within the malformation, so that angiography fails to reveal any trace of it (Kamrin and Buchsbaum, 1965; Sukoff et al., 1972).

(4) Signs of hydrocephalus: ventricular blood or engorged varices may occlude the aqueduct of Sylvius or posthemorrhagic basal arachnoiditis may lead to a tentorial-block hydrocephalus. Although best demonstrated by computed tomography, the angiograms will usually reveal evidence of hydrocephalus. Preoperative or postoperative angiography is essential for successful angioma surgery, since any remnants left behind will continue to grow and may re-rupture.

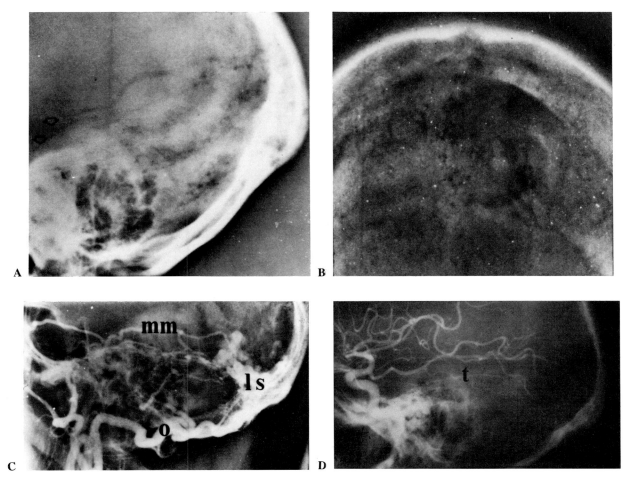

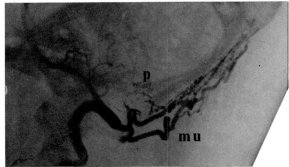

Fig. 3–28 Dural arteriovenous malformation shown by selective angiography to be supplied by branches of the external and internal carotid and vertebral arteries, and draining into the lateral sinus. The occipital and other extracranial feeding arteries penetrate the skull through a maize of "pepperpot" translucencies. (A and B) Plain radiographs of the skull showing widened grooves of the posterior branches ôf both middle meningeal arteries *(open arrows)* leading to the occiput which has a "motheaten" texture due to the numerous arteries perforating it. (C) External carotid angiograms, showing hypertrophied feeding branches draining into the lateral sinus (ls). (mm) Middle meningeal arteries; (o) occipital artery. (D) Internal carotid angiogram. (t) Tentorial artery. (E) Vertebral angiogram, showing hypertrophied muscular branches (mu) perforating the skull (p).

Pneumography: Following the introduction of computed tomography, the bizarre deformities and displacements of the ventricles demonstrable by pneumoencephalography in cases of large arteriovenous malformation are largely irrelevant (McRae and Valentino, 1958).

INTRACEREBRAL HEMATOMA

Nontraumatic rupture of a blood vessel into the brain produces blood stained cerebrospinal fluid in 70 to 80 percent of cases (McKissock et al., 1961). In all such disasters, the pathological lesion is an intraparenchymal hematoma which displaces as well as destroys the white matter. About two-thirds of hematomas involve the basal ganglia and most of the remainder lie in the adjacent parts of the brain. Brainstem and cerebellar hemorrhage is far less common.

Etiology
The causes of intraparenchymal hematomas are particularly relevant to the investigating radiologist,

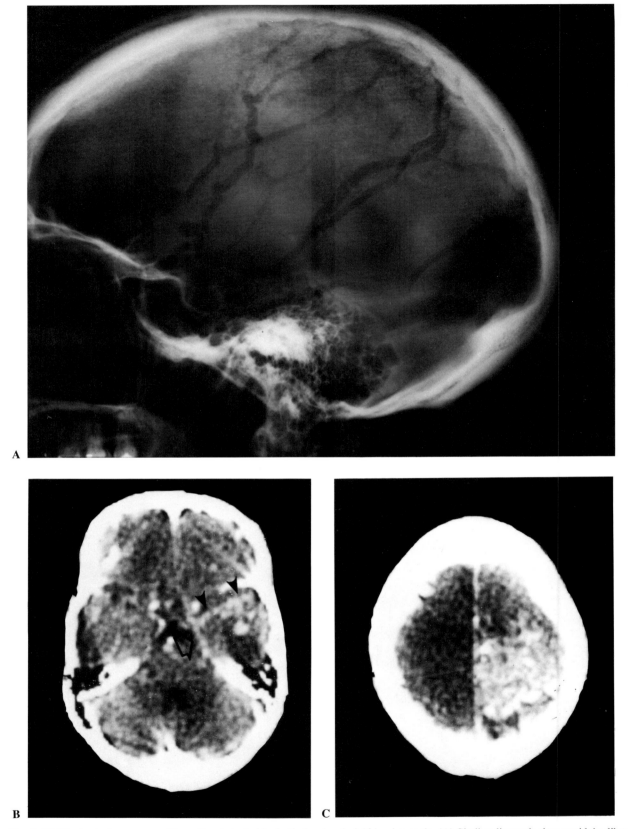

Fig. 3−29 Giant arteriovenous malformation irrigated by both dural and pial blood vessels. (A) Skull radiograph shows widely dilated "corkscrew" grooves of both middle meningeal arteries and floccular calcification in the posterior half of the right cerebral hemisphere. Appearances 20 years after initial presentation, reflecting the continuing growth of the dural and internal carotid feeding arteries (Porter and Bull, 1969). (B) Computed tomogram, showing that the lesion is too extensive for radical surgery, being supplied via the right posterior cerebral artery *(open arrow)*, in addition to the middle cerebral *(arrowheads)* and probably the anterior cerebral arteries. Therefore, investigation by angiography is superfluous for management.

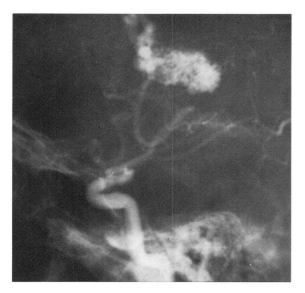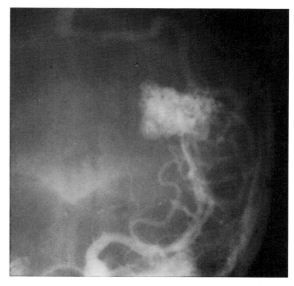

Fig. 3–30 A typical example of the common variety of intracranial arteriovenous malformation, made up of three components, viz., large feeding artery(ies), a tangle of blood vessels, and dilated draining vein(s).

who usually provides the etiological diagnosis. He can expect to find that in about one-half of the patients the hematoma is the result of a ruptured aneurysm or—much less frequently—a pial arteriovenous malformation; other very rare causes of secondary intracerebral hemorrhage are hypocoagulation states and bleeding into a necrotic glioma. In the remaining half, the hematoma is described as a primary intracerebral hemorrhage, and the majority of these patients suffer from systemic arterial hypertension. A hypertensive stroke is synonymous with hemorrhage into the basal ganglia, and destruction of the pyramidal tract. The careful work of Ross Russell (1963) has revealed that such hemorrhages are caused by rupture of microaneurysms situated on the small perforating arteries of the circle of Willis. A small proportion of younger patients in this group, in whom angiography fails to reveal an underlying lesion, are found at autopsy to harbor arteriovenous malformations or aneurysms which were obliterated at the time of rupture.

Plain skull radiographs usually show no abnormality. Minor degrees of lateral displacement of the pineal calcification are significant if the direction is clinically appropriate in the acute phase, but often a devastating capsular hemorrhage may not be sufficiently space-occupying to dislodge it from the midline. In survivors, the blood clot may calcify and be encountered by chance years later, as an asymptomatic "brain stone."

Radiological Investigation

Computed tomography is the primary investigation in the diagnosis of brain hemorrhage in adults and children. Ambrose in 1974 demonstrated that blood clot has a significantly higher photon absorp-

tion coefficient than brain substance, and appears as a "white" area on the computed tomogram (Fig. 3–37). Experience of the method has confirmed that the site and extent of a hematoma can be demonstrated accurately, and that often the nature and location of the underlying lesion, particularly aneurysms, can be determined. The transverse axial plane is the most favorable one for differentiating between primary intracerebral hematomas which involve the basal ganglia (thalamus and caudate nucleus, internal and external capsules), and ruptured aneurysms which may exhibit characteristic site-dependent patterns. It is clear that computed tomography, which has confirmed the statistical findings of earlier autopsy and angiographic studies of brain hemorrhage, yields much of the information necessary for clinical management (Crompton, 1962; Paxton and Ambrose, 1974; Hayward and O'Reilly, 1976; Berger et al., 1976; Terbrugge et al., 1977).

Within a month of suffering a hypertensive hemorrhage, the surviving patient may exhibit focal atrophy or hydrocephalus.

Angiography: Appropriate carotid and vertebral angiography retains an investigative role in demonstrating the underlying etiological lesion, and to provide answers to specific technical questions, e.g., the presence of spasm, aneurysm size and its relationship to adjacent vessels. Compared to computed tomography, angiography is a crude and unreliable method of imaging the hematoma, and it may expose the hypertensive patient to unnecessary hazard.

The angiographic appearances of a basal ganglion hematoma will depend on its size, the direction in which it has split (outward into the temporal lobe,

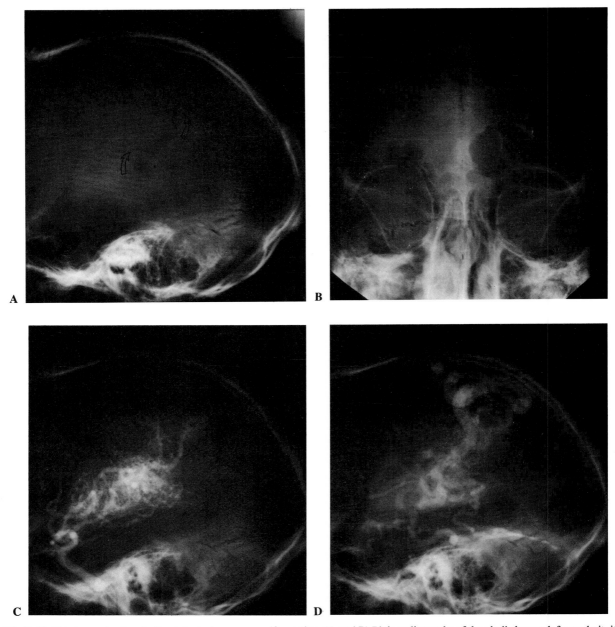

Fig. 3–31 Giant vessels of a wholly pial arteriovenous malformation. (A and B) Plain radiographs of the skull show a deformed pituitary fossa and deepened carotid sulcus, caused by hypertrophy of the carotid siphon *(arrow)*, and venous grooving of the inner surface of the parietal bone made by a dilated surface vein *(open curved arrows)*, and abnormal heaping up of inner table of the skull vault. (C and D) Left carotid angiogram shows the malformation with its hypertrophied feeding arteries and draining veins.

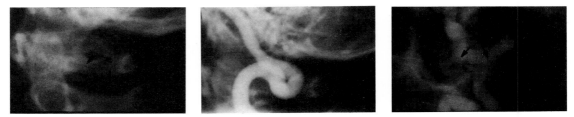

Fig. 3–32 Arteriovenous malformation of the posterior fossa. Pressure erosion of the superior surface of the arch of the atlas, caused by hypertrophy of the vertebral artery. Same patient as illustrated in Figure 3–11.

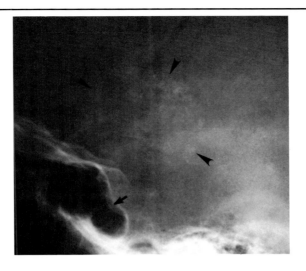

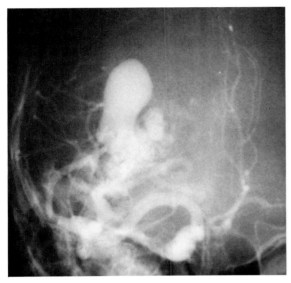

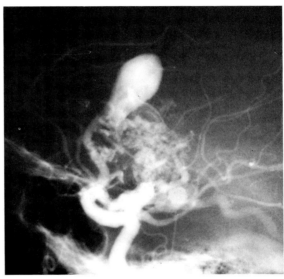

Fig. 3–33 Calcified arteriovenous malformation in the deep frontal region. Delicate, fluffy deposits of calcium *(arrowheads)*. Deepened, asymmetrical pituitary fossa is caused by a hypertrophied carotid siphon *(arrow)*.

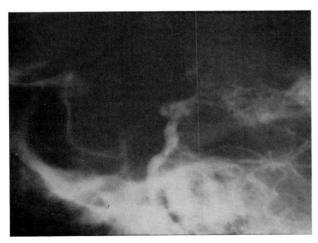

Fig. 3–34 Tentorial arteriovenous malformation producing obstructive hydrocephalus. The pituitary contour reflects prolonged pressure erosion by a dilated third ventricle.

medially into the ventricular system, downward into the midbrain), and the severity of structural complications such as obstructive hydrocephalus and tentorial herniation. The hematoma itself, an avascular mass, is limited by its intra-axial position in the extent to which it is space-occupying. The one constant angiographic sign is contralateral displacement of the internal cerebral vein (Fig. 3–3), and this may be the solitary abnormality. Other venous signs are: medial and upward displacement of the thalamostriate vein (accompanying the midline shift of the internal cerebral vein); and well-visualized subependymal veins. Arterial features are: medial displacement of the lenticulostriate arteries, lateral displacement and stretching of the sylvian arteries (and also elevation if the hematoma extends into the temporal lobe), and slight contralateral displacement of the anterior cerebral artery. Parenchymal contrast extravasation may be present.

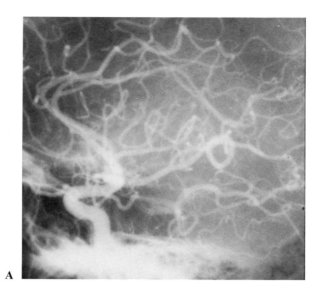

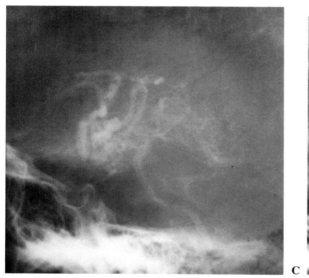

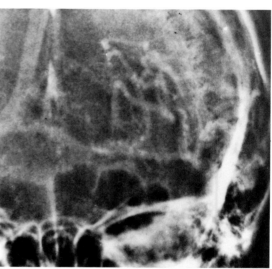

Fig. 3–35 Rare venous type of pial arteriovenous malformation. The abnormal vessels appeared only 8 seconds after contrast injection, stressing the importance of adequate serial angiography if such lesions are not to be missed (Isler, 1971; Scotti et al., 1975).

Rupture into the ventricular system alters the picture: for the angiographic appearances of obstructive hydrocephalus, see Chapter 6 (Odom et al., 1966; Huckman et al., 1970; Scott et al., 1974).

Scintigraphy: The results of static radioisotope imaging of intracranial hematomas are disappointing, and this method has been superceded.

OTHER LESIONS

Trauma
At least 10 percent of patients with severe craniocerebral trauma show an accompanying subarach-noid hemorrhage. Trauma should be suspected wherever an unconscious patient exhibits blood-stained cerebrospinal fluid even if carotid angiography reveals no structural abnormality. See Chapter 4.

Moya Moya Disease
A significant proportion of patients with this disease present with subarachnoid hemorrhage — see Chapter 2.

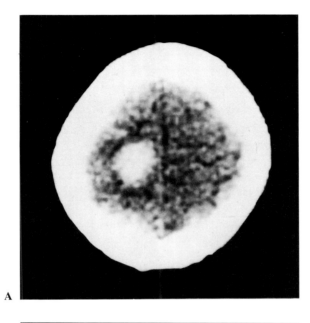

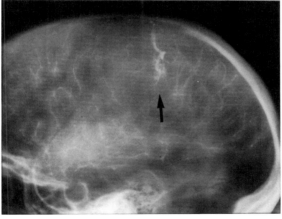

Fig. 3–36 "Cryptic" arteriovenous malformation of parietal cortex. An 11-year-old girl who was rescued unconscious from the sea. (A) Computed tomogram. (B) Left carotid angiogram: venous phase shows a solitary early draining vein *(arrow)* which strengthened the diagnosis, made from the history and computed tomography, of subarachnoid hemorrhage due to ruptured angioma.

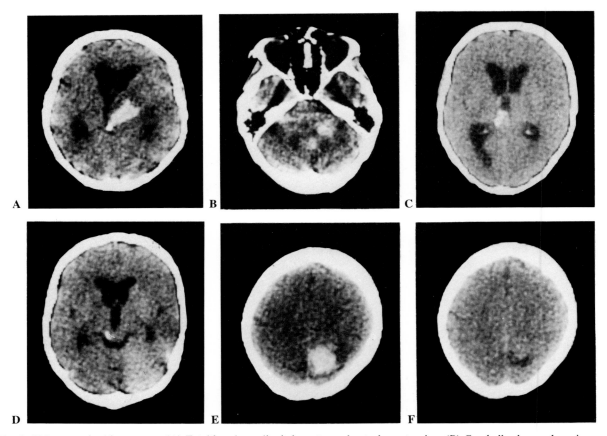

Fig. 3–37 Intracerebral hematoma. (A) Fatal basal ganglionic hematoma due to hypertension. (B) Cerebellar hemorrhage in a young subject, no cause found. (C) Hypertensive midbrain hemorrhage. (D) Same patient, 13 days later: the hematoma has resolved but the pineal remains displaced. (E) Occipital hematoma presenting clinically as a homonymous field defect of sudden onset; CSF clear. No cause found. (F) Same case, 3 months later: resolution of blood but residual low-density lesion. Homonymous hemianopia still present.

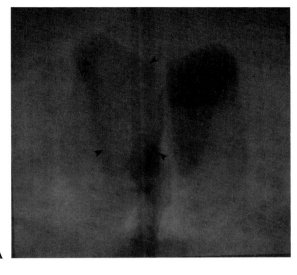

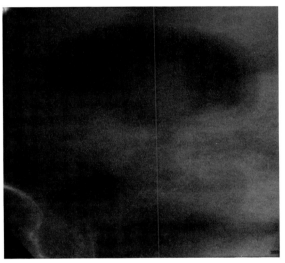

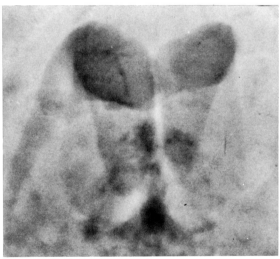

Fig. 3–38 Intraventricular hemorrhage in an 8-year-old boy; 4-vessel angiography was negative. (A and B) A filling defect is present in the right lateral ventricle *(arrows),* unaccompanied by any displacement. (C) Two months later, a return to normal appearances.

REFERENCES

Allcock, J. M.: Aneurysms. In Newton T. H. and Potts, D. G., Eds.: Radiology of the Skull and Brain. Vol. 2, book 4. St. Louis: C. V. Mosby, 1974.

Allcock, J. M. and Drake, C. G.: Postoperative angiography in cases of ruptured intracranial aneurysm. Journal of Neurosurgery, *20*, 752–759, 1963.

Amacher, A. L. and Shillito, J.: The syndromes and surgical treatment of aneurysms of the great vein of Galen. Journal of Neurosurgery, *39*, 89–98, 1973.

Aminoff, M. J. and Kendall, B. E.: Asymptomatic dural vascular anomalies. British Journal of Radiology, *46*, 662–667, 1973.

Anderson, R. McD. and Blackwood, W.: The association of arteriovenous angioma and saccular aneurysm of the arteries of the brain. Journal of Pathology and Bacteriology, *77*, 101–110, 1959.

Berger, P. E., Harwood-Nash, D. C. and Fitz, C. R.: Computerized tomography: Abnormal intracerebral collections of blood in children. Neuroradiology, *11*, 29–33, 1976.

Bingham, W. G., Jr., and Hayes, G. J.: Persistent carotid-basilar anastomosis: report of two cases, Journal of Neurosurgery, *18*, 29–32, 1961.

Björkesten, G. and Halonen, V.: Incidence of intracranial vascular lesions in patients with subarachnoid hemorrhage investigated by four-vessel angiography. Journal of Neurosurgery, *23*, 29–32, 1965.

Bull, J. W. D.: Contribution of radiology to the study of intracranial aneurysms. British Medical Journal, *2*, 1701–1708, 1962.

Bull, J. W. D.: Massive aneurysms at the base of the brain. Brain, *92*, 535–570, 1969.

Burrows, E. H.: Intracranial calcification. In Newton, T. H. and Potts, D. G., Eds.: Radiology of the Skull and Brain. Vol. 1, book 2. St. Louis: C. V. Mosby, 1971.

Crompton, M. R.: The pathology of ruptured middle-cerebral aneurysms with special reference to the differences between the sexes. The Lancet, *2*, 421–425, 1962.

Crompton, M. R.: The pathogenesis of cerebral aneurysms. Brain, 89, 797–814, 1966

Crompton, M. R.: Recurrent haemorrhage from cerebral aneurysms and its prevention by surgery. Journal of Neurology, Neurosurgery and Psychiatry, 29, 164–170, 1966b.

Cronqvist, S.: Encephalographic changes following subarachnoid haemorrhage. British Journal of Radiology, 40, 38–42, 1967.

Cronqvist, S. and Troupp, H.: Intracranial arteriovenous malformation and arterial aneurysm in the same patient. Acta Neurologica Scandinavica, 42, 307–316, 1966.

Cummins, B. H., Griffith, H. and Thomson, J. L. G.: Per-operative cerebral angiography. British Journal of Radiology, 47, 257–260, 1974.

Danziger, J. and Bloch, S.: Intracranial aneurysms presenting as mass lesions. Clinical Radiology, 26, 267–273, 1975.

Davies, E. R. and Sutton, D.: Pseudo-occlusion of the internal carotid artery in raised intracranial pressure. Clinical Radiology, 18, 245–252, 1967.

Donaldson, A. A.: Total angiography in spontaneous intracranial haemorrhage. Acta Radiologica Diagnosis, 5, 163–167, 1966.

Drake, C. G. and Allcock, J. M.: Postoperative angiography and the "slipped" clip. Journal of Neurosurgery, 39, 683–689, 1973.

Du Boulay, G., Edmonds-Seal, J. and Bostick, T.: The effect of intermittent positive pressure ventilation upon the calibre of cerebral arteries in spasm following subarachnoid haemorrhage – a preliminary communication. British Journal of Radiology, 41, 46–48, 1968.

Du Boulay, G. and Gado, M.: The protective value of spasm after subarachnoid haemorrhage. Brain, 97, 153–156, 1974.

Fein, J. M. and Rovit, R. L.: Interhemispheric subdural hematoma secondary to hemorrhage from a callosomarginal artery aneurysm. Neuroradiology, 1, 183–186, 1970.

Forbus, W. D.: On the origin of miliary aneurysms of the superficial cerebral arteries. Bulletin of Johns Hopkins Hospital, 47, 239–284, 1930.

Fox, J. L. Baiz, T. C. and Jakoby, R. K.: Differentiation of aneurism from infundibulum of the posterior communicating artery. Journal of Neurosurgery, 21, 135–138, 1964.

Galera, R. and Greitz, T.: Hydrocephalus in the adult secondary to the rupture of intracranial aneurysms. Journal of Neurosurgery, 32, 634–641, 1970.

Griffith, H. B., Cummins, B. H. and Thomson, J. L. G.: Cerebral arterial spasm and hydrocephalus in leaking arterial aneurysms. Neuroradiology, 4, 212–214, 1972.

Handa, J., Matsuda, M., Koyama, T., Handa, H, Kikuchi, H. and Hiyashi, K.: Internal carotid aneurysm associated with multiple anomalies of cerebral arteries. Neuroradiology, 2, 230–233, 1971.

Hassler, O.: On the etiology of intracranial aneurysms. In Fields, W. S. and Sahs, A. L., Eds.: Intracranial Aneurysms and Subarachnoid Hemorrhage. Springfield: Charles C Thomas, 1965.

Hassler, O. and Saltzman, G. F.: Angiographic and histologic changes in infundibular widening of the posterior communicating artery. Acta Radiologica Diagnosis, 1, 321–327, 1963.

Hayward, R. D. and O'Reilly, G. C. A.: Intracerebral haemorrhage. Accuracy of computerised transverse axial scanning in predicting the underlying aetiology. The Lancet, 1, 1–4, 1976.

Huckman, M. S., Weinberg, P. E., Kim, K. S. and Davis, D. O.: Angiographic and clinico-pathologic correlates in basal ganglionic hemorrhage. Radiology, 95, 79–92, 1970.

Isler, W.: Acute Hemiplegias and Hemisyndromes in Childhood. London: William Heinemann Medical Books, 1971.

Kamrin, R. B. and Buchsbaum, H. W.: Large vascular malformations of brain not visualized by serial angiography. Archives of Neurology, 13, 413–420, 1965.

Kaplan, H. A., Aronson, S. M. and Browder, E. J.: Vascular malformations of the brain: an anatomical study. Journal of Neurosurgery, 18, 630–635, 1961.

Kendall, B. E. and Claveria, L. E.: The use of computed axial tomography (CAT) for the diagnosis and management of intracranial angiomas. Neuroradiology, 12, 141–160, 1976.

Kendall, B. E., Lee, B. C. P. and Claveria, E.: Computerized tomography and angiography in subarachnoid haemorrhage. British Journal of Radiology, 49 483–501, 1976.

Krayenbühl, H. and Siebenmann, R.: Small vascular malformations as a cause of primary hemorrhage. Journal of Neurosurgery, 22, 7–20, 1965.

Liliequist, B., Lindqvist, M. and Valdimarsson, E.: Computed tomography and subarachnoid hemorrhage. Neuroradiology, 14, 21–26, 1977.

Lin, J. P. and Knicheff, I. I.: Angiographic investigation of cerebral aneurysms (techical aspects). Radiology 105, 69–76, 1972.

Locksley, H. B., Sahs, A. L. and Knowler, L.: Report on the cooperative study of intracranial aneurysms and subarachnoid hemorrhage. Section 2. General survey of cases in the central registry and characteristics of the sample population. Journal of Neurosurgery, 24, 922–932, 1966.

Lyall, A.: Large aneurysm of the circle of Willis with spontaneous cure by thrombosis. British Medical Journal, 2, 282–284, 1966.

McKissock, W., Richardson, A. and Walsh, L.: Spontaneous intracerebral haemorrhage. The Lancet, 2, 221–226, 1961.

McKissock, W., Richardson, A., Walsh, L. and Owen, E.: Multiple intracranial aneurysms. The Lancet, 1, 623–626, 1964.

McRae, D. L. and Valentino, V.: Pneumographic findings in angiomata of the brain. Acta Radiologica, 50, 18–26, 1958.

Matson, D. D.: Intracranial arterial aneurysms in childhood. Journal of Neurosurgery, 23, 578–583, 1965.

Michael, W. F.: Posterior fossa aneurysms simulating tumours. Journal of Neurology, Neurosurgery and Psychiatry, 37, 218–223, 1974.

Moody, R. A. and Poppen, J. L.: Arteriovenous malformations. Journal of Neurosurgery, 32, 503–511, 1970.

Newton, T. H. and Cronqvist, S.: Involvement of dural arteries in intracranial arteriovenous malformations. Radiology, 93, 1071–1078, 1969.

Nishimura, K. and Hawkins, T. D.: Cerebral vasospasm with subarachnoid haemorrhage from arteriovenous malformations of the brain. Neuroradiology, 8, 201–207, 1975.

Odom, G. L., Tindall, G. T., Cupp, H. B. and Woodhall, B.: Neurosurgical approach to intracerebral hemorrhage. Research Publications, Association for Research in Nervous and Mental Disease, 46, 145–168, 1966.

Oldberg, E.: Hemorrhage into gliomas. A review of 832 consecutive verified cases of glioma. Archives of Neurology and Psychiatry, 30, 1061–1073, 1933.

Padget, D. H.: The circle of Willis: its embryology and anatomy. In Dandy, W. E., Ed.: Intracranial Arterial Aneurysms. Ithaca, N.Y.: Comstock Publishing Company, 1944.

Paxton, R. and Ambrose, J.: The EMI scanner. A brief review of the first 650 patients. British Journal of Radiology, 47, 530–565, 1974.

Perret, G. and Nishioka, H.: Report on the cooperative study of intracranial aneurysms and subarachnoid hemorrhage. Section 4. Cerebral angiography, an analysis of the diagnostic value and complications of carotid and vertebral angiography in 5,484 patients. Journal of Neurosurgery, 25, 98–114, 1966.

Porter, A. J. and Bull, J. W. D.: Some aspects of the natural history of cerebral arteriovenous malformation. British Journal of Radiology, 42, 667–675, 1969.

Pressman, B. D., Kirkwood, J. R. and Davis, D. O.: Computerized transverse tomography of vascular lesions of the brain. Part 1: Arteriovenous malformations. American Journal of Roentgenology, 124, 208–214, 1975.

Pribram, H. F. W., Hudson, J. D. and Joynt, R. J.: Posterior fossa aneurysms presenting as mass lesions. American Journal of Roentgenology, *105*, 334–340, 1969.

Roberson, G. H., Kase, C. S. and Wolpow, E. R.: Telangiectases and cavernous angiomas of the brainstem: "cryptic" vascular malformations. Report of a case. Neuroradiology, *8*, 83–89, 1974.

Ross Russell, R. W.: Observations on intracerebral aneurysms. Brain, *86*, 425–442, 1963.

Rumbaugh, C. L. and Potts, D. G.: Skull changes associated with intracranial arteriovenous malformations. American Journal of Roentgenology, *98*, 525–534, 1966.

Russell, W. and Newton, T. H.: Aneurysm of the vein of Galen: case report and review of literature. American Journal of Roentgenology, *92*, 756–760, 1964.

Sarwar, M., Batnitzky, S. and Schechter, M. M.: Tumorous aneurysms. Neuroradiology, *12*, 79–97, 1976.

Schunk, H.: Spontaneous thrombosis in intracranial aneurysms. American Journal of Roentgenology, *91*, 1327–1338, 1964.

Scott, W. P., New, P. F. J., Davis, K. R. and Schnur, J. A. Computerized axial tomography of intracerebral and intraventricular hemorrhage. Radiology, *112*, 73–80, 1974.

Scotti, G., Ethier, R., Melancon, D. and Tchang, S.: Computed tomography in the evaluation of intracranial aneurysms and subarachnoid hemorrhage. Radiology, *123*, 85–90, 1977.

Scotti, L. N., Goldman, R. L., Rao, G. R. and Heinz, E. R.: Cerebral venous angioma. Neuroradiology, *9*, 125–128, 1975.

Sharr, M. M. and Kelvin, F. M.: Vertebrobasilar aneurysms. Experience with 27 cases. European Neurology, *10*, 129–143, 1973.

Soni, S. R.: Aneurysms of the posterior communicating artery and oculomotor paralysis. Journal of Neurology, Neurosurgery and Psychiatry, *37*, 475–484, 1974.

Steven, J. L.: Postoperative angiography in treatment of intracranial aneurysms. Acta Radiologica Diagnosis, *5*, 536–548, 1966.

Sukoff, M. H., Barth, B. and Morant, T.: Spontaneous occlusion of a massive arteriovenous malformation—case report. Neuroradiology, *4*, 121–123, 1972.

Sutton, D.: The vertebro-basilar system and its vascular lesions. Clinical Radiology, *22*, 271–287, 1971.

Sutton, D. and Trickey, S.: Subarachnoid haemorrhage and total cerebral angiography. Clinical Radiology, *13*, 297–303, 1962.

Terbrugge, K., Scotti, G., Ethier, R., Melancon, D., Tchang, S. and Milner, C.: Computed tomography in intracranial arteriovenous malformations. Radiology, *122*, 703–705, 1977.

Tindall, G. T., Goree, J. A., Lee, J. F. and Odom, G. L.: Effect of common carotid ligation on size of internal carotid aneurysms and distal intracarotid and retinal artery pressures. Journal of Neurosurgery, *25*, 503–511, 1966.

Turnbull, I. W.: Computed tomographic pointers to the prognosis of subarachnoid haemorrhage. British Journal of Radiology, *53*, 416–420, 1980.

Waltino, O., Eistola, P. and Vuolio, M.: Brain scanning in the detection of intracranial arterio-venous malformations. Acta Neurologica Scandinavica, *49*, 434–442, 1973.

Wood, E. H.: Angiographic identification of the ruptured lesion in patients with multiple cerebral aneurysms. Journal of Neurosurgery, *21*, 182–198, 1964.

4 Head Injuries

A wide variety of injuries may be demonstrable radiologically after severe head trauma (see Table 4–1).

SKULL RADIOGRAPHY

Timing of Examination
Skull radiographs should be made on every patient with definite cerebral concussion or a deep scalp contusion. Apart from medicolegal requirements, "early radiography is an essential part of the diagnosis of head injury, and frequently determines the pattern of further managment" (Lewin, 1966). Routine or basic views ("skull trauma series," see below) should be taken as soon as the initial clinical assessment in the accident room has been completed, and possible shock and airway obstruction have been treated. If the patient is too restless to cooperate, less is lost by delaying examination for a few hours than by producing substandard radiographs. More detailed study, e.g., special views of the temporal bones or facial skeleton, is best deferred until more favorable conditions prevail, although emergency radiography of the optic canals is essential in patients with traumatic visual loss.

Reasons for immediate examination include the following. (1) A traumatic aerocele—which may be the only visible sign of a fracture of the base of the skull—usually disappears within a few days, especially if small. (2) A subsequent deterioration in the patient's clinical state may be accompanied by pineal shift, and this change can be documented if baseline radiographs are available for comparison. (3) Adequate examination of the skull may be impossible after other injuries have been treated, e.g., splinting of the jaw or femur. (4) Rarely, intracranial gas may appear subsequently as a result of clostridial infection of a compound fracture.

Interpretation—What Is Important?
Interpretation must be directed to providing the surgeon or clinician with the information that he requires for the patient's management. The radiolo-

Table 4–1 Radiology of Head Injury (after Gabrielsen and Seeger, 1975)

Acute	
Scalp	– Hematoma
Skull	– Fracture, suture diastasis
Meningeal	– Leptomeningeal cyst ("growing fracture")
	– Hygroma
Vascular	– Hematoma (epidural, subdural, intracerebral)
	– Fistula (carotid-cavernous, carotid-jugular)
	– Aneurysm (dissecting, pseudoaneurysm)
	– Occlusion, arterial and venous (cerebral veins and dural sinuses)
	– Infarction
	– Arterial spasm
Cerebral	– Edema (focal, multifocal or generalized)
	– Contusion (focal or multifocal, hemorrhagic)
	– Herniations (cingulate, uncal, tonsillar)
	– Brain death (see Ch. 7, Fig. 7–60)
	– Atrophy (see Delayed, below)
Delayed	
Fistula (otorrhea, rhinorrhea)	
Pneumocephalus	
Meningitis	
Hydrocephalus	
	– Convexity-block, tentorial adhesions
	– Normal (low) pressure
Loss of brain substance ("atrophy")	
	– Focal, hemispherical or generalized
	– Porencephaly

gist's report should include the answers to the following questions, which are listed in order of importance:

1. Is the brain displaced? (pineal shift)
2. Is the dura torn? (intracranial gas, medially directed fragments of a comminuted fracture)
3. Is there a fracture? On what side is it, and is the fracture compound/comminuted/depressed? (fracture lines, displacements, opaque paranasal sinuses)
4. Other associated injuries of the face or neck, or chest organs? (fractures of the mandible, cervical spine or ribs, pulmonary contusion or collapse).

1. Pineal Shift: The radiologist's most important contribution to the management of a patient with a severe head injury is to identify the position of the pineal gland — and to relate it to any fracture of the vault that may be present — see Ch. 1, p. 11. These two radiological signs, if present, may indicate an intracranial situation that requires urgent neurosurgical intervention. For example, usually

fracture + contralateral pineal shift = extradural hematoma and/or contusion,

fracture + ipsilateral pineal shift = subdural hematoma and/or contusion. The warning should be stressed that the pineal may retain its normal position in the presence of a devastating or rapidly fatal head injury, and bilateral subdural hematomas of equal thickness may "tether" it to the midline. Following successful evacuation of a unilateral extracerebral hematoma, the displaced pineal may take several weeks to return to the midline. Downward dislocation of the midline pineal of an unconscious head-injured patient should prompt thought of bilateral supratentorial space-occupying lesions — or of an infratentorial hematoma causing obstructive hydrocephalus.

2. Aerocele: Fractures of the base of the skull that cross an air-filled space and rupture the dura cause pneumocephalus. Apart from iatrogenic causes, such as spinal puncture or postoperative craniotomy, recent trauma is the most frequent cause of intracranial aerocele. Since fractures of the base of the skull are notoriously difficult to demonstrate, aerocele may be the only visible radiological evidence of a penetrating injury. The commonest type is the frontal aerocele, complicating a fracture through the frontoethmoidal cells. Perisellar cisternal air may accompany fracture of the base of the skull through the sphenoidal sinus (Fig. 4–1). Mastoid fractures are less commonly penetrating. In infants, sharp objects such as a pencil tip may accidentally penetrate the orbital plate, producing a frontal aerocele. The risk of intracranial infection and cerebrospinal-fluid leakage such as rhinorrhea always accompanies a severe head injury, and it may require neurosurgical correction.

3. Fracture: The presence of a fracture is objec-

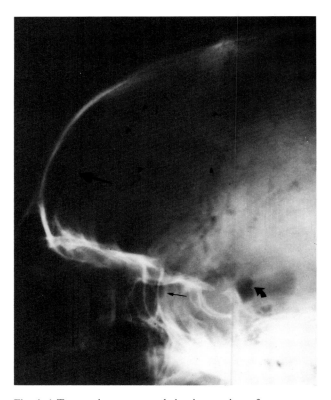

Fig. 4–1 Traumatic pneumocephalus in a patient after a severe head injury. Air is present in the subdural and subarachnoid spaces and an air-fluid level is visible in the sphenoidal sinus *(small arrow)*, suggesting a fracture of the base of the skull. Subdural air covers the frontal lobes *(large arrow)* and subarachnoid air outlines cortical sulci *(small arrowheads)* and the prepontine cistern *(curved arrow)*. A frontoethmoidal fracture was present, which is not visible. What are the advantages of the brow-up position for the lateral view of the skull?

tive documentation of an injury to the protective covering of the brain, and it should serve as a warning of the possibility of damage to the brain itself. However, the brain may sustain devastating and fatal damage without the skull being fractured.

Fractures of the skull vault may be linear or comminuted, compound and/or depressed. Simple linear fractures are usually of no consequence, unless they cross a vascular groove; they may then be responsible for an epidural hematoma (Cronqvist and Köhler, 1963). Thus, a fracture must always be correctly sited, and failure of the radiologist to identify the particular side of the vault may lead to surgical disaster. Fractures are best lateralized by a coronal view which is made with a central ray directed along the line of the fracture (see below). A compound fracture may be diagnosed by placing a metal marker over the scalp laceration, and verifying by means of a radiograph that the fracture is situated beneath it. Radiological initiative in confirming the compound nature of a brain injury may eliminate

hematomas depends on three factors, viz., location, shape and density, and all of these depend on the age of the clot (Svendsen, 1976). (A) Location. Subdural hematomas usually cover the convexity of a hemisphere (Fig. 4–12) but they may extend beneath the temporal lobe, or into the interhemispheric fissure; occasionally they will be confined to the interhemispheric surface (Fig. 4–13). Epidural hematomas are confined to the convexity, almost invariably beneath the fracture of the vault which may be visible. (B) Shape. The epidural hematoma has a lentiform shape which is localized to a part of the convexity. Consequently it produces very little midline displacement, in contrast to the dislocation produced by subdural collections, which are more extensive. (C) Density. The density of clotted blood diminishes in the course of a few weeks, consequently the appearances will depend on the age of the lesion. According to Scotti et al. (1977) subdural hematomas exhibit an increased density (Figs. 4–12 and 4–13) during the first week and a low density after the third week (Fig. 4–15). In the intervening period, when the lesion is isodense with normal brain, the diagnosis may be suspected if midline displacement or ventricular compression is present without a mass being identified (Fig. 4–14). Patients with a chronic subdural hematoma may undergo repeated trauma, so an acute and chronic lesion may be identified, the rebleed subdural. Contrast enhancement may reveal com-

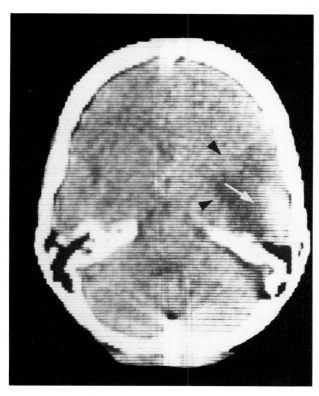

Fig. 4–8 Hemorrhagic contusion. A heterogeneous density of the right temporal lobe represents a contusion *(arrowheads)* with associated hemorrhage *(arrow)* abutting on the brain surface.

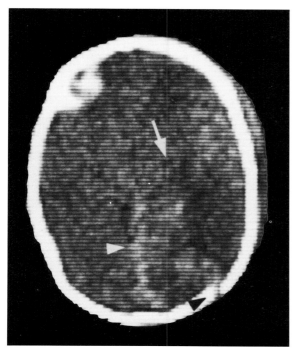 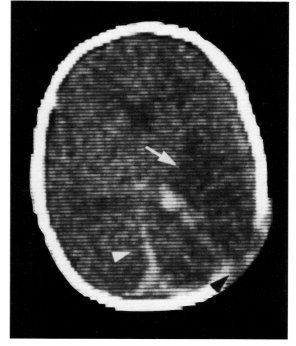

Fig. 4–9 Battered child. A hematoma of the right temple is visible, and the right parietal bone is fractured *(black arrowhead)*. Hemorrhagic contusion of the underlying hemisphere is present *(arrow)*, and there is blood in the interhemispheric fissure, indicating subarachnoid hemorrhage *(white arrowhead)*. The midline is displaced.

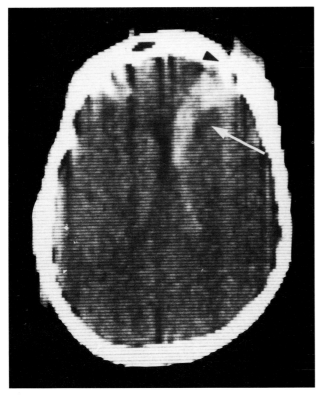

Fig. 4–10 "Dive-bomber" injury; this child fell from a height directly onto the frontal bone. There is a fracture of the right frontal bone *(arrowhead)*, with a crescentic hematoma dissecting through the cortex to the right lateral ventricle *(arrow)*.

pressed cortical sulci of the underlying hemisphere, or an opacifying membrane (Figs. 4–14 and 4–17). Experience with computed tomography has revealed that subdural hematomas of different ages

not infrequently coexist, sometimes over the same hemisphere (Fig. 4–16). Buckling of the white matter indicates the presence of an extracerebral mass (Fig. 4–14).

2. Vault Fracture: The variable window-width facility of most apparatus for computed tomography enables fractures of the vault to be identified and related to complicating intracranial lesions such as epidural hematoma and aerocele (Figs. 4–18 through 4–20).

3. Aerocele—see Figure 4–20.

4. Scalp Hematoma—see Figure 4–21.

Chronic Lesions and Sequelae

The pattern of these lesions varies greatly, depending on the particular part of the brain, its coverings or blood vessels injured. Damage to cerebral parenchyma results in cortical atrophy and gliosis. Stenosis or occlusion of the carotid or vertebral arteries in the neck may lead to cerebral infarction, atrophy, focal ventricular dilatation or porencephaly. Damage to periventricular white matter causes focal enlargement of the adjacent ventricle. Obliteration of the basal cisterns or convexity sulci, often associated with subarachnoid hemorrhage, may lead to hydrocephalus.

The importance of computed tomography in the management of head-injured patients is enhanced by the accuracy with which sequential changes and the late effects of trauma on the brain can be studied. Figure 4–24 illustrates the evolution of the process from the acute post-injury phase to the end result, which is dilatation of the ventricles and subarachnoid spaces due to brain atrophy or convexity blockage. In other instances, gliosis or atrophy may be observed to follow cortical injury—probably as a result of arterial or cortical damage, or both

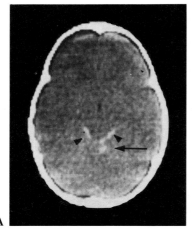
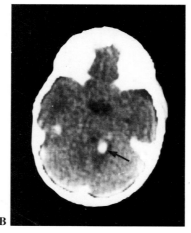
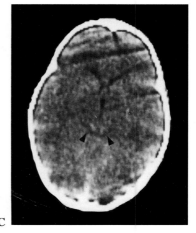

Fig. 4–11 Brainstem damage in an unconscious patient following a traffic accident. (A) Initial examination, showing a focal hemorrhage in the right cerebellar peduncle *(arrow)* and subarachnoid blood in the quadrigeminal plate cistern *(arrowheads)*. (B and C) Two days later, the peduncular hematoma has enlarged *(arrow)* and there is a surrounding low-density zone of contusion. Blood has cleared from the quadrigeminal plate cistern *(arrowheads)*.

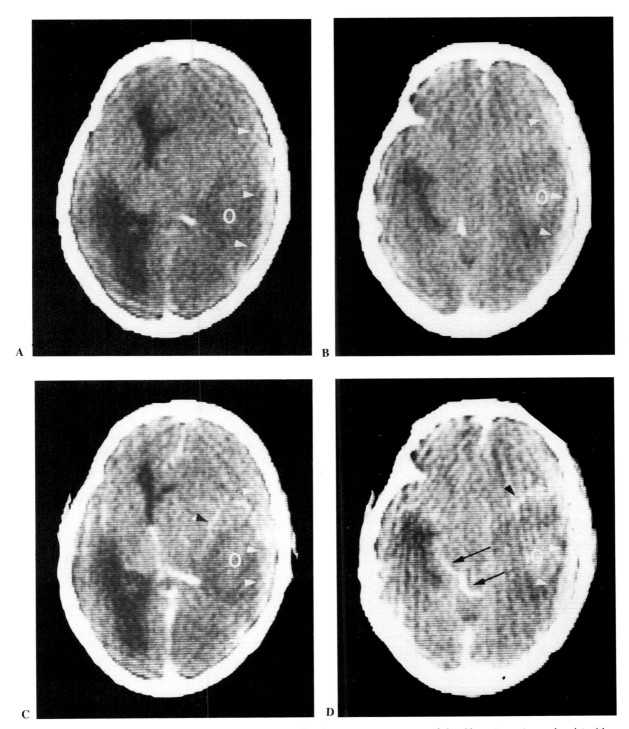

Fig. 4–12 Acute subdural hematoma. (A and B) Noncontrast slice demonstrates an acute subdural hematoma *(arrowheads)* with a crescentic border and an underlying hemorrhagic contusion (O). Considerable ventricular displacement is present—greater than the thickness of the hematoma, which confirms the presence of an additional, i.e., intracerebral mass lesion. (C and D) Contrast enhancement reveals that the midbrain, although incompletely outlined, is compressed and rotated *(arrows)*, indicating incisural herniation. A prominent draining vein is visible, representing hyperperfusion *(arrowhead)*.

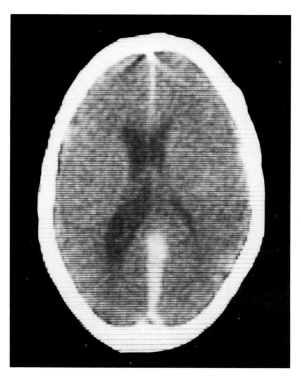
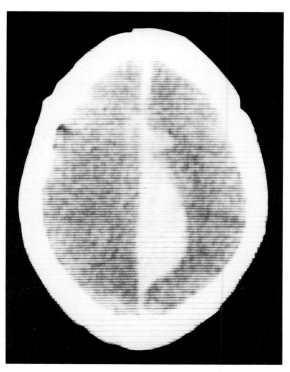

Fig. 4–13 Interhemispheric subdural hematoma. The ventricular system is not displaced from the midline and there is no evidence of a convexity hematoma.

(Figs. 4–25 and 4–26). In the case illustrated in Figure 4–27, a solitary contusion of the right frontal lobe, a repeat examination 6 months later showed considerable progression of the lesion, implying arterial compromise at the outset. Ventricular dilatation may commence as early as 10 days after a head injury (Fig. 4–28). Porencephaly is the end result of cerebral damage or vascular injury, sometimes perinatal (Fig. 4–29).

An epidural or subdural hematoma, if unrecognized or if treated conservatively, may be identified as a lentiform extracerebral collection of lower density than normal brain (Figs. 4–15 and 4–16). An enhancing membrane may delineate it (Fig. 4–17). The end-result, an extracerebral hygroma, if it develops sufficiently early in life may deform the skull (Figs. 4–30 and see 1–37). Intracranial hematomas once hypodense lose their space-

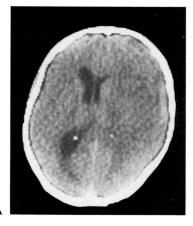
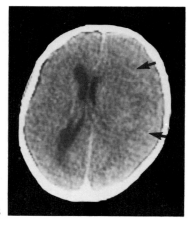
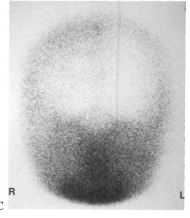

Fig. 4–14 Isodense subdural hematoma (19 days old). (A) Nonenhanced and (B) enhanced slices at ventricular level demonstrate marked midline displacement without underlying abnormality. The enhanced slice outlines deformed cortical sulci, thus indicating the thickness of the lesion. Buckling of the white matter is noted *(arrows)*. (C) The diagnosis of a subdural collection was confirmed by radionuclide imaging and the lesion was evacuated surgically.

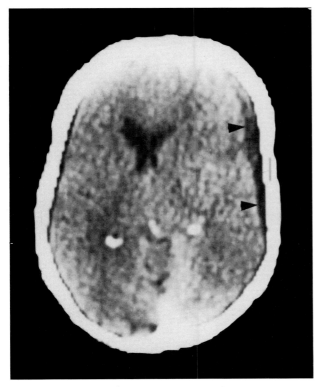

Fig. 4–15 Chronic subdural collection. A low-density lesion is visible over the convexity of the right hemisphere *(arrowheads)*, displacing the ventricular system.

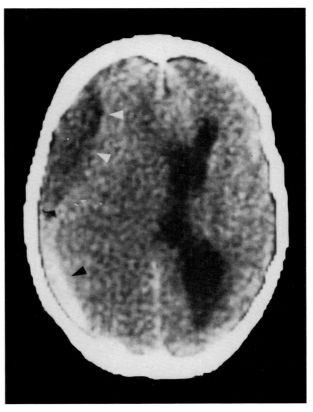

Fig. 4–16 Acute and chronic subdural hematomas. Anteriorly a chronic subdural collection is present, a low-density lesion with a lentiform outline *(white arrowheads)*. Posteriorly there is an acute collection, a high-density lesion with a crescentic outline *(black arrowhead)*. Marked midline displacement is shown.

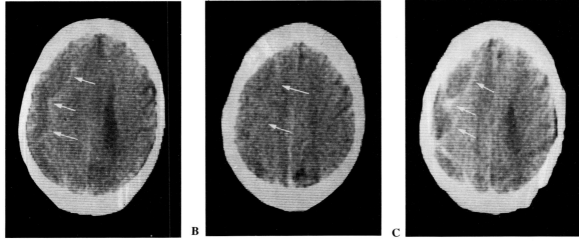

Fig. 4–17 Chronic subdural collection with enhancing membrane. (A and B) Noncontrast slices show a lentiform chronic subdural collection over the left convexity, with a thin medial density suggesting a membrane *(arrows)*. Ventricular displacement is present. (C) Following contrast injection, the membrane enhances *(white arrows)*.

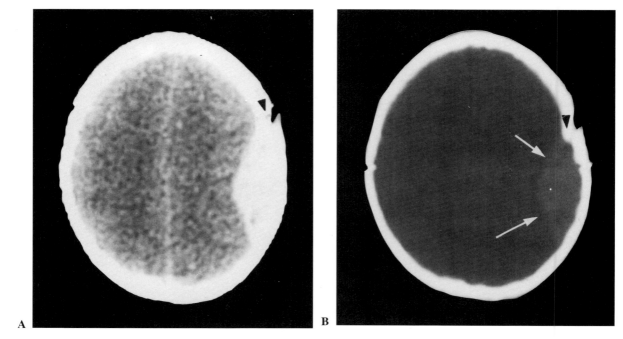

Fig. 4–18 Epidural hematoma with fracture. (A) A high-density lentiform opacity is present over the surface of the right hemisphere. At its anterior end, a fracture is visible *(arrowhead)*. (B) Same slice, with the window-width adjusted to bone density, confirms the presence of a depressed fracture *(arrowhead)* in the region of the epidural collection *(arrows)*. The fracture had torn the middle meningeal artery, producing the hematoma.

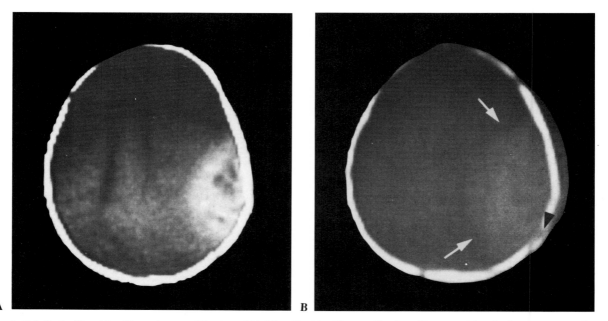

Fig. 4–19 Infant with epidural hematoma and fracture. (A) A localized lentiform collection of increased density is present over the surface of the right hemisphere. The patchy low-density areas within it probably represent trapped subarachnoid fluid or tissue. There is marked displacement of the midline structures. (B) Vertex slice with window adjusted again demonstrates the epidural collection *(arrows)* and also a fracture of the right parietal bone *(arrowhead)*.

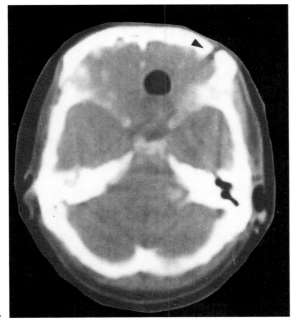 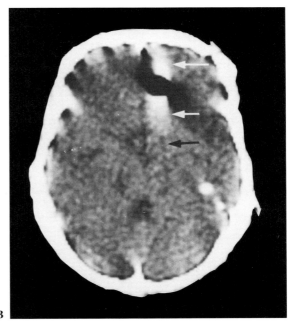

A   B

Fig. 4–20 A patient with visual deterioration and rhinorrhea following an automobile accident. (A) Basal slice, with the window adjusted for better visualization of bone, demonstrates the presence of a right frontal fracture *(arrowhead)* and pneumocephalus manifested by a well-defined, low-density focus in the midline of the anterior cranial fossa. (B) A slightly higher slice, showing a parasagittal hematoma *(white arrows)*. The hematoma extends posteriorly to deform the right side of the suprasellar "star" *(black arrow)*, accounting for the clinical signs of chiasmal involvement. The pocket of air appears as a sharply-circumscribed low density bisecting the hematoma.

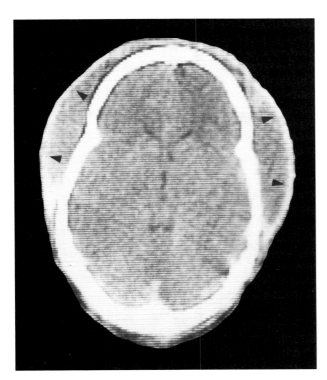

Fig. 4–21 Bilateral cephalhematomas *(arrowheads)* without underlying damage to the brain or calvarium, in a child involved in a traffic accident.

occupying property, and fail to show enhancement; they may be indistinguishable from chronic cerebral infarction (Fig. 6–19). Occasionally resolving hematomas exhibit a ring blush: Zimmerman et al. (1978) showed that this appearance may appear from 6 days to several months after the original ictus and that it resembles the enhancing ring blush of metastatic malignancy, glioblastoma multiforme or pyogenic abscess.

At an interval of weeks to years from the original injury, the following lesions may be present:

Foreign material: bullet, air (Fig. 4–20)

Fracture (Figs. 4–19 and 4–22)

Subdural collection: hygroma (Figs. 4–22 and 4–30), enhancing membranes (Fig. 4–15 and 4–23).

Cerebral atrophy: focal, multifocal, hemispherical or generalized (Fig. 4–24)

Hydrocephalus, probably due to extraventricular obstruction (Figs. 4–23 and 4–28)

Cerebral infarction (Figs. 4–26 and 4–27)

Porencephalic cyst (Fig. 4–29)

Deformity of the skull caused by extracerebral collections in early life (Fig. 4–30)

The role and appearances of computed tomography in head injuries and their sequelae have been described by several authors, including the following: Richardson, 1975; Ambrose et al. 1976; Berger

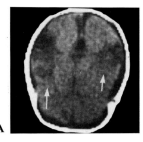
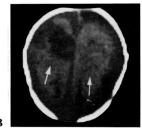
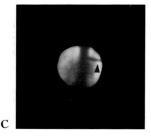
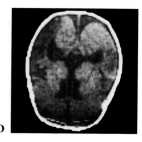

Fig. 4—22 Battered child with subdural hygroma, contusions and multiple fractures. (A) A low-density collection completely envelops the brain, which is denser than normal as a result of compression by the fluid envelope. The bilateral low-density intracerebral lesions are contusions *(arrows)*. (B) Slice at a higher level shows a thicker fluid envelope and further contusions *(arrows)*. (C) Fracture of the left parietal bone *(arrowhead)*. (D) Three weeks later: the ventricles have enlarged and the fluid envelope after repeated tapping has diminished in volume. The brain remains denser than normal.

et al. 1976; Merino-de-Villasante and Taveras 1976; Davis et al. 1977; Dublin et al. 1977; Koo and LaRoque 1977.

ANGIOGRAPHY

Extracranial Carotid and Vertebral Injuries (Table 4—4)

Blunt trauma or a nonpenetrating blow to the neck may damage the carotid artery (Fig. 4–31). Bleeding into the soft tissues of the neck as a consequence of external trauma may lead to stenosis or occlusion through external compression (Fig. 4–32). Another mechanism is sudden forced stretching of the internal carotid artery in the region of the vertebral axis by hyperextension of the neck combined with contralateral rotation of the head (New and Momose, 1969; Sullivan et al., 1973). Arterial stretching may rupture the intima and media and leave the adventitial layer intact (Bergan, 1963). The other lesion associated with this type of injury is initial rupture of the media, with dissection of blood into the intimal and adventitial layers (Northcroft and Morgan, 1944; Brown and Armitage, 1973). Such damage to a cervical carotid artery may result in ischemic swelling or infarction of the ipsilateral cerebral hemisphere; often a latent interval is present before a clinical deficit appears (Zilkha, 1970).

The angiographic appearances vary greatly. If the intimal and medial layers are elevated by a hematoma, then in addition to encroachment on the lumen an intimal flap may be recognized. An intimal tear or thrombus may serve as a site for further thrombus development or as a source of emboli, and either of these lesions may be responsible for intracranial complications such as infarction (Acosta et al., 1972; Loar et al., 1973; Friedenberg et al., 1973). Besides stenosis and occlusion, an aneurysmal sac may form on the cervical carotid artery, and sometimes the segments of the artery proximal and distal to it are narrowed (Margolis et al., 1972; Teal et al., 1973). If the aneurysm is not treated surgical-

ly, subsequent angiography may show that it has enlarged, or that it has healed by thrombosis (McDonald et al., 1976).

A direct blow to the scalp, such as a fall downstairs onto the head, may damage the scalp arteries. Pseudoaneurysm or arteriovenous fistula may develop on the scalp or neck (Figs. 4–33 and 4–34).

Penetrating injuries to the neck may be similar to

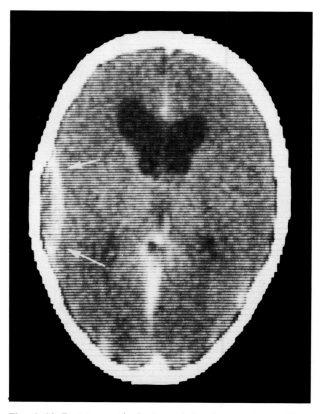

Fig. 4—23 Post-traumatic hydrocephalus in a patient with a chronic subdural collection. A circumscribed cortical collection is outlined by an enhancing membrane *(white arrows)*. There is no midline displacement. The cause of the hydrocephalus was presumed to be tentorial or convexity adhesions.

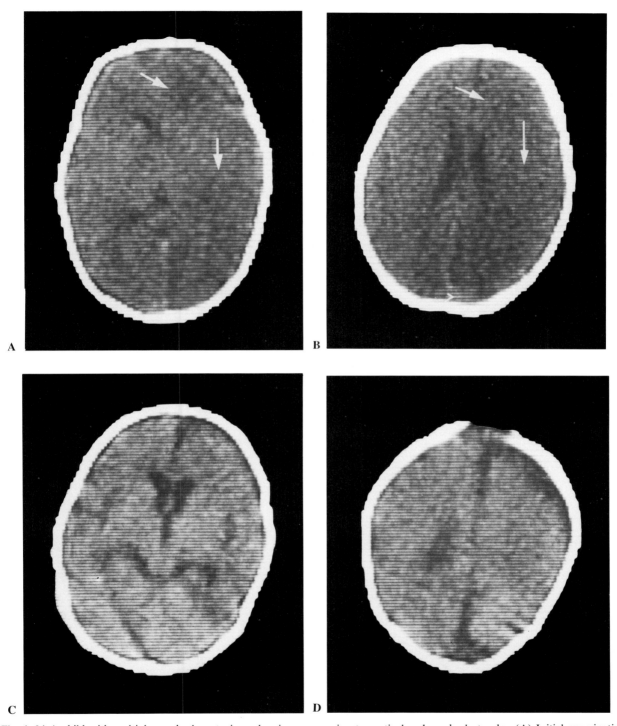

Fig. 4–24 A child with multiple cerebral contusions showing progression to cortical and cerebral atrophy. (A) Initial examination. There are low-density lesions in the right hemisphere *(arrows)*, the right lateral ventricle is compressed and the midline is displaced to the left side. (B) Nine days later: the contusions are less marked *(arrows)*, the right lateral ventricle is less compressed and the midline displacement has diminished. (C and D) One month later: the ventricles have enlarged and the subarachnoid spaces and interhemispheric fissure have widened, due to atrophy.

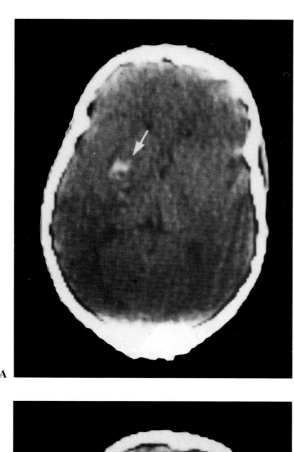

A

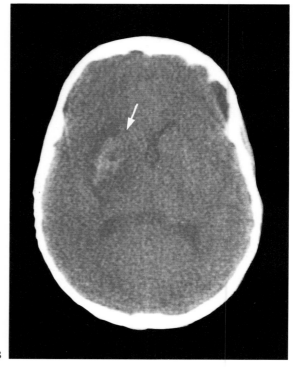

B

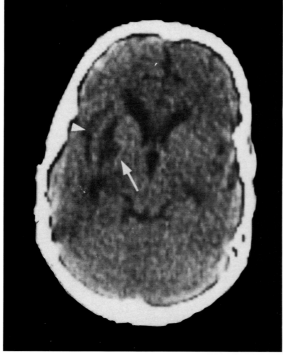

C

Fig. 4–25 The changing pattern of an intracerebral hemotoma. (A) A noncontrast slice reveals clotted blood in the lateral ganglionic region of the left hemisphere—probably a result of traumatic damage to the lenticulostriate arteries. No midline displacement is present. (B) Four days later. The ganglionic hematoma is still present *(arrow)* but it is now surrounded by a lucent zone and the right lateral ventricle is compressed. There may also be minimal midline displacement. (C) One month later a low-density lesion is present in the area of the hematoma *(white arrow)*. The sylvian fissure is wide *(arrowhead)* and the ventricles are dilated, compared to the initial appearance.

nonpenetrating ones, because the mechanism of their production is similar (Figs. 4–35 and 4–36). However, several additional abnormalities may occur (Table 4–3). These include arteriovenous fistula (Fig. 4–37; Chou and French, 1965) and laceration of the artery, with extravasation and the formation of a periarterial hematoma. The commonest penetrating injuries are stab wounds, but iatrogenic arterial damage may be produced in the course of arterial punctures or catheterization, or during the placement of central venous catheters.

The vertebral artery may be damaged as it lies in the foramen transversarium by the same mechanism that accounts for traumatic occlusion of the carotid artery. It is most vulnerable at the atlantoaxial level, and traumatic damage at this site is usually the result of forced extension and contralateral rotation of the cervical spine. The injuries include dissecting aneurysm and/or thrombosis. Chiropractic manipulation may account for this type of injury (Miller and Ayers, 1967; Davidson et al., 1975).

Intracranial Lesions

Damage to Blood Vessels

(1) **Carotid-Cavernous Fistula:** Traumatic damage to the base of the skull accompanying nonpenetrating or penetrating injuries may occasionally lead to the formation of aneurysms of the petrous or cavernous portions of the internal carotid artery. No fracture may be demonstrable. However, the more usual vascular complication of fracture of the base of the skull is carotid-cavernous fistula (Figs. 4–38 and 4–39; Janon et al., 1967; Clemens and Lodin, 1968A and 1968B). Carotid-cavernous fistulae may be recognized on carotid angiography by the extravasation of contrast medium into the cavernous sinus, with venous discharge along one or more of several routes (Table 4–5; Fig. 4–40). An important anastomotic communication to identify between the external and internal carotid arteries is that via the middle meningeal artery and the artery of the inferior cavernous sinus (Fig. 4–39, Wallace et al., 1967). Selective or superselective external carotid injection as well as internal carotid examination is necessary in all patients with carotid-cavernous fistulae to exclude this potential pathway. Conventional surgical techniques may fail because the external carotid communicates with the cavernous part of the internal carotid artery. Floatation of a muscle embolus or a balloon catheter to the site of the fistula is now the therapeutic technique of choice (Pickard et al., 1974; Debrun et al., 1975).

(2) **False Aneurysm of the Internal Carotid Branches:** Post-traumatic aneurysms are either true aneurysms or so-called false aneurysms (Miller and Ayers, 1967; Handa et al., 1970; Lukin and Cham-

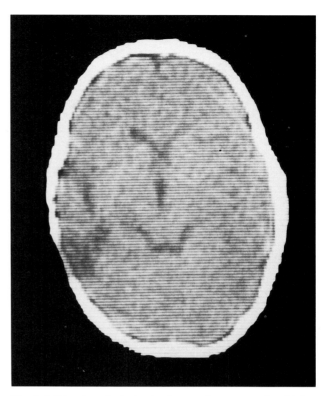

Fig. 4–26 Focal cortical atrophy 1 year after a severe head injury. A low-density lesion with irregular margins is present in the posterior half of the left hemisphere. This area represents a focal post-traumatic cerebral infarct.

bers, 1974). The true variety is a localized dilatation of the arterial wall which is frequently associated with fracture of the skull and underlying damage to the cerebral cortex (Gurdjian et al., 1971). The arterial wall may be damaged in closed head injuries as well. A false aneurysm or pseudoaneurysm is the term used to describe the cavity that develops within an encapsulated hematoma communicating with the lumen of an artery. Intracranially it is most commonly observed along the distribution of the middle cerebral artery (Fig. 4–41) and there are often contiguous extracerebral collections (Rudikoff et al., 1968; Rumbaugh et al., 1970). Fractures are not invariably observed. Various mechanisms have been implicated, which include the following: (A) a rotatory type of motion causing a shearing force, which tears the arachnoid and ruptures the artery (Rudikoff et al., 1968); (B) a yielding rotatory movement of the brain within the skull upon impact, causing an artery to tear from its dural attachment and producing a small defect in its wall; (C) if a fracture occurs, the underlying dura may be lacerated, and the cerebral cortex and cortical vessels may momentarily herniate into the fracture site; (D) another mechanism that may be responsible for tearing of peripheral branches of the middle

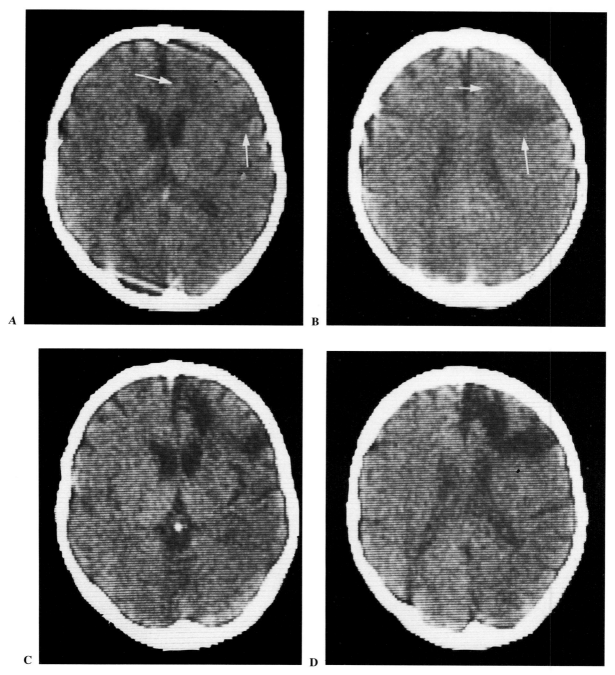

Fig. 4–27 Acute contusion followed up 6 months later. (A and B) Initial examination shows a poorly defined, low-density lesion in the right frontal lobe *(arrows)*. (C and D) Repeat examination 5 months later shows two low-density areas at the level of the anterior horns, which probably represent cerebral infarcts, secondary to vascular damage at the time of the original injury. Both lateral ventricles are slightly dilated.

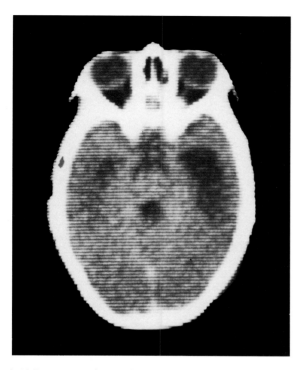
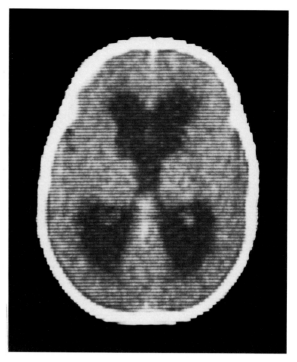

Fig. 4–28 Post-traumatic ventricular dilatation in a baby, 2 weeks after a contusional injury of the brain. The cause of the hydrocephalus is not shown.

cerebral artery is the fact that the trunk is relatively fixed proximally at the carotid bifurcation and distally at the sylvian point. Consequently the shearing force imparted to the brain at the time of injury is greatest on the peripheral branches, particularly those with vascular plaques. Most patients with arterial tears are beyond middle age. Rarely a traumatic fistulous connection with surface veins may be identified as a result of shearing of cortical arteries. Leakage of contrast medium into the brain may occur as a result of trauma without the site of arterial rupture being identifiable. No false aneurysm need be present (Fig. 4–42; Rumbaugh et al., 1970; Benoit and Wortzman, 1973).

(3) Trauma to the External Carotid Branches: The middle meningeal artery may be damaged as a result of fracture of the vault crossing a meningeal groove (Cronqvist and Köhler, 1963). Rupture of the middle meningeal artery may give rise to a variety of abnormal vascular patterns, almost always in association with an epidural hematoma (Schechter et al., 1966; Sones et al., 1970). These abnormalities include the following: (A) pseudoaneurysm of the middle meningeal artery; (B) stenosis of the superficial temporal artery due to injury (Fig. 4–43); (C) medial displacement of the middle meningeal artery by the epidural collection (Fig. 4–44); (D) tearing of the two meningeal veins which run parallel to the artery in the groove and, if accompanied by tearing of the artery, arteriovenous fistula—so-called rail-

road tracks (Figs. 4–45 and 4–46; Schechter et al., 1966).

Epidural collections may displace the venous sinuses from the inner table (Fig. 4–47). An epidural hematoma may be distinguished from a subdural collection by demonstrating any of the abnormalities mentioned above, which indicate involvement of the middle meningeal artery. In addition, an epidural collection because of its location tends to be *localized* or confined, and to have a lentiform configuration. Midline displacement is minimal. Damage to the venous sinuses may produce tearing of a sinus with leakage or an infratentorial epidural mass (Fig. 4–48).

(4) Arterial Occlusion (Thrombosis, Embolism, Spasm): Intracranial arterial occlusion may be the result of *thrombosis* due to propagation of clot from injured extracranial arteries or as a consequence of intimal or medial damage to the vulnerable parts of the intracranial carotid tree. The two intracranial sites most easily injured are the supraclinoid segment just distal to the point of dural penetration and the intracranial carotid bifurcation. Shearing forces within the cranial cavity exert the greatest effect on cortical branches and on the supraclinoid carotid and carotid bifurcation. Dissecting aneurysms and/or intramural thrombi may also form at these sites as a result of intimal injury (Fig. 4–49; Wolpert and Schechter, 1966; Loar et al., 1973).

Fat emboli may be released at the site of a frac-

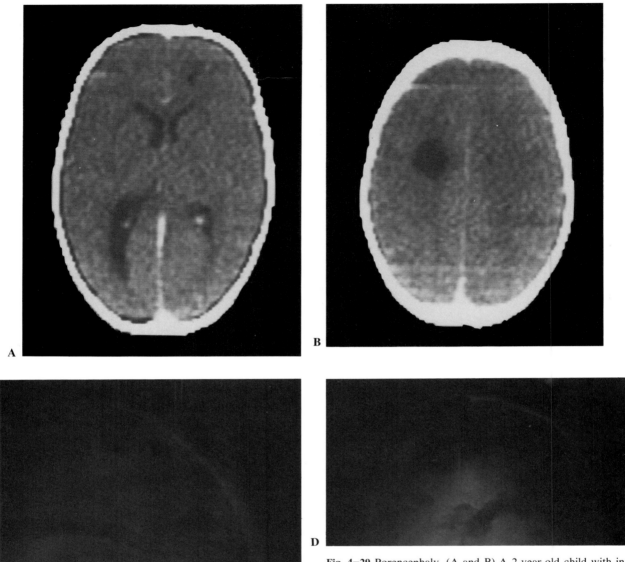

Fig. 4–29 Porencephaly. (A and B) A 2-year-old child with increasing spasticity of the right limbs and ataxia. Protracted birth with forceps delivery: ? perinatal brain damage. (C and D) A 46-year-old policeman with left homonymous hemianopia. The cystic cavity at the right occipital pole communicates with the ventricular system and *replaces* normal brain.

ture elsewhere in the body, and may cause stenosis or occlusion of the intracranial arteries (Fig. 4–50). Trauma to the extracranial carotid may cause intimal rupture with hematoma or aneurysm formation, which may act as a source of emboli (Fig. 4–51). Any alterations in caliber due to trauma may be hemodynamically significant and produce turbulent flow which may also be a source of emboli (Fig. 4–36).

Trauma is a common cause of *subarachnoid*

hemorrhage, of which over 10 percent of cases show arterial vasospasm (Freidenfelt and Sunström, 1963). Arterial vasoconstriction secondary to subarachnoid hemorrhage should be distinguished from other causes of arterial narrowing at the base of the brain where the blood accumulates. The commonest site of involvement is the point at which the internal carotid artery penetrates the dura and is most vulnerable to subarachnoid blood. Spasm may also be present in the vicinity of an intracranial

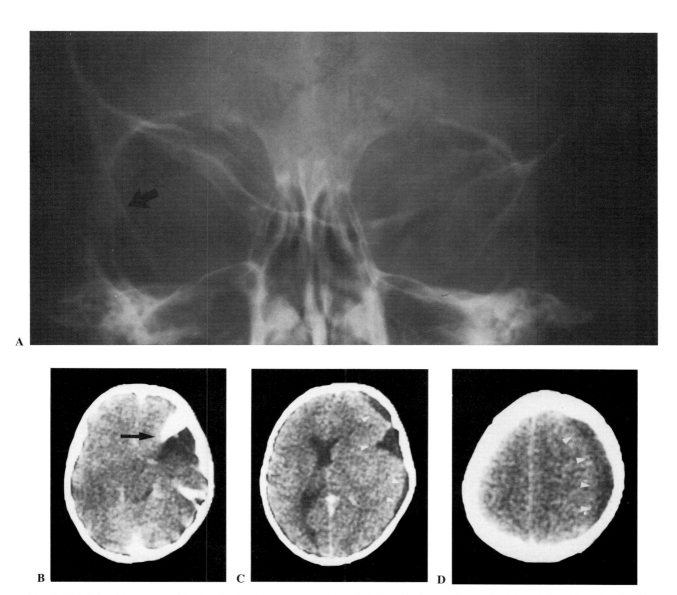

Fig. 4–30 Subdural hygroma deforming the skull in a 9-year-old boy. (A) Perorbital view shows elevation of the right sphenoid ridge and lateral displacement of the innominate line *(arrow)*. (B) Basal slice shows a collection of fluid beneath the elevated right sphenoid ridge *(arrow)*. (C) Ventricular slice shows marked ventricular displacement by the irregular extracerebral collection of fluid *(white arrows)*. (D) A higher slice shows greater thickness of the collection which explains the marked degree of ventricular displacement.

hematoma (Fig. 4–52) or affect peripheral vessels beneath an extracerebral collection (Fig. 4–53).

Alterations in the Cerebral Circulation

As with other mass lesions, space-occupying traumatic lesions within the skull—both cerebral and extracerebral—may upset the circulatory dynamics (Leeds et al., 1966). The cerebral circulation time may be prolonged, especially the arterial and intermediate phases. Cerebral compression also results in delayed venous filling. Acute arterial trauma may produce a loss of cerebral autoregulation due to the accumulation of acid metabolites (see Ch. 6, p. 31).

The resulting abnormal vascular pattern may include hyperperfusion, which is observed immediately after acute trauma as opposed to the slight delay in patients with vascular disease. An area of vascular disarray with a hyperemic blush and early filling veins may be seen (Fig. 4–54). This appearance should not be confused with the hypervascularity of a cerebral neoplasm: no abnormal vessels are visible and the opacified veins are the normal regional veins which fill early and more densely, because of shunting through the open capillary bed.

Another feature is the occurrence of a "pseudocapsule" surrounding normal brain compressed by

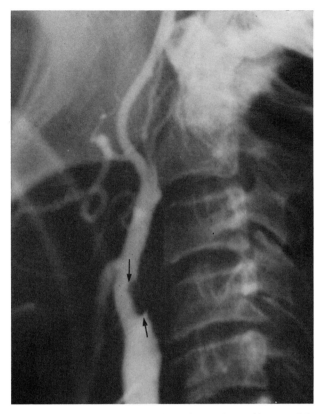

Fig. 4–31 Complete occlusion of the internal carotid artery following a blow on the neck, without external evidence of injury. The patient, a young soldier, was found unconscious some hours later. The carotid angiogram shows a radiolucent defect *(arrows)* along the posterior wall of the common carotid artery — subintimal hematoma occluding the internal carotid artery.

Table 4–4 Trauma to Extracranial Vessels

Nonpenetrating or Blunt Trauma
True or post-traumatic ("false") aneurysm
Dissecting aneurysm
Thrombosis
   Luminal blood clot
   Extrinsic compression
Extravascular hematoma
Penetrating Injury Including Iatrogenic Lesions, e.g., Needle Punctures
May produce all of the above
Arteriovenous fistula
Extravascular hematoma with or without continued leakage

an intracranial mass such as a hematoma. The stain of a pseudocapsule, as opposed to a true capsule, lasts briefly, being only observed in the intermediate phase. Early draining veins or delayed filling veins may be seen. A striking finding after severe head trauma is the occurrence of arteries that fill late and slowly, as a result of severe damage to the brain, cerebral edema, or the presence of subarachnoid blood (Fig. 4–54).

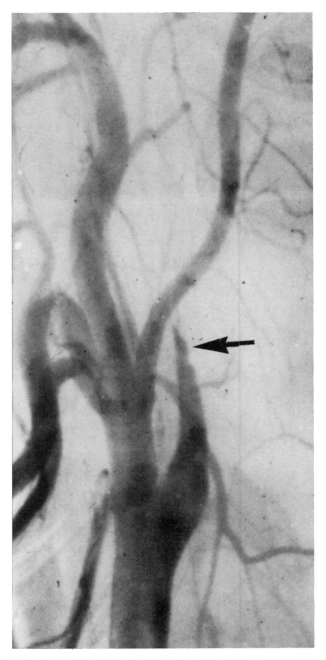

Fig. 4–32 Complete occlusion of the internal carotid artery as a result of direct trauma. The patient was a teenager who was struck by a wave during waterskiing, and developed symptoms 10 days later. The arrow points to a tapering occlusion of the proximal internal carotid artery, and slight irregularity of its margins.

Mass Effects of Trauma

1. Epidural Hematoma. Epidural hematomas are confined in extent, being limited by the dura which is tightly adherent to the endosteum of the skull. In contrast to subdural hematomas, they are: (A) always lentiform in cross-section, (B) nearly always

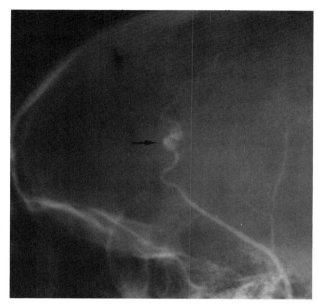

Fig. 4–33 Traumatic aneurysm of the superficial temporal artery found in a middle-aged patient after a fall. Palpation revealed a lump on the temple, which was shown by external carotid arteriography to correspond to an aneurysmal dilatation of the superficial temporal artery *(arrow).*

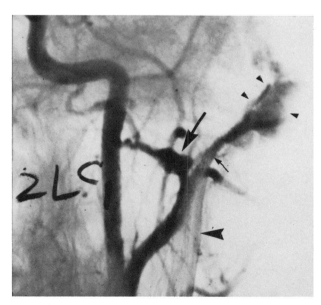

Fig. 4–34 Traumatic arteriovenous fistula of the superficial temporal artery *(small arrow)* in a patient sustaining a blow to the left side of the face. The extravasated contrast medium *(small arrowheads)* drains superiorly via the facial vein and inferiorly to the external jugular vein *(large arrowhead).* The large arrow points to a false aneurysm of the internal maxillary artery.

associated with an overlying fracture or suture diastasis, and (C) unlikely to displace the midline structures, such as the pineal gland, as much as a subdural hematoma (Norma, 1956; Cronqvist and

Köhler, 1965; May, 1974). Figures 4–18 and 4–55 illustrate these features.

Carotid angiography may reveal one or more of the following signs of epidural hematoma:

Medial displacement of the middle meningeal artery (Fig. 4–44)

Pseudoaneurysm or extravasation of contrast medium (Fig. 4–45)

Arteriovenous fistula of the middle meningeal artery (Fig. 4–46)

Separation of the inner table from the venous sinuses (Fig. 4–47; Columella et al., 1963)

Compression or spasm of superficial sylvian arteries (Glickman et al., 1976).

Tearing of the venous sinus may accompany its separation from the inner table, causing contrast extravasation (Fig. 4–48). Since extradural hematomas tend to be localized, the anteroposterior projection may not demonstrate the avascular component at all, revealing only dislocated vessels and midline displacement to indicate an abnormality. Oblique projections are necessary to demonstrate the maximal thickness of the hematoma.

2. Subdural Hematoma. Unlike extradural hematoma, a history of and a direct association with recent injury is not always a feature of patients with a subdural hematoma; sometimes the diagnosis when made comes as a surprise to the neurologist. The majority represent contre-coup damage, the subdural hematoma being either the total injury or combined with a focal contusion of the underlying brain substance. A small proportion are nontraumatic collections, caused by ruptured aneurysm or arteriovenous malformation or excessive anticoagulant therapy. As many as one-third of supratentorial acute subdural hematomas exhibit false-lateralizing clinical signs due to the "notch effect" (Kernohan and Woltman, 1929); therefore skull radiography is important prior to angiography, to determine the direction of displacement of the pineal gland (see p. 11).

Norman (1956) postulated that, although epidural hematomas form a lentiform shape, subdural hematomas alter from a crescentic shape in the first two weeks, through an intermediate stage, to a lentiform shape after the first month (Fig. 4–56). These configurations, which are illustrated in Figures 4–56, 4–57, 4–58 and 4–59, respectively, have been accepted as a useful way of dating a subdural collection. Several authors have questioned the reliability of Norman's findings (Zingesser et al., 1965; Radcliffe et al., 1972), but experience of computed tomography has on the whole confirmed them. The following conclusions are based on the studies of Gilday and his colleagues (1974) and of May (1974), and on the authors' personal experience: (A) all, or nearly all, acute subdural hematomas have a crescentic shape (Fig. 4–57). (B) If a subdural

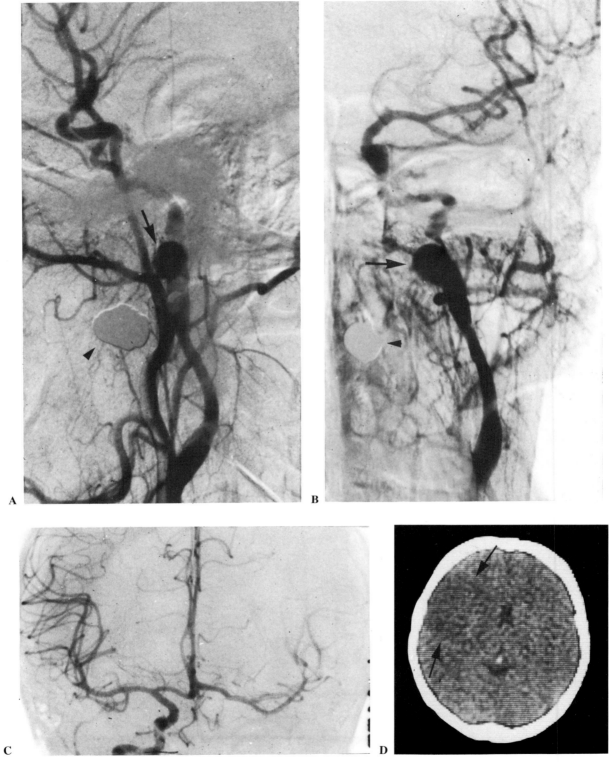

Fig. 4–35 Aneurysm of the neck and impaired cerebral perfusion caused by a gunshot wound. (A and B) An aneurysm of the distal cervical segment of the internal carotid artery is present *(arrow)*. The bullet projects as a gray image on the subtraction views *(arrowhead)*. The internal carotid artery has a reduced lumen above and below the bullet due to reduced flow, which is caused by compression of the artery by the aneurysm. The aneurysm is therefore hemodynamically significant, and intracranial perfusion is reduced. (C) Injection into the right common carotid artery demonstrates spontaneous cross-flow to the left to compensate for the reduced flow. (D) Noncontrast computed tomogram shows a low-density lesion in the left hemisphere *(arrows)* — cerebral infarction resulting from ischemia.

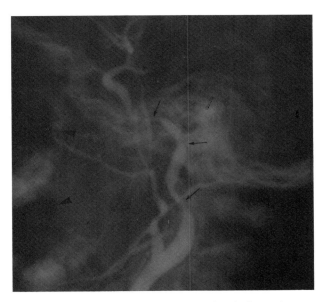

Fig. 4–36 Hematoma of the neck compressing the internal carotid artery, which complicated a stab wound. A large soft-tissue mass of the nasopharynx and neck is visible *(arrowheads)*. The cervical, petrous and extradural portions of the internal carotid artery *(small arrows)* are constricted. These luminal changes are the result of external compression of the arterial wall and/or vasospasm.

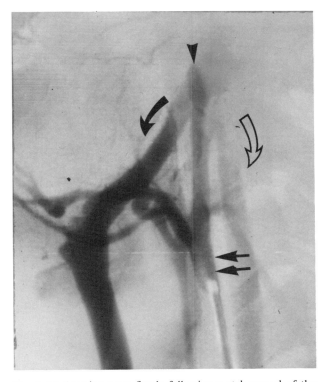

Fig. 4–37 Arteriovenous fistula following a stab wound of the neck. Selective injection of the external carotid artery *(two arrows)* shows an arteriovenous fistula *(arrowhead)*. The black curved arrow is the external jugular vein and the open curved arrow is the internal jugular vein.

hematoma is lentiform, it is chronic (Fig. 4–59), but (C) a subdural hematoma with a crescentic shape may be acute or chronic. Gilday and his colleagues identified a third pattern which they referred to as transitional and which the present authors call subacute (Fig. 4–58): it really includes all cases without distinctive crescentic or lentiform outlines. Rumbaugh et al. (1970) has pointed out the exceptional occurrence of "lentiform" patterns in patients with acute and subacute subdural hematomas, due to adhesions between the dural and arachnoid layers.

Anteroposterior angiography in patients with subdural hematomas will reliably confirm the presence of a superficial space-occupying lesion, but it may not always be obvious that the mass is extracerebral. In such instances oblique projections are necessary to demonstrate the avascular component, and they are always useful in determining its shape, size and extent (Fig. 4–57). Frontal collections are best examined by lateral and frontal ipsilateral oblique projections which will reveal displacement of the frontalpole vessels from the inner table. Posterior collection may require a contralateral oblique.

Nelson and Freimanis (1965) studied the possibility of diagnosing bilateral subdural hematomas from a unilateral carotid angiogram, from the nature of the angiographic abnormality as seen on the anteroposterior view. They showed that if the midline displacement of the anterior cerebral artery is 50 percent or less of the maximum width of the collection, then a subdural hematoma on the opposite side should be suspected. In large trauma series examined by computed tomography and angiography, bilateral lesions have been reported in 25 percent of cases (Dublin et al., 1977).

Subdural collections in infants and young children may cover the entire surface of both hemispheres and encase the brain in an envelope of fluid (Fig. 4–22; Leeds et al., 1968). Angiography in such cases reveals, in addition to the avascular lesion and displacements described above, a "brain stain" on the frontal and lateral convexities. This appearance arises from an excessive accumulation of contrast medium, as a result of the prolonged circulation time, caused by compression of the cortex by the subdural collection (Leeds et al., 1966). In children and young adults a chronic subdural collection (hygroma) may accumulate, usually in a middle cranial fossa (Fig. 4–60; Davidoff and Dyke, 1938; Robinson, 1964; Cronqvist and Efsing, 1970). The distinctive deformity of the skull produced by this collection is illustrated in Figure 1–37 and described on page 39. A rare lesion is the acute post-traumatic subdural hygroma (Winestock et al., 1975). These collections are said to develop following tearing of the arachnoid membrane, with unidirectional flow of cerebrospinal fluid into the subdural space. They have the angiographic appear-

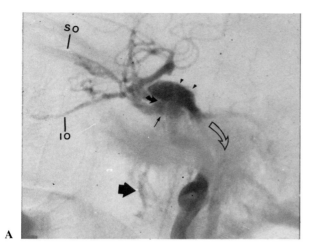

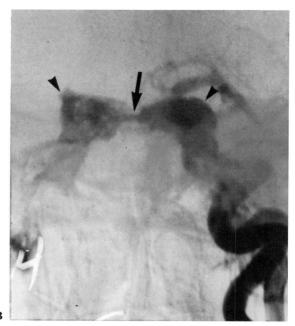

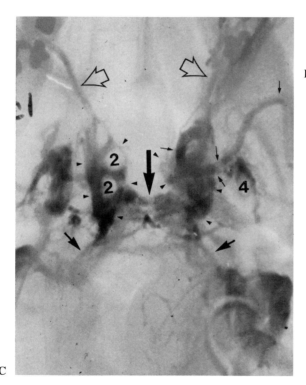

Fig. 4–38 Carotid-cavernous fistula filling only via the internal carotid artery. (A and B) Selective injection into the left internal carotid artery with excellent filling of the cavernous portion *(small arrow)* opacifies the fistula superiorly *(solid curved arrow)* early in the arterial phase. The following structures are visualized: cavernous sinus *(small arrowheads)*, superior ophthalmic vein (SO), inferior ophthalmic vein (IO), pterygoid venous plexus *(large arrow)* and the internal jugular vein *(curved open arrow)* filling via the superior petrosal sinus. The frontal projection shows a well-opacified cavernous sinus *(left arrowhead)* with drainage across the midline via the circular sinus *(arrow)* into the right cavernous sinus *(right arrowhead)*. (C) Full-axial projection of the same angiogram demonstrates the venous anatomy to advantage. The cavernous part of the left internal carotid and the middle cerebral arteries are visualized *(small black arrows)* with the left cavernous sinus superimposed *(small black arrowheads)*. Venous discharge from the left cavernous sinus takes place across the midline via the circular sinus *(large black arrow)* to the right cavernous sinus *(small black arrowheads)*. Two negative shadows within the opacified right cavernous sinus *(each marked 2)* represent the two loops of the cavernous part of the internal carotid artery. Venous discharge from the cavernous sinuses occurs backward through the superior petrosal sinus *(medium black arrows)* to the jugular veins; outward and downward to the pterygoid venous plexus *(marked 4 on the left)* and forwards via the ophthalmic veins *(open arrows)*.

ances of acute subdural hematomas, but appear hypodense on computed tomography.

Vasoconstriction of the basal and peripheral vessels may be seen in proximity to an extracerebral collection, because of the sensitivity of the intracranial circulation to the presence of subarachnoid blood (Fig. 4–52). False, i.e., post-traumatic aneurysms of the internal carotid tree (see p. 173) and other intrinsic vascular causes of subarachnoid hemorrhage should be sought and identified, since treatment in such cases by simple burrhole evacuation of the hematoma will prove inadequate.

Extracerebral collections simulating subdural hematomas, so-called pseudosubdural hematomas, are listed in Table 4–6 (Bergström and Lodin, 1967; Ferris et al., 1967). One such lesion is the hemispherical atrophy and thickened dural membrane of encephalotrigeminal angiomatosis (Sturge-Weber's syndrome; Fig. 4–61).

3. Cerebral Contusion and Hematoma. The commonest intracranial lesion observed after head trauma is cerebral contusion. Any severe head injury produces movement of the brain within the cranial cavity. In addition to the violent impact and com-

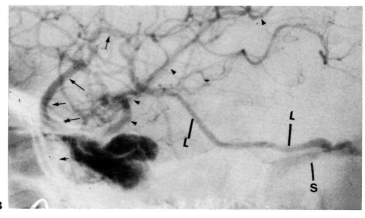

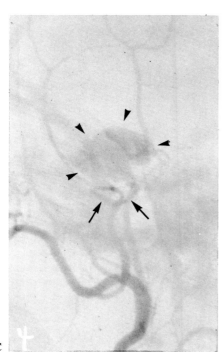

Fig. 4–39 Carotid-cavernous fistula filling from both internal and external carotid arteries. (A and B) Internal carotid angiogram showing the fistula between the cavernous part of the internal carotid artery *(arrow)* and the cavernous sinus *(arrowheads)*. In the late arterial phase, the cavernous sinus opacifies densely and venous drainage occurs via the superficial sylvian vein *(arrows)* and the vein of Labbé (L) into the lateral sinus (S). The arrowheads identify the middle cerebral artery. (C) Ipsilateral external carotid angiogram. The middle meningeal artery *(arrows)* fills the cavernous sinus *(arrowheads)* via the artery of the inferior cavernous sinus.

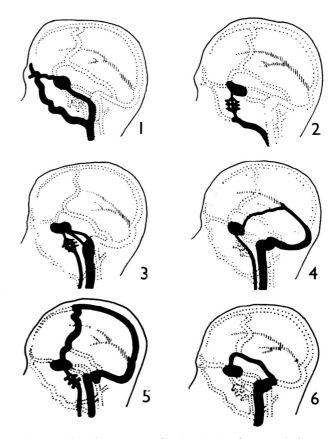

Table 4–5 Routes of Venous Discharge in Carotid-Cavernous Fistula (see Fig. 4–40; Biolcati and Barisini, 1966)

1. Cavernous sinus—superior ophthalmic vein—facial vein—internal jugular vein
2. Cavernous sinus—inferior ophthalmic vein—pterygoid venous plexus—internal jugular vein
3. Cavernous sinus—basilar venous plexus—superior petrosal sinuses—sigmoid sinuses—internal jugular vein
4. Cavernous sinus—basal vein of Rosenthal—vein of Galen—straight sinus—internal jugular vein
5. Cavernous sinus—sylvian veins, vein of Trolard—superior sagittal sinus—transverse sinus—internal jugular vein
6. Cavernous sinus—sylvian veins—vein of Labbé—transverse sinus—internal jugular vein
7. A combination of more than one of the above
8. From one cavernous sinus to the other through the circular sinuses, and a combination of more than one of the above

Fig. 4–40 Carotid-cavernous fistula. Routes of venous drainage according to Biolcati and Barisini (1966). See Table 4–5 for anatomical details.

Table 4–6 Angiographic Differential Diagnosis of Subdural Hematoma (after Ferris et al., 1967)

Epidural hematoma
Subdural hygroma
Temporal contusion
Tuberculoma
Cortical atrophy
Occlusion of the middle cerebral artery
"Cortical steal"
Subdural empyema
Meningeal neoplasms
  Avascular meningioma
  Meningeal carcinomatosis, lymphoma (including Hodgkin's disease), leukemia, sarcoma
  Meningeal melanoma
Subdural invasion by glioma
Meningeal thickening
  Traumatic
  Inflammatory, including syphilitic meningitis
Neoplasms of bone infiltrating the dura
  Epidermoids
  Reticulosis
  Sarcomas and metastatic carcinoma of the calvarium

pression against adjacent bony structures, acceleration and deceleration of the brain occurs, with an implosion within it due to transmitted vector of force. The resulting trauma patterns depend on the degree of force and its effect on the brain cells. Extracellular fluid (edema) may accumulate in a focal, multifocal or diffuse pattern. If in addition there are petechial hemorrhages or small hemorrhagic areas, a cerebral contusion is present. Such contusions are usually multiple and when found at the poles of the frontal, temporal and occipital lobes, represent contre-coup lesions.

Intracerebral hematomas also are common following head injury, they can be demonstrated by computed tomography in about 25 percent of severe cases (Koo and LaRoque, 1977). While computed tomography can distinguish easily between hematoma, contusion and hemorrhagic contusion, angiographic differentiation between these traumatic entities is always difficult and it may be impossible—notably between polar contusion and extracerebral collections. Cerebral edema may be recognisable when confined to a solitary focus and distinguishable from a hematoma because the vascular changes are usually diffuse or regional in distribution, Columella et al., 1963; Leeds et al., 1966). Without supporting evidence of arterial rupture, e.g., extravasated contrast medium (Fig. 4–42) or segmental vasoconstriction due to spasm

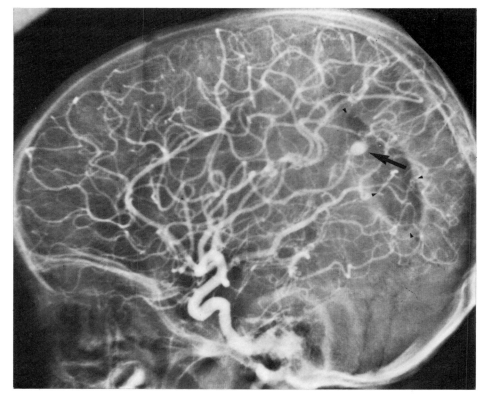

Fig. 4–41 False-aneurysm and "growing skull fracture" in a 9-year-old child. An aneurysm is present on a peripheral branch of the middle cerebral artery *(arrow)*, at the margin of a leptomeningeal cyst *(arrowheads)*. The proximity of the fracture to the aneurysm suggests a direct relationship. This case was described and illustrated by L. Rothman et al. in Pediatrics, *57,* 26–31, 1976; copyright American Academy of Pediatrics 1979.

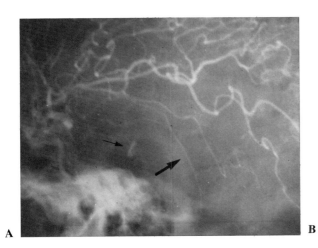

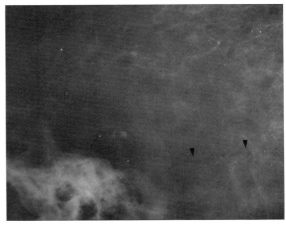

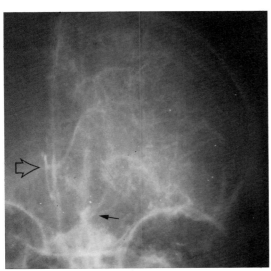

Fig. 4–42 Severe head injury with leakage of contrast medium into the contused brain. (A and B) Lateral views show an irregular collection of contrast medium in the middle of the temporal lobe *(small arrow)*. The sylvian branches of the middle cerebral artery are "draped" *(large arrow)*, indicating a mass within the temporal lobe. A fracture of the temporal bone is visible *(arrowheads)*. The collection of contrast medium persists during the intermediate phase. (C) Frontal view, venous phase, showing contralateral displacement of the internal cerebral vein *(open arrow)*. The collection of contrast medium is visible in the medial part of the temporal lobe *(small arrow)*.

(Fig. 4–52), there is no angiographic feature to distinguish an intracerebral hematoma from any other focal mass (Fig. 4–62).

Extracerebral collections in the temporal fossa may sometimes be excluded by utilizing the full-axial projection, which reveals sylvian branches reaching the inner table of the skull in temporal-pole lesions (Fig. 4–63; Glickman et al., 1971).

SCINTIGRAPHY

Static radionuclide imaging of the brain remains a useful examination in patients suspected of a chronic subdural hematoma. However, in the acute situation cerebral angiography is the alternative to computed tomography, and radionuclide imaging fails to be satisfactory for two reasons, viz., it does not provide the information required for surgical management, and there are too many false-negative results.

Subdural Hematoma

A peripheral crescentic rim of increased radioactivity, demonstrated in the anterior, posterior or vertex views, is usually a chronic subdural hematoma (Fig. 4–64). However, it is by no means specific of this entity, and a variety of other lesions may present a similar scintigraphic appearance: scalp trauma and infection, surgical defects, neoplastic infiltration or Paget's disease of the skull vault, epidural or subdural empyema, and cortical infarction or metastases (Williams and Beiler, 1966). In the frontal view a zone of high radioactivity between the hematoma and the compressed brain — the socalled "rim sign" — may impart some specificity in chronic subdural hematomas. This sign according to Penning and Front (1975), is due to crowding of the cortical vessels.

Various series indicate a diagnostic accuracy of 70 to 80 percent, both false-negative and false-positive interpretation being responsible for the error. There is some evidence that only subdural hematomas more than 1 cm. in thickness will be visible; that lesions older than 10 days are more likely to be seen than acute hematomas; and that delayed scanning and other technical considerations are important (Cowan et al., 1970; Apfelbaum et al., 1973; Gilday et al., 1973).

Cerebral Contusion and Infarction

Focal damage as a result of a direct blow, contre-coup injuries and infarction secondary to arterial

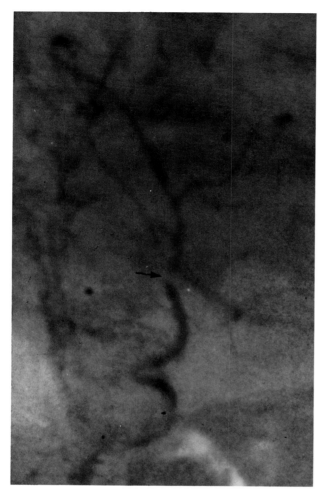

Fig. 4–43 A patient with severe scalp injury in whom there was delayed filling and emptying of the superficial temporal artery. In the intermediate phase shown here, segmental stenosis of the artery is present, indicating arterial damage *(arrow)*.

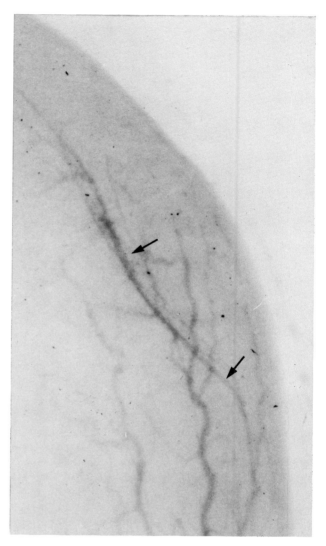

Fig. 4–44 Epidural hematoma, outlined by a medially displaced middle meningeal artery. The hematoma has the typical lentiform medial border of an epidural hematoma *(arrows)*. (See Fig. 4–18.)

occlusion is demonstrable scintigraphically (Fig. 4–65), but external lesions of the skull and scalp may be impossible to differentiate.

Radiography of the skull should always be viewed as an integral part of the scintigraphic examination of the brain. In doubtful cases the presence of a fracture and/or lateral displacement of the pineal gland may be decisive.

Cerebrospinal Fluid Rhinorrhea

Fractures through the floors of the anterior or middle cranial fossae in which the dura and arachnoid are torn may be complicated by leakage of cerebrospinal fluid in about 2 percent of head-injured patients. Up to one-quarter of such cases become infected (meningitis), and in another 20 percent gas can be demonstrated radiologically within the skull. The site of the leak may be demonstrable by in-

trathecally injected radionuclide such as RIHSA (radioiodinated human serum albumin), which accumulates selectively around it (Fig. 4–66). Such activity may be encountered in patients submitted immediately after a head injury to this examination, due to leakage of radionuclide-containing cerebrospinal fluid into the soft tissues of the face; and in more chronic cases a similar appearance may be given by a leptomeningeal or porencephalic cyst at the pole of the frontal lobe (Penning and Front, 1975). CSF cisternography may also prove helpful.

Hydrocephalus and Other Abnormalities of Flow and Absorption of Cerebrospinal Fluid

See Chapter 10.

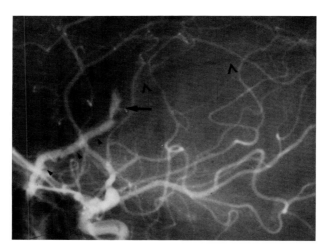

Fig. 4–45 Fracture, epidural hematoma and traumatic fistula. Contrast medium outlines the middle meningeal artery *(arrow)* and fills the meningeal vein *(arrowhead)*, which runs parallel to it. Open arrowheads point to the fracture of the overlying vault.

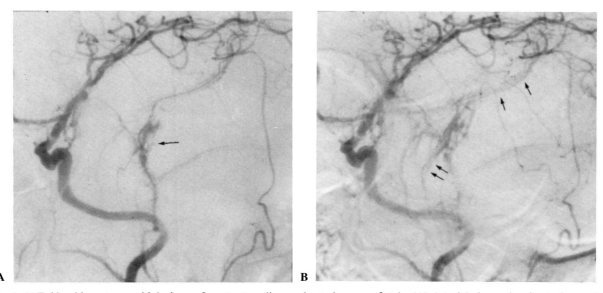

A   B

Fig. 4–46 Epidural hematoma with leakage of contrast medium and arteriovenous fistula. (A) Arterial phase, showing leakage of contrast medium around the middle meningeal artery *(arrow)*. (B) Two seconds later, filling of meningeal veins is visible, i.e., an arteriovenous fistula *(arrows)*.

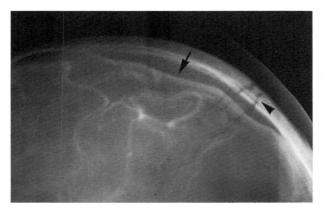

Fig. 4–47 Epidural hematoma displacing the superior sagittal sinus. A fracture of the parietal bone is present *(arrowhead)*, and beneath it an epidural collection which displaces the sinus from the inner table of the vault *(arrow)*.

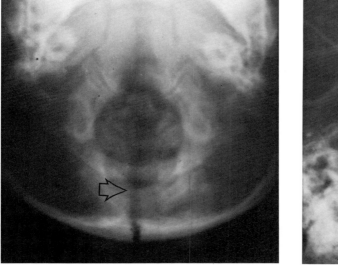

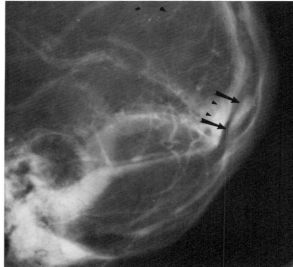

Fig. 4–48 Fracture of the base of the skull with torn torcular. A diastatic fracture of the occipital bone is present in the midline *(open arrow)*. (B) The superior sagittal sinus is displaced from the inner table by a localized epidural collection *(arrows)*, as a result of tearing of the torcular herophili *(arrowheads)*.

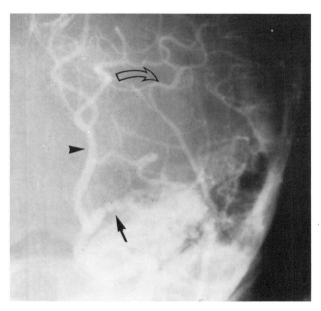

Fig. 4–49 Dissecting aneurysm of the middle cerebral artery. The proximal part of the artery is corrugated (large arrow) and the sylvian branches opacify poorly. The posterior cerebral artery is well filled *(arrowhead)* and compensatory leptomeningeal collateral channels deliver blood from it to the deprived middle cerebral territory *(open curved arrows)*.

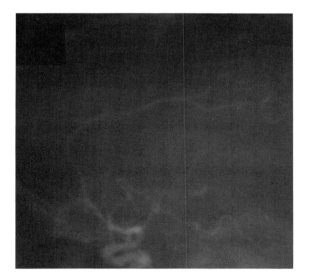
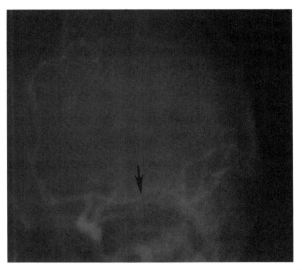

Fig. 4–50 Fat emboli occluding the middle cerebral artery, with cerebral infarction, in a 25-year-old man with fracture of a femur, who became suddenly aphasic and hemiplegic. The arrow points to the site of occlusion of the arterial trunk; several small branches remain patent. Falcine herniation in the presence of a major-artery occlusion indicates an infarcted hemisphere.

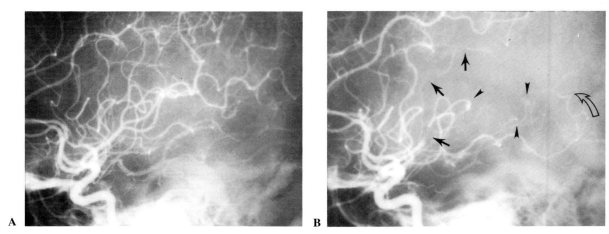

Fig. 4–51 Post-traumatic hemiplegia due to microembolism, caused by damage to the internal carotid artery in the neck, in a 25-year-old girl injured in an automobile accident. (A) Initial examination, normal appearances. (B) repeat examination one week later, after onset of weakness, reveals multiple occlusions *(arrowheads)*, arterial irregularity *(arrows)* and collateral channels *(open arrows)*.

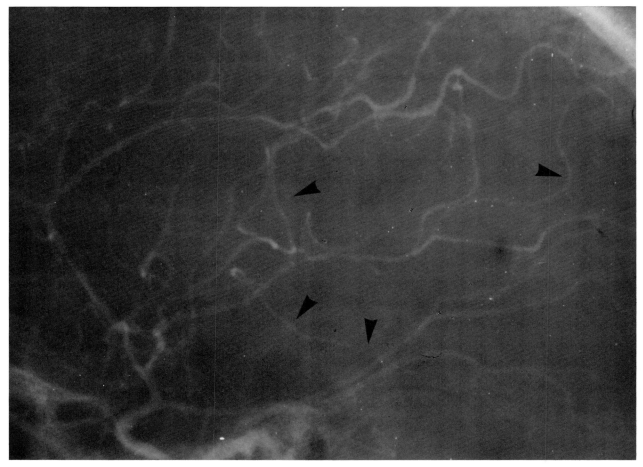

Fig. 4–52 Vasospasm accompanying intracerebral hemorrhage. A large avascular mass is present, displacing the parietotemporal part of the hemisphere *(arrowheads)*. The siphon and proximal branches of the internal carotid artery show marked spasm, which can be appreciated by comparison with the caliber of the convexity vessels.

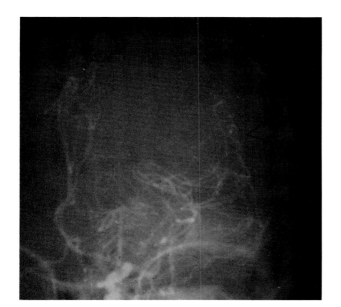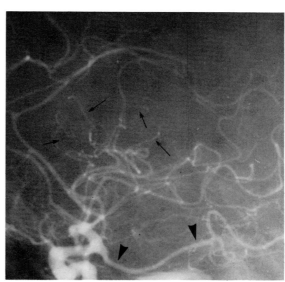

Fig. 4–53 Vasospasm associated with an extracerebral collection. A subdural hematoma is present *(open arrow)*. The carotid angiogram demonstrates irregularity and constriction of branches of the middle cerebral artery *(small arrows)*, with consequent reduced flow through the middle cerebral territory, compared to the anterior cerebral territory. Downward and medial displacement of the posterior communicating artery indicates incisural herniation *(arrowheads)*.

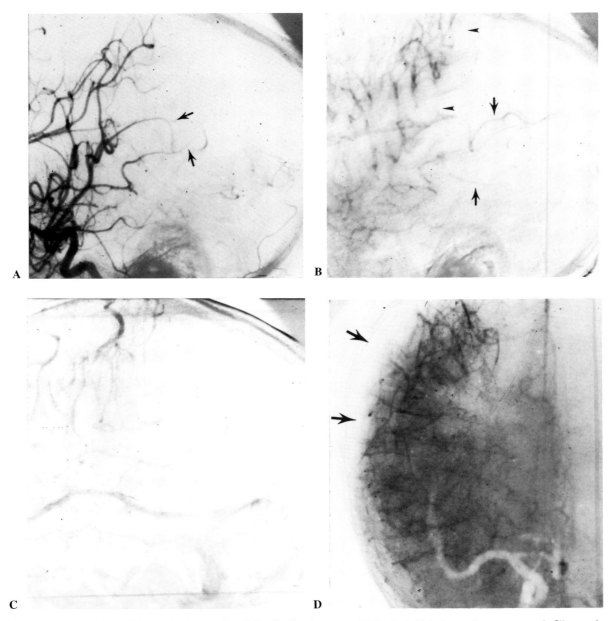

Fig. 4–54 A child with multiple cerebral contusions following head trauma. (A) In the initial phase, almost no vessels fill over the posterior third of the hemisphere. Distal branches of the middle cerebral artery in this region fill slowly and appear thinned and stretched *(arrows)*. (B) Two seconds later, the intermediate phase shows a zone of hyperperfusion blush *(arrowheads)* in the circulation adjoining the avascular zone. The branches of the middle cerebral artery within the damaged parietal lobe show delayed filling *(arrows)*. (C) In the venous phase, the relative avascularity persists. There is a profusion of cortical veins on the cortex anterior to the avascular zone. (D) Frontal view, intermediate phase, shows a lack of filling of surface branches of the middle cerebral artery *(arrows)*, simulating a subdural collection. (See Table 4–6.)

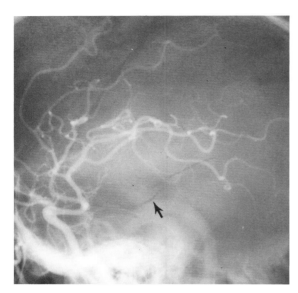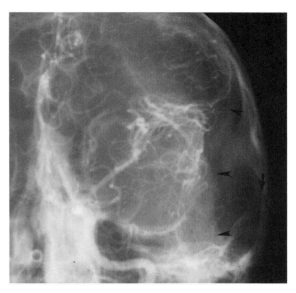

Fig. 4–55 Subtemporal epidural hematoma with fracture in a 19-year-old youth who had crashed his motorcycle 20 hours previously. The trunk and sylvian branches of the middle cerebral artery are elevated and the anterior cerebral artery is contralaterally displaced by a lentiform extracerebral collection *(arrowheads)*. The fracture *(arrow)* could be lateralized only in the perorbital projection; none of the other frontal views showed it.

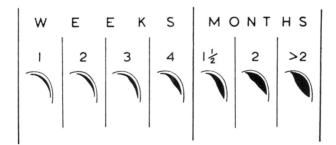

Fig. 4–56 The relationship of a subdural hematoma to its duration (after Norman, 1956). The acute hematoma follows the line of the skull in a crescentic shape since the hemisphere floats in the blood. The chronic subdural hematoma is more confined and expands into a lentiform shape thus resembling an epidural hematoma.

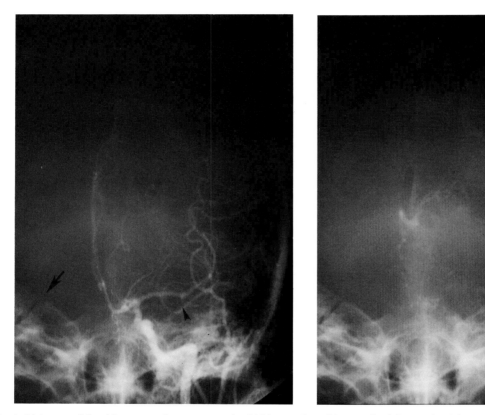

Fig. 4–57 Acute subdural hematoma in a man examined 15 hours after a blow on the right temple. A layer of liquid blood 1 cm. in thickness separates the cortical arteries and veins from the inner table of the vault *(open arrows)*, and the middle cerebral arteries are elevated indicating a subtemporal extension *(arrowhead)*. Uniform displacement of the midline structures (anterior cerebral artery and deep veins) reflects the diffuse nature of the space-occupying lesion. The black arrow points to a fracture of the right petrous pyramid — indicating the contre-coup nature of the injury.

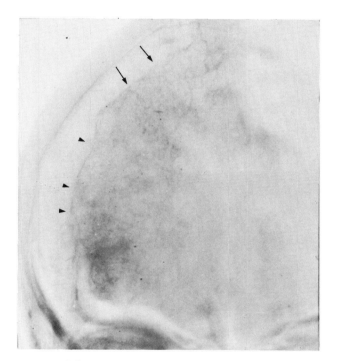

Fig. 4–58 Subacute subdural collection. This case is an example of the mixed type, lentiform above *(arrows)* and crescentic below *(arrowheads)* and separated by an irregular outline. This mixed pattern is unlikely in the acute phase.

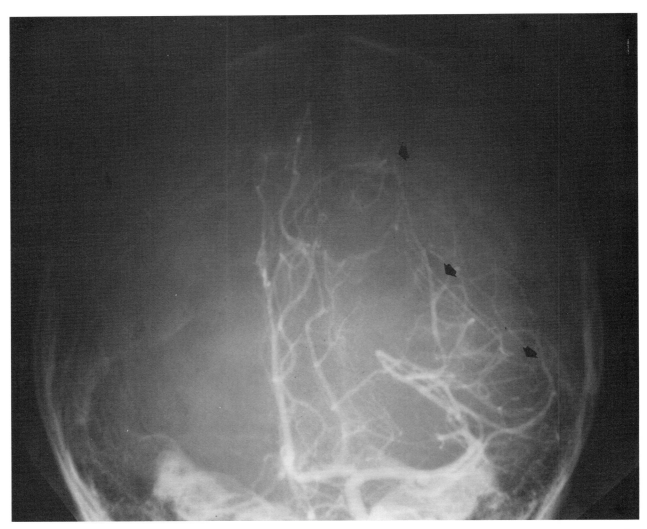

Fig. 4–59 Chronic subdural hematoma. A lentiform avascular mass displaces the hemisphere from the inner table *(arrows)*, producing medial dislocation of the angiographic U-loop and subfalcine herniation. The patient had fallen downstairs five weeks previously, injuring his head.

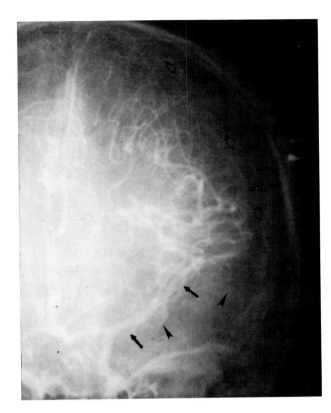

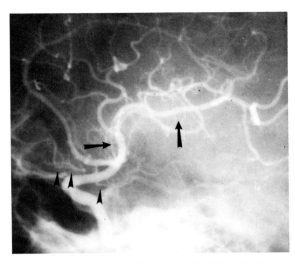

Fig. 4−60 Temporal subdural hygroma of childhood. The trunk and sylvian branches of the middle cerebral artery are elevated (*arrows*). The arrowheads point to elevated anterior temporal branches which, together with the "naked" appearance of the artery in the lateral view, indicate the presence of an extracerebral mass in the temporal fossa. As a rule, temporal hygromas displace the midline structures only slightly, due to bulging of the middle cranial fossa (see Fig. 1−37). In this patient, a 21-year old man, the hygroma was a chance finding. He had been injured 3 days previously in a traffic accident and the acute convexity hematoma (*open arrows*) accounted for the contralateral displacement of the anterior cerebral artery.

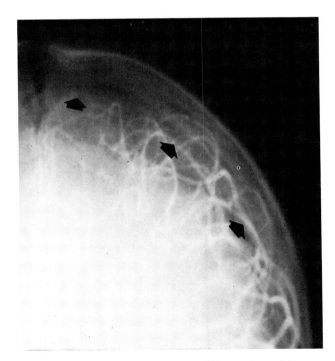

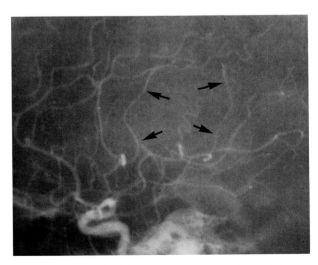

Fig. 4−61 "Pseudo-subdural hematoma" in a patient with encephalotrigeminal angiomatosis (Sturge-Weber's syndrome), in whom a combination of thickened meninges and cortical atrophy simulated an extracerebral collection (*arrows*).

Fig. 4−62 Intracerebral hematoma. An avascular posterior suprasylvian mass is outlined by displaced cortical vessels (*arrows*) and a depressed sylvian triangle. There is no angiographic clue to the nature of the mass.

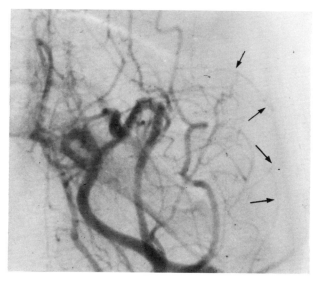

Fig. 4–63 Temporal contusion. Carotid angiography using routine projections in this patient indicated the presence of a temporal mass. But is it intracerebral (contusion) or extracerebral (subdural hematoma)? The submentovertical projection shows stretched temporal branches reaching the inner table of the skull *(arrows)*, confirming the presence of a contusion.

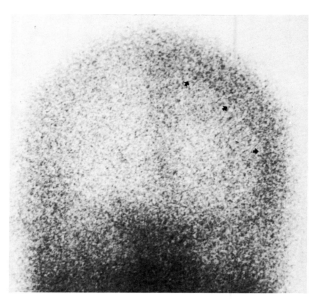

Fig. 4–64 Chronic subdural hematoma *(arrows)* shown by static scintigraphic imaging using radiopertechnetate. For the differential diagnosis of a peripheral crescentic pattern of radioactivity, see page 260.

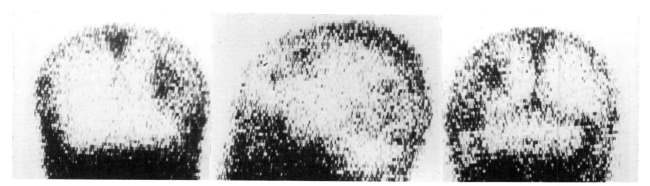

Fig. 4–65 Multiple cerebral contusions in an acutely head-injured subject. (Reproduced by kind permission by Dr. M. Maisey, Guy's Hospital, London.)

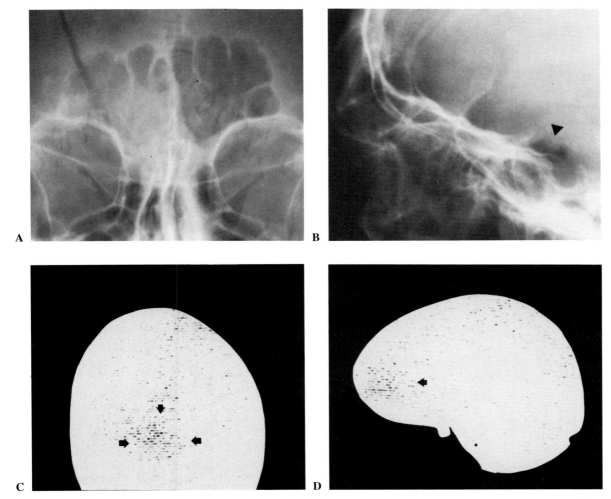

Fig. 4–66 Penetrating frontoethmoidal fracture causing delayed leakage of cerebrospinal fluid. A 20-year-old man returned 3 months after an automobile accident, complaining of rhinorrhea, and subsequently he developed a meningitis. (A and B) Initial examination of the skull revealed the fracture of the frontal squame and a right frontal sinus filled with blood. A suprasellar aerocele *(arrowhead)* in the lateral view indicates that a dural tear is present. (C and D) Radiocisternography reveals the site of leakage *(arrows)* to be in the vicinity of the fracture and not through the sphenoidal sinus.

REFERENCES

Acosta, C. Williams, P. E. Jr. and Clark, K.: Traumatic aneurysms of the cerebral vessels. Journal of Neurosurgery, *36*, 531–536, 1972.

Ambrose, J. Gooding, M. R. and Uttley, D.: E.M.I. scan in the management of head injuries. The Lancet, *1*, 847–848, 1976.

Andrew, W. K.: The soft tissue sign: A new parameter in the diagnosis of the fracture of the base of the skull. Clinical Radiology, *29*, 443–446, 1978.

Apfelbaum, R. I., Newman, S. and Zingesser, L. H.: Dynamics of technetium scanning of subdural hematomas. Radiology, *107*, 571–576, 1973.

Benoit, B. and Wortzman, G.: Traumatic cerebral aneurysms: Clinical features and natural history. Journal of Neurology, Neurosurgery and Psychiatry, *36*, 127–138, 1973.

Bergan, F.: Traumatic intimal rupture of the popli·
with acute ischaemia of the limb in cases with supracondylar fracture of the femur. Journal of Cardiovascular Surgery, *4*, 300–302, 1963.

Berger, P. E., Harwood-Nash, D. C. and Fitz, C. R.: Computer-

ized tomography: Abnormal intracerebral collections of blood in children. Neuroradiology, *11*, 29–33, 1976.

Bergström, K. and Lodin, H.: An angiographic observation in intracerebral haematoma. British Journal of Radiology, *40*, 228–229, 1967.

Biolcati, A. and Barisoni, D.: Considerazioni sull'evoluzione di una fistola carotido-cavernosa. Quaderni di Radiologia, *31*, 643–662, 1966.

Brown, O. L. and Armitage, J. L.: Spontaneous dissecting aneurysms of the cervical internal carotid artery. American Journal of Roentgenology, *118*, 648–653, 1973.

Chou, S. N. and French, L. A.: Arteriovenous fistula of vertebral vessels in the neck. Journal of Neurosurgery, *22*, 77–80, 1965.

Clemens, F. and Lodin, H.: Some viewpoints in the venous outflow pathways in cavernous sinus fistulas. Clinical Radiology, *19*, 196–200, 1968–A.

Clemens, F. and Lodin, H.: Non-traumatic external carotid-cavernous sinus fistula. Clinical Radiology, *19*, 201–203, 1968B.

Columella, F., Delzanno, G. B., Gaist, G. and Piazza, G.: Angiography in traumatic cerebral lacerations with special regard to some less common aspects. Acta Radiologica Diagnosis, 1, 239–247, 1963.

Columella, F., Gaist, G., Piazza, G. and Caraffa, T.: Extradural haematoma at the vertex. Journal of Neurology, Neurosurgery and Psychiatry, 31, 315–320, 1968.

Cowan, R. J., Maynard, C. D. and Lassiter, K. R.: Technetium 99^m pertechnetate brain scans in the detection of subdural hematomas: A study of the age of the lesion as related to the development of a positive scan. Journal of Neurosurgery, 32, 30–34, 1970.

Cronqvist, S. and Efsing, H. O.: Roentgendiagnosis of subdural hygroma in infants. Neuroradiology, 1, 61–67, 1970.

Cronqvist, S. and Köhler, R.: Angiography in epidural haematomas. Acta Radiologica Diagnosis, 1, 42–52, 1963.

Davidoff, L. M. and Dyke, C. G.: Relapsing juvenile chronic subdural hematoma and a clinical and roentgenographic study. Bulletin of the Neurological Institute of New York, 7, 95–111, 1938.

Davidson, K. C., Weiford, E. C. and Dixon, G. D.: Traumatic vertebral artery pseudoaneurysm following chiropractic manipulation. Radiology, 115, 651–652, 1975.

Davis, K. R., Taveras, J. M., Roberson, G. H., Ackerman, R. H. and Dreisbach, J. N.: Computed tomography in head trauma. Seminars in Roentgenology, 12, 53–62, 1977.

Debrun, G., Lacour, P., and Caron, J. P.: Treatment of arteriovenous fistulas and aneurysms with an inflatable released balloon. Experimental work – application in man. In Salamon, G., Ed.: Advances in Cerebral Angiography. Berlin: Springer, 1975.

Dolinskas, C. A., Zimmerman, R. A. and Bilaniuk, L. T.: A sign of subarachnoid bleeding on cranial computed tomograms of pediatric head trauma patients. Radiology, 126, 409–412, 1978.

Dublin, A. B., French, B. N. and Rennick, J. M.: Computed tomography in head trauma. Radiology, 122, 365–369, 1977.

Ferris, E. J., Lehrer, H. and Shapiro, J. H.: Pseudo-subdural hematoma. Radiology, 88, 75–84, 1967.

Friedenberg, M. J., Lake, P. and Landau, S.: Bilateral incomplete traumatic occlusion of internal carotid arteries. American Journal of Roentgenology, 118, 546–549, 1973.

Freidenfelt, H. and Sunström, R.: Local and general spasm in the internal carotid system following trauma. Acta Radiologica Diagnosis, 1, 278–283, 1963.

Gabrielsen, T. O. and Seeger, J. F.: Radiodiagnosis of brain injury. In Vinken, P. J. and Bruyn, G. W. Eds.: Handbook of Clinical Neurology, 23, 239–253, 1975.

Gilday, D. L., Coates, G. and Goldenberg, D.: Subdural hematoma — what is the role of brain scanning in its diagnosis? Journal of Nuclear Medicine, 14, 283–287, 1973.

Gilday, D. L., Wortzman, G. and Reid, M.: Subdural hematoma: Is it or is it not acute? Radiology, 110, 141–145, 1974.

Glickman, M. G., Gletne, J. S. and Mainzer, F.: The basal projection in cerebral angiography. Radiology, 98, 611–618, 1971.

Glickman, M. G., Mandel, S. F., Hoff, J. T., and Coulson, W.: Cerebral cortical arteries in the diagnosis of epidural hematoma. Neuroradiology, 10, 187–195, 1976.

Gurdjian, E. S.: Spasm of the extracranial internal carotid artery resulting from blunt trauma demonstrated by angiography. Case report. Journal of Neurosurgery, 35, 742–747, 1971.

Handa, J., Shumizu, Y., Matsuda, M. and Handa, H.: Traumatic aneurysm of the middle cerebral artery. American Journal of Roentgenology, 109, 127–129, 1970.

Janon, E. A.: Traumatic changes in the internal carotid artery associated with basal skull fractures. Radiology, 96, 55–59, 1970.

Kernohan, J. W. and Woltman, H. W.: Incisura of the crus due to contralateral brain tumor. Archives of Neurology and Psychiatry, 21, 274–287, 1929.

Kimber, P. M.: Radiography of head injury patients. Radiography (London), 42, 173–175, 1976.

Koo, A. H. and LaRoque, R. L.: Evaluation of head trauma by computed tomography. Radiology, 123, 345–350, 1977.

Leeds, N. E., Reid, N. D. and Rosen, L. M.: Angiographic changes in cerebral contusions and intracerebral hematomas. Acta Radiologica, 5, 320–327, 1966.

Leeds, N. E., Shulman, K., Borns, P. F. and Hope, J. W.: The angiographic demonstration of a "brain stain" in infantile subdural hematoma. American Journal of Roentgenology, 104, 66–70, 1968.

Lewin, W.: Radiology in acute head injury. British Journal of Radiology, 39, 168–171, 1966.

Loar, C. R., Chadduck, W. M. and Nugent, G. R.: Traumatic occlusion of the middle cerebral artery. Journal of Neurosurgery, 39, 753–756, 1973.

Lukin, C. and Chambers, A.: Traumatic aneurysm of peripheral cerebral artery. Neuroradiology, 8, 1–3, 1974.

McDonald, E. J., Winestock, D. P. and Hoff, J. T.: The value of repeat cerebral arteriography in the evaluation of trauma. American Journal of Roentgenology, 126, 792–797, 1976.

Margolis, M. T., Stein, R. L. and Newton, T. H.: Extracranial aneurysms of the internal carotid artery. Neuroradiology, 4, 78–89, 1972.

May, B. R.: Radiological differentiation of extracerebral haematomas. British Journal of Radiology, 47, 742–746, 1974.

Merino-de Villasante, J. and Taveras, J. M.: Computerized tomography (CT) in acute head trauma. American Journal of Roentgenology, 126, 765–778, 1976.

Miller, J. D. R. and Ayers, T. N.: Post-traumatic changes in the internal carotid artery and its branches: An arteriographic study. Radiology, 89, 95–100, 1967.

Nelson, S. W. and Freimanis, A. K.: Angiographic features of convexity subdural hematomas with emphasis on the differential diagnosis between unilateral and bilateral hematomas. American Journal of Roentgenology, 90, 445–461, 1963.

New, P. F. J. and Momose, K. J.: Traumatic dissection of the internal carotid artery at the atlanto-axial level. Secondary to nonpenetrating injury. Radiology, 93, 41–49, 1969.

Norman, O.: Angiographic differentiation between acute and chronic subdural and extradural haematomas. Acta Radiologica, 46, 371–378, 1956.

Northcroft, G. B. and Morgan, A. D.: A fatal case of traumatic thrombosis of the internal carotid artery. British Journal of Surgery, 32, 105–107, 1944.

Penning, L. and Front, D.: Scintigraphy in brain injury. In Vinken, P. J. and Bruyn, G. W., Eds.: Handbook of Clinical Neurology, 23, 287–315, 1975.

Picard, I., Lepoire, J., Montaut, J., Hepner, H., Roland, J., Guyonnaud, J. C., Jacob, F. and André, J. M.: Endarterial occlusion of carotid-cavernous sinus fistulas using a balloon tipped catheter. Neuroradiology, 8, 5–10, 1974.

Radcliffe, W. B., Guinto, F. C. Jr., Adcock, D. F. and Krigman, M. R.: Subdural hematoma shape. A new look at an old concept. American Journal of Roentgenology, 115, 72–77, 1972.

Richardson, A.: Computerised transverse axial scanning in the management of head injured patients. In Vinken, P. J. and Bruyn, G. W., Eds.: Handbook of Clinical Neurology, 23, 255–264, 1975.

Robinson, A. E., Meares, B. M. and Goree, J. A.: Traumatic sphenoid sinus effusion. American Journal of Roentgenology, 101, 795–801, 1967.

Robinson, R. G.: The temporal lobe agenesis syndrome. Brain, 87, 87–106, 1964.

Rothman, L., Rose, J. S., Laster, D. W., Quencer, R. and Tenner, M.: The spectrum of growing skull fracture in children. Pediatrics, 57, 26–31, 1976.

Rudikoff, J. C., Ferris, E. J. and Shapiro, J . H.: Intracerebral vascular rupture. Radiology, 90, 288–291, 1968.

Rumbaugh, C. L., Bergeron, R. T. and Kurze, T.: Intracranial

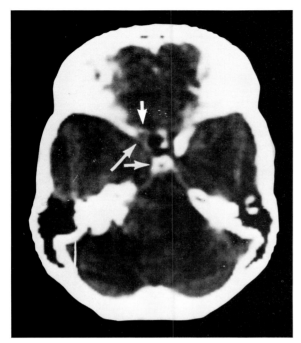

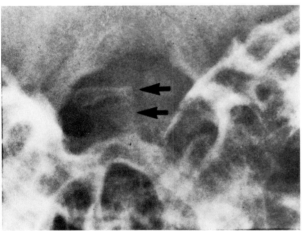

Fig. 5–2 Bone destruction in parasellar masses. Erosion of the left anterior and posterior clinoid processes and the left half of the sphenoid body and dorsum sellae *(arrows)* by a chondrosarcoma of the left temporal fossa (for enhanced computed tomogram of this patient, see Fig. 5–20).

cal methods exist of measuring the pituitary fossa, both in profile and volumetrically. The most logical profile measurements are: the widest anteroposterior diameter (measured parallel to a line between the nasion and tuberculum sellae) = 8 – 15 mm; and the greatest vertical diameter (drawn perpendicular to that line) = 6.5 – 12.5 mm (Joplin and Fraser, 1960). Sellar volume is given by the formula of Di Chiro and Nelson (1962), viz.:

$$\tfrac{1}{2}\,\text{length} \times \text{depth} \times \text{width} = 340 - 1092 \text{ mm}^3$$

Such wide variations largely negate the clinical value of these measurements, and the authors support the view expressed nearly 20 years ago by Mahmoud (1958) in his important monograph: "Measurement of the sella turcica is more of academic than clinical importance."

Cortical Lining: The sella turcica is lined by a single layer of cortical bone, often referred to as the "lamina dura of the pituitary fossa." After pineal identification, this lining is the most important feature for the radiologist to evaluate during skull interpretation, since its appearances may directly mirror the state of health of the intracranial compartment. In healthy adults the lamina dura is intact: a useful way of confirming this is to verify that it is *as dense as the roof of an orbit in lateral projection.* Cortical thinning or demineralization are early signs of raised intracranial pressure (see below), and this diagnosis can be made confidently in young or middle-aged individuals. Since the pituitary cortex loses calcium as part of the normal process of aging, the borderline between normal and early pathological change is impossible to define in elderly subjects and especially in postmenopausal women. Similar appearances are seen in a small proportion of arterial hypertensives and chronic alcoholics (Fry and Du Boulay, 1965; Albert and LeMay, 1968).

Raised Intracranial Pressure, Including "Pressure Sella"

Several specific deformities of the pituitary fossa accompany raised intracranial pressure (Fig. 5–3). El Gammal and his colleagues (Du Boulay and El Gammal, 1966; El Gammal and Allen, 1972a and 1972b) have shown that pressure erosion of the cortical lining is caused by subarachnoid cisterns that herniate into the pituitary fossa or, if hydrocephalus is present, by the dilated anterior end of the third ventricle.

The speed of onset of the raised intracranial pressure is probably responsible for the particular pattern of radiological abnormality. If the syndrome is *acute,* i.e., weeks or months, the following sellar changes are seen, irrespective of whether the third ventricle is dilated or normal: (1) The earliest perceptible change is erosion of the posterior part of the lamina dura, a sign which may precede clinical evidence of a raised intracranial pressure syndrome by several weeks. (2) Next the dorsum sellae decalcifies, and its cortical lining and the posterior clinoid processes become indistinct ("ghosted"). An important diagnostic feature, differentiating the "pressure sella" from sellar erosion due to an adjacent tumor, is the fact that the fossa *retains its normal size.* (3) Total disappearance of the lamina dura and the dorsum sellae, finally producing appearances indistinguishable from local tumor destruction.

If the intracranial pressure syndrome runs a *chronic* course, e.g., in nontumor hydrocephalus due to aqueduct stenosis or a phakomatosis or poly-

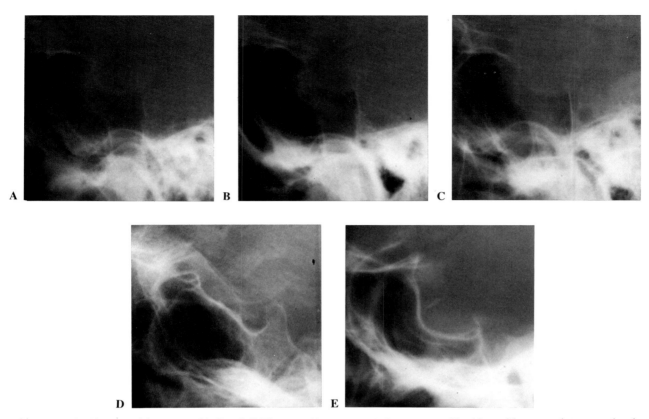

Fig. 5–3 Raised intracranial pressure. (A, B and C) The acute "pressure sella." A 50-year-old subject with metastatic cancer, showing progressive loss of the cortical lining over 4 months. (Below) Chronic hyperpressure states. (D) Typical flattened, well-corticated chiasmatic sulcus of low-grade hydrocephalus. (E) Characteristic sellar deformity of nontumor aqueduct stenosis. See Figure 5–43. (Lewtas, 1966; Du Boulay and Trickey, 1970).

saccharidosis: one of two deformities is found. The commonest is the typical pituitary shape seen in benign aqueduct stenosis, in which the superior surface of the sphenoid body is re-molded by the dilated fluid-filled cavities compressing it. The second is rare: the deep, thin-walled pituitary fossa, with changes so subtle as often to escape recognition.

Pituitary-Fossa and Adjacent Lesions (Fig. 5–5)

Intrasellar: Tumors confined wholly to the pituitary fossa are usually adenomas of the chromophobe or acidophil cells; about one-third of the latter are accompanied by signs of acromegaly. Both types of adenoma expand the fossa uniformly in all directions and erode its walls, producing a "balloon" or "cup-shaped" sella. These terms describe abnormally large fossae, in which the widest anteroposterior diameter lies, respectively, below or at the level of the diaphragma sellae. In the absence of acromegaly, there are no plain-film appearances which permit differentiation between eosinophil and chromophobe adenomas (Ross and Greitz, 1969). Unusual features in adenomas are a normal-sized pituitary fossa or amputation of the dorsum sellae.

Prolactin-secreting pituitary microadenomas may be responsible for the syndrome of amenorrhea or galactorrhea—a source of infertility (Vezina and Sutton, 1974). These adenomas may be too small to enlarge the pituitary fossa, but they can produce local thinning, erosions or bulging which may be detected only with multidirectional tomograms (Fig. 5–5; Robertson and Newton, 1978). Post-mortem studies have failed to show any convincing correlation between pituitary gland dimensions and radiographic sellar appearances (McLachlan et al., 1968).

Proven primary intrasellar masses other than chromophobe and acidophil adenomas are rare, e.g., aneurysm (Keller and Galatius-Jensen, 1975).

Suprasellar Midline: The commonest mass found in the suprasellar midline is a primary pituitary tumor that has grown upwards, funnelling the sella so that its widest anteroposterior diameter corresponds to the level of its diaphragm. An identical shape may be produced by a downward-growing craniopharyngioma, one of the two common primary suprasellar masses. The other is meningioma, which is far less likely to deform the pituitary fossa. Posterior-lying or large midline suprasellar tumors exert their pressure effects on the dorsum sellae: usually they erode it from above ("sawn-off" dorsum) but they may, by thinning its anterior walls,

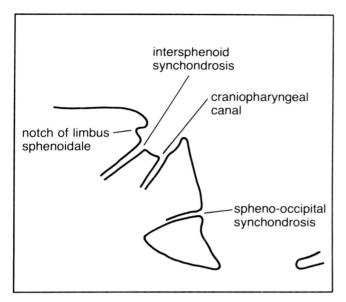

Fig. 5–4 The infantile sella. The intersphenoid synchondrosis separates the presphenoid and postsphenoid parts of the bone until ossification is complete in the third year of life. The craniopharyngeal canal may be confused with it. The spheno-occipital synchondrosis fuses by the twenty-fifth year. Both synchondroses tend to remain patent in chronic hydrocephalus. The notch caused by a non-ossified (cartilaginous) limbus sphenoidale must not be confused with the sclerotic margin of the normal optic canal or the J sella configuration (Shopfner et al., 1968).

actually elongate it ("high-riding" dorsum). Anterior-lying suprasellar tumors typically pressure-erode the chiasmatic sulcus without affecting the dorsum sellae. A statistic to remember: every fifth craniopharyngioma and every third suprasellar meningioma shows a normal pituitary fossa.

The J sella is an easily-recognizable deformity found in a large proportion of patients with optic gliomas or low-grade communicating hydrocephalus, especially dysostosis multiplex (Martin and Cushing, 1923; Burrows, 1964; Kier, 1969). It is produced by chronic molding of the superior surface of the sphenoid body by the optic pathway tumor or the dilated third ventricle. The J sella, while not pathognomonic of these conditions and liable to misinterpretation in infants (Fig. 5–4), is invaluable in differential diagnosis if properly defined, viz.: a forward extension of the pituitary fossa beyond the tuberculum sellae, the anterior compartment thus formed being as large as the fossa itself and sometimes possessing a cortical lining thicker than normal (Fig. 5–5).

Parasellar: Parasphenoid and other medial temporal masses may deform the pituitary fossa through asymmetrical erosion of the ipsilateral carotid sulcus. The true extent of this erosion is revealed by computed tomographic scanning and conventional tomography—it may not be visible on the lateral skull radiograph. A characteristic tomographic deformity of the sulcus, which may involve

the pituitary fossa itself, is produced by enlargement of the infraclinoid part of the internal carotid artery due to atherosclerotic ectasia, aneurysm or hypertrophy accompanying an arteriovenous malformation (Rådberg, 1963a; Anderson, 1976).

Retrosellar: Other than the changes of generalized raised intracranial pressure, no early abnormality of the pituitary fossa is seen in these lesions. Destructive tumors such as chordomas may sweep away the dorsum sellae and pituitary fossa in their path, if they grow forward.

Infrasellar: Nasopharyngeal carcinomas, sphenoid mucoceles and other processes involving the body of the sphenoid bone may alter the appearances of the fossa or destroy it. Osseous lesions such as fibrous dysplasia transform the texture of the sphenoid body and obliterate the sinus: the sellar lamina dura disappears and the outline of the fossa may be destroyed (Fig. 5–7).

CALCIFICATION

Physiological ligamentous calcification is discussed above.

The commonest pathological intracranial calcification are the curvilinear deposits of calcium in the carotid siphons of elderly atherosclerotic subjects. Typically they are concave to the skull base and overlie the pituitary fossa in lateral projection. Their juxtasellar position is best confirmed on the anteroposterior 20° view or by coronal tomograms, when they may appear as complete ring shadows.

Pituitary adenomas calcify only rarely. "Burnt-out" tumors may be responsible for intrasellar deposits ("pituitary calculi," Mascherpa and Valentino, 1959).

Three morphological types of suprasellar calcification occur (Fig. 5–6): (1) Curvilinear calcification in the wall of a cystic cavity, e.g., the outline of a partly thrombosed giant carotid aneurysm, cystic craniopharyngioma. Vascular curvilinear calcification has a peculiarly delicate appearance: the rings of Albl, so-called after the German physician who described them. (2) Granular deposits, often tightly packed—commonly in craniopharyngioma or meningioma. (3) Amorphous deposits in a variety of neoplastic or non-neoplastic conditions, including successful antituberculous treatment.

No histological diagnosis can ever be made on the basis of the morphological appearances of the calcium deposits alone, but the total radiological picture—sellar profile, type of calcification, and the nature of any adjacent bone changes—frequently narrows the possibilities to one or more specific entities. For example: granular deposits above a normal pituitary fossa in a middle-aged subject with visual deterioration prompts the diagnosis of meningioma, and the radiologist should search diligently

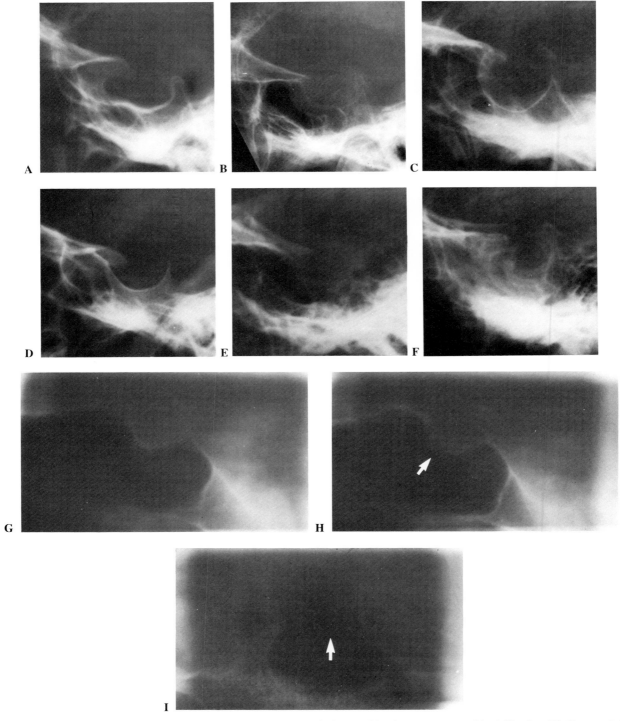

Fig. 5–5 The pituitary profile. (A) Optic glioma. (B) Parasellar meningioma, with atheromatous carotid calcification. (C) Chromophobe adenoma. (D) Craniopharyngioma. (E) End-stage acute raised intracranial pressure. (F) Postoperative pituitary adenoma following (transsphenoidal hypophysectomy (Rådberg, 1963b). (G, H, I) Patient with elevated prolactin and galactorrhea with normal-appearing sella turcica on plain radiographs, but complex-motion tomography demonstrates the presence of a pituitary microadenoma. (G) Section on the right is normal. (H) Section on the left demonstrates cortical thinning and bulging of the anterior inferior aspect of the sella *(arrow)* at the site of the microadenoma. (I) Coronal section shows tilting of the floor of the sella turcica with thinning on the left *(arrow)*.

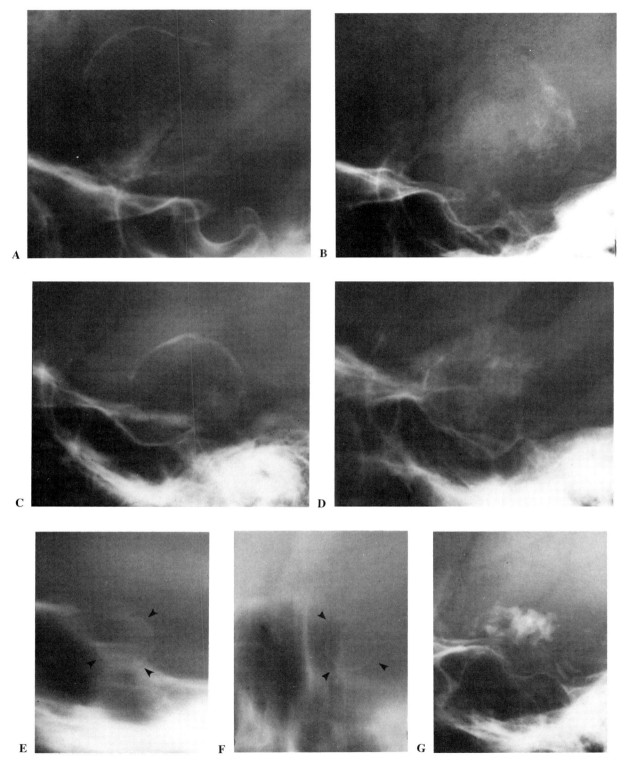

Fig. 5–6 Pathological calcification in the pituitary region. Curvilinear (A, C and E, F) and nodular (B, D and G) types. (A) Giant supra-clinoid aneurysm. (B) Hypothalamic glioma. (C) Cystic craniopharyngioma. (D) Craniopharyngioma. (E and F) Thrombosed infracli-noid aneurysm. (G) After tuberculous meningitis.

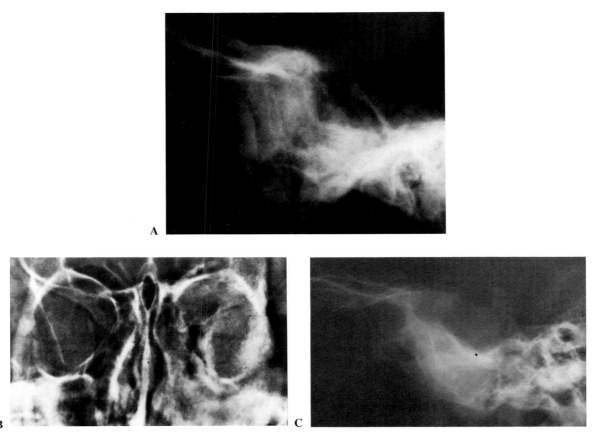

Fig. 5–7 Sphenoid sclerosis. *En plaque* lesions of the sphenoid bone deforming the pituitary fossa. (A and B) Sphenoid wing meningioma (postoperative growth). (C) Fibrous dysplasia of bone.

for focal bone changes to confirm it. Suprasellar calcification in a child is only rarely caused by any lesion other than craniopharyngioma. Calcified debris situated above, beside or behind the pituitary fossa and associated with bone destruction suggests chordoma.

ADJACENT BONE CHANGES

Two types of focal change occur, sclerosis or erosion, and the pattern is important because it possesses pathognomonic diagnostic value. Virtually only one tumor produces a well-defined area of sclerosis of the superior surface or wings of the sphenoid bone, namely meningioma. Meningioma hyperostosis may vary from a small nodule on the tuberculum sellae, planum sphenoidale, cribriform plate or an anterior clinoid process, to sclerosis of an entire lesser or greater sphenoid wing. A condition simulating meningioma hyperostosis is the *en plaque* type of fibrous dysplasia (Fig. 5–7, see also Fig. 1–29). Metastatic deposits may occasionally produce patchy sclerosis of a sphenoid wing (Fig. 1–60) or body (see Fig. 9–28). Sclerosis of

the body also accompanies mucoceles of the sphenoidal sinus and a small proportion of nasopharyngeal carcinomas.

Tumors of the skull base, sometimes indicated by widening of the nasopharyngeal soft tissues, may invade the sphenoid body or wings and destroy them. Parasellar masses such as giant infraclinoid aneurysms, chromophobe adenomas or trigeminal neuromas may pressure-erode the walls of a middle fossa and produce a characteristic pattern: destruction of the bony strut between the superior orbital fissure and the optic canal so that the two orifices communicate; sometimes destruction of the floor of the fossa; and asymmetrical erosion of the pituitary fossa producing a sloping sellar floor (Fig. 5–8). In infraclinoid aneurysms and rarely also in tumors, erosion of the optic strut may be the only plain-film abnormality (Rischbieth and Bull, 1958). Other parasellar masses may destroy a wider area of the sphenoid wing, including an anterior clinoid process. Such erosion may be difficult or impossible to identify on routine views of the skull, and special views or coronal or axial tomography is required (Fig. 5–2).

Optic Canals: Special projections of the optic

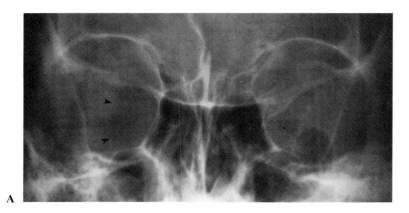

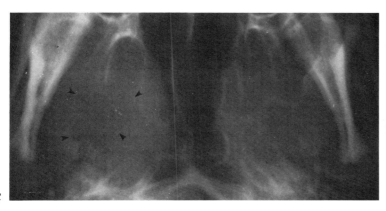

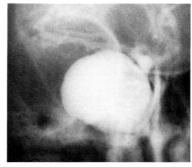

Fig. 5–8 Sphenoid destruction in parasellar masses. Giant infraclinoid aneurysm of the right carotid artery eroding the superior orbital fissure (*arrowheads*, A) and the floor of the right temporal fossa (*arrowheads*, C).

canals are an integral part of the plain-film examination of any patient with visual failure or upper cranial nerve involvement (anosmia, ptosis, proptosis or unilateral ophthalmoplegia) in whom a pituitary mass is suspected. Alone of all the plain films, the optic nerve views may yield the diagnosis (Fig. 5 – 9).

Optic gliomas in children usually enlarge one optic canal which, in the absence of sellar deformity, is the only abnormality present. Asymmetrically enlarged optic canal with a well-preserved corticated lining has virtually one cause only, viz., optic nerve glioma. Sometimes the optic canal may show irregular enlargement as part of the general orbital hypertrophy of neurofibromotosis, in the absence of a tumor of the optic nerve. Rarely, orbital neurofibromas or retinoblastomas growing inward, and suprasellar cholesteatomas growing outward, may enlarge one optic canal (Evans et al., 1963). Bilaterally enlarged canals are pathognomonic of glioma of the anterior optic pathway. Perioptic meningiomas seldom enlarge the canal, instead the enostosis deforms a segment of its bony wall and constricts it. A constricting effect is also produced by fibrous dysplasia and other rare bone dysostoses such as osteopetrosis involving a sphenoid wing. Enucleation at an early age for trauma or tumor stunts orbital growth, and the optic canal may be half the adult diameter.

Erosion of the inferolateral segment of the canal margin, i.e., the strut between the optic canal and the superior orbital fissure, is a common feature of parasellar masses such as giant infraclinoid aneurysm (invariably), chromophobe adenoma (25%) and chordoma; it is rare in craniopharyngioma. Sphenoid neoplasms and granulomas may erode the inferomedial segment. Loss of definition of the cortical margins of both canals is a pathognomonic and an invariable feature of chronic generalized raised intracranial pressure — analagous to the "pressure sella." The canals are usually not enlarged and, if the high pressure is relieved, their appearances return to normal. Complete disappearance of an optic canal accompanies destruction of the lesser sphenoid wing by invasive or erosive tumor such as histiocytosis-X, lytic metastases, chromophobe adenoma and neoplasms of the skull base.

Orbitocranial Asymmetry: A variety of unrelated conditions may deform or erode the bony orbit and adjacent cranium, producing remarkably uniform clinical pictures, yet producing radiological features which may be distinctive (Table 5 – 1). A deformed orbital rim that is smaller than normal invariably follows enucleation of the eyeball in early life, producing an obvious asymmetry. Processes involving the adjacent skeleton may also reduce the diameter of the rim by deforming it, e.g., fibrous dysplasia of bone, frontal chronic subdural hygroma, giant os-

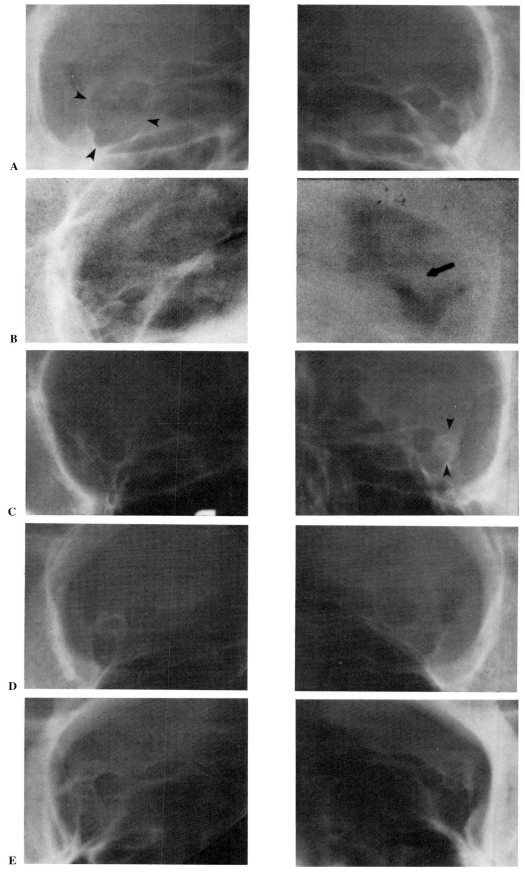

Fig. 5–9 Optic canal involvement. (A) Right parasellar lesion (chromophobe adenoma). (B) Fibrous dysplasia of bone narrowing the left optic canal *(arrow)*. (C) Left perioptic meningioma *(arrowhead)*. (D) Chiasmal glioma involving left optic nerve. (E) Atrophy of the left optic nerve following childhood enucleation for a penetrating injury.

Table 5-1 Orbitocranial Asymmetry

Encephalocele
Generalized neurofibromatosis
Plagiocephalic craniostenosis
Congenital facial hemihypertrophy
Intraorbital lesions, primary and secondary, causing proptosis
Paranasal sinus and nasopharyngeal lesions invading the orbit
Intracranial lesions invading the orbit
Skeletal lesions invading the orbit

teoma of the frontal sinus (Burrows, 1978).

Orbital enlargement denotes a benign lesion of the orbital cavity which is of long standing (Lloyd, 1967). However, this rule does not apply in children, in whom raised intraorbital pressure more quickly enlarges the orbit. Symmetrical enlargement points to a tumor within the muscle cone, causing an even distribution of intraorbital pressure, e.g., glioma of the optic nerve. Tumors outside the muscle cone tend to produce asymmetrical enlargement of the rim, sometimes with focal erosion, indentation and a reaction of the bony wall adjacent to the mass, e.g., epidermoid, lacrimal gland tumor. Intraorbital tumors that enlarge the rim without eroding it seldom deform the oblique line or sphenoid ridge, although the optic canal may be enlarged through spread of a retinoblastoma to involve the intracanalicular part of the optic nerve. The three causes of orbital enlargement in generalized neurofibromatosis are discussed in Chapter 1 (see Fig. 1-66).

Hemicoronal synostosis (plagiocephalic craniostenosis) enlarges the bony orbit by distorting it, the outer and upper corner being drawn up towards the tethered coronal suture — the so-called harlequin deformity. Another rare cause of an asymmetrical bony orbit is congenital facial hemihypertrophy.

Proptosis: Plain radiographs fail to reveal the cause in about 50 percent of cases of unilateral proptosis (Lloyd, 1967). Radiological examination is usually diagnostic in lesions spreading from adjacent structures to involve the orbit, e.g., mucocele, infection or carcinoma of the paranasal sinuses; meningioma, fracture or other bony abnormality of the sphenoid ridge; and aneurysm, carotid-cavernous fistula or tumor of the parasellar part of the intracranial compartment. On the contrary, plain radiography is likely to be unhelpful in primary lesions of the intraorbital tissues, which include the following:

Dysthyroidism: the cause of 80 percent of cases of unilateral proptosis (Hanafee, 1972)

Inflammatory or autoimmune reaction: orbital cellulitis or pseudotumor

Retro-orbital hematoma

Primary neoplasms: lacrimal gland carcinoma, optic glioma, neurofibroma, orbital meningioma, rhabdomyosarcoma, dermoid, retinoblastoma

Secondary deposits: carcinoma, lymphoma, histiocytosis-X, leukemia

In such lesions, computed tomography of the orbits nearly always demonstrates the reason for the proptosis, and sometimes yields appearances that are diagnostic, e.g., retro-orbital hematoma, dysthyroidism and pseudotumor oculi.

COMPUTED TOMOGRAPHY

The axial plane of computed tomography is especially useful in identifying bone destruction or sclerosis in the pituitary region, which may be invisible on the routine skull radiographs. The total information accruing from computed tomography frequently enable a tissue diagnosis to be made.

Technique: There are two essentials. (1) "Overlapping" or thin tomographic slices must be made at successive levels, viz., through the pituitary fossa, the suprasellar cistern and the anterior end of the third ventricle. This technique ensures that the pituitary region will be visualized adequately in 98 percent of cases (Naidich et al., 1976; Leeds and Naidich, 1977; Gyldensted and Karle, 1977). Thin slices at three- or four-millimeter intervals allow for computer reconstruction of the image in lateral and coronal planes (Maravilla, 1978). (2) Contrast enhancement by means of the intravenous injection of a meglumine salt, and repetition of the "overlapping" tomographic slices.

Anatomy: Figure 5-10 shows the symmetrical arrangement of anatomical structures at the level of the sella turcica and sphenoid sinus revealed by the appropriate slice. As a rule, focal bone lesions, e.g., an eroded anterior clinoid process, are better demonstrated by this method than by conventional radiography of the skull. The axial plane is also the ideal projection for evaluating the extent of parasellar and other masses which spread horizontally at this level.

On slices made at a slightly higher level (Fig. 5-10, B and C), the cerebrospinal fluid within the chiasmatic and interpeduncular cisterns produces a distinctive low-density configuration which is the key to diagnostic interpretation of the suprasellar region. This is the 5- or 6-pointed "suprasellar star" (Naidich et al., 1976). The anterior point of the star lies in the interhemispheric fissure, the anterolateral points represent the origins of the sylvian fissures and the posterolateral points the crural cisterns, and the posterior point of the star lies between the cerebral peduncles. After contrast injection, the blood vessels of the circle of Willis outline the star.

In slices obtained just above the star, the anterior recesses of the third ventricle and the foramina of Monro will be shown.

Pattern of Pathology:

Bone Changes (Fig. 5-11). Correct evaluation of any accompanying bone changes or tumor calcification and their correlation with the computed

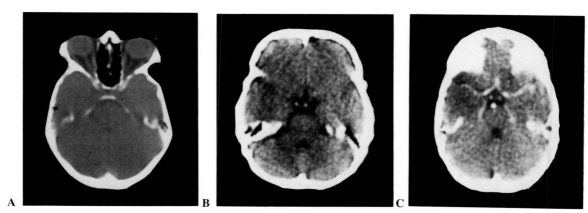

Fig. 5–10 Computed tomography of the normal sella turcica and suprasellar region. (A) Noncontrast slice made at the level of the pituitary fossa, showing the anterior clinoid processes forming the lateral walls of the optic canals, and the dorsum sellae with the posterior clinoid processes. (B) Suprasellar "star," situated 8 mm. above the sella turcica. The anterior part is bounded by the frontal lobes and its anterior point lies in the interhemispheric fissure. The lateral margins are defined by the temporal lobes. The posterior margins are formed either by the midbrain, when there is a 6-pointed "star," or by the pons, when a 5-pointed "star" is present (as in this example). The two radiodensities visible within the star are the optic nerves. (C) Same slice as (B), after contrast enhancement, showing the "star" framed by the anterior and posterior cerebral arteries and the trunk of the basilar artery.

images of the brain may be the key to successful differential diagnosis. Enlargement of the pituitary fossa is the commonest finding, reflecting the predominating incidence of pituitary tumors, which only rarely grow without pressure-eroding the adjacent bone. Predominantly intrasellar tumors produce symmetrical biconcave excavation of the fossa, while parasellar extensions typically show sideways funnelling, i.e., a sloping floor, an angled dorsum sellae and an eroded anterior clinoid process. A well-defined hyperostosis confined to the planum or medial part of a sphenoid wing is almost pathognomonic of meningioma, especially if the adjacent tumor mass contains speckled psammoma-body calcification. Bone erosion, caused either by pressure or invasive destruction, may be dramatically revealed in the axial plane, especially if it involves the parasellar region, the clinoid processes or the medial part of the sphenoid ridge.

Deformed Suprasellar Star (Fig. 5–12). The symmetrical configuration of the suprasellar star may be deformed, or the cisterns obliterated, by adjacent tumors. The anterior half of the star may be indented by subfrontal tumors, its lateral margin by parasellar or temporal tumors. Pituitary adenomas and optic gliomas, in the course of their growth upwards, may first obliterate its center while preserving a circumferential ring of cerebrospinal fluid intact, prior to obliterating the star completely. If the lesion has a less dense core, e.g., craniopharyngioma or arachnoid cyst, the replacing cyst may be mistaken for a suprasellar star, but careful study will usually show that it lacks the symmetry and anatomical points of the normal configuration.

Because the star lies at a higher level than the pituitary fossa, it will remain intact in the presence

of a purely intrasellar tumor, or an intrasellar tumor that grows only sideways.

Masses Shown by Contrast Enhancement: Lesions in the pituitary region classified according to their postenhancement appearances fall into three groups:

1. Round masses of homogeneous density (Fig. 5–13)
2. Ring lesions, i.e., round masses with a low-density core (Fig. 5–14)
3. Irregularly-shaped masses (Fig. 5–15)

Study of the examples in these three figures will show that computed tomography provides the following: (1) A perfect image of the size and position of the mass, relative to the pituitary fossa and its cisterns—intrasellar, suprasellar, parasellar, subfrontal or retrosellar. (2) Details of the effect of the mass upon adjacent structures. Thus, the third ventricle may be indented or obliterated, producing obstructive hydrocephalus A part of the circle of Willis, usually an internal carotid artery, may be displaced or entrapped (craniopharyngioma, chromophobe adenoma or meningioma) or the mass may arise from it (aneurysm). (3) No certain information on the histological nature of a mass. However, a specific disease pattern may emerge when the computed tomographic appearances are correlated with the findings of conventional radiography.

Pituitary adenomas enhance vividly and homogeneously after contrast injection. Usually the tumor is asymmetrical, lobulated or irregular, and spreads upward and forward over the planum. However, a suprasellar meningioma, craniopharyngioma or hypothalamic glioma may produce similar appearances, and the radiological diagnosis will depend on the type of plain-film abnormality present. Ring

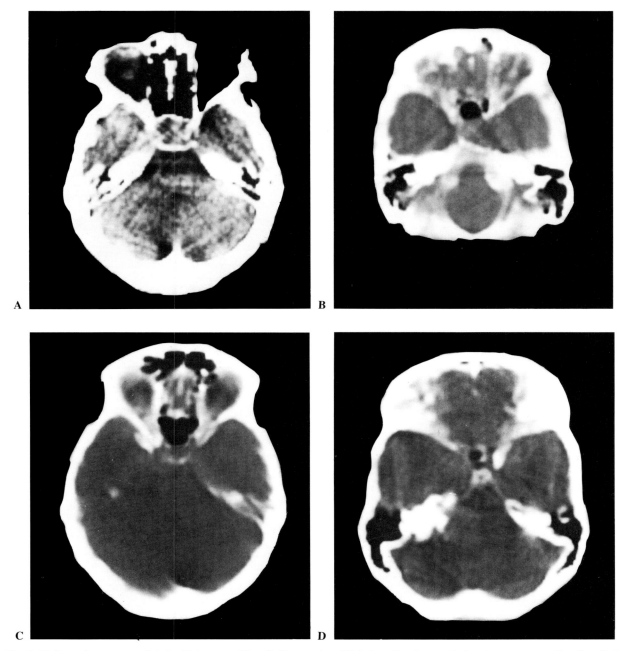

Fig. 5–11 Bone changes associated with tumors of the pituitary region. (A) Intrasellar chromophobe adenoma excavating the pituitary fossa. (B) Chromophobe adenoma spreading sideways as a parasellar mass, funnelling the pituitary fossa to the right side. (C) Sphenoid meningioma arising from an enostosis of the left anterior clinoid process. (D) Chondroma of the left temporal fossa, destroying the left anterior and posterior clinoid processes and deforming the medial half of the left sphenoid ridge. Same case as Figures 5 – 2 and 5 – 20.

shadows represent cystic degeneration or necrosis within a tumor, or a cystic lesion such as an aneurysm or cystic craniopharyngioma; in the latter, cholesterol salts may produce a core of very low density. Aneurysm and colloid cyst of the third ventricle should be considered if the suprasellar lesion is geometrically round; curiously, both these lesions more often cast homogeneous than ring shadows.

The Negative Result: Computed tomography has replaced angiography and pneumography as the primary investigation in patients suspected of harboring a pituitary-region tumor. Plain radiography is an integral part of the study, undertaken to search for relevent features such as sellar enlargement, suprasellar calcification and focal bone changes. If computed tomography shows no abnormality,

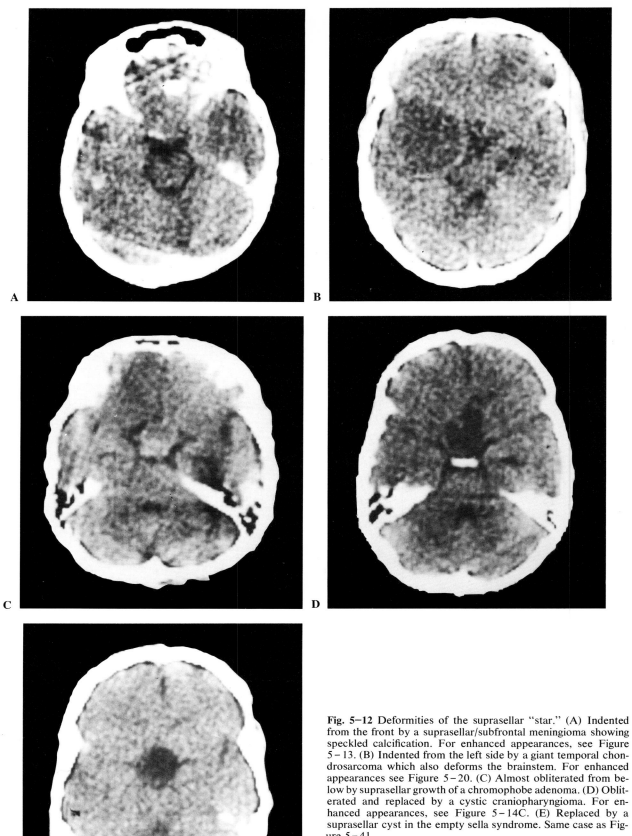

Fig. 5–12 Deformities of the suprasellar "star." (A) Indented from the front by a suprasellar/subfrontal meningioma showing speckled calcification. For enhanced appearances, see Figure 5–13. (B) Indented from the left side by a giant temporal chondrosarcoma which also deforms the brainstem. For enhanced appearances see Figure 5–20. (C) Almost obliterated from below by suprasellar growth of a chromophobe adenoma. (D) Obliterated and replaced by a cystic craniopharyngioma. For enhanced appearances, see Figure 5–14C. (E) Replaced by a suprasellar cyst in the empty sella syndrome. Same case as Figure 5–41.

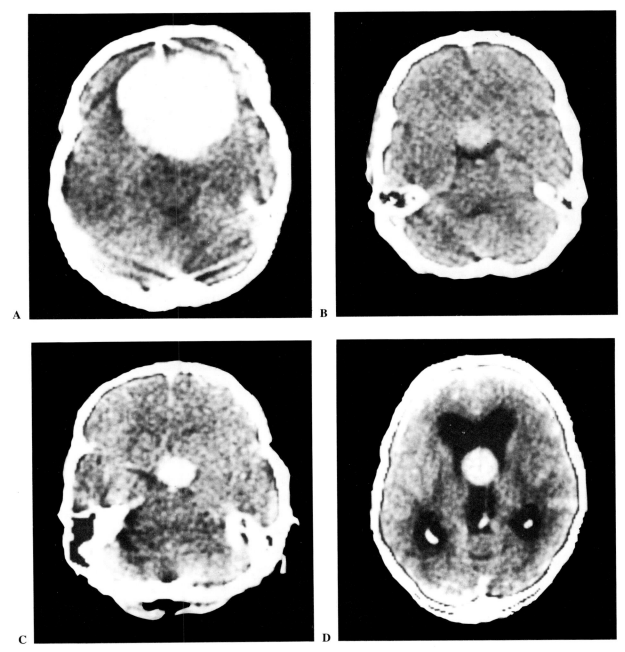

Fig. 5–13 Contrast-enhanced pituitary masses. (1) Round lesions of homogeneous density. (A) Meningioma. (B) Chromophobe adenoma. (C) Giant aneurysm of the anterior communicating artery. (D) Colloid cyst of the third ventricle producing massive obstructive hydrocephalus.

pneumography is probably inevitable in those patients in whom the clinical suspicion of a lesion is strong, e.g., progressive visual failure. But the yield of positive results from air injection is low (Leeds and Naidich, 1977). Many prolactin-secretors show no abnormality with either computed tomography or conventional radiographs because of their small size; an exception is shown in Figure 5–29, unless high-resolution scans are obtained at 1.5 mm. inter-

vals through the sella turcica in the coronal plane (Syvertsen et al., 1979).

If an operable tumor is shown, appropriate angiography is indicated. Thus, both carotids should be opacified in suprasellar lesions, only the ipsilateral carotid in parasellar lesions, and the vertebrobasilar tree in all suprasellar masses and particularly those that extend behind the dorsum sellae.

The commonest causes of an enhancing mass

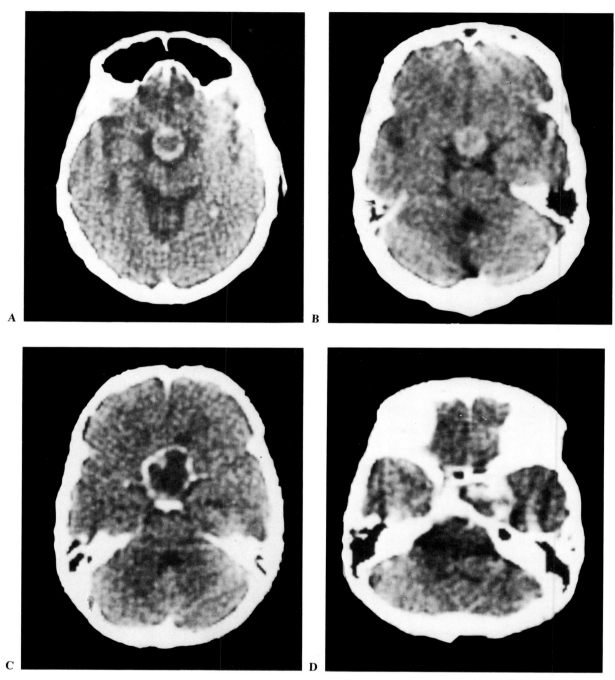

Fig. 5–14 Contrast-enhanced pituitary masses (continued). (2) Ring lesions. (A) Chromophobe adenoma. (B) Metastatic deposit from bronchial carcinoma. (C) Craniopharyngioma, cystic with mural nodule. Same case as Figure 5–12D. (D) Parasellar aneurysm of the infraclinoid carotid artery, with blood clot within the irregular lumen.

above an abnormal pituitary fossa are chromophobe adenoma and craniopharyngioma, and rarely chordoma or glioma; and of an enhancing mass above a normal pituitary fossa the commonest causes are meningioma or aneurysm, either of which may calcify.

ANGIOGRAPHY

Cerebral angiography is indispensable in the investigation of masses in the pituitary region. The purposes, as defined by Chase and Taveras (1963), are to rule out aneurysm and perhaps to enable a histo-

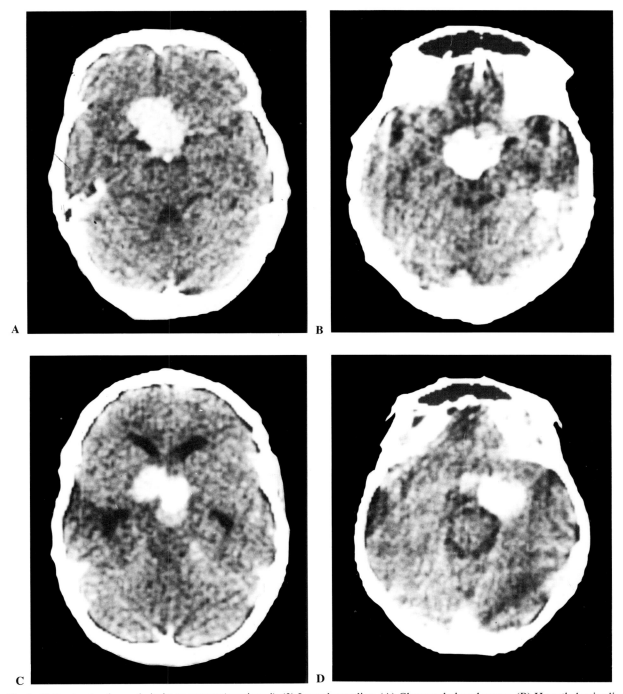

Fig. 5–15 Contrast-enhanced pituitary masses (continued). (3) Irregular outline. (A) Chromophobe adenoma. (B) Hypothalamic glioma (calcified). (C) Craniopharyngioma (calcified). (D) Parasellar meningioma.

logical diagnosis to be made. In this respect, angiography complements computed tomography or pneumography, and it yields essential information which no other investigative method can provide. Bilateral carotid and vertebral angiography are necessary for the following reasons:

1. To exclude carotid or basilar aneurysm.

2. To determine the extent of displacement of the cavernous part of the internal carotid artery in parasellar masses, and of the anterior cerebral arteries in suprasellar masses, and the precise position of the arteries.

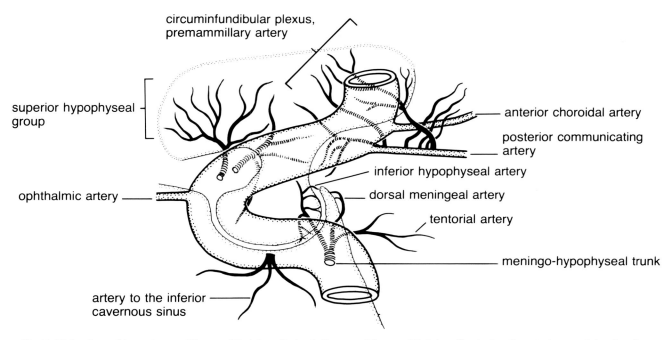

Fig. 5–16 Angiographic anatomy of the carotid siphon. Lateral diagram of the carotid siphon illustrating the arteries supplying the pituitary gland and stalk, optic pathway, mammillary bodies and hypothalamus.

3. To exclude circumferential entrapment (narrowing) of the artery by parasellar neoplasms or granulomas.

4. Sometimes to provide a histological diagnosis, through the presence of a characteristic pattern of staining and of feeding arteries, e.g., hypertrophied recurrent dural branch of the ophthalmic artery in sphenoid meningioma.

5. To reveal displacement of the thalamoperforator vessels in suprasellar or retrosellar extension.

Interest in the angiography of the pituitary region has intensified since the introduction of serial magnification combined with the subtraction technique and tomography, which add refinement to angiographic diagnosis. These technical advances have revealed that the small parasellar branches of the carotid siphon, already known to anatomists (Fig. 5–16; McConnell, 1953), are relevant in diagnosis and possess recognizable angiographic patterns in certain types of tumor (Baker, 1972; Palacios et al., 1975). The *cavernous (infraclinoid) branches* consist of the following: twigs to the pituitary capsule (not shown in Fig. 5–16), the meningohypophyseal (dorsal mainstem) trunk and the artery to the inferior cavernous sinus (Wallace et al., 1967). All except the last-named artery communicate across the midline with their contralateral namesake to form an anastomotic network. The normal posterior pituitary "blush" reflects the high vascularity of the neurohypophysis. The *supraclinoid group* consists of the superior hypophyseal arteries and various unnamed branches of the posterior communicating (including the premammillary artery, which is larg-

er). An anastomosis of these vessels, the circuminfundibular network, supplies the anterior lobe and stalk of the pituitary, the optic nerves and chiasm, and part of the hypothalamus. All these vessels are under 0.5 mm. in diameter but when hypertrophied they are easily demonstrable by direct magnification.

Abnormal Feeding Arteries: The angiographic appearances depend on whether the lesions are predominantly expansile, i.e., displacing and compressing normal structures, or whether they attract a greater blood supply (arteriovenous malformations, some meningiomas and malignant neoplasms). In expansile lesions, the normal posterior pituitary "blush" and cavernous sinus filling are absent; even the cavernous branches of the internal carotid may be obliterated and fail to fill. The hypervascular group of tumors exhibit, apart from sometimes an abnormal blush, hypertrophied feeding vessels. (1) Meningohypophyseal trunk and other cavernous branches (Fig. 5–17): lesions on the floor of the middle cranial fossa, e.g., dural venous malformations (Schnürer and Stattin, 1963), meningiomas, gasserian ganglion neuromas (Westberg, 1963), also pituitary adenomas (Powell et al., 1974). The tentorial branch may be enlarged by arteriovenous malformations or by several types of neoplasm, and its dorsal meningeal branch by meningiomas or other lesions attached or adjacent to the clivus. (2) Ophthalmic artery: meningeal branches—particularly the recurrent meningeal which supplies the dura of the sphenoid ridge (Stattin, 1961; Kuru, 1967)—hypertrophy regularly in meningiomas of

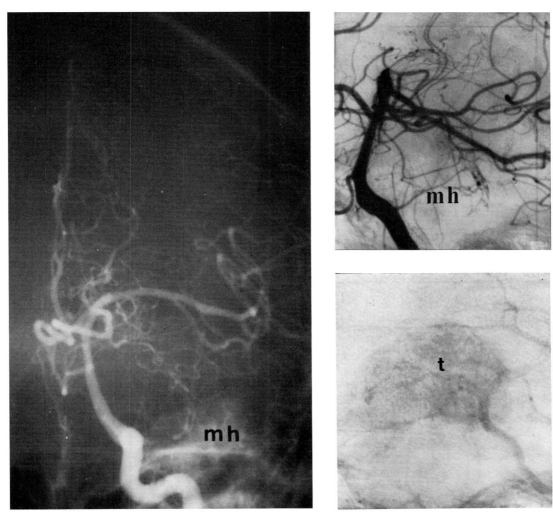

Fig. 5—17 Three angiographic features of the blood supply of a tumor are illustrated, viz., hypertrophied feeding arteries, displaced vessels and pathological tumor staining. Hypothalamic glioma. The supraclinoid carotid is straightened, elevated and stretched. (mh) Meningohypophyseal trunk, which is stretched, enlarged and displaced laterally; (t) tumor stain.

the medial third of the sphenoid ridge (Fig. 5 – 34). (3) Supraclinoid branches of the internal carotid artery (circuminfundibular plexus) feed the pathological circulation found in a small proportion of suprasellar masses — pituitary adenoma, meningioma, optic glioma (Baker, 1972).

"Tumor Blush": The above-named branches of the internal carotid artery, sometimes invisible without magnification, may contribute to a "tumor blush", although they do not always do so. This feature is not difficult to differentiate from normal capillary staining of the neurohypophysis and basal nuclei (Fig. 5 – 17). Pituitary adenomas may occasionally exhibit delicate tumor staining (Fig. 5 – 28); the prognostic significance of this feature is uncertain (Roth et al., 1971). Meningiomas of the parasellar and presellar regions as a rule show distinctive abnormal staining which is well circumscribed, persistent and dense, but an adjacent enostosis is probably necessary to confirm a specific diagnosis (Figs. 5 – 34 and 5 – 35). Similar staining may be present in other tumors in this location, such as sarcoma or neurinoma (Hasso et al., 1975).

Carotid Entrapment: Compressive narrowing or occlusion of the cavernous part of the internal carotid artery due to encasement by tumor is an unfavorable sign for successful surgery, indicating involvement of the cavernous sinus. It is a feature of parasellar meningiomas but it is not infrequently seen in other laterally spreading masses such as pituitary adenoma (Fig. 5 – 18; Epstein and Epstein, 1968), craniopharyngioma and also nasopharyngeal carcinoma. Similar appearances are seen in nonspecific inflammatory lesions which are reversible by steroid therapy (Tolosa, 1954; Hallpike, 1973).

Displacement: Computed tomography has largely eliminated the need for angiography to assess the size of pituitary-region tumors. However, vital

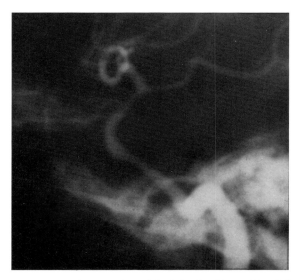
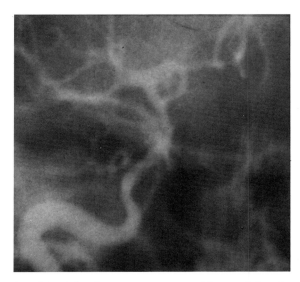

Fig. 5–18 Concentric narrowing of the infraclinoid carotid and distortion of the siphon by tumor entrapment. Chromophobe adenoma extending laterally into the left cavernous sinus and also upward to compress the optic nerves. A 51-year-old woman complaining of visual deterioration.

preoperative information on the precise extent of displacement or other involvement of the internal carotid, anterior cerebral and/or basilar trunk demands angiography, the appearances of which may also indicate the nature of the tumor (Hilal, 1971).

1. Intrasellar Masses (chiefly chromophobe adenoma, but also craniopharyngioma). The carotid siphon may be displaced laterally, and this is evaluated on the frontal view. The lateral view may be normal, although the siphon may be depressed, elevated or stretched (Fig. 5–19).

2. Parasellar Masses (Fig. 5–20). They grow in three sites: medial side and floor of the temporal fossa (giant infraclinoid carotid aneurysm, gasserian ganglion neuroma, extradural epidermoid and cartilaginous tumors); medial half of the sphenoid ridge (meningioma); and midline, growing to one side (nasopharyngeal carcinoma and other lytic basal processes, sphenoid mucocele, pituitary adenoma, chordoma). Medial and lateral displacement of the cavernous part of the internal carotid artery possess more differential-diagnostic value than a shift ante-

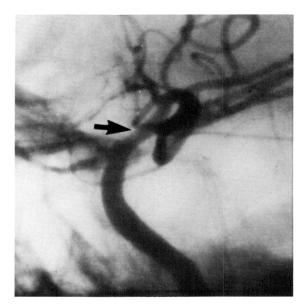
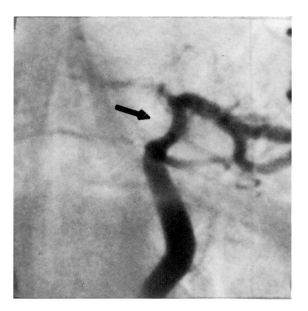

Fig. 5–19 Distortion and lateral displacement of the internal carotid artery by an intrasellar and parasellar chromophobe adenoma. No suprasellar extension, but entrapment of the supraclinoid carotid *(arrow)*. A 45-year-old army sergeant with hypopituitary signs but normal visual fields.

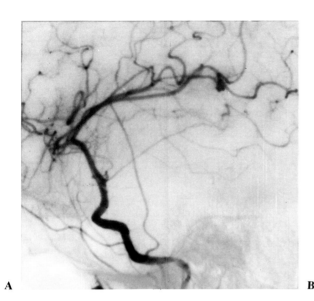 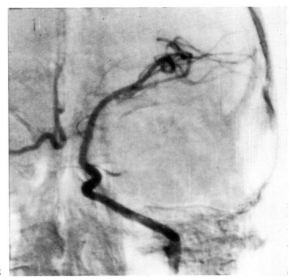

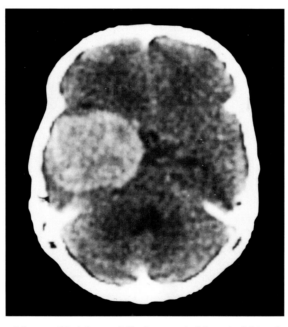

Fig. 5–20 (A and B) Medial dislocation of the carotid siphon and displacement of the arterial tree by a large extradural mass of the temporal fossa. (C) Chondrosarcoma imaged by computed tomography. Same patient as Figures 5 – 2 and 5 – 12B.

riorly or posteriorly (Bull and Schunk, 1962). Intracerebral temporal masses such as hematomas or gliomas usually do not displace the cavernous carotid medially, but extradural masses may do so, e.g., medial sphenoid meningiomas (Fig. 5 – 34) and cartilaginous tumors (Fig. 5 – 20). The following masses are said to cause characteristic displacements (Westberg, 1969):

gasserian ganglion neuroma   – medial and anterior

cavernous carotid aneurysm   – medial and posterior

chordoma   – anterior

pituitary adenoma, sphenoid   – lateral mucocele

3. Suprasellar – Subfrontal Masses (usually chromophobe adenoma or craniopharyngioma, Fig. 5 – 21). The angiographic appearances of suprasellar masses depend on their precise location in the median sagittal plane: the further forward the mass lies, the greater the likelihood of its being outlined by carotid angiography. The typical finding is elevation, and especially upward bowing, of the proximal parts of both anterior cerebral arteries from their

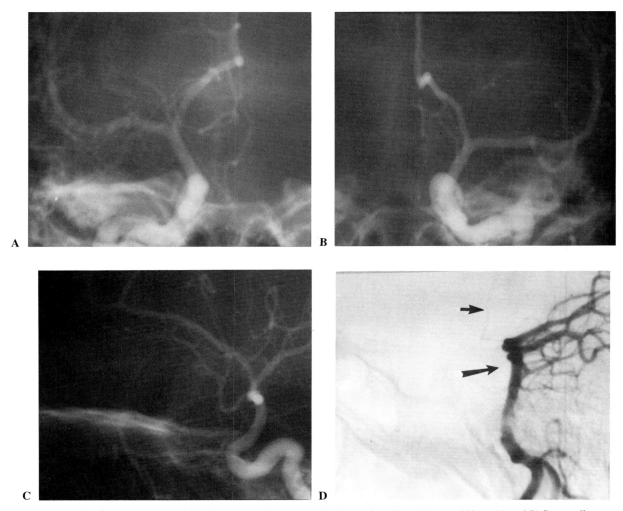

Fig. 5–21 Arterial displacements outlining the extent of a large craniopharyngioma in an 8-year-old boy. (A and B) Suprasellar: upward displacement of the proximal anterior cerebral arteries. (C) Subfrontal: upward bowing of the subcallosal part of the anterior cerebral artery. (D) Retrosellar: posterior displacement of the distal basilar trunk *(arrow)* and thalamoperforator branches *(short arrow)*.

normal horizontal positions—best shown by a cross-compression anteroposterior carotid angiogram; the perorbital projection is preferable to the anteroposterior-20° view (Gado and Bull, 1971). The lateral angiographic series may be normal. A thrombosed aneurysm of the supraclinoid carotid, presenting clinically as visual failure, may appear as an avascular mass in the suprasellar midline, although usually contralateral carotid angiography will reveal an aneurysmal sac. In some instances the mass may only be identified by displacement of anterior thalamoperforators related to the third ventricle (George et al., 1975).

4. Subfrontal Masses (meningioma arising from the cribriform plate, planum sphenoidale or tuberculum sellae, Fig. 5–22, chromophobe adenoma, optic glioma). The lateral series usually shows elevation of the infracallosal part of the anterior cerebral artery over the surface of the tumor. A diagno-

sis of meningioma is provided by one or more specific features such as enostosis, wide base of implantation of the tumor, hypertrophied feeding artery or a "tumor blush." The supraclinoid carotid is displaced laterally and posteriorly, closing the siphon (Fig. 5–22).

5. Retrosellar Masses (chromophobe adenoma, craniopharyngioma, clivus meningioma or chordoma, etc.). Retrochiasmal suprasellar masses may not be demonstrable at all by carotid angiography. The retrosellar limits of a suprasellar mass are revealed by vertebral angiography: the distal trunk of the basilar artery is displaced backward and the posterior cerebral and thalamoperforator arteries are elevated (Fig. 5–21; George et al., 1975; Lin and Kricheff, 1974). The thalamoperforating arteries are often stretched and retrodisplaced.

Direct magnification and subtraction techniques in suprasellar tumors may reveal diagnostically rel-

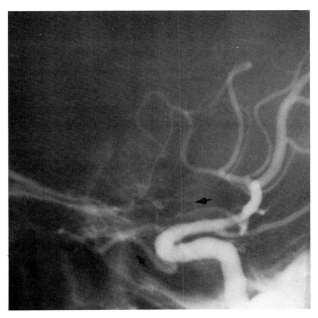 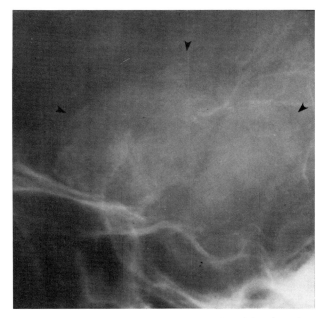

Fig. 5–22 Closing of the carotid siphon by a presellar meningioma. Note feeding vessels from the ophthalmic and other siphon branches *(arrows),* and the persistent, homogeneous stain *(arrowheads).* Nonopacifying anterior cerebral artery.

evant displacements of the supraclinoid branches of the internal carotid artery, notably the circuminfundibular plexus. If the suprasellar tumor is large enough or strategically placed to cause obstructive hydrocephalus, angiographic evidence of dilated

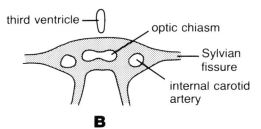

Fig. 5–23 Normal anatomy of the optochiasmatic cisterns. (A) Lateral view: relation of the chiasmal point (●) to the tuberculum sellae and optic canal (*). (B) Frontal view: relation of the internal carotid arteries to the optic nerves and chiasm. (After Caille et al., 1971, and McLachlan et al., 1971.)

lateral ventricles will be present. For the angiographic appearances of colloid cyst of the third ventricle, see Figure 7 – 14.

PNEUMOGRAPHY

Pneumoencephalography and ventriculography (gas or water-soluble contrast media) continue to be relevant investigations for tumors of the pituitary region, because lateral and frontal views of the brain are necessary to study morphological details of the anterior end of the third ventricle and adjacent cisterns. These invasive procedures are now indicated mostly as an aid to the surgeon, but they may be the only diagnostic method of revealing perioptic or chiasmal lesions that are too small to be detected with current scanning techniques. The converse is also true: small perioptic meningiomas may occasionally be present, despite normal tomopneumographic appearances of the pituitary region. The wise radiologist is aware that in patients with visual failure and normal plain radiographs, a combination of technical enthusiasm and interpretative caution – and not the reverse – prevents errors in diagnosis.

Third Ventricle: The most important anatomic landmark to identify is the *chiasmal point,* i.e., the point of insertion of the optic chiasm into the wall of the third ventricle between the optic and infundibular recesses (Fig. 5 – 23). With the exception mentioned below, it is impossible to diagnose a suprasellar mass if this point occupies a normal position and if the two recesses are not deformed. According

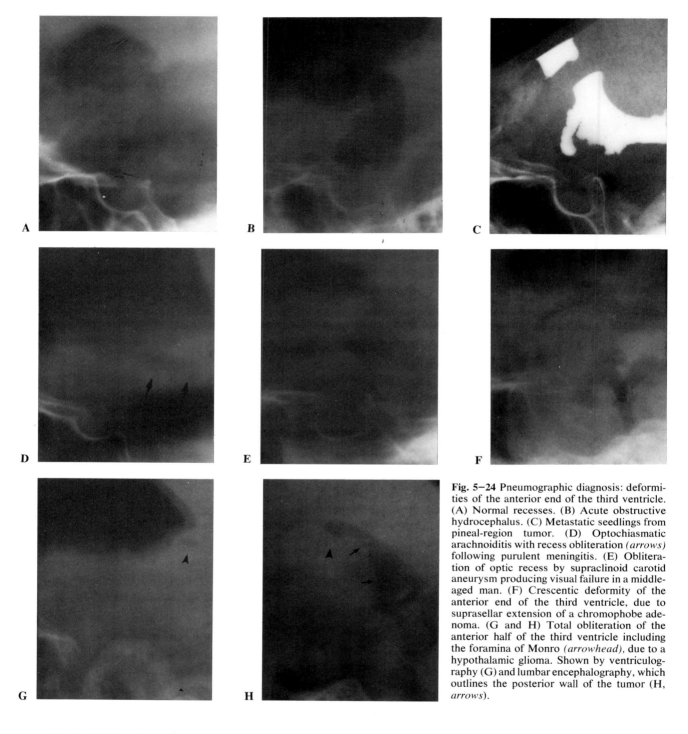

Fig. 5–24 Pneumographic diagnosis: deformities of the anterior end of the third ventricle. (A) Normal recesses. (B) Acute obstructive hydrocephalus. (C) Metastatic seedlings from pineal-region tumor. (D) Optochiasmatic arachnoiditis with recess obliteration *(arrows)* following purulent meningitis. (E) Obliteration of optic recess by supraclinoid carotid aneurysm producing visual failure in a middle-aged man. (F) Crescentic deformity of the anterior end of the third ventricle, due to suprasellar extension of a chromophobe adenoma. (G and H) Total obliteration of the anterior half of the third ventricle including the foramina of Monro *(arrowhead)*, due to a hypothalamic glioma. Shown by ventriculography (G) and lumbar encephalography, which outlines the posterior wall of the tumor (H, *arrows*).

to Bull (1956), the distance from the tuberculum sellae to the chiasmal point, i.e., the intracranial length of the optic nerves, varies between 10 and 23 mm. (in only 5 percent of normal subjects does it exceed 15 mm.). The only exception to this rule is the individual with a post-fixed chiasm, i.e., the chiasmal point lies behind the level of the dorsum

sellae; he may harbor a large suprasellar or subfrontal mass yet show a normal ventriculogram.

The commonest extra-axial tumors (chromophobe pituitary adenoma, craniopharyngioma, meningioma, Fig. 5–24) lie as a rule in the suprasellar midline. Depending on the size of the mass, the anterior end of the third ventricle exhibits three stages of deformity in lateral view, viz.: 1. Obliteration or deformity of one recess only, either the infundibular or the optic recess; the chiasmal point is not displaced. Deformity of a recess in a patient with visual failure calls for bilateral carotid angiography to exclude a supraclinoid "berry" aneurysm. Another nontumoral cause is optochiasmatic arachnoiditis. 2. Upward and backward displacement of the anterior end of the third ventricle, in a deformity that has a sharp crescentic outline. 3. Complete obliteration of the third ventricle to the height of the foramina of Monro, with resultant obstructive hydrocephalus of the lateral ventricles.

Massive dilatation of the lateral ventricles in the presence of a third ventricle of normal size (sometimes obscured by the hydrocephalus) always merits a careful search for an obstructive lesion. Colloid cysts of the third ventricle arise in the *roof* of the lateral ventricle behind the foramina of Monro, upon which they exert an intermittent ball-valve action. Metastatic deposits, or an aneurysm of the termination of the basilar artery, or an ectatic atherosclerotic basilar artery, indent the *floor* of the third ventricle (Scatliff and Bull, 1965; Greitz et al., 1969).

The midline position of the anterior end of the third ventricle is useful in differentiating between intra-axial tumors such as hypothalamic gliomas or metastases and extrinsic suprasellar masses. Gliomas usually grow eccentrically and displace the third ventricle to one side; in lateral view, the compressed chamber fills poorly and may show "thumb-printing." Extrinsic masses on the other hand, indent the anterior end of the third ventricle and widen it, converting it in frontal view from a keyhole appearance to a tent-like structure. In addition the margins of the ventricle juxtaposed to the mass may be blurred with an intrinsic mass and sharp with an extrinsic mass.

Optochiasmatic Cisterns: Meticulous biplanar multisection tomography following lumbar injection of gas (tomopneumoencephalography) is essential to identify the internal carotid arteries and optic pathway, and the integrity of the cisterns in which they lie (Caille et al., 1971; Johnson et al., 1975). This ensures that any mass deforming these cisterns will be outlined, especially the upper and lateral limits of tumors rising up from the superior surface of the sphenoid bone, e.g., pituitary adenoma and optic glioma. The true extent of encroachment of the parasagittal mass upon the lateral cisterns can only be evaluated by successful coronal tomopneumography: exceptional tumors are sufficiently large to spread across the middle fossa and deform and dislocate the temporal horn. Suprasellar anatomy is frequently obscured in lateral view by collections of gas situated around the supraclinoid portions of the carotid arteries on each side. The dimensions of

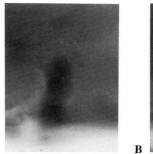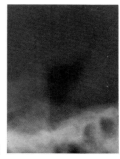

Fig. 5–25 The "tough" membrane of Liliequist (1959). (A) Normal membrane with outline convex upward. (B) Retrosellar craniopharyngioma, membrane inverted.

these so-called carotid cisterns (Lewtas and Jefferson, 1966) are well illustrated by computed tomography of the suprasellar region (see Fig. 5–10).

Occasionally, filling of the optochiasmatic cisterns will fail to occur, due to an arachnoid membrane that covers the midline between the oculomotor nerves. Liliequist (1959) first pointed out this anatomical variant, which is identified by its concave-downward outline, behind the dorsum sellae (Fig. 5–25.).

SCINTIGRAPHY

Most pituitary-region tumors occupy a mediobasal location within the skull. For this reason, a large proportion are likely to remain undetected by the scintigraphic method, irrespective of their size or histological nature. In the series of one of the authors, only 7 out of 20 (35 percent) gave positive results (Burrows, 1972). One of these was a 2.5 cm-diameter suprasellar meningioma, while the suprasellar component of a pituitary adenoma and an optic glioma, both of similar size, were false-negative. Positive results not significantly better were produced by Sauer, Otto and their colleagues (1971, 1972) in a large review of the scintigraphic literature, viz.:

Pituitary adenoma	80/167
Craniopharyngioma	38/59
Optic glioma	7/9

They reported that the diagnosis remained in doubt in the majority of their own 24 cases, and another contrast investigation was required to confirm the presence of tumor. Meningiomas are the suprasellar tumors most likely to be demonstrated: in an adult with failing vision and a normal-sized pituitary fossa, an abnormal accumulation of radionuclide in the suprasellar midline points to meningioma or giant carotid aneurysm (see Fig. 3–25). Cerebral scintigraphy, because of its diagnostic unreliability in the sellar region, is no longer justified in the investigation of patients with visual failure or endocrine disorders.

OTHER METHODS

Cavernous Sinus Venography: This is a refined modification of retrograde jugular venography, and has been used to study tumors in the sellar region (Hanafee et al., 1965; Waga et al., 1970).

Computed Metrizamide Cisternography: This technique may prove useful in outlining suprasellar tumors by computed tomography, following metrizamide opacification of the interpeduncular and suprasellar cisterns (Fig. 5-26, Drayer et al., 1977a, 1977b; Sheldon and Molyneux, 1979).

SPECIAL PATHOLOGY

Over a 10-year period in the Wessex Neurological Centre, more tumors of the pituitary gland were seen than all the other sellar-region masses added together:

Primary pituitary tumors	131
(chromophobe 106, acidophil 25)	
Craniopharyngioma	21
Meningioma	15
Giant aneurysm	10
Glioma (optic, hypothalamic)	12
Colloid cyst of the third ventricle	7
Malignant metastases	5
Chordoma	3
Other	5

Pituitary Tumors

These are the commonest tumors by far. Chromophobe pituitary adenomas are tumors of adults, but occasionally acidophil tumors start earlier, producing teenage giants rather than true agromegalics. Adenomas of the chromophil cells account for the majority of primary pituitary tumors and they have a tendency to spread upward (Fig. 5-27). Most acidophil tumors, on the other hand, remain confined to the sella turcica. Unless clinical signs of acromegaly are present, it is impossible to predict the cellular origin of a pituitary adenoma from its radiological appearances.

Plain Radiographs: Pituitary tumors typically enlarge the pituitary fossa by pressure-eroding all its walls equally, producing a "balloon" sella. This process includes thinning of the dorsum sellae (Fig. 5-5) and in about 25 percent of cases erosion of the lesser sphenoid wing and optic canal. In only 3 (2 percent) of the 131 Southampton patients was the pituitary fossa called normal. Calcification is rare.

Computed Tomography: Diagnostic and differential-diagnostic aspects have been discussed above in the section on Computed Tomography. The statistical predominance of pituitary tumors must be

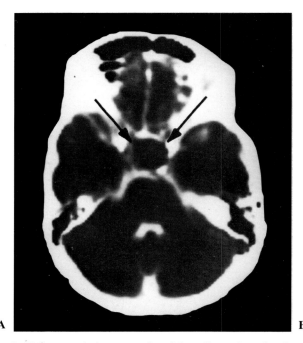
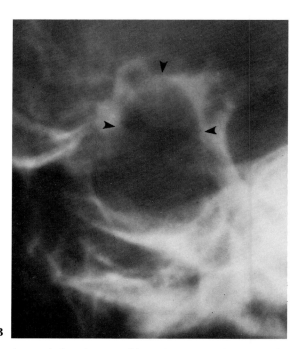

A   B

Fig. 5-26 Computed cisternography of the sellar region, showing a chromophobe adenoma with moderate suprasellar extension. (A) Horizontal computed tomogram, imaging the round filling defect in the suprasellar region *(arrows)*. (B) Lateral view, showing an enlarged pituitary fossa with the upper limit of the mass outlined by metrizamide *(arrowheads)*. (Reproduced by courtesy of Dr. V. McAllister, Newcastle General Hospital, Newcastle-upon-Tyne.)

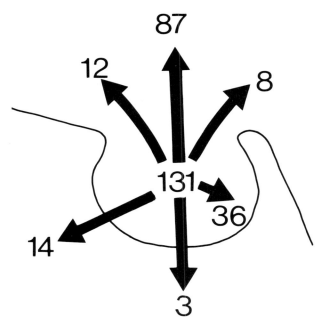

Fig. 5–27 The direction of spread of pituitary tumors, based on radiological and surgical findings in 131 cases seen in the Wessex Neurological Centre, Southampton. In 36, including the majority of the acromegalic patients, the tumor was confined to the pituitary fossa. The majority spread upwards, at least 14 spread sideways only.

stressed, in respect of an enhancing lesion in the sellar region: the diagnosis becomes almost certain if the patient is an adult and the plain radiographs show an enlarged pituitary fossa and no suprasellar calcification (Naidich et al., 1976; Leeds and Naidich, 1977). The use of computed reconstruction permits complete outlining of the neoplasm (Maravilla, 1978).

Angiography: The commonest feature is displacement of the juxtapituitary vessels around the mass, and bowing of the anterior cerebral arteries upward, of one carotid siphon outward (Fig. 5–19) or of the basilar artery (thalamoperforator branches) backward (Fig. 5–21); displacement depends on the location of the tumor. More refined techniques such as magnification with subtraction and angiotomography may reveal subtle and more specific changes which are constantly produced by pituitary tumors. For example, the capsule of both chromophobe and acidophilic adenomas is supplied by dilated vessels arising from the extradural part of the carotid siphon. This is a characteristic angiographic feature of such tumors, which is unusual in craniopharyngiomas or meningiomas. In tumors showing asymmetrical growth, the cavernous branches of the carotid artery are more prominent on the side where the growth is largest. In tumors with large suprasellar extensions, the superior hypophyseal artery and the circuminfundibular plexus are invariably displaced. Rarely, a diffuse pituitary "blush" is found (Fig. 5–28), which may sometimes be mistaken for the richer blood supply of a meningioma (Westberg and Ross, 1967; Hatam, 1971; Powell et al., 1974; Bonneville et al., 1976).

Pneumography: Pneumographic examination if properly performed remains useful, particularly in the surgical management of pituitary tumors. It may reveal the following: (1) Small tumors in which computed tomography gives a doubtful or negative result (Fig. 5–29). (2) The extent of vertical growth of a tumor, which is difficult to judge on axial computed tomograms. The surgeon's decision regarding his approach, viz., conventional craniotomy or transsphenoidal hypophysectomy, depends on the precise relation of the upper and posterior margins

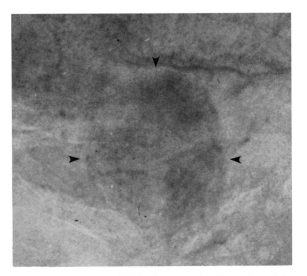

Fig. 5–28 Chromophobe adenoma with a delicate homogeneous "blush" *(arrowheads)*, supplied by hypertrophied branches of the cavernous carotid including the inferior hypophyseal artery *(arrows)*.

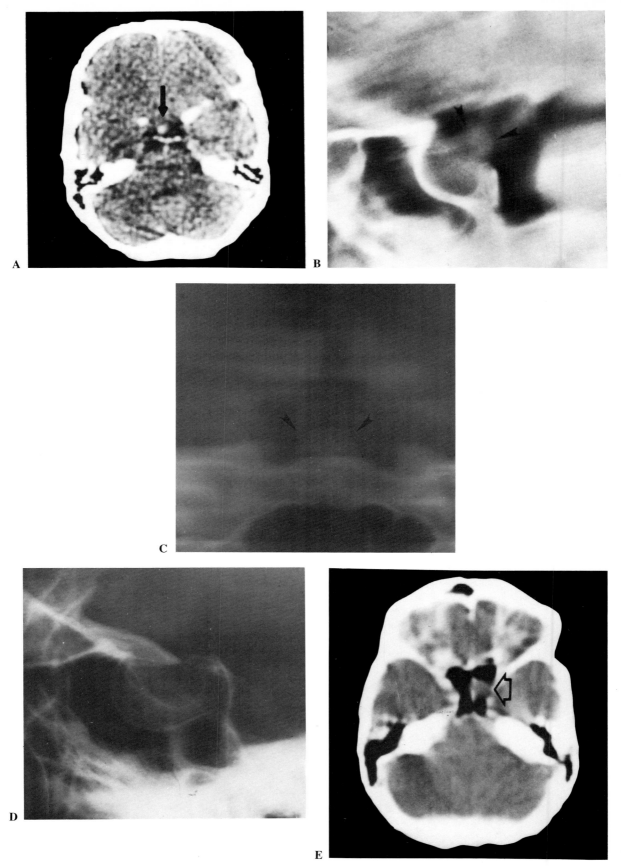

Fig. 5–29 Two patients with pituitary tumors submitted to computed tomography, in whom additional investigation was required for diagnosis. (A, B and C) A 14-year-old boy with hypopituitarism. A solitary white shadow is visible on the enhanced slice *(arrow)*, which tomopneumography revealed to be a small suprasellar extension of an intrasellar tumor *(arrowheads)*. (D and E) A 50-year-old hyperprolactinemic woman with an abnormally large, asymmetric pituitary fossa. The low slice of the computed tomogram shows a small intrasellar mass excavating the right sphenoidal sinus *(open arrow)*.

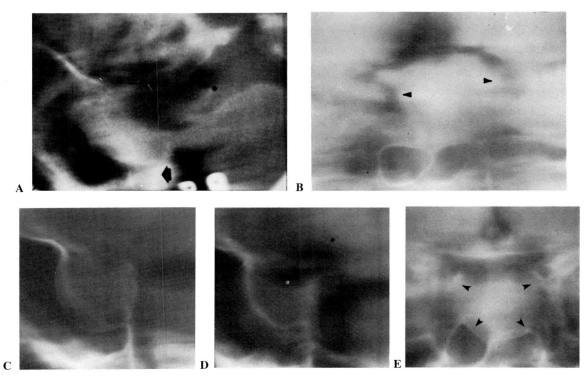

Fig. 5—30 The post-fixed chiasm and pituitary tumors. (A and B) A middle-aged man with visual failure. The lateral tomogram appears to reveal no suprasellar growth—the chiasmal point *(black dot)* and recesses are not deformed, but they lie behind the level of the clivus *(arrow).* The coronal tomogram shows a suprasellar extension of the mass bounded by gas-filled carotid cisterns *(arrowheads).* (C, D, and E) A 35-year-old man with hypopituitarism but intact visual fields. Lateral tomograms, made in the midline (C) and 1 cm. to the right side (D), show a sloping sellar floor; the chiasmal point *(black dot),* which is post-fixed, is not distorted. The apparent sloping floor suggests a left parasellar mass, and the post-fixed position of the normal chiasmal point does not rule out a suprasellar mass. The coronal tomogram (E) outlines a wholly intrasellar mass which is scalloping the sellar floor *(lower arrowheads).*

of the mass to the dorsum sellae. The three-dimensional view of the tumor surrounded by cisternal gas remains a most complete examination (Fig. 5–30). (3) Postoperative evaluation (Fig. 5–31): clinical recurrence may be mimicked by scarring, radiation damage or intrasellar cisternal herniation (see Empty Sella Syndrome, below; McLachlan et al., 1971). Another rare occurrence following the treatment of a pituitary tumor is a symptomatic suprasellar aerocele (Sage and McAllister, 1974).

Craniopharyngioma

A typical case is a child or youth with failing vision and signs of raised intracranial pressure, whose skull radiographs show suprasellar calcification and an abnormal pituitary fossa. Although craniopharyngiomas are traditionally tumors of childhood, 6 of the 21 Southampton patients (25 percent) were aged over 35 years when first seen. Banna (1976a) in a retrospective study of 160 cases, demonstrated that the radiological appearances of the tumor will depend on its site of origin. If arising below the dorsum sellae from the lower layer of squamous epithelial cells, the tumor tends to expand the pituitary fossa uniformly and resemble a chromophobe adenoma. More frequently it arises from the upper lay-

er of cells and then widens the sellar outlet and erodes the dorsum sellae from above (Fig. 5–5). Tumor calcification and pituitary changes are commoner in children than in adults: calcification in 80 percent (compared to 40 percent in adults), and pituitary changes, usually a flattened sellar profile, in 70 percent (adults 50 percent). Thus, the plain skull radiographs are normal in 50 percent of adults but in only one out of 5 children. Causes of suprasellar calcification in children other than craniopharyngioma are rare.

All types of pathological calcification occur and none is specific. Curvilinear calcification, which is rare, indicates that the tumor is cystic: it is less delicate than aneurysmal calcification and outlines the true extent of the tumor (Lindgren and Di Chiro, 1951). Deposits of granular calcification, on the other hand, do not reveal the full extent of the tumor (Fig. 5–32).

Computed tomography provides an accurate view of the size and nature of the mass, notably cystic craniopharyngiomas with intramural nodules (Fig. 5–14). It also shows the extent of retrosellar spread, which previously required pneumoencephalography or vertebral angiography (Fig. 5–21).

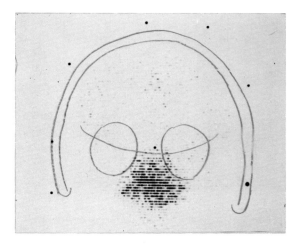

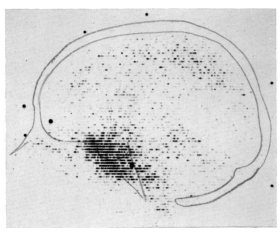

Fig. 5–31 A middle-aged woman with a pituitary tumor developed severe rhinorrhea following transsphenoidal hypophysectomy. RIHSA imaging revealed the sphenoidal sinus as the site of leakage of cerebrospinal fluid.

Secondary obstructive hydrocephalus is common — usually due to obstruction of the third ventricle or blockage of the foramina of Monro. Specific angiographic features are unusual and carotid angiography merely outlines an avascular mass, but the major reason for performing angiography in all cases is the frequency of involvement of the supraclinoid internal carotid artery.

Meningioma

A middle-aged woman with a normal pituitary fossa who complains of visual failure or a painless proptosis is likely to harbor a presellar or suprasellar meningioma. If computed tomography reveals an enhancing mass, the plain radiographs usually contribute toward confirming this diagnosis — by revealing a pituitary fossa of normal size (thus excluding a chromophobe adenoma) or by demonstrating a meningioma enostosis.

The majority of sphenoid meningiomas possess enostoses at their point of attachment. However, the changes may be slight and they are easily missed on plain radiographs unless supplemented by optic canal views and tomography (Sansregret and Ledoux, 1971; Gregorius and Bentson, 1975; Lee, 1976). This applies particularly to perioptic meningiomas attached by a small bony nodule to the tuberculum sellae. On the sphenoid jugum the enostosis is usually larger, resembling a piece of chewing gum flattened on a table-top. A specific clue to meningioma is the combination of bony deformity and pneumosinus dilatans, so-called blistering (Fig. 5–33; Wiggli and Oberson, 1975). "Blistering" appears to be a presclerotic stage of the meningioma hyperostosis which thickens the greater or lesser wings in a characteristic way (Fig. 5–7; see also Fig. 1–26). Tumor calcification is present in less than 5 percent of juxtasellar meningiomas.

The most specific contrast investigation is carotid angiography. In parasellar meningiomas, correct diagnosis of the mass shown by vessel displacements rests on the presence of a combination of features, viz., hypertrophied feeding vessels (a single meningohypophyseal trunk or numerous dural branches — Handa et al., 1967) and a distinctive stain. In medial sphenoid meningiomas, the principal source of supply is an hypertrophied ophthalmic artery through its recurrent dural branches (Fig. 5–34). Of the 28 presellar meningiomas submitted to angiography by Gregorius and Bentson (1975), 21 exhibited typical staining on selective internal carotid injection. Tumors attached more laterally on the sphenoid ridge are supplied by the external carotid artery through its middle meningeal branch (Fig. 5–35). Vessel displacement, although providing a reliable, albeit indirect indication of the size of the tumor, gives no clue to its nature.

Computed tomography and pneumoencephalography, while invariably imaging the mass, do not always provide the specific diagnosis of meningioma, for which plain-film changes or angiography are necessary. A little more than half of presellar meningiomas give positive scintigraphic results, presumably because of the small average size of these tumors, viz., 1.7 cm. (Gregorius and Bentson, 1975).

Giant Aneurysm

Space-occupying giant intracranial aneurysms, most of which are lesions of the pituitary region, have been discussed in Chapter 3. They develop in two sites: (1) On the infraclinoid or cavernous part of the internal carotid artery, being extradural masses lying on the medial side of the temporal fossa. Such aneurysms erode the superior orbital fissure, optic canal and sometimes the skull base in a characteristic way (Fig. 5–8). (2) Within the subarachnoid space, either on the supraclinoid part of the internal carotid or its major branches, or on the bas-

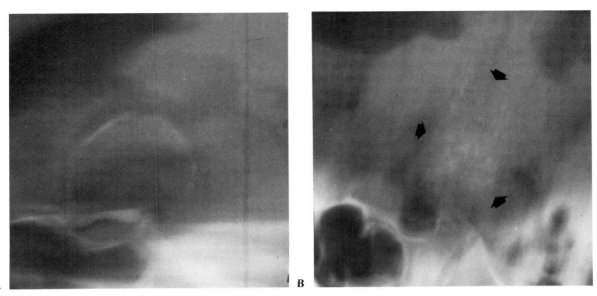

Fig. 5—32 Two cases of calcified craniopharyngioma. (A) Curvilinear deposits outlining the tumor. (B) Nodular deposits within the tumor, outlined by arrows.

ilar artery. They frequently calcify. The importance is stressed of carrying out vertebral and bilateral carotid angiography to exclude aneurysm, in any unexplained suprasellar mass, and especially if it contains curvilinear calcification.

Optic Glioma
Piloid astrocytomas of the anterior optic pathway form a distinct clinical entity—perhaps accounting

for as many as 7 percent of the gliomas of childhood (Fowler and Matson, 1957; Tym, 1961). Characteristically they are slow-growing tumors—at least some are present at birth—and their clinical picture may be so ill-defined that the burden of diagnosis is radiological. Malignant optic gliomas of adulthood, also, tend to present with vague symptoms and signs (Hoyt et al., 1973).

The plain skull radiographs may have a distinc-

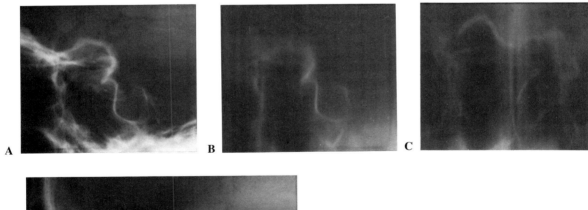

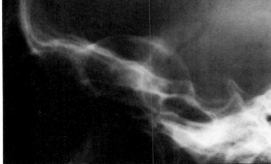

Fig. 5—33 Meningioma "blisters." (A, B, C) Typical pneumosinus dilatans of a planum meningioma. (D) Blister-like hyperostosis transforming the right half of the sphenoid ridge—a precursor of the typical hyperostotic sphenoid wing meningioma.

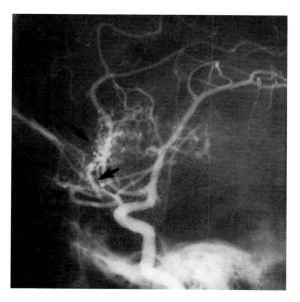
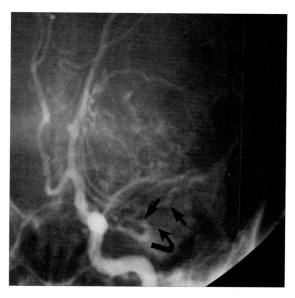

Fig. 5—34 Hypertrophied recurrent dural branches *(arrows)* of the left ophthalmic artery *(curved arrows)* supplying a large medial-third sphenoid meningioma. Note also the characteristic medial dislocation of the carotid siphon associated with an extradural mass in the temporal fossa (Compare with Fig. 5–20).

tive appearance in reflecting both the site and slow growth of these tumors. The superior surface of the sphenoid bone (including the optic canal) and the bony orbit may show a deformed appearance, as if molded into abnormality by the enlarged optic nerve (s) and chiasm. Thus, one or both optic canals may enlarge geometrically to two or four times the normal size, with the cortical outline preserved. The chiasmatic sulcus is deepened to the **J** sella deformity described above. Evans et al. (1963)

found the following defects in their 56 children with optic gliomas.:

J sella	20/55 (36 percent)
Enlarged optic canal	38/51 (74 percent)
Both canals enlarged	7/27 (26 percent)
Enlarged orbit	11/55 (20 percent)

One optic canal was enlarged in 83 percent of children with tumors of the optic nerve, and in 62 percent of children with tumors of the optic chiasm.

Important negative findings were the absence of

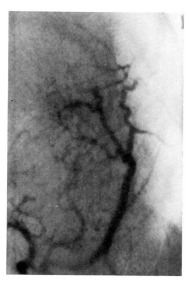
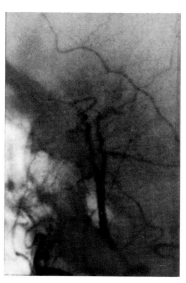
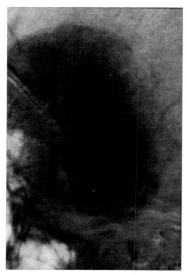

Fig. 5—35 Hypertrophied middle meningeal branch of the left external carotid artery, supplying a pterional meningioma through its pedicle of attachment. The middle meningeal was largely responsible for the characteristic "blush" of the tumor, and selective internal carotid injection revealed merely displaced vessels.

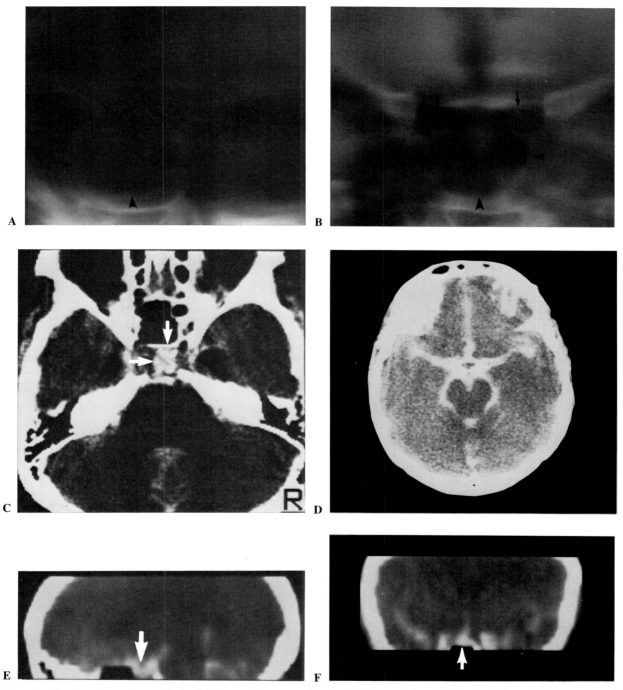

Fig. 5–40 Empty sella syndrome. (A, B) A 51-year-old woman with visual failure and signs of chronic pituitary deficiency, with a ballooned sella. Tomopneumography in coronal and lateral planes revealed intrasellar herniation of the pituitary cistern *(arrowheads)*. The anterior ecesses of the third ventricle, the optic nerves *(arrows)* and the pituitary stalk appeared to be undisplaced. (C, D, E, F) Metrizamide cisternography in patient with empty sella syndrome. (C) On axial scan, metrizamide is observed *(arrows)* occupying the sella turcica. (D) Normal suprasellar cistern. (E, F) Sagittal and corona reconstructions confirm presence of metrizamide *(arrows)* within the sella turcica and an absence of mass.

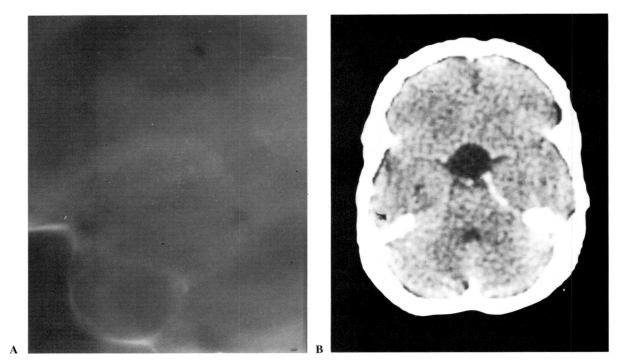

Fig. 5–41 Suprasellar arachnoid cyst of the noncommunicating variety in a 23-year-old man with bitemporal hemianopia. (A) Pneumographic diagnosis: primary pituitary tumor growing upward. (B) Computed tomogram of this patient.

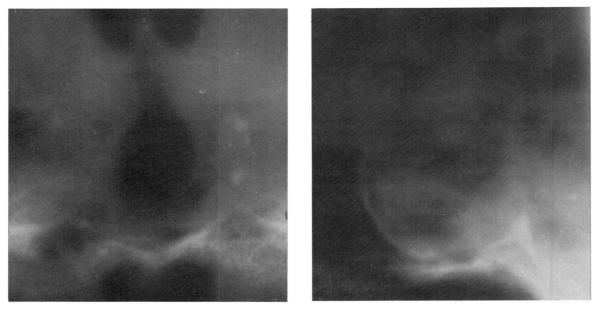

Fig. 5–42 Intrasellar third-ventricle herniation (empty sella syndrome) — a postoperative complication. A 58-year-old woman with a history of craniotomy for chromophobe adenoma 20 years previously, complained of progressive visual loss for 6 months. Biplanar tomopneumography revealed a dilated third ventricle, with its anterior end herniated into an enlarged pituitary fossa; no evidence was present of a suprasellar mass. Exploratory craniotomy: empty sella, with optic nerves carried into the fossa as part of the process of herniation.

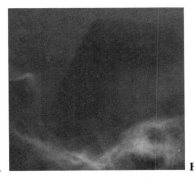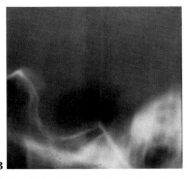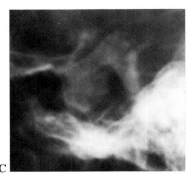

A   B   C

Fig. 5–43 Intrasellar cisternal and third-ventricle herniation (empty sella syndrome), complicating nontumor aqueduct stenosis in a 12-year-old boy. (A) Ventriculogram showing anterior end of the dilated third-ventricle occupying the pituitary fossa, which shows typical deformity. (B) Pneumoencephalogram showing herniation of the pontine cistern into the pituitary fossa. (C) Another patient with the empty-sella syndrome, confirmed by metrizamide cisternography. (Reproduced by courtesy of Dr. V. McAllister, Newcastle General Hospital, Newcastle-upon-Tyne.)

REFERENCES

Albert, M. and LeMay, M.: Demineralisation of the dorsum sellae associated with alcoholism. British Journal of Radiology, *41*, 331–332, 1968.

Anderson, R. D.: Tortuosity of the cavernous carotid arteries causing sellar expansion simulating pituitary adenoma. American Journal of Roentgenology, *126*, 1203–1210, 1976.

Bajraktari X., Grepe, A. and Goulatia, R. K.: Pneumoencephalographic changes with intrasellar cisternal herniation (primary empty sella). Neuroradiology, *13*, 97–106, 1977.

Baker, H. L., Jr.: The angiographic delineation of sellar and parasellar masses. Radiology, *104*, 67–78, 1972.

Banna, M.: Arachnoid cysts in the hypophyseal region. Clinical Radiology, *25*, 323–326, 1974.

Banna, M.: Craniopharyngioma: based on 160 cases. British Journal of Radiology, *49*, 206–223, 1976a.

Banna, M.: Arachnoid cysts on computed tomography. American Journal of Roentgenology, *127*, 979–982, 1976b.

Banna, M.: Arachnoid cysts on computed tomography. American Journal of Roentgenology, *127*, 979–982, 1976c.

Binet, E. F., Kieffer, S. A., Martin, S. H. and Peterson, H. O.: Orbital dysplasia in neurofibromatosis. Radiology, *93*, 829–833, 1969.

Bonneville, J. F., Bugault, R., Van Effenterre, R., Pertuiset, B. and Metzger, J.: Delineation of pituitary adenomas by angiotomography. Neuroradiology, *11*, 49–51, 1976.

Bull, J.: The normal variations of the position of the optic recess of the third ventricle. Acta Radiologica, *46*, 72–80, 1956.

Bull, J. W. D. and Schunk, H.: The significance of displacement of the cavernous portion of the internal carotid artery. British Journal of Radiology, *35*, 801–814, 1962.

Burrows, E. H.: The so-called J-sella. British Journal of Radiology, *37*, 661–669, 1964.

Burrows, E. H.: False-negative results in brain scanning. British Medical Journal, *1*, 473–476, 1972.

Burrows, E. H.: Intracranial calcification. In Newton, T. H. and Potts, D. G., Eds.: Radiology of the Skull and Brain, Vol. 1, St. Louis: C. V. Mosby, 1971.

Burrows, E. H.: Orbitocranial asymmetry. British Journal of Radiology, *51*, 771–781, 1978.

Caille, J. M., Piton, J., Basseau, J. P., Gerves, P. and Broussin, J.: Cisterno-tomographie de la région opto-chiasmatique dans l'etude du syndrome chiasmatique. Journal de Radiologie et d'Electrologie, *52*, 663–668, 1971.

Castroviejo, I. P., Martin, V. L., Knapp, K. and Costa, R. T.: Examen radiologique des tumeurs de la région du chiasma et de l'hypothalamus. Annales de Radiologie, *13*, 149–155, 1970.

Chase, N. E. and Taveras, J. M.: Carotid angiography in the diagnosis of extradural parasellar tumors. Acta Radiologica Diagnosis, *1*, 214–224, 1963.

Danziger, J. and Bloch, S.: Hypothalamic tumours presenting as the diencephalic syndrome. Clinical Radiology, *25*, 153–156, 1974.

Danziger, J. and Bloch, S.: The radiology of arachnoid pouches. Clinical Radiology, *26*, 275–283, 1975.

Di Chiro, G. and Nelson, K. B.: The volume of the sella turcica. American Journal of Roentgenology, *87*, 989–1008, 1962.

Drayer, B. P., Rosenbaum, A. E. and Higman, H. B.: Cerebrospinal fluid imaging using serial metrizamide CT cisternography. Neuroradiology, *13*, 7–17, 1977a.

Drayer, B. P., Rosenbaum, A. E., Kennerdell, J. S., Robinson, A. G., Bank, W. O. and Deeb, Z. L.: Computed tomographic diagnosis of suprasellar masses by intrathecal enhancement. Radiology, *123*, 339–344, 1977b.

Du Boulay, G. and El Gammal, T.: The classification, clinical value and mechanism of sella turcica changes in raised intracranial pressure. British Journal of Radiology, *39*, 421–442, 1966.

Du Boulay, G. and Trickey, S.: The sella in aqueduct stenosis and communicating hydrocephalus. British Journal of Radiology, *43*, 319–326, 1970.

El Gammal, T. and Allen, M. B.: Further consideration of sellar changes associated with increased intracranial pressure. British Journal of Radiology, *45*, 561–569, 1972a.

El Gammal, T. and Allen, M. B.: The intrasellar subarachnoid recess. Some clinical and radiologic observations. Acta Radiologic Diagnosis, *13*, 401–412, 1972b.

Epstein, B. S. and Epstein, J. A.: The angiographic demonstration and surgical implications of imbedding of the carotid syphons by a large pituitary adenoma. American Journal of Roentgenology, *104*, 162–167, 1968.

Evans, R. A., Schwartz, J. F. and Chutorian, A. M.: Radiologic diagnosis in pediatric ophthalmology. Radiologic Clinics of North America, *1*, 459–495, 1963.

Fowler, F. D. and Matson, D. D.: Gliomas of the optic pathways in childhood. Journal of Neurosurgery, *14*, 515–528, 1957.

Fry, I. K. and Du Boulay, G.: Some observations on the sella in old age and arterial hypertension. British Journal of Radiology, *38*, 16–22, 1965.

Gado, M. and Bull, J. W. D.: The carotid angiogram in suprasellar masses. Neuroradiology, *2*, 136–153, 1971.

George, A. E., Raybaud, C., Salamon, G. and Kricheff, I. I.: Anatomy of the thalamoperforating arteries with special emphasis on arteriography of the third ventricle: Part 1. American Journal of Roentgenology, *124*, 220–230, 1975a.

George, A. E., Salamon, G. and Kricheff, I. I.: Pathologic anatomy of the thalamoperforating arteries in lesions of the third ventricle: Part II. American Journal of Roentgenology, *124*, 231–240, 1975b.

Goalwin, H. A.: One thousand optic canals: clinical anatomic and roentgenologic study. Journal of the American Medical Association, *89*, 1745–1748, 1927.

Gregorius, F. K. and Bentson, J. R.: Comparison of radiological tests in the detection of presellar meningiomas. Neuroradiology, *8*, 267–274, 1975.

Greitz, T., Ekbom, K., Kugelberg, E. and Breig, A.: Occult hydrocephalus due to ectasia of the basilar artery. Acta Radiologica Diagnosis, *9*, 312–316, 1969.

Gyldensted, C. and Karle, A.: Computed tomography of intra- and juxtasellar lesions. A radiological study of 108 cases. Neuroradiology, *14*, 5–13, 1977.

Hallpike, J. F.: Superior orbital fissure syndrome. Some clinical and radiological observations. Journal of Neurology, Neurosurgery and Psychiatry, *36*, 486–490, 1973.

Hanafee, W.: Plain views of the orbit. Radiologic Clinics of North America, *10*, 167–179, 1972.

Hanafee, W., Rosen, L. M., Weidner, W. and Wilson, G. H.: Venography of cavernous sinus, orbital veins and basal venous plexus. Radiology, *84*, 751–753, 1965.

Handa, J., Kikuchi, H. and Handa, H.: Angiographic demonstration of dural branches of the internal carotid artery in sphenoid ridge meningiomas. American Journal of Roentgenology, *101*, 28–33, 1967.

Hasso, A. N., Bentson, J. R., Wilson, G. H. and Vignaud, J.: Neuroradiology of the sphenoidal region. Radiology, *114*, 619–627, 1975.

Hatam, A.: The vascular supply of eosinophilic and mixed pituitary adenomas in acromegalic patients. Neuroradiology, *3*, 4–7, 1971.

Hilal, S. K.: Angiography in juxtasellar masses. Seminars in Roentgenology, *6*, 75–88, 1971.

Holman, C. B.: Roentgenologic manifestations of glioma of the optic nerve and chiasm. American Journal of Roentgenology, *82*, 462–471, 1959.

Hoyt, W. F., Meshel, L. G., Lessell, S., Schatz, N. J. and Suckling, R. D.: Malignant optic glioma of adulthood. Brain, *96*, 121–132, 1973.

Johnson, J. C., Lubow, M. and Stears, J.: Polytomoencephalography of the optic chiasm and adjacent structures. Radiology, *114*, 629–132, 1973.

Johnson, J. C., Lubow, M. and Stears, J.: Polytomoencephalography of the optic chiasm and adjacent structures. Radiology, *114*, 629–634, 1975.

Joplin, G. F. and Fraser, R.: Cited by Oon, C. L. The size of the pituitary fossa in adults. British Journal of Radiology, *42*, 845–847, 1963.

Kaufman, B.: The "empty" sella – a manifestation of the intrasellar subarachnoid space. Radiology, *90*, 931–941, 1968.

Kaufman, B. and Chamberlin, W. B. Jr.: The ubiquitous "empty" sella turcica. Acta Radiologica Diagnosis, *13*, 413–425, 1972.

Keller, N. and Galatius-Jensen, F.: Enlarged sella turcica associated with a rare vascular anomaly. British Journal of Radiology, *48*, 936–937, 1975.

Kier, E. L.: 'J' and 'omega' shape of sella turcica. Anatomic clarification of radiologic misconceptions. Acta Radiologica Diagnosis, *9*, 91–94, 1969.

Kosowicz, J. and Rzymski, K.: Radiologic features of the skull in Klinefelter's syndrome and male hypogonadism. Clinical Radiology, *26*, 371–378

Kuru, Y.: Meningeal branches of the ophthalmic artery. Acta Radiologica Diagnosis, *6*, 241–251, 1967.

Lee, K. F.: The diagnostic value of hyperostosis in midline subfrontal meningioma. An analysis of 66 cases. Radiology, *119*, 121–130, 1976.

Leeds, N. and Naidich, T. P.: Computerized tomography in the diagnosis of sellar and parasellar lesions. Seminars in Roentgenology, *12*, 121–135, 1977.

Lewtas, N. A.: Symposium on pituitary tumours. (2) Radiology in diagnosis and management. Clinical Radiology, *17*, 149–153, 1966.

Lewtas, N. A. and Jefferson, A. A.: The carotid cistern. A source of diagnostic difficulties with suprasellar extensions of pituitary adenomata. Acta Radiologica Diagnosis, *5*, 675–690, 1966.

Liliequist, B.: The subarachnoid cisterns. Acta Radiologica Supplementum, *185*, 1959.

Lin, J. P. and Kricheff, I. I.: Displacement of the anterior cerebral artery complex by intracranial masses. In Newton, T. H. and Potts, D. G., Eds.: Radiology of the Skull and Brain, Vol. 2, St. Louis: C. V. Mosby, 1974.

Lindgren, E. and Di Chiro, G.: Suprasellar tumours with calcification. Acta Radiologica, *36*, 173–195, 1951.

Lloyd, G. A. S.: Radiological signs in proptosis. Transactions of the Ophthalmological Society of the United Kingdom, *87*, 375–383, 1967.

McConnell, E. M.: The arterial supply of the human hypophysis cerebri. Anatomical Record, *115*, 175–203, 1953.

McLachlan, M. S. F., Lavender, J. P. and Edwards, C. R. W.: Polytome-encephalography in the investigation of pituitary tumours. Clinical Radiology, *22*, 361–369, 1971.

McLachlan, M. S. F., Williams, E. D., Fortt, R. W. and Doyle, F. H.: Estimation of pituitary gland dimensions from radiographs of the sella turcica. A post-mortem study. British Journal of Radiology, *41*, 323–330, 1968.

Mahmoud, M. E. S.: The sella in health and disease. British Journal of Radiology, Supplement 8, 1958.

Maravilla, K. R.: Computer reconstructed sagittal and coronal computed tomography head scans: clinical applications. Journal of Computer Assisted Tomography, *2*:189–198, 1978.

Marshall, D.: Glioma of the optic nerve (as a manifestation of von Recklinghausen's disease). American Journal of Ophthalmology, *37*, 15–36, 1954.

Martin, P. and Cushing, H.: Primary gliomas of chiasm and optic nerves in their intracranial part. Archives of Ophthalmology, *52*, 209–241, 1923.

Mascherpa, F. and Valentino, V.: Intracranial Calcification. Springfield: Charles C Thomas, 1959.

Naidich, T. P., Pinto, R. S., Kushner, M. J., Lin, J. P., Kricheff, I. I., Leeds, N. E. and Chase, N. E.: Evaluation of sellar and parasellar masses by computed tomography. Radiology, *120*, 91–99, 1976.

Otto, H., Fiebach, O., Sauer, J., Bettag, W., Löhr, E. and Strötges, M. W.: Cerebral scintigraphy in relation to roentgenological methods for detection of tumours situated in the sellar region and the posterior fossa. Neuroradiology, *4*, 30–35, 1972.

Overbeek, W. J., Front, D. and Penning, L.: Primary enlarged "empty" sella. Neurochirurgia, *14*, 110–115, 1971.

Palacios, E., Azar-Kia, B., Williams, V.: The significance of the dural supply from the carotid siphon. American Journal of Roentgenology, *125*, 816–822, 1975.

Powell, D. F., Baker, H. L. and Laws, E. R.: The primary angiographic findings in pituitary adenomas. Radiology, *110*, 589–595, 1974.

Rådberg, C.: Some aspects of the asymmetric enlargement of sella turcica. Acta Radiologica Diagnosis, *1*, 152–163, 1963a.

Rådberg, C.: Appearance of sella turcica following transsphenoidal hypophysectomy. Acta Radiologica Diagnosis, *1*, 140–151, 1963b.

Rischbieth, R. H. C. and Bull, J. W. D.: The significance of enlargement of the superior orbital (sphenoidal) fissure. British Journal of Radiology, *31*, 125–135, 1958.

Roberson, C. and Till, K.: Hypothalamic gliomas in children. Journal of Neurology, Neurosurgery and Psychiatry, *37*, 1047–1052, 1974.

Robertson, W. D. and Newton, T. H.: Radiologic assessment of pituitary microadenomas. American Journal Roentgenology, *131*:489–492, 1978.

Ross, R. J. and Greitz, T. V. B.: Changes of the sella turcica in chromophobic adenomas and eosinophilic adenomas. Radiology, *86*, 892–899, 1966.

Roth, D. A., Ferris, E. J. and Tomiyasu, U.: Prognosis of pituitary adenomas with arteriographic abnormal vascularization. Journal of Neurology, Neurosurgery and Psychiatry, *34*, 535–540, 1971.

Rozario, R., Hammerschlag, S. B., Post, K. D., Wolpert, S. M. and Jackson, I.: Diagnosis of empty sella with CT scan. Neuroradiology, *13*, 85–88, 1977.

Sage, M. R. and McAllister, V. L.: Spontaneous intracranial "aerocoele" with chromophobe adenoma. British Journal of Radiology, *47*, 727–729, 1974.

Sansregret, A. and Ledoux, R.: Lesser wing meningiomas: A few unfamiliar differential diagnoses. Neuroradiology, *2*, 9–14, 1971.

Sauer, J., Fiebach, O., Otto, H., Löhr, E., Strötges, M. W. and Bettag, W.: Comparative studies of cerebral scintigraphy, angiography and encephalography for detection of meningiomas. Neuroradiology, *2*, 102–106, 1971.

Scatliff, J. H. and Bull, J. W. D.: The radiological manifestations of suprasellar metastatic disease. Clinical Radiology, *16*, 66–70, 1965.

Schnürer, L-B. and Stattin, S.: Vascular supply of intracranial dura from internal carotid artery with special reference to its angiographic significance. Acta Radiologica Diagnosis, *1*, 441–450, 1963.

Schuster, G. and Westberg, G.: Gliomas of the optic nerve and chiasm. Acta Radiologica Diagnosis, *6*, 221–232, 1967.

Sheldon, P. and Molyneux, A.: Metrizamide cisternography and computed tomography in the investigation of pituitary lesions. Neuroradiology, *17*:83–87, 1979.

Shopfner, C., Wolfe, T. W. and O'Kell, R. T.: The interspehenoid synchondrosis. American Journal of Roentgenology, *104*, 184–193, 1968.

Stattin, S.: Meningeal vessels of the internal carotid artery and their angiographic significance. Acta Radiologica, *55*, 329–336, 1961.

Swanson, H. A. and Du Boulay, G.: Borderline variants of the normal pituitary fossa. British Journal of Radiology, *48*, 366–369, 1975.

Syvertsen A., Haughton V. M., Williams L. and Cusick J. E.: The computed tomographic appearance of the normal pituitary gland and pituitary microadenomas. Radiology, *133*, 385–392, 1979.

Tolosa, E.: Periarteritic lesions of the carotid siphon with the clinical features of a carotid infraclinoid aneurysm. Journal of Neurology, Neurosurgery and Psychiatry, *17*, 300–302, 1954.

Tym, R.: Piloid gliomas of the anterior optic pathway. British Journal of Surgery, *49*, 322–331, 1961.

Underwood, L. E., Radcliffe, W. B. and Guinto, F. C.: New standards for the assessment of sella turcica volume in children, Radiology, *119*, 651–654, 1976.

Vezina, J. L. and Sutton, T. J.: Prolactin-secreting pituitary microadenomas, roentgenologic diagnosis. American Journal of Roentgenology, *120*, 46–54, 1974.

Waga, S., Kikuchi, H., Handa, J. and Handa, H.: Cavernous sinus venography. American Journal of Roentgenology, *109*, 130–137, 1970.

Wallace, S., Goldberg, H. I., Leeds, N. E. and Mishkin, M. M.: The cavernous branches of the internal carotid artery. American Journal of Roentgenology, *101*, 34–46, 1967.

Westberg, G.: Angiographic changes in neurinoma of the trigeminal nerve. Acta Radiologica Diagnosis, *1*, 513–520, 1963.

Westberg, G. and Ross, R. J.: The vascular supply in chromophobe adenomas. Acta Radiologica Diagnosis, *6*, 475–480, 1967.

Wiggli, U. and Oberson, R.: Pneumosinus dilatans and hyperostosis: Early signs of meningiomas of the anterior chiasmatic angle. Neuroradiology, *8*, 217–221, 1975.

6 Supratentorial Hemispherical Lesions

The two radiological techniques best suited to study the cerebral hemispheres are computed tomography and carotid angiography. Cerebral scintigraphy is a reliable noninvasive method for verifying the presence of a lesion and demonstrating its location and size, but it is inferior to computed tomography in information yield. Angiography frequently provides a type diagnosis when noninvasive methods fail to do so, and it may be a preoperative requirement. Vertebral injection is necessary to examine the cortex of the occipital lobe by angiography in patients with signs such as homonymous hemianopia, if the posterior cerebral artery fails to fill during carotid injection.

INTRODUCTION

This chapter deals with the radiological investigation of lesions of the cerebral hemispheres and their coverings, excluding trauma (Ch. 4). Most such lesions affect the cerebral cortex and subcortical white matter of the four lobes: frontal, parietal, temporal and occipital. Involvement of the basal ganglia, ventricles and other deep structures is covered in Chapter 7. Degenerative diseases of the white matter are dealt with in Chapter 10.

Because important functional parts of the brain lie in the hemispheres, such as the motor and sensory cortex, higher cortical centers for vision and hearing and the optic radiations, the clinical picture is often dominated by "hard" signs. These include hemiparesis, apraxia, aphasia or homonymous hemianopia which always lateralize the lesion, and may localize it within a particular hemisphere. Often the questions for the neuroradiologist to answer are not so much, Is there a lesion present? as, What is the likely histological diagnosis, and, Is the lesion space-occupying and therefore potentially treatable surgically?

COMPUTED TOMOGRAPHY

Computed tomography is an important first step in demonstrating the presence of an intracranial lesion. This examination usually proves sufficient for primary diagnosis, i.e., whether or not an abnormality is present, and whether it is space-occupying. It outlines the extent and location of mass lesions in a satisfactory way, although surgical requirement in some patients may demand the additional use of angiography or even pneumography to achieve a more precise diagnosis and localization.

The advantage of computed tomography over other imaging techniques is that the anatomy of the brain is displayed, and its relationship to pathological findings can be visualized. Horizontal slices are particularly useful in the supratentorial compartment, in which the lateral and third ventricles, gray matter, white matter and ganglionic substance can be demonstrated to advantage (Du Boulay and Marshall, 1975; New et al., 1975).

Accuracy and Diagnostic Patterns
The remarkable accuracy of this revolutionary diagnostic weapon virtually restricts false-negative or false-positive results to the realm of observer error and or technical inadequacy (Paxton and Am-

brose, 1974). The abnormalities that should be searched for include:

1. Midline shift: septum pellucidum, pineal calcification, and sometimes opacified arteries or veins.

2. Displacements other than the midline: displacement, compression or obliteration of the ventricles, displacement or dislocation of the calcified glomus bodies of the choroid plexus, displacement of vessels.

3. Parenchymal abnormalities: alterations in density (low-density lesions, high-density lesions, mixed-density lesions), shape and outline of lesions, and obliteration of tissue planes.

4. Contrast enhancement: abnormal pooling of contrast medium, enhancement of existing lesions, abnormal vessels.

5. Pathological calcification: site, nature, unifocal or multifocal.

6. Abnormalities of the skull: defects, destruction, expansion or thickening.

The diagnostic specificity depends on the nature of the lesion demonstrated. For example, collections of clotted blood and most arteriovenous malformations are recognizable without difficulty; however, solitary metastatic deposits can seldom be distinguished from malignant gliomas. Claveria and his colleagues (1977b) reported a series of 66 patients in whom they had made a diagnosis of supratentorial metastasis, of whom 41, i.e., over two-thirds, were subsequently confirmed as having some other pathology.

"Doughnut" Lesion: This term, which possesses no specific etiological connotation, describes a solitary mass with an enhancing capsular ring and a low-density core (Fig. 6–6). It occurs in a variety of lesions and represents either a tumor with a necrotic or cystic center, or it may be a nonspecific re-

sponse of the brain to cerebral insults. The center or lucent zone represents a cyst or an area of hemorrhage, infarction or necrosis. The peripheral ring of increased attenuation may be a zone of marginal hyperperfusion due to a loss of autoregulation, or it may consist of tumor or granulation tissue, or tissue undergoing regeneration. A "doughnut lesion" may represent any of the following:

1. Glioblastoma multiforme
2. Metastasis
3. Pyogenic, tuberculous or fungal abscess
4. Lymphoma or leukemia
5. Pituitary adenoma
6. Craniopharyngioma
7. Resolving hematoma
8. Resolving infarct
9. Postoperative deformity
10. Radiation necrosis
11. Post-traumatic cerebral damage
12. Multiple sclerosis
13. Giant aneurysm
14. Pseudo-ring

Solid Lesion: This term also is descriptive and nonspecific etiologically, but it differs in one important respect from ring lesions, in that it includes meningioma. Meningiomas exhibit fairly uniform characteristics, namely a tissue attenuation slightly higher than that of normal brain combined with the frequent presence of calcified deposits and hyperostotic bone. Contrast injection produces a dense and homogeneous image with well-defined margins.

Multiplicity: Such a wide variety of lesions, including non-neoplastic conditions, simulate multiple neoplastic metastases of the brain, that multiplicity *per se* possesses very little diagnostic value. Several foci within the territory of the same cere-

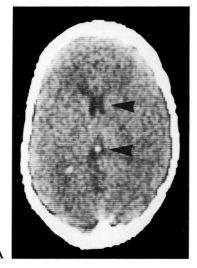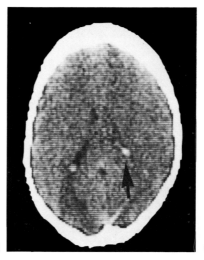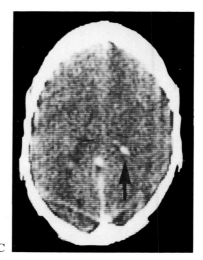

A   B   C

Fig. 6–1 Infiltrating low-grade astrocytoma. (A and B) Noncontrast slices show minimal displacement of the septum pellucidum and slight pineal shift (*arrowheads*). Slice A shows the left calcified glomus body only, while slice B (13 mm. higher) shows the right glomus displaced forward and upward (*arrow*). (C) Postcontrast slice shows that the mass is isodense, and fails to enhance.

bral artery are usually cortical infarcts from a shower of emboli, bland or infected, and rarely neoplastic metastases (Fig. 6–13). However, multiple infarcts may be distributed over both hemispheres and the cerebellum, and unlike metastases they may not all date from the same illness (see Fig. 6–20). The experience of computed tomography has confirmed that multiple neoplastic deposits are more frequent than has been demonstrated by conventional neuroradiological procedures in the past, and their incidence exceeds the 6 percent of all fatal cases of malignant disease reported by Willis (1967).

Glioma

Low-grade astrocytomas may show merely space-occupying properties if their tissue density corresponds to that of normal brain; even contrast enhancement may fail to outline them. Thus, displacement of the pineal and choroid calcification, of the ventricles or tissue planes, may be the only abnormality (Fig. 6–1). Tumor calcification or cystic change may aid in localization (Fig. 6–2 and 6–9). Cystic gliomas may show layering upon enhancement (Kingsley and Kendall, 1977).

Examination before as well as after contrast injection is important in diagnosis and differential diagnosis: foci of calcification, altered blood or other high-density lesions can be identified only if noncontrast slices are available. Low-grade gliomas appearing as low-density lesions may upon enhancement be isodense (Fig. 6–3; New et al., 1975) or show a mixed-density pattern. Most gliomas show enhancement and provoke surrounding ede-

ma (Figs. 6–4 and 6–5). Ventricular displacement may be minimal, especially in vertex tumors (Fig. 6–5). Surface lesions tend to efface cortical sulci and if very slow-growing, they may produce localized thinning of the skull.

Malignant glial tumors (glioblastoma multiforme, astrocytoma grades 3–4) enhance vividly upon the injection of contrast medium. Peritumoral edema is a prominent feature which usually displaces, compresses or obliterates the ventricles. Three patterns of enhancement are recognized (Figs. 6–6, 6–7 and 6–8) but none permits a specific diagnosis of glioma or malignancy. "Doughnut" and ring lesions are not always cystic, since this appearance may represent necrosis (Figs. 6–9 and 6–10; Kramer et al., 1975; Thomson, 1976a; Steinhoff et al., 1977; Norman et al. 1978). An unusual feature is subependymal contrast enhancement, a sign indicating spread to the periventricular region (McGeachie et al., 1977).

Metastasis

A solitary deposit may be indistinguishable from a malignant glioma. Edema is usually present, and the lesion is round and well-defined with or without a lucent center (Figs. 6–11 and 6–12). Hematomas characterize metastases from melanoma, choriocarcinoma and sometimes also breast and lung (Mandybur, 1977). Multiplicity is not infrequent (Fig. 6–13). Kramer and his colleagues (1975) stressed the importance of an enhancement technique in such cases, to demonstrate all lesions, and the need of high slices to identify small vertex me-

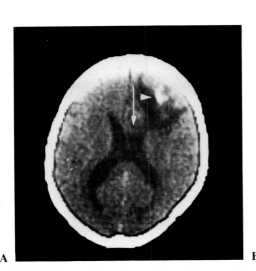
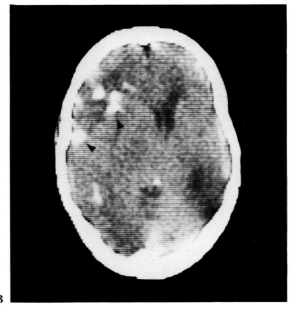

A   B

Fig. 6–2 Calcified gliomas shown by unenhanced computed tomography. (A) An irregular low-density mass is present in the right frontal lobe, obliterating the frontal horn and producing falcine herniation *(arrow)*. The high-density area within the mass *(arrowhead)* is a calcified deposit. (B) A 50-year-old chronic epileptic in whom examination showed marked midline displacement and ventricular compression. The mass contains discrete nodular deposits of calcium *(arrowheads)*. The low-density area in the right temporal region is an artifact.

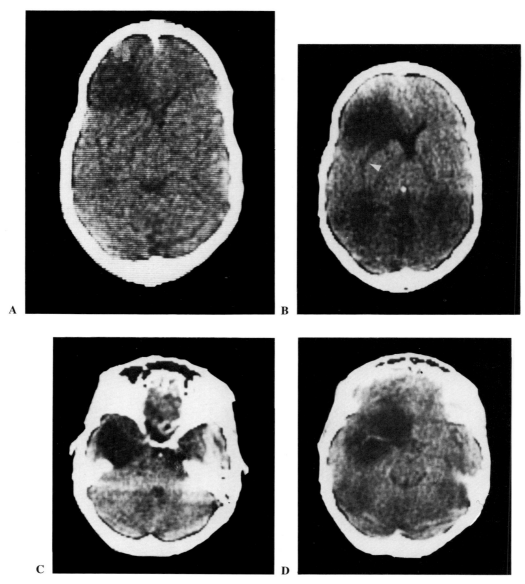

Fig. 6–3 Low-grade astrocytomas. (A and B) A 55-year-old woman had a generalized seizure. The initial examination (A) revealed a low-density lesion in the left frontal lobe which did not enhance with contrast medium. Slight compression and ventricular displacement was noted, but the patient was treated conservatively. Re-examination 14 months later (B) showed considerable midline displacement due to spread of edema into the lateral ganglionic region *(arrowhead)*, but no enhancement occurred. Operation: astrocytoma, grade 1. (C and D) A glioma, grade 2, in a 31-year-old woman with temporal-lobe epilepsy, in whom examination showed a well-defined low-density lesion in the left temporal lobe which failed to enhance.

tastases (Fig. 6–11). Computed tomography is particularly useful in revealing small multiple lesions, especially in the posterior fossa, which scintigraphy fails to demonstrate (Bardfeld et al., 1977).

Metastases are often dural based and thus may be difficult to differentiate from a meningioma. Hyperemia of the dura and tentorium can occur.

Meningioma

Meningiomas occur in particular locations—parasagittal (Fig. 6–14), cortical convexity (Fig. 6–15), sphenoid wing (Fig. 6–16), falx (Fig. 6–17), floor of the anterior cranial fossa (Fig. 6–18). The ap-

pearances on computed tomography are uniform and often characteristic: in unenhanced slices the tumor is usually slightly denser than the normal parenchyma, with well-defined round or lobulated margins and often containing psammomatous calcification. Enhancement produces uniformly dense intensification, which accentuates the sharp edges of the tumor. The surrounding edema present in most meningiomas may be a thin halo (Fig. 6–18) or hemispherical in extent (Fig. 6–16) (Vassilouthis and Ambrose, 1979). Figure 6–15 shows that ventricular displacement or compression depends on the amount of edema present, since meningiomas

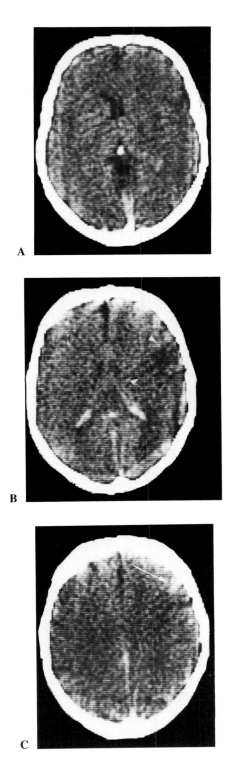

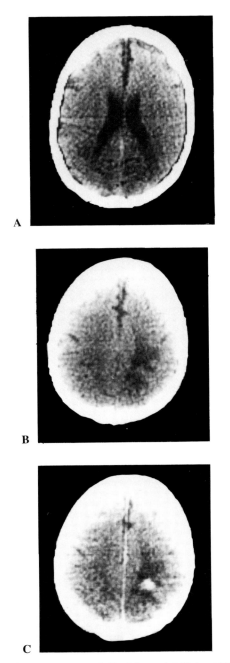

Fig. 6−5 Astrocytoma, grade 3, of the parietal lobe. (A) Ventricular slice shows no displacement or deformity of the lateral ventricles. (B) An unenhanced slice at a higher level shows an irregular low-density lesion in the right parietal lobe — an appearance which represents peritumoral edema. (C) Slice at the same level after contrast injection, reveals an enhancing mass surrounded by edema.

Fig. 6−4 Astrocytoma, grade 2, of the right frontal lobe, post-enhancement slices. (A) The anterior horn of the right lateral ventricle is deformed and there is slight midline displacement. (B) Slice 26 mm. higher, showing an irregular, low-density lesion (arrowheads). (C) Slice 13 mm. higher still, a triangular area of enhancement (arrow) is present in the cortex of the frontal lobe.

themselves cause minimal dislocation. The supratentorial lesions are border forming on convexity or parasagitally with a broad base and sharp margins. Adjacent bone thickening adds a pathognomonic dimension to the diagnosis in those cases in which the computed tomographic ap-

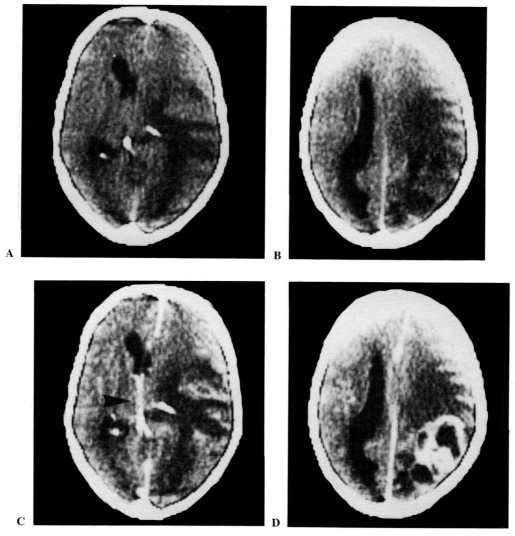

Fig. 6–6 Glioblastoma multiforme of the parietal lobe: "doughnut" lesion. (A and B) Unenhanced ventricular slices show a low-density lesion of the posterior half of the right hemisphere, with finger-like projections into the cortex that indicate edema. There is marked midline displacement and the right glomus body is dislocated forward and medially. (C and D) Enhancement shows a "doughnut" lesion of the parietal lobe surrounded by extensive edema. The arrowhead points to the displaced internal cerebral vein. Surrounding gyri are enhanced as a result of a loss in cerebral auto-regulation.

pearances suggest a meningioma. In its absence, lesions with a propensity to affect the dura, such as solitary metastasis, astrocytoma or lymphoma, may be mistaken for meningioma (Claveria et al., 1977). Only exceptionally do meningiomas have a cystic or low-density core.

Other Lesions

Intracerebral Hematoma: See Chapter 3

Cerebral Infarction: Computed tomography is probably the most sensitive existing method for diagnosing cerebral infarction. Within 24 hours of the ictus the lesion will outline as a homogeneous low-density area, and the diagnosis of infarction is usually suggested by the absence of any mass effect such as midline displacement (Fig. 6–19). However, a proportion of infarcts show the following: (1)

Some infarcts may show no abnormality for 1 to 3 days. (2) For a brief period—which includes the 8th to the 18th days after the ictus, according to Yock and Marshall (1975)—infarcts may enhance with contrast injection. The enhancement corresponds to the area of damaged cortex, and often a pattern of abnormal gyri and sulci can be seen, a pattern which is dissimilar to neoplastic enhancement. (3) Large infarcts may be space-occupying, and these usually involve the white matter as well as the cortex. In the small proportion of infarcts that both enhance and displace the brain, other radiological investigations are required to prove the diagnosis, since they are indistinguishable from malignant gliomas or metastases.

Beyond the first 24 hours or after enhancement ceases, the appearances of cerebral infarcts do not

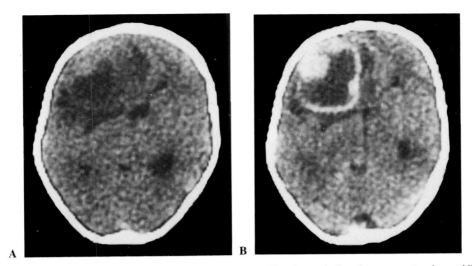

Fig. 6–7 Glioblastoma multiforme of the frontal lobe: "ring" lesion. (A) Unenhanced slice shows an extensive and ill-defined low-density mass in the left frontal lobe, displacing the anterior parts of the lateral ventricles. (B) Same slice after the injection of contrast medium shows the enhancing capsule of a necrotic tumor. This glioblastoma provoked less surrounding edema than that in Figure 6–6.

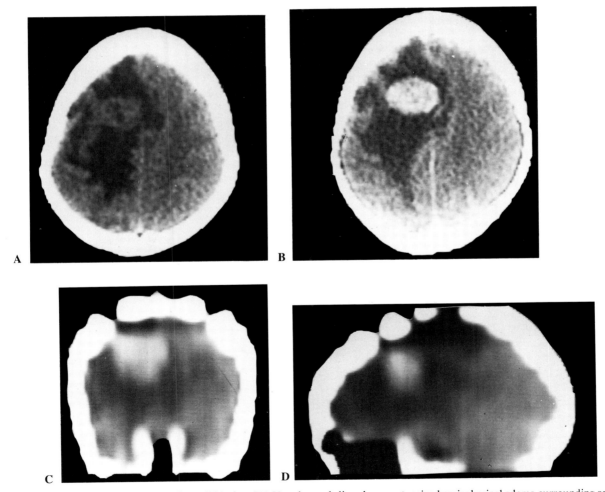

Fig. 6–8 Glioblastoma of the frontal lobe: solid lesion. (A) Unenhanced slice shows extensive hemispherical edema surrounding an isodense mass. (B) After contrast injection, the same slice displays the mass which enhances richly and homogeneously. (C and D) Reconstructed coronal and sagittal views provide localization for burrhole biopsy and accurately outline the extent of the surrounding edema.

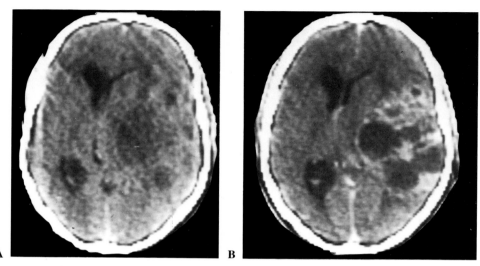

Fig. 6–9 Glioblastoma multiforme of the parietal lobe: cystic lesion. (A) The unenhanced slice shows a large mixed-density mass in the posterior frontal and parietal parts of the right hemisphere, displacing the midline structures. Most of the lateral ventricle has been obliterated. (B) An injection of contrast medium produces vivid enhancement of the multicystic tumor.

alter much. Focal atrophy of the adjacent cerebral substance leads to ipsilateral ventricular enlargement and midline displacement, but the low-density scar remains present for years (Fig. 6–20). Identical low-density areas are seen in patients who survive intracerebral hematomas, and the nature of the original ictus cannot be predicted from the computed tomographic appearance (Cronqvist et al. 1975; Messina and Chernik, 1975; Davis et al., 1975). Resolving hematomas and infarcts both occasionally present as "doughnut" lesions (Zimmerman et al., 1977).

Intracranial Infection Including Brain Abscess: Pyogenic, tuberculous or fungal organisms may produce an abscess or meningitis, and the herpes simplex virus may cause a focal or multifocal encephalitis. The greater diagnostic value of computed tomography in these lesions has been established, compared to the indifferent yield obtained from carotid angiography and scintigraphy. The early diagnosis and precise localization of abscesses has always been important to the neurosurgeon, but promising new chemotherapeutics have added a fresh urgency to the diagnosis of herpes simplex encephalitis.

A purulent brain abscess is recognized by its distinctive capsule—a smooth, ring-like structure of uniform thickness recognized only after contrast

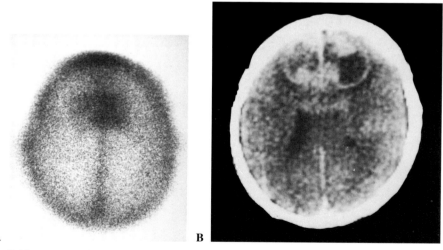

Fig. 6–10 Bifalcine glioblastoma multiforme. A 55-year-old man with mental deterioration and papilledema, in whom scintigraphic examination suggested the presence of a bifalcine meningioma (A, vertex view). (B) Enhanced computed tomographic slice shows obliteration of both lateral ventricles by a bifrontal necrotic mass. The glioblastoma probably arose in the corpus callosum and spread into the medial parts of both frontal lobes.

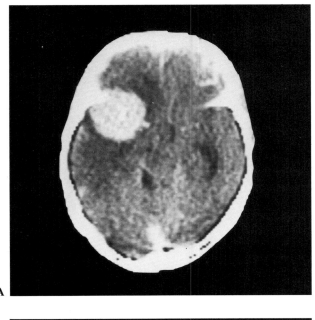

A

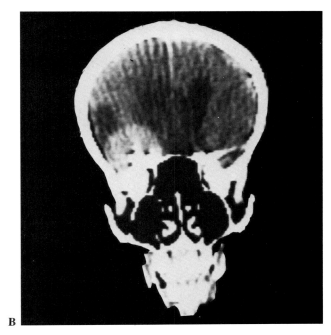

B

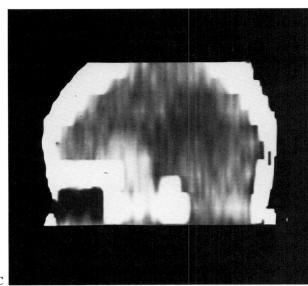

C

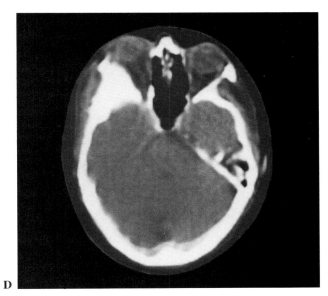

D

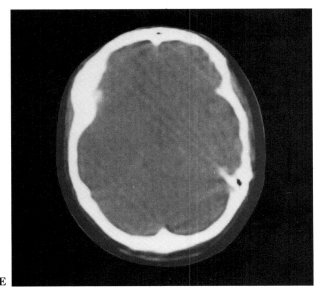

E

Fig. 6−16 Pterional meningioma in a 55-year-old woman. (A and B) Horizontal and coronal slices made after contrast injection show a tumor that is perfectly round, homogeneously enhancing and arising from a thickened left pterion. A halo of edema surrounds the tumor. The coronal view indicates the extent of ventricular deformity and midline displacement. (C) Reconstructed sagittal view. (D and E) Another outer-wing sphenoid meningioma. The patient, a 60-year-old woman, complained of a progressive painless left proptosis. The thickened bone and the extent of its encroachment upon the left orbital cavity and pterygomandibular fossa can be appreciated by comparison with the normal anatomy of the right side. The eyeball is displaced forward and the optic nerve is stretched and dislocated medially by the abnormal bony buttress.

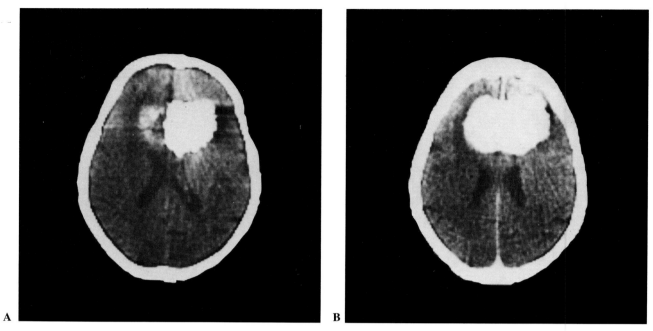

A   B

Fig. 6–17 Calcified falx meningioma. (A) The unenhanced slice shows a bifalcine mass of which the right half is solidly calcified. A halo of edema is visible. (B) After the injection of contrast medium, the rest of the tumor attenuates the beam almost as greatly as the calcified part.

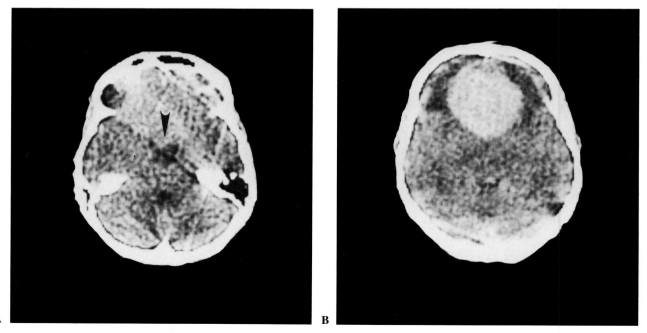

A   B

Fig. 6–18 Subfrontal meningioma arising from the cribriform plate. (A) Unenhanced slice reveals a mass deforming the anterior aspect of the suprasellar "star" *(arrowhead)*. The mass is slightly denser than normal brain. (B) Postcontrast slice made at a higher level, showing a giant, homogeneously-enhancing midline tumor surrounded by a thin rim of edema.

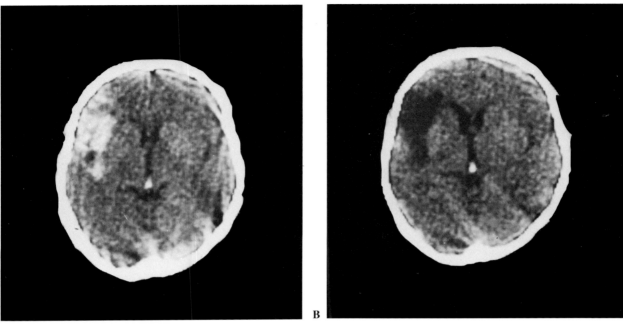

A   B

Fig. 6–19 Cerebral infarction in a 34-year-old man with atrial fibrillation who suddenly developed a right hemiplegia. Arteriography showed an embolus obstructing the mouth of the left middle cerebral artery. (A) Enhanced computed tomogram made 12 days after the ictus showing cortical hyperperfusion. (B) Repeat examination, same enhanced slice, 46 days later, i.e., 58 days after the ictus. Ipsilateral midline displacement due to atrophy is now present. For the time sequence of the hyperperfusion pattern, see Yock and Marshall (1975). For serial scintigrams of this patient, see Figure 6–29.

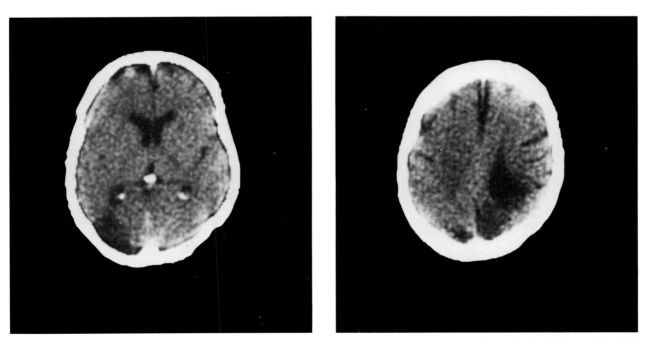

Fig. 6–20 Bilateral cerebral infarcts of 13 years' standing. The patient at the age of 32 years, seven days after the delivery of her fifth child, suddenly became drowsy and complained of blindness; subsequently she partly recovered her sight. Two years later, in 1965, on the basis of the history and clinical signs then present, a neurologist diagnosed visual disorientation due to bilateral parieto-occipital lesions and published a report of the case in a journal (Godwin-Austen, 1965). Computed tomography in 1976 confirmed the neurologist's diagnosis: in the slices demonstrated here, a low-density lesion is present in the parieto-occipital cortex of each hemisphere, without displacement of the brain.

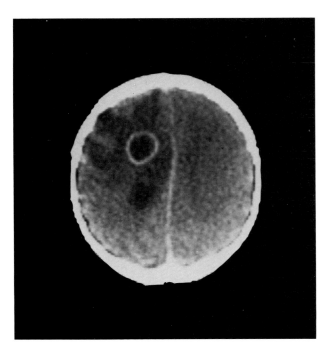

Fig. 6–21 Cerebral abscess secondary to pyogenic sinusitis in a 12-year-old boy. The abscess, once formed, has a tense capsule which enhances vividly upon contrast injection. Note the wide area of edema.

ferential-diagnostic clues: convexity masses usually displace the pineal from the midline, while most patients with cerebral infarction retain a central pineal because the cortical lesion does not take up space. Surface meningiomas usually present as a uniformly dense, well-defined and round area of abnormal uptake, and in more than 50 percent focal plain-film changes are present at the site of attachment of the tumor (Fig. 6 – 26). This combination is sufficient to establish the diagnosis of meningioma. A scintigraphic diagnosis of meningioma should not be ventured in the absence of focal bone changes, if the uptake is not in a characteristic location, i.e., abutting on the surface of the brain in two projections, and especially in the parasagittal gutter (Stannard, 1975). The "doughnut" scintigraphic lesion, a solitary ring of abnormal uptake with a less dense center, is a descriptive term without diagnostic significance. This appearance may be produced by neoplasms which are cystic or necrotic, abscess, resolving subdural hematoma or infarction, empyema, etc. (Fig. 6 – 27; Tarcan et al., 1976).

Crescent: Although a peripheral crescent on frontal or vertex scans is highly suggestive of a subdural hematoma or empyema, these conditions should not be diagnosed until two points have been verified from the radiographs, namely that the pineal is contralaterally displaced and that the calvarium is free from disease. In uncomplicated extracerebral collections the lateral scan may not be convincingly positive, while it is usually abnormal in the conditions that mimic the crescent of a subdural hematoma, namely scalp neoplasms or contusions, neoplasms or Paget's disease of the vault, or cerebral infarction (Fig. 6 – 28).

Linear: A solitary focus that connects by linear abnormal uptake with the superior sagittal sinus is usually a giant unruptured arteriovenous malformation. Any irregular forms of cortical uptake, i.e., not round in shape, should prompt thought of this condition, but a type diagnosis is impossible without the linear component (Fig. 3 – 4). Sylvian infarctions caused by occlusion of branches of the middle cerebral artery also may give rise to irregular, bizarre cortical foci.

Multiple: The causes of several foci of abnormal uptake confined to one hemisphere are: multiple infarction, regrowth of a partly treated meningioma or glioma, multifocal glioma, and only rarely metastatic abscess or neoplasm. Multiple lesions that lie in the same plane are usually sylvian infarcts (6 – 29) or craniotomy artifacts (Fig. 6 – 30). This appearance is unusual in multiple cerebral metastases, which seldom are confined to one hemisphere and may involve the posterior fossa as well. Symmetrical temporal lobe uptake strongly favors herpes simplex encephalitis, and this diagnosis should always be considered in the presence of multiple lesions. For scintigraphy in meningiomas, see Sauer et al. (1971) and Stannard (1975); oligodendrogliomas, see Schall et al. (1975); metastatic malignancy, see Sellwood (1972); childhood cancer, see Gilday and Ash (1975); clinical utility and false-negative results, see Burrows (1972a and 1972b).

ANGIOGRAPHY

Although replaced by computed tomography as the first step in supratentorial diagnosis, carotid angiography remains an investigation that may be essential for accurate diagnosis. The failure of computed and radioisotope imaging to provide information concerning the nature or histology of a lesion may be dramatically rectified by carrying out technically adequate angiography. For descriptive diagnostic purposes, the topographical arrangement proposed by Taveras and Wood (1976) is valuable because it corresponds to the conventional projections used for carotid angiography (Fig. 6 – 31).

Measurements
In lateral view the sylvian part of the middle cerebral artery is projected as an inverted triangle formed inferiorly by the main branch of the middle cerebral artery, anteriorly by the orbitofrontal branch within the sylvian fissure, and superiorly by

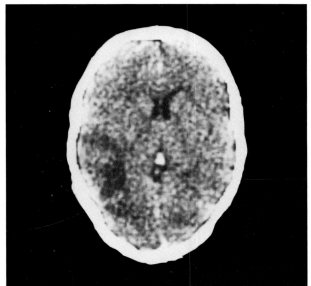

A

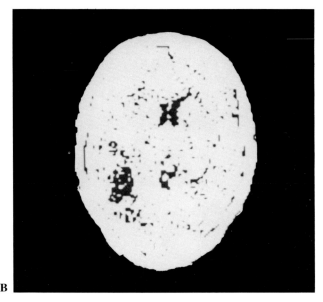

B

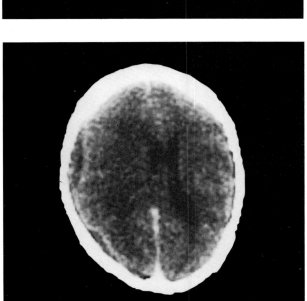

C

Fig. 6–22 Other inflammatory lesions. (A and B) "Cerebritis". A 23-year-old Algerian student with hyperpyrexia, stiff neck and headache for three days, who was admitted with a suspected brain abscess. The low-density lesion in the left parietal lobe is not accompanied by pineal displacement. Massive antibiotic therapy aborted the infection. (C) Subdural empyema secondary to pyogenic otitis media in a 25-year-old man. Following contrast enhancement, superficial extracerebral pockets are visible which may be mistaken for chronic extracerebral collections of blood.

a line joining the cranial loop of each ascending frontoparietal branch in the sylvian fissure to the ascending parietal branch as it emerges from the sylvian fissure *(sylvian point)*. The area thus outlined is called the *sylvian triangle* (Fig. 6–32). Deformity or dislocation of this triangle aids in the localization of supratentorial masses (Figs. 6–33 through 6–36).

The clinoparietal line is drawn from the tuberculum sellae to a point 9 cm. above the internal occipital protuberance or 2 cm. above the bregma. In the adult the axis of the middle cerebral artery in lateral projection should lie on this line or within 1 cm. above or below it. However, in children the middle

cerebral artery lies 2 cm. above the line, never on it.

The frontal view is essential for localizing masses; in some areas it is of greater value than the lateral. An important landmark is the angiographic sylvian point, i.e., the point at which the middle cerebral artery emerges from the sylvian fissure. It is projected in anteroposterior projection as the highest point within the sylvian fissure, and several branches arise from it and run superficially (Fig. 6–32). This point, which corresponds to point "B" of Taveras and Wood (1976), lies between 30 and 43 mm. from the inner table. These authors' other measurement, point "A," is also made on the anteroposterior view. It represents the central part of the insular segment of the middle cerebral artery, and lies between 20 and 30 mm. from the inner table.

Displacements

Arterial Dislocations in Lateral View: Frontal-lobe or frontal-pole lesions displace the sylvian triangle backwards and they may straighten the ascending frontoparietal branches as they emerge onto the surface of the hemisphere (Fig. 6–33).

Suprasylvian masses, i.e., those situated in the frontal, posterior frontal or parietal region of the convexity, depress or flatten the sylvian triangle and stretch or spread surface branches (Lehrer,

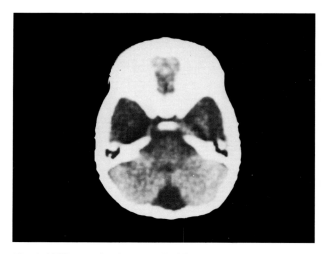 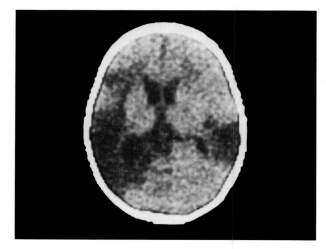

Fig. 6—23 Herpes simplex encephalitis in an 18-month-old boy. Both temporal lobes and the left parietal lobe are involved. A large cisterna magna is a normal variant.

1967). If the entire sylvian triangle is depressed, the lesion is described as suprasylvian (Fig. 6–34). Otherwise lesions are anterior mid, or posterior suprasylvian.

Retrosylvian lesions, i.e., those situated in the occipital or posterior temporoparietal region, telescope the sylvian triangle or compress it forward. Distal hemispherical and convexity branches may be stretched or spread. These changes are also observed when the atrium of the lateral ventricle enlarges and simulates a mass (Fig. 6–35, and see Fig. 7–9). Infrasylvian lesions, i.e., those situated within the temporal lobe, raise the sylvian triangle by elevating the main branch of the middle cerebral artery, and they stretch the temporal branches in a characteristic way (Fig. 6–36). This appearance is called "draping" and indicates the presence of an infrasylvian mass (Chase and Taveras, 1963). Such lesions must be differentiated from ones arising *within* the sylvian fissure, i.e., intrasylvian, which merely spread the temporal branches. Intrasylvian masses, although rare, are usually meningiomas and rarely astrocytomas.

Arterial Dislocations in Frontal View: The sylvian

point is displaced by convexity masses, being depressed by frontoparietal lesions and elevated by temporal lesions. Anterior suprasylvian or frontal masses, because of their distance, do not usually displace the sylvian point.

The anterior cerebral artery is an important indicator of the midline of the brain, and a carotid angiogram is incomplete if the artery is not opacified. In the presence of space-occupying lesions, the proximal part may be displaced beneath the falx cerebri to the contralateral side (subfalcine herniation), but it is forced back to the ipsilateral side in the parietal part of its course, being constrained by the obliquity of the free edge of the falx. It should be noted that the pericallosal artery as it passes around the genu of the corpus callosum is free to move to either side anatomically; therefore, a slight off-center position of the mid-segment should not be construed as an abnormal sign (Fig. 6–37). Callosomarginal branches arise from the pericallosal artery and extend laterally into the sulci from the

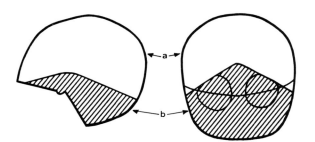

Fig. 6—24 Diagnostic accuracy of cerebral scintigraphy: the site of the lesion. a. Vertex and cerebral hemispheres: equal or superior to carotid angiography. b. (Hatched area): unreliable, far inferior to computed tomography or pneumography.

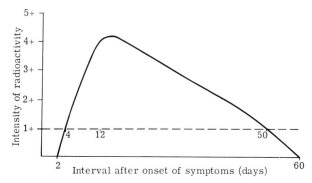

Fig. 6—25 Scintigraphy in cerebrovascular accidents. Intensity of radioactivity plotted against the interval after the onset of symptoms (after Williams and Beiler, 1966). The hatched line represents the level at which a positive diagnosis is usually possible.

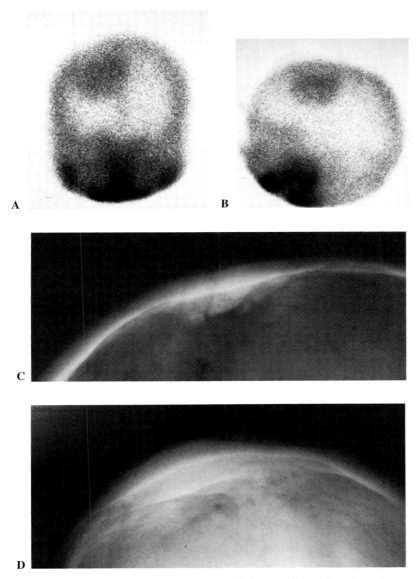

Fig. 6–26 Parasagittal meningioma. This example illustrates the specificity afforded to the solitary "hot spot" by adjacent calvarial changes. (A and B) Frontal and lateral scintigrams, showing a well-rounded area of hyperactivity in the parasagittal gutter (C and D). Well-marked thickening of the vault in the vicinity of the enostosis. The combination of calvarial enostosis and dense, well-defined uptake is pathognomonic of meningioma.

medial surface of the hemisphere. These branches may be stretched or spread by masses situated in the parasagittal region, either on the surface or within the brain (Fig. 6–38B, C).

Several types of displacement of the anterior cerebral artery are found, most of which are variations of two patterns, namely round or square shifts of the artery. *Round shifts* are caused by low-lying or midfrontal lesions within the anterior or middle part of the hemisphere. This term indicates that the contralaterally displaced pericallosal artery has returned to the midline proximal to the falx and derives from the configuration of the pericallosal

artery as it reaches the midline. If the lesion is low-lying, i.e., frontal, subfrontal or temporal, a low round shift is present (Fig. 6–38A). A diffuse round shift is present with midfrontal or deeply situated frontal lesions (Fig. 6–38B). High anterior frontal or frontal-pole lesions produce a high round (distal) shift (6–38C). Thus the center of the segment of the displaced artery indicates the level of the lesion in the brain and it can be used as a guide to the level of the mass on the lateral view. A lesion producing a distal shift will be either on a line with the point of maximum shift or above that level (Fig. 6–38C).

A *square shift* indicates that the contralaterally

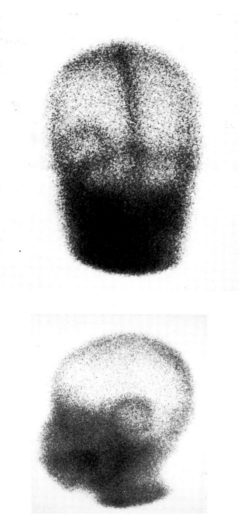

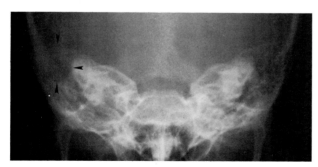

Fig. 6–27 Otogenic cerebral abscess in a 5-year-old girl with a "doughnut" lesion of the right posterior temporal region, complicating acute otitis media *(arrowheads)*.

displaced pericallosal artery is forced back to the midline by the restraining effect of the rigid falx (Fig. 6–39A). An acute- or right-angled junction of the pericallosal artery with the falx is caused by

herniation of the cingulate gyrus beneath the falx (subfalcine herniation). This contour produces a square configuration, and is caused by a low-lying mass situated in the posterior half of the hemisphere. If the mass is high rather than low, a triangular configuration is present—strictly speaking, a triangular shift, but commonly called a distal square shift (Fig. 6–39B).

The type of displacement of the anterior cerebral artery and the point of maximum displacement serves as an accurate guide to the position of the mass in the hemisphere and aids in localizing the level of the lesion in the lateral projection. Deeply situated or posterior masses may spare the pericallosal artery and displace only the internal cerebral vein (Fig. 6–40).

The internal cerebral vein is the other important indicator of the midline. Lateral displacement of the vein has the same significance as displacement of the pineal gland. The internal cerebral vein will be displaced by posterior-lying masses but it may not be affected by anterior lesions which exert their major effect on the pericallosal artery.

Abnormalities of Capillaries and Veins: A non-homogeneous cast of the brain is obtained during the intermediate (capillary) phase, when contrast medium opacifies the arterioles, capillaries and venules (Liliequist, 1967). This vascular opacification of the brain is best studied by means of subtraction and magnification techniques. Any space-occupying lesion may compress the brain and produce an avascular zone (Fig. 6–42). This sign when present is the most reliable in localizing a mass within the brain.

The superficial cortical veins drain superiorly and empty into the superior sagittal sinus (Fig. 6–41). These veins have a slight posterior bow, and curve forward as they join the superior sagittal sinus. Di Chiro (1962) demonstrated frequent variations of the venous filling between two hemispheres. The anterior segment of the superior sagittal sinus may be absent and replaced by an anastomotic vein (Kaplan et al., 1975). Segmental absence of filling without collateral or anastomotic veins may be produced by dilution or wash-out with nonopacified blood from the opposite side (Marc and Schechter, 1974). If occlusion of the superior sagittal sinus is suspected, repeat examination with cross-compression is necessary to visualize the sinus. The cortical superficial veins fill in a caudad direction: thus parietal veins *never* fill before frontal or sylvian veins (Leeds and Taveras, 1969) (Fig. 6–41).

The pattern of venous filling may be a more reliable indicator of the presence of a mass than arterial abnormalities, because the veins are more sensitive to compression and displacement. Displaced surface veins will be found in almost all cases in which the intermediate (capillary) phase is abnormal.

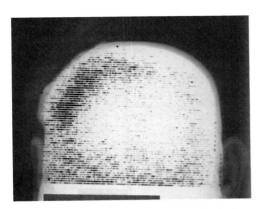
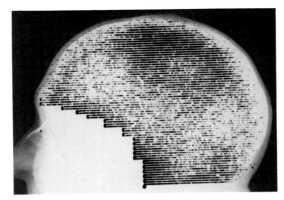

Fig. 6–28 Squamous carcinoma of the scalp, imaged in the frontal scintigram as a peripheral crescent of hyperactivity. The technique of superimposing a soft-tissue radiographic exposure of the head on the rectilinear scan shows up the tumor as an irregularity of the scalp.

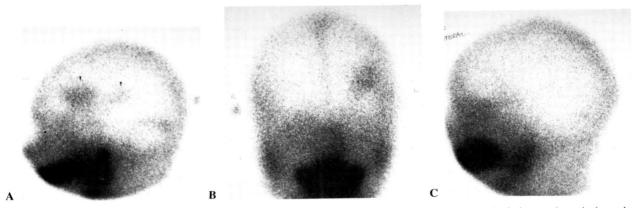

A   B   C

Fig. 6–29 Sylvian infarction. (A and B) Scintigram made 12 days after the stroke, showing two foci of abnormal cortical uptake *(arrowheads)* corresponding to the ascending frontoparietal and angular branches of the middle cerebral artery. (C) Repeat examination 48 days later, i.e., 60 days after the stroke. By that time the patient, a 48-year-old man, had recovered function, and the scan was normal. For serial computed tomograms of this patient, see Figure 6–19.

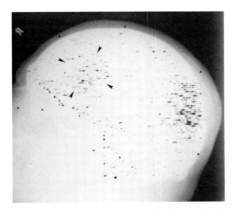

Fig. 6–30 Tumor and artifact. Lateral scintigram of a 55-year-old with a glioma of the corpus callosum *(arrowheads)*, performed 48 hours after unsuccessful ventriculography via posterior parietal burrholes. The surgical trauma shows denser activity than the neoplasm! See Hurley (1973).

Accompanying cerebral edema produces swelling of the sulci, resulting in bowing of the veins within the sulci. Heinz and Cooper (1968) referred to localized stretching of veins as the "ripple sign" and believed it to be a feature of brain abscess. Bowing of veins, particularly in the parietal region, is actually a nonspecific observation in any lesion that produces gyral swelling and stretching of sulci (Fig. 6–42). The swelling points to the area of involvement but it does not serve to identify the precise location of the lesion. This may be recognized within a diffuse area of swelling if the local arteries or veins are displaced or if a tumor stain is present. Such changes in the venous phase are an accurate guide to localization but they offer no clue to possible histology.

Frontal Masses: Space-occupying lesions or collections within or covering a frontal lobe may displace the anterior cerebral artery complex both sideways and backward. In the frontal projection, contralateral displacement of the artery from the

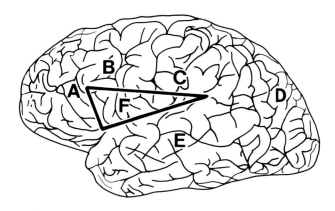

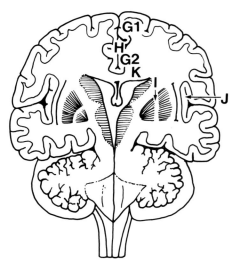

Fig. 6–31 Locations of supratentorial masses by means of carotid angiography, according to Taveras and Wood (1976).
  A. Frontal.
  B. Anterior suprasylvian.
  C. Posterior suprasylvian.
  D. Retrosylvian.
  E. Infrasylvian (temporal).
  F. Intrasylvian.
  G. Parasagittal,
     1. Frontal
     2. Parietal.
  H. Interhemispherical.
  I. Ganglionic.
  J. Centrosylvian.
  K. Enlargement of lateral ventricles.

midline takes the form of a round or a square shift, as discussed above; see Figures 6–38 and 6–39. In lateral projection, the important diagnostic feature is dislocation of the pericallosal artery: masses at or covering the frontal pole displace the pericallosal artery backward (Fig. 6–43), and higher; frontal-parasagittal masses displace it downward (Fig. 6–44). Once an abnormal position of this artery has established the presence of a mass, dislocation or stretching of smaller arteries such as the frontopolar, frontal gyral and orbital branches should be

sought. These displacements may indicate whether the mass covers or lies within the frontal lobe (see Fig. 6–43).

Temporal Masses: The anterior temporal arteries (Dahlström et al., 1969) may be recognized by means of good subtraction and magnification angiograms as they course around the anterior pole of the temporal lobe. Displacement of these arteries (Fig. 6–45) will be helpful in revealing location of mass as opposed to draping with an intra-axial lesion (Figs. 6–36, 6–47, 6–48). A full-axial projection may be useful in distinguishing an extracerebral subtemporal mass from one which is intra-axial, by means of displacement of these branches (Glickman et al., 1973).

The "naked middle cerebral artery" is a simple and helpful sign for identifying lesions adjacent to, arising within or extending into the anterior pole of the temporal lobe. In the normal lateral carotid angiogram the intracranial carotid bifurcation is hidden from view by overlapping of the anterior and middle cerebral arteries. Any mass within or adjacent to the anterior temporal pole elevates the trunk of the middle cerebral artery and displaces it backward, so that the carotid bifurcation is visible (Fig. 6–46). This observation is helpful in identifying anterior temporal tumors that spread into the ganglionic region, particularly when the temporal component is overshadowed by the larger ganglionic mass. In these cases a "naked middle cerebral artery" confirms the presence of tumor in the anterior temporal lobe (Fig. 6–47). However, this sign does not aid in distinguishing between intra-axial and extra-axial lesions. It has been recognized in the following:

Extra-axial mass in the middle fossa, e.g. meningioma, subdural collection.

Sphenoid ridge meningioma.

Intra-axial mass in the temporal lobe: anterior part alone, combined with other parts of the temporal lobe, combined with a ganglionic mass.

Dilatation of the temporal horn.

Cysts of the sylvian fissure.

Mid- and posterior-temporal lesions do not produce a "naked middle cerebral artery" sign; instead, they distort the sylvian branches of the middle cerebral artery (Fig. 6–48). In frontal view, the sylvian point is often elevated and displaced medially, and the midline structures are contralaterally displaced.

Posterior temporal masses elevate the sylvian point. The frontal view shows a square shift with minimal or no arterial displacement. The internal cerebral vein is displaced more than the anterior cerebral artery, because of the posterior location of the mass.

The "draping" sign (Fig. 6–48) is a valuable means of distinguishing an intracerebral from an extracerebral lesion in the temporal fossa (Chase and Taveras, 1963). This sign when present indi-

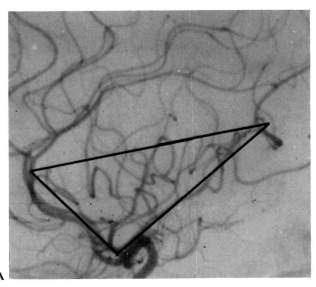

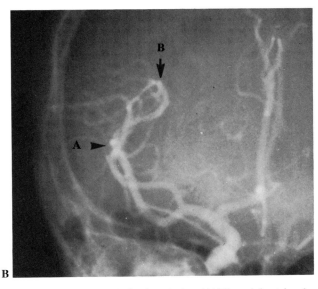

Fig. 6–32 Angiographic measurements according to Taveras and Wood (1976) — see page 261 for description. (A) The sylvian triangle. (B) Points A *(arrowhead)* and B *(arrow)*. Point B is also called the sylvian point.

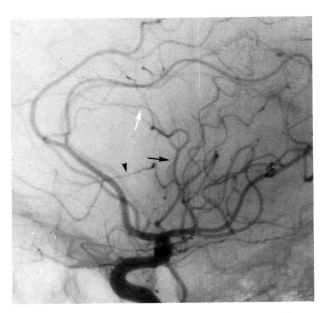

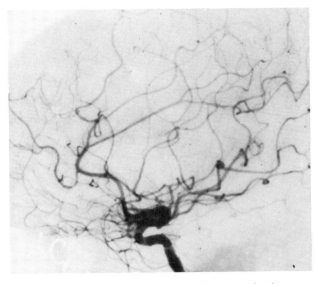

Fig. 6–33 The sylvian triangle: backward displacement by an anterior sylvian mass *(black arrow)*. A prerolandic branch *(arrowhead)* is straightened and indicates the center of the mass. Another prerolandic branch is curved *(white arrow)*, and defines the upper extent of the mass. Diagnosis: low-grade astrocytoma of the frontal lobe.

Fig. 6–34 The sylvian triangle (continued): depression by a suprasylvian mass. Ascending rolandic and prerolandic surface branches are separated. Diagnosis: bronchial metastasis.

cates an intra-axial lesion: the arteries, though displaced by a mass, must navigate around the mass to nourish the brain, and they become draped around its margins (see also Fig. 6–36). If the mass is extracerebral, the arteries are arched and do not course around the mass (6–45): the "draping" sign, while reliable in most instances, does not hold if an intracerebral lesion is situated too medially or if

chronic extracerebral lesions invaginate the brain and mimic a "draped" appearance.

Occipital Masses: Occipital lesions may be detected only with vertebral angiography, which will show the displaced posterior parietal and calcarine arteries. The displacement is more apparent in the anteroposterior projection, in which the asymmetry can be easily appreciated by comparing the two sides (Fig. 6–49). A square shift of the anterior cerebral artery may be present, and the internal cerebral vein is displaced more than the artery (see Figs. 6–39 and 6–40). In some instances the artery

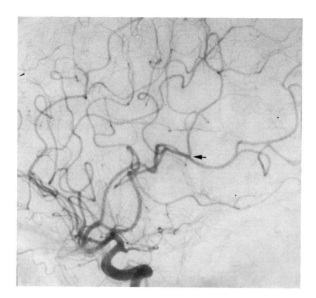

Fig. 6–35 The sylvian triangle (continued): forward displacement. The triangle is telescoped forward and surface vessels arising from the sylvian point *(arrow)* are abnormally spread. Diagnosis: dilated atrium of the lateral ventricle, caused by glioblastoma multiforme.

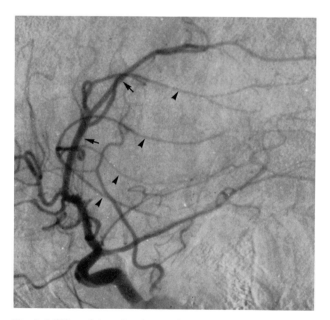

Fig. 6–36 The sylvian triangle (continued): elevation and forward displacement of the trunk *(arrows)*, with characteristic deformity of the temporal-lobe branches of the middle cerebral artery *(arrowheads)*—so-called "draping," indicating an infrasylvian intracerebral mass.

is not displaced at all, only the internal cerebral vein is shifted from the midline.

Convexity and Parasagittal Masses: Convexity lesions in the frontal and parietal regions affect the sylvian triangle as described above; the depth of the lesion may be assessed by the type of shift of the

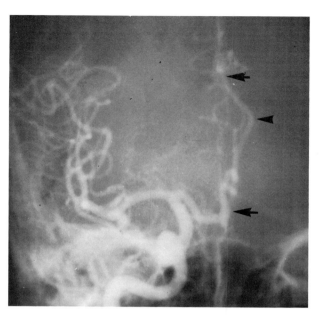

Fig. 6–37 "Wandering" anterior cerebral artery—a normal variant. Normally the mid-segment of the pericallosal artery *(arrowhead)* lies free on the genu of the corpus callosum, not necessarily in the midline. The important parts of the artery to evaluate are the proximal segment *(lower arrow)* and the parietal segment at the free border of the falx cerebri *(upper arrow)*.

midline structures. Parasagittal masses are more apparent on the anteroposterior projection because they tend to displace the anterior cerebral artery laterally. Also, local stretching and spreading of callosomarginal branches of the anterior cerebral artery may aid in accurate localization of the mass (Fig. 6–44; see also Fig. 6–38). Parasagittal lesions produced secondary effects on the sylvian triangle as a consequence of the vector of force exerted by the mass, and errors in localization may occur because of this displacement (Fig. 6–44).

Other useful arterial displacements discussed elsewhere are:

1. Separation or spreading of pericallosal arteries by interhemispherical collections of blood or pus.

2. Displacement of arteries above the corpus callosum ("moustache").

3. Spreading of the intrasylvian branches of the middle cerebral artery caused by ganglionic or intrasylvian masses.

4. Displacements of the sylvian point: elevated in temporal mass, depressed in posterior frontal masses or telescoped forward in occipital or posterior temporal masses.

Intrinsic Abnormalities of Vessels

Arteries on the medial and lateral surfaces of the hemisphere may be observed to undulate as they course in and out of sulci (see Fig. 6–32); an artery that is straight should be viewed with suspicion and the radiographs carefully scrutinized for other signs

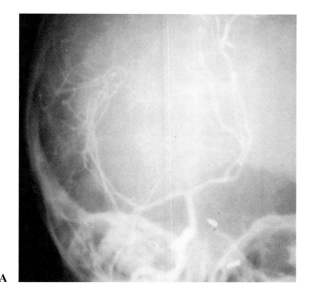

A

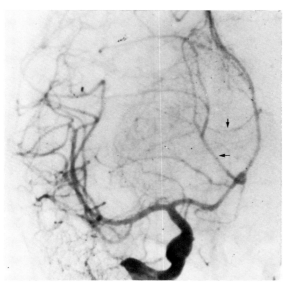

B

Fig. 6-38 Round shifts of the anterior cerebral artery. (A) Low round shift from medulloblastoma seedlings in the subfrontal region. Occipital craniotomy. (B) Diffuse round shift with stretched and deviated branches of the callosomarginal artery *(arrows)*. Diagnosis: lymphoma deposits in the frontal parasagittal region. (C) Distal round shift *(arrowhead)* caused by a high-lying tumor. The small arrows point to stretched convexity branches of the middle cerebral artery outlining the tumor. Diagnosis: glioblastoma multiforme.

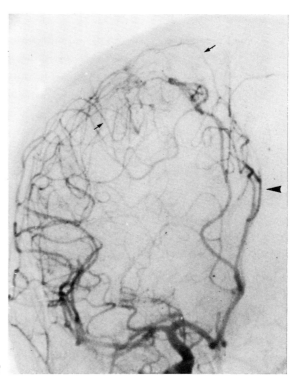

C

of a mass. The peripheral margins of the lesion are defined by curved branches, the circumferential arteries (Fig. 6-50; Kricheff and Taveras, 1964). Circumferential branches are curved and bowed either forward or backward as they relate to the mass. The bowing is due to tumor involvement or swelling of the adjacent sulci (see Fig. 6-42). The straight artery usually indicates the center of the mass and has been called the axis artery by Kricheff and Taveras.

A shaggy or irregular artery has been identified in a variety of lesions. The appearance is caused by actual involvement of the arterial wall in the pathological process or through edema (Figs. 6-45C, 6-50). Neoplasms involving the arterial wall include glioblastoma multiforme, astrocytoma, metastasis, lymphoma and sarcoma (Leeds et al.,

1971). The numerous causes of such changes in the arterial wall are discussed in Chapter 2.

Hypertrophied middle meningeal branches of the external carotid artery most commonly supply meningiomas (see p. 35) and arteriovenous malformations involving the dura (see p. 146), but any lesion of the dura may receive a direct meningeal supply or a parasitized blood supply because of its proximity or because of dural invasion (Silverberg and Hanbery, 1971). This is particularly likely in the temporal region, but it may also occur on the convexity (Steven, 1961). Branches of the internal carotid artery also may enlarge and supply blood to an arteriovenous malformation, malignant glioma or a meningioma.

Other angiographic abnormalities of mass lesions include occlusion or delayed filling of veins. Occlu-

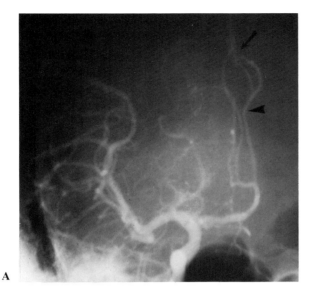

A

Fig. 6–39 Square shifts of the anterior cerebral artery. (A) Square shift with subfalcine herniation *(arrow)*, caused by a temperoparietal mass. Diagnosis: neoplastic metastasis. Note the "wandering" mid-segment of the anterior cerebral artery *(arrowhead)* — of no diagnostic significance. (B and C) Another case. Distal square shift due to a high posterior mass. The sylvian point (B, *arrow*) is depressed. The internal cerebral vein (C, *arrowhead*) is also displaced — but less than the pericallosal artery, indicating that the mass is high, rather than low-lying in the hemisphere. Diagnosis: parietal astrocytoma.

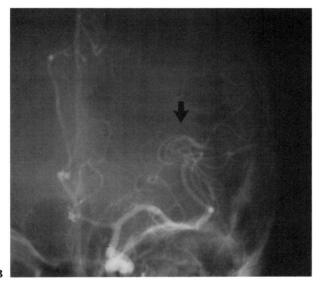

B

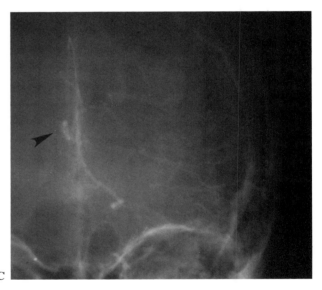

C

sion may be recognized by noting non-filling of a vein in the presence of opacified adjacent veins, or a redirection or reversal of flow. Venous obstruction is commonest with meningiomas but it has been observed in glioblastoma multiforme. It is also seen in inflammatory lesions and arteritis (see Ch. 2).

Alterations in Circulation Time and Dynamics
Changes in circulatory dynamics are an important guide to the presence of an intracranial mass, since more than 90 percent of supratentorial mass lesions exhibit them (Leeds and Taveras, 1969).

Normal Circulation Time: Circulation time reflects the interval taken for a bolus of contrast medium injected into the cervical part of the carotid artery to travel from the carotid siphon to the parietal veins (Greitz, 1956). The mean arteriove-

nous circulation time is 4.35 seconds (± SD 0.83 seconds). It is reduced in children (to 2.5 – 3 seconds) and in adults with arterial hypertension, and it is physiologically prolonged in advanced age. Pathological causes of prolonged circulation time are raised intracranial pressure including neoplasms and cerebrovascular degenerative disease.

The arterial circulation time varies from 1 to 2.5 seconds, irrespective of whether the hemisphere or a local area is studied. The pattern of arterial filling is determined by the distance of the vessels from the carotid siphon; therefore, proximal vessels appear first and the filling is sequential. Any alteration in this pattern is pathological.

The intermediate (capillary) phase is recorded from the moment of arterial emptying to the start of venous filling. It measures 0.5 to 1 second.

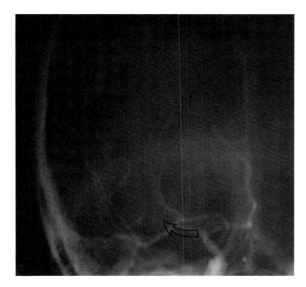

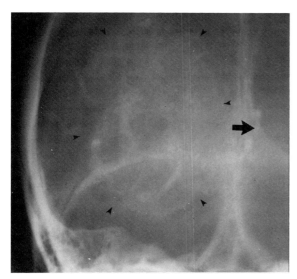

Fig. 6-40 Supratentorial mass without midline arterial displacement. The anterior cerebral artery is undisplaced but the venous phase reveals that a large tumor stain *(arrowheads)* dislocates the internal cerebral vein contralaterally *(arrow)*. The open arrow points to a hypertrophied anterior choroidal artery supplying the tumor. Diagnosis: intraventricular meningioma.

The venous circulation time varies so widely — from 6 to 12 seconds — that its measurement has doubtful value; therefore, the arteriovenous circulation time is considered more useful for practical purposes. Normal hemispherical venous filling takes place from the frontal to the occipital region. Frontal or sylvian veins opacity first; parietal veins *never* fill before frontal veins. Superficial veins usually fill before deep veins, but in one-third of subjects the deep veins are seen first. The point to observe is that the actual sequence of filling is more important than the acutal size of veins (White and Greitz, 1972): parietal-lobe veins are always larger

than frontal or sylvian veins, so they are more readily visualized (Fig. 6-41). A search may be required to observe the frontal veins. Difficulty may arise if the sequence is altered, in deciding whether the first veins recognized are early-filling veins or whether the more proximal veins are filling late.

Abnormal Patterns: According to Leeds and Taveras (1969), abnormalities in circulation time include the following:
1. Delayed arterial filling
2. Prolonged intermediate (capillary) phase
3. "Tumor blush" with early venous filling
4. Early venous filling
5. Delayed venous filling
6. "Tumor blush" with delayed venous filling
7. More than one of the above
8. No abnormality in the local circulation.

1. Delayed Arterial Filling: Delayed filling of a local artery is uncommon, because the muscular walls of arteries are difficult to compress. Neoplasms may affect the wall of the blood vessel by direct spread or through perivascular edema — changes which result in delayed filling and/or emptying of the artery. Delayed arterial filling is more frequently seen in intra-axial than extra-axial lesions (Fig. 6-51). It is also encountered in patients with atherosclerotic vascular disease: after a shower of emboli, the arteries involved fill and empty slowly. Arterial spasm following severe head trauma or intracerebral hemorrhage may provoke similar slow-filling and emptying of the distal arteries.

2. Prolonged Intermediate (Capillary) Phase: Any lesion which evokes cerebral edema or raises intracranial pressure may prolong the intermediate phase. Slowing of the circulation time is frequently accentuated during this phase (Fig. 6-52).

3. "Tumor Blush" With Early Venous Filling: The combination of neovascularity with pathological arteries and early-filling draining veins, appearing in the midarterial or late arterial phase and before the normal veins, is usually the signature of a glioblastoma multiforme (Fig. 6-53; Cronqvist, 1969). Huang and Wolf (1964) pointed out that early filling of the medullary veins draining deeply, appearing as a spray of vessels into the white matter, is an indication that the tumor is almost certainly a glioblastoma, seldom a metastasis and only rarely another lesion. This sign has been reported in normal subjects, in arteriovenous malformations, atherosclerotic vascular disease and lymphoma (Stein and Rosenbaum, 1974).

4. Early Venous Filling: The observation of early-filling veins without neovascularity in a tumor patient was originally thought to be a sign of a malignant lesion, but it is now recognized to be more commonly associated with benign lesions (Leeds and Goldberg, 1973; Bradac et al., 1975). Since the introduction of the direct magnification and subtrac-

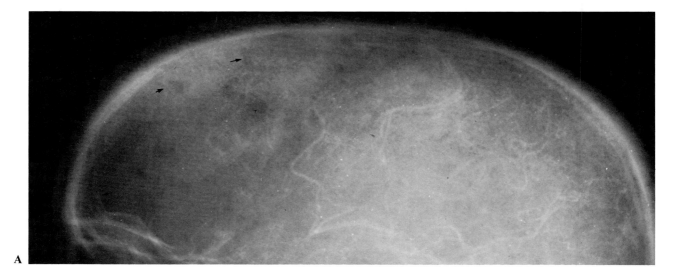

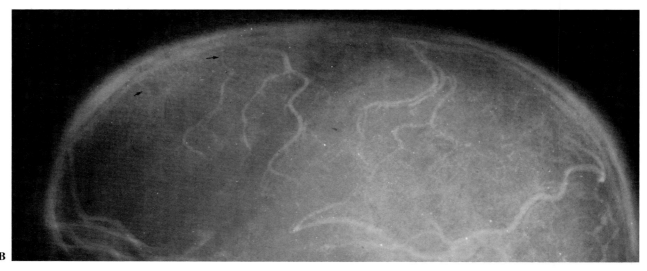

Fig. 6–41 Normal venous discharge. (A) The frontal veins appear to be filling later than the parietal cortical veins, but careful scrutiny shows that the frontal veins are actually present *(arrows)*, overlooked merely because of their small caliber. (B) One second later the frontal veins are better filled *(arrows)*.

tion techniques in angiography, it is unusual to find such veins without concomitant neovascularity in neoplasms. Because the tumor causes cerebral compression and because veins are thin-walled structures that are easily obliterated, the paradox of the early-filling of tumor-draining veins combined with delayed filling of normal veins may be observed (Fig. 6 – 55).

5. *Delayed Venous Filling:* Delayed filling of veins is a common finding during cerebral angiography in the investigation of a mass lesion. The delay may be polar or focal, and may affect only one or two veins (Fig. 6 – 54). Rapid serial angiography is required to identify delayed filling of only a few veins, and the radiographs must be carefully studied sequentially forward and backward, to identify

such an abnormality. Although delayed filling confirms the presence and location of the mass, it provides no clue to possible histology.

Delayed filling in the intermediate (capillary) phase may also be present. The brain opacifies during this phase, and the avascular filling defect of a tumor readily becomes apparent, particularly with subtraction. As the sequence of vascular opacification progresses in such cases, delay in venous filling is also revealed. Occasionally, delayed filling is confined to the intermediate phase (Fig. 6 – 52).

6. *"Tumor Blush" With Delayed Venous Filling:* There may be delayed filling of normal veins in the vicinity of a neoplasm, for the reasons given in the section above, *after* the tumor-draining veins have emptied (Fig. 6 – 55).

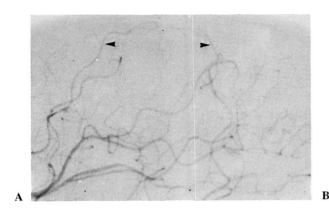

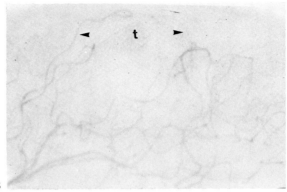

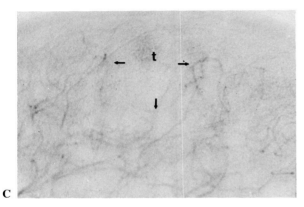

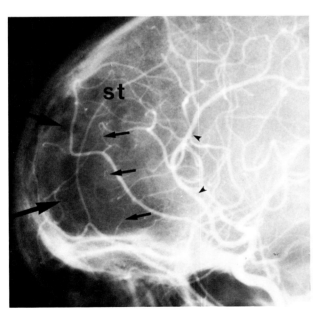

Fig. 6–42 Gyral swelling producing an avascular zone outlined by circumferential vessels. (A) Stretched branches of the callosomarginal artery define the anterior and posterior borders of the lesion *(arrowheads)*. (B) 0.5 seconds later: a tumor blush (t) is visible in the center of the mass, surrounded by edema. (C) Intermediate phase: the tumor blush (t) is surrounded by a vascular zone of edema *(arrows)*. Diagnosis: bronchial metastasis.

Fig. 6–43 Frontal-fossa mass. The pericallosal artery *(arrowhead)* is displaced backward, and the frontopolar is stretched. The frontal gyral branches *(arrows)* are displaced from the inner table, indicating an extracerebral collection over the frontal lobe. The large arrows point to an osteomyelitis of the frontal bone. A branch of the superficial temporal artery (st) is stretched over a subgaleal collection of pus. Diagnosis: subdural empyema secondary to post-traumatic osteomyelitis.

7. More Than One of The Above: More than one of these changes was identified in one-third of the patients with local circulatory changes examined by Leeds and Taveras (1969).

"Tumor Blush"

The time of appearance, duration, configuration, vascular supply and the relations of the neovascularity to the normal phases of the circulation time is often a guide to the histology of the lesion.

Glioblastoma Multiforme. One-third of brain tumors are glioblastomas, and about one half of these show tumor circulation. The "blush" appears in the early arterial or midarterial phase, consisting of pathological arteries and veins, and disappears before or just after the normal veins opacify (Figs. 6–48 and 6–56; Leeds and Taveras, 1969). The arteries within the tumor may have irregular walls or be occluded (Fig. 6–52). Deep medullary veins may be present (6–53). Early draining veins are a hallmark of glioblastoma multiforme. Cerebral edema is often extensive and largely responsible for the midline displacement which is usually present. Abnormal vascularity is absent in 30–40% of patients.

Metastases. About one-third of brain tumors are neoplastic secondary deposits, the majority arising from bronchial carcinoma. They appear later in the sequence of the circulation time than

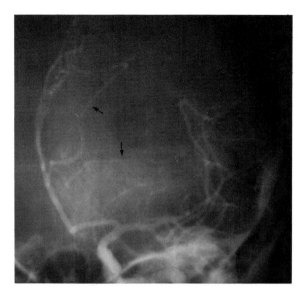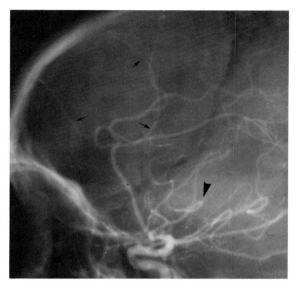

Fig. 6—44 High frontal mass. The diffuse round shift of the pericallosal artery with laterally elevated and stretched callosomarginal arteries indicates a frontal parasagittal mass. In lateral view the callosomarginal artery is depressed and its callosomarginal branches are displaced and stretched *(arrows)*. The arrowhead points to flattening of the sylvian triangle—a false sign, due to the vector of force of the mass. Diagnosis: frontal parasagittal meningioma.

glioblastomas, being seen in the late arterial, intermediate (capillary) and/or venous phase, and persistence late into the venous phase. The area of neovascularity is often well circumscribed ("coin" lesion Fig. 6–57). Occasionally a diffuse "blush" is present (Fig. 6–42). Extensive surrounding edema is common. Multiple deposits are frequent. Solitary lesions may be indistinguishable from glioblastoma multiforme (Trevisian and Dettori, 1972).

Meningiomas. Intracranial meningiomas are slightly less common than neoplastic metastases, accounting for 15 to 20 percent of brain tumors. In about half of these tumors the angiographic appearances are pathognomonic, possessing a distinctive blood supply and/or a "tumor blush."

The distinctive blood supply of meningiomas consists of hypertrophied arterial branches, usually derived from the external carotid artery. This frequently encountered pathological pattern underlines the importance of routinely examining the common carotid artery, or selectively injecting the external carotid artery, in the investigation of supratentorial space-occupying lesions by carotid angiography (Danziger and Bloch, 1975). Convexity and parasagittal meningiomas almost always exhibit an external carotid supply, which arises partly from branches of this artery to the scalp that perforate the skull and partly from its middle meningeal branch (Figs. 6–58, 6–59). As a rule the surface of the tumor is supplied by the internal carotid and the core by the external carotid branch (Fig. 6–58).

Frontobasal meningiomas have a variable blood supply, depending on their location. Pterional and lateral sphenoid meningiomas are supplied by the anterior branch of the middle meningeal artery (Fig. 6–59). Medial sphenoid and parasellar meningiomas are supplied by cavernous branches of the internal carotid and meningeal branches of the ophthalmic artery (Fig. 6–60; see Ch. 5), and occasionally by the middle meningeal artery (Sansregret and Ledoux, 1971). Meningiomas arising from the planum sphenoidale and ofactory groove have a similar blood supply, although 20 to 30 percent will show no neovascularity with high-grade angiography including subtraction and magnification techniques. Anterior falcine meningiomas are supplied by a hypertrophied anterior falcine artery, either the ipsilateral or the contralateral one. This vessel is usually a branch of the ophthalmic artery, but it may arise from the middle meningeal artery (Fig. 6–61; Pollock and Newton, 1968). Meningiomas within the sylvian fissure may insinuate themselves around branches of the middle cerebral artery and cause arterial irregularity or occlusion.

The typical "tumor blush" of a meningioma is homogeneous and prolonged, starting in the midarterial or later arterial phase and ending in or beyond the late venous phase. More than one-third of meningiomas exhibit no tumor circulation—notably those in the suprasellar and parasagittal regions (Wickbom, 1953; Banna and Appleby, 1969; Stannard, 1975). Such meningiomas may have prominent capsular veins which define the margin of the lesion as a consequence of venous thrombosis (Fig. 6–62). Early-filling veins of the type seen in glioblastoma multifo.

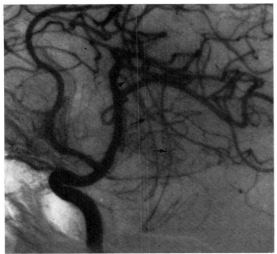

A

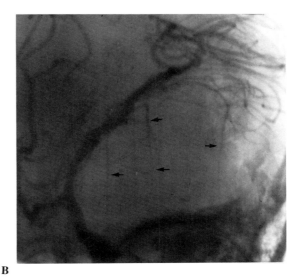

B

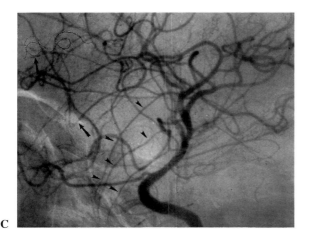

C

Fig. 6–45 Temporal-fossa mass. (A and B) The anterior temporal branches of the middle cerebral artery *(arrows)* are stretched, elevated, and retrodisplaced by the mass, and do not reach the floor of the middle fossa. A "naked" middle cerebral artery is present. Diagnosis: *pterional meningioma* examined by selective internal carotid angiography. External carotid injection revealed a tumor blush — see Figure 6–62. (C) Stretched and elevated anterior temporal branches *(arrowheads)* indicate an extra-axial mass. Several arterial branches are encased *(arrows)*, indicating an intra-axial mass. Diagnosis: *malignant glioma of the frontal lobe*, spreading into the temporal lobe and also extra-axially.

claimed in up to 20–30% of cases (see Fig. 6–59B; Stattin, 1961; El Banhawy and Walter, 1962; Kieffer et al., 1963). Parasagittal meningiomas often have no demonstrable abnormal feeding arteries, but they may invade the superior sagittal sinus, and compress or occlude it (Fig. 6–63). Venous thrombosis occurs frequently with meningiomas accounting for the capsular veins frequently observed (Fig. 6–62).

"Doughnut" or "Ring" Lesions. An angiographic ring lesion is characteristic of three entities, viz, glioblastoma multiforme, neoplastic metastasis and brain abscess. Occasionally meningiomas and other lesions produce similar appearances. In glioblastoma and metastasis, the peripheral vascular zone is usually thick-walled, but it may be thin-walled (Fig. 6–64). The hypervascular zone is caused by tumor neovascularity, and the core is necrotic or cystic. In an abscess, the enhancing rim is caused by the vascularity of the abscess wall (Fig. 6–65; Nielsen and Halaburt, 1976). The ring lesion

usually persists well into the venous phase. A "doughnut" lesion may also be seen in the luxury perfusion syndrome — see below. Apparent ring lesions of meningiomas are caused by capsular veins which envelop the tumor in the form of a ring (Fig. 6–66).

Hyperperfusion and Cerebral Infarction. A variety of benign conditions cause increased vascularity. In 1966 Lassen introduced the concept of loss in cerebral autoregulation. This mechanism is believed to be responsible for the changes in cerebral blood flow caused by the shunting of blood through an open capillary bed and resulting in veins filling early (hyperperfusion, luxury perfusion). This loss in cerebral autoregulation is a complication of the accumulation of acid metabolites and carbon dioxide in the brain. Leeds and Goldberg (1973) identified the various abnormalities that may exhibit a luxury perfusion:

1. Cerebral infarction (Llenas and Tortella, 1972)
2. Cerebral trauma

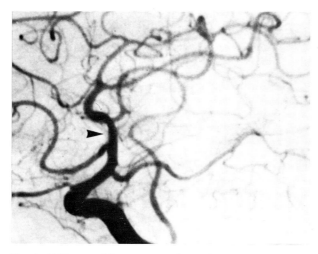

Fig. 6—46 Temporal-fossa mass. The "naked" middle cerebral artery. The bifurcation of the internal carotid artery as well as the abnormally elevated trunk of the middle cerebral artery are visible *(arrowhead)*. The sign indicates the presence of a mass of the anterior temporal pole, either intracerebral or extracerebral. Diagnosis: pterional meningioma.

3. Inflammatory diseases of the brain: meningitis, encephalitis, "cerebritis," abscess.

4. Arteritis

5. Parenchymal degenerative disease

6. Encephalopathy, idiopathic and toxic

7. Compression of the brain by a space-occupying lesion

8. Vascular spasm secondary to subarachnoid hemorrhage

9. Repeated seizures or status epilepticus (Farrell and Taveras, 1974; McDonald et al., 1975).

The appearances of this condition as revealed by cerebral angiography or computed tomography vary greatly and depend on the stage at which the examination is performed in the course of the lesion, since the pathological process is an evolutionary rather than a static one (Cronqvist and Laroche 1967). During the initial phase, i.e., up to the 10th day, a proliferation of arteries or arterioles may be recognized in the region of involvement. A stippled blush is identified, consisting of dilated perforating arterioles parallelling large second- or third-order cortical arteries; there may be early-filling veins. This profusion of dilated vessels produces a punctate perivascular stain (Fig. 6–67). The pattern alters during the second and third week when an abnormal zone of hypervascularity develops, which conforms to the pattern of a gyrus and the lesion is cortically oriented. A dense early-filling draining vein may be present, which is denser than the neighboring veins (Fig. 6–68). During the succeeding 3 to 6 weeks, the gyral "blush" and early-filling vein become less perceptible and gradually fade until a normal appearance is again observed (Leeds and Goldberg, 1973).

The importance of identifying the stain caused by luxury perfusion is to avoid the need for unnecessary surgery or radiation in such patients. A hyperperfusion lesion may at times be difficult to distinguish from a malignant tumor. For example, the phenomenon of hyperperfusion may be associated with a mass lesion: when the mass causes cerebral

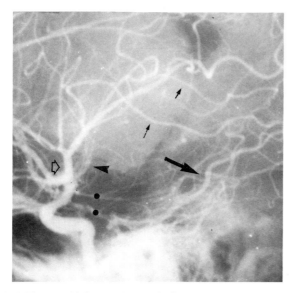

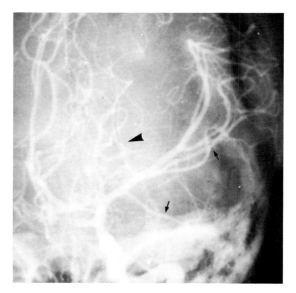

Fig. 6—47 Temporal-lobe neoplasm. The following signs are present: elevated sylvian triangle, "draping" of the temporal arteries *(small arrows)*, "naked" middle cerebral artery *(open arrow)*. Deep extension is indicated by posterior and medial displacement of the lenticulostriate arteries *(arrowhead)*. Incisural herniation is manifested by downward and medial displacement of the anterior choroidal and posterior communicating arteries *(black spots)*. The large arrow points to a tentorial step of the posterior cerebral artery at the incisural edge. Diagnosis: recurrent glioblastoma multiforme.

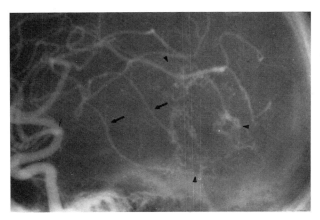

Fig. 6–48 Temporal-fossa mass. The "draping" sign. Elevation of the sylvian triangle and draping of the temporal branches of the middle cerebral artery *(small arrows)* are signs that indicate the presence of an intra-axial tumor in the posterior temporal region. The arteries are draped over a hypervascular mass *(arrowheads)*. Diagnosis: glioblastoma multiforme.

compression, a loss in autoregulation at the margins of the mass may account for a peripheral zone of hypervascularity. This may manifest by the presence of an early-filling vein or a pseudocapsule due to vascular compression. The pseudocapsule—unlike a true vascular capsule (Leeds and Goldberg, 1973)—is transient and opacifies only in the intermediate phase (Fig. 6–66). Hyperperfusion pat-

terns may be differentiated from neoplastic lesions and arteriovenous malformations by the following: (1) There is usually very little mass present, except for swelling; shifts are unusual and, when present, minimal (Fig. 6–69). (2) The veins filling early are normal draining veins which opacify earlier and more densely than neighboring veins because of rapid shunting through the open capillary bed. (3) No true neovascularity is present—all the dilated arteries, arterioles and draining veins are the normal vascular structures of the area. (4) The hypervascularity occurs only in the cortical gray matter, the island of Reil and the basal ganglia. (5) Three specific vascular patterns are recognized, which are time-dependent and transient. (6) Since the vascular changes are transient, repeat examination will demonstrate an evolution of the process under investigation.

It must be stessed that the hypervascular pattern depends on the stroke-angiogram interval and is unrelated to the underlying pathology. Secondly, there must be flow for these changes to occur: no hyperperfusion will occur in the presence of vascular occlusion, except at the margin of the lesion.

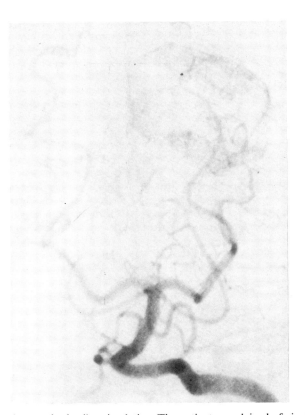

Fig. 6–49 Occipital-lobe tumor with an exclusive blood supply from the vertebrobasilar circulation. The patient complained of visual symptoms and exhibited a right homonymous hemianopia. The left carotid angiogram (not shown here) revealed a slight lateral displacement of the internal cerebral vein but no pathological circulation; however, the posterior cerebral artery did not opacify. Vertebral angiography reveals a hypervascular neoplasm in the left occipital lobe.

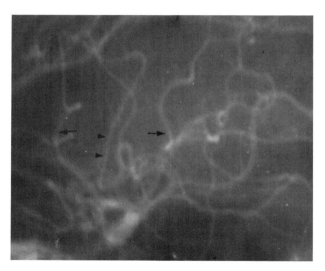

Fig. 6–50 Neoplastic involvement of arteries. The axis artery *(arrowheads)* has shaggy walls, indicating tumor encasement. The arrows point to circumferential arteries defining the anterior and posterior borders of the tumor. The sylvian triangle is displaced backward and is depressed by temporal spread of a frontal tumor. Diagnosis: glioblastoma multiforme.

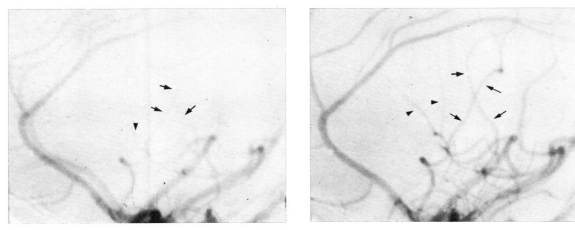

Fig. 6–51 Delayed filling of arteries. Lateral angiograms, made 0.5 seconds apart, show slight delay in opacification of the anterior prerolandic branches *(arrowheads)*, compared to the more posterior prerolandic branches *(arrows)*. Diagnosis: hematoma of the frontal lobe.

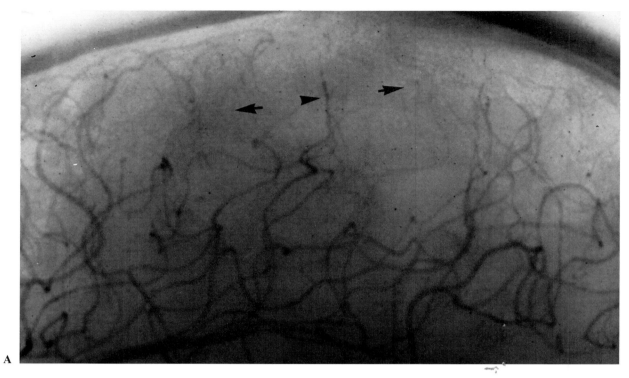

A

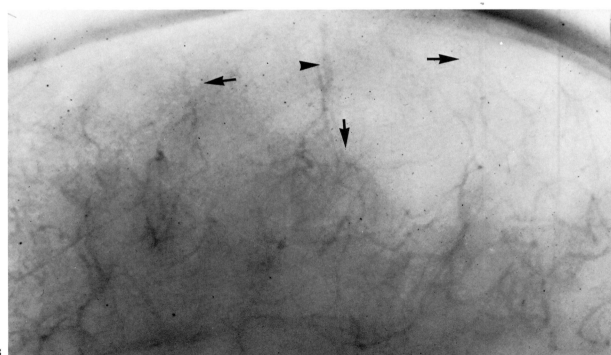

B

REFERENCES

Banna, M. and Appleby, A.: Some observations in the angiography of supratentorial meningiomas. Clinical Radiology, 20, 375–386, 1969.

Bardfeld, P. A., Passalaqua, A. M., Braunstein, Raghavendra, B. N., Leeds, N. E. and Kricheff, I. I.: Journal of Computer Assisted Tomography, 1, 315–318, 1977.

Bradac, G. B., Simon, R. S., and Fiegler, W.: The early filling of a vein in the carotid angiogram. Neuroradiology, 9, 13–19, 1975.

Brismar, J., Roberson, G. H. and Davis K. R.: Radiation necrosis of the brain. Neuroradiological considerations with computer tomography. Neuroradiology, 12, 109–113, 1976.

Burrows, E. H.: The clinical utility of brainscanning in nuclear medicine. Progress in Nuclear Medicine, 1, 287–335, 1972a.

Burrows, E. H.: False-negative results in brain scanning. British Medical Journal, 1, 473–476, 1972b.

Chase, N. E. and Taveras, J. M.: Temporal tumors studied by serial angiography: A review of 150 cases. Acta Radiologica Diagnosis, 1, 225–235, 1963.

Claveria, L. E., Du Boulay, G. H. and Moseley, I. F.: Intracranial infections: Investigation by computerized axial tomography. Neuroradiology, 12, 59–71, 1976.

Claveria, L. E., Sutton, D. and Tress, B. M.: The radiological diagnosis of meningiomas. The impact of EMI scanning. British Journal of Radiology, 50, 15–22, 1977a.

Claveria, L. E., Kendall, B. E. and Du Boulay, G. H.: Computed axial tomography in supratentorial gliomas and metastases. In Du Boulay, G. H. and Moseley, I. F., Eds.: Computed Axial Tomography in Clinical Practice. Berlin: Springer, 1977b.

Cronqvist, S.: Angiography and cerebral blood flow in malignant glioma. Acta Radiologica Therapy, 8, 78–85, 1969.

Cronqvist, S., Brismar, J., Kjellin, K. and Söderström, C. E.: Computer assisted axial tomography in cerebrovascular lesions. Acta Radiologica Diagnosis, 16, 135–145, 1975.

Cronqvist, S. and Laroche, F.: Transitory hyperaemia in focal cerebral vascular lesions studied by angiography and regional cerebral blood flow measurements. British Journal of Radiology, 40, 270–274, 1967.

Dahlström, L. Fagerberg, G., Lanner, L. and Stattin, S.: Anatomical and angiographic studies of arteries supplying anterior part of temporal lobe: a preliminary report. Acta Radiologica Diagnosis, 9, 257–263, 1969.

Danziger, J., and Bloch, S.: The value of the external carotid circulation in the assessment of intracranial lesions. Clinical Radiology, 26, 261–266, 1975.

Davis, K. R., Taveras, J. M., New, P. F. J., Schnur, J. A. and Roberson, G. H.: Cerebral infarction diagnosis by computerized tomography. American Journal of Roentgenology, 124, 643–660, 1975.

DiChiro, G.: Angiographic patterns of cerebral convexity veins and superficial dural sinuses. American Journal of Roentgenology, 87, 308–321, 1962.

Du Boulay, G. H. and Marshall, J.: Comparison of E. M. I. and radioisotope imaging in neurological disease. The Lancet, 2, 1294–1297, 1975.

El-Banhawy, A. and Walter, W.: The incidence and significance of the early filling of veins in carotid angiography of supratentorial meningiomas. Acta Neurochirurgica, 10, 247–267, 1962.

Farrell, F. W., and Taveras, J. M.: Case reports: Angiographic stain produced by seizures. Neuroradiology, 8, 49–53, 1974.

Gilday, D. L. and Ash, J.: Accuracy of brain scanning in pediatric craniocerebral neoplasms. Radiology, 117, 93–97, 1975.

Glickman, M. G., McNamara, T. O., and Margolis, M. T.: Arteriographic diagnosis of subtemporal subdural hematoma. Radiology, 109, 607–615, 1973.

Godwin-Austen, R. B.: A case of visual disorientation. Journal of Neurology, Neurosurgery and Psychiatry, 28, 453–458, 1965.

Greitz, T.: A radiologic study of the brain circulation by rapid serial angiography of the carotid artery. Acta Radiologica Supplementum, 140, 1956.

Heinz, E. R. and Cooper, R. D.: Several early angiographic findings in brain abscess including "the ripple sign". Radiology, 90, 735–739, 1968.

Huang, Y. P. and Wolf, B. S.: Veins of the white matter of the cerebral hemispheres (the medullary veins). Diagnostic importance in carotid angiography. American Journal of Roentgenology, 92, 739–755, 1964.

Hurley, P. J.: Effect of craniotomy on the brainscan related to the time elapsed after surgery. Journal of Nuclear Medicine, 13, 156–158, 1973.

Kaplan, H. A., Browder, J., and Krieger, A. J.: Venous channels within the intracranial dural partitions. Radiology, 115, 641–645, 1975.

Kaufman, D. M. and Leeds, N. E.: Computed tomography (CT) in the diagnosis of intracranial abscesses–brain abscess, subdural empyema and epidural empyema. Neurology, 27, 1069–1073, 1977.

Kazner, E., Wilske, J., Steinhoff, H. and Stochdorph, O.: Computer assisted tomography in primary malignant lymphomas of the brain. Journal of Computer Assisted Tomography, 2, 125–134, 1978.

Kieffer, S. A., Larson, D. A., Gold, L. H. A., Prentice, W. B., Stadlan, E. M. and Seyfert, S.: Rapid circulation in intracranial meningiomas. Radiology, 106, 575–580, 1973.

Kingsley, D. and Kendall, B. E.: Dependent layering of contrast medium in cystic astrocytomas. Neuroradiology, 14, 107–110, 1977.

Kramer, R. A., Janetos, G. P., and Perlstein, G.: An approach to contrast enhancement in computed tomography of the brain. Radiology, 116, 641–647, 1975.

Kricheff, I. I. and Taveras, J.M.: The angiographic localization of suprasylvian space-occupying lesions. Radiology, 82, 602–614, 1964.

Lassen, N. A.: The luxury perfusion syndrome and its possible relation to acute metabolic acidosis localized within the brain. The Lancet, 2, 1113–1115, 1966.

Leeds, N. E. and Goldberg, H. I.: Abnormal vascular patterns in benign intracranial lesions: Pseudotumors of the brain. American Journal of Roentgenology, 118, 576–585, 1973.

Leeds, N. E., Rosenblatt, R. and Zimmerman, H. M.: Focal angiographic changes of cerebral lymphoma with pathologic correlation. Radiology, 99, 595–599, 1971.

Leeds, N. E. and Taveras, J. M.: Dynamic Factors in Diagnosis of Supratentorial Brain Tumors by Cerebral Angiography. Philadelphia: W. B. Saunders Company, 1969.

Lehrer, H.: Mechanism in indirect arterial displacements over cerebral convexities accompanying cerebral mass lesions. Acta Radiologica Diagnosis, 6, 233–240, 1967.

Liliequist, B.: Capillary phase in cerebral angiography. Acta Radiologica Diagnosis, 6, 113–125, 1967.

Llenas, J. S. and Tortella, E. P.: Correlation between pathologic and angiographic findings in so-called "incomplete cerebral infarct". Neuroradiology, 4, 108–113, 1972.

McDonald, E. J., Goodman, P. C., Nielsen, S. L. and Winestock, D. P.: Cerebral hypervascularity and early venous opacification in status epilepticus. Radiology, 117, 87–88, 1975.

McGeachie, R. E., Gold, L. H. A. and Latchaw, R. E.: Periventricular spread of tumor demonstrated by computed tomography. Radiology, 125, 407–410, 1977.

Mandybur, T. I.: Intracranial hemorrhage caused by metastatic tumors. Neurology, 27, 650–655, 1977.

Marc, J. A. and Schechter, M. M.: Cortical venous rerouting in parasagittal meningiomas. Radiology, 112, 85–92, 1974.

Messina, A. V. and Chernik, N. L.: Computed tomography: the "resolving" intracerebral hemorrhage. Radiology, 118, 609–613, 1975.

New, P. F. J., Scott, W. R. Schnur, J. A., Davis, R. R., Taveras, J. M. and Hochberg, F. H.: Computed tomography with the E. M. I. scanner in the diagnosis of primary and metastatic intracranial neoplasms. Radiology, *114*, 75–87, 1975.

Nielsen, H. and Gyldensted, C.: Computed tomography in the diagnosis of cerebral abscess. Neuroradiology, *12*, 207–217, 1977.

Nielsen, H. and Halaburt, H.: Cerebral abscess with special references to the angiographic changes. Neuroradiology, *12*, 85–88, 1976.

Norman, D., Enzmann, D. R., Levin, V. A., Wilson, C. B. and Newton, T. H.: Computed tomography in the evaluation of malignant glioma before and after therapy. Radiology, *121*, 85–88, 1976.

Paxton, R. and Ambrose, J.: The E. M. I. scanner. A brief review of the first 650 patients. British Journal of Radiology, *47*, 530–565, 1974.

Pay, N. T., Carella, R. J., Lin, J. P., and Kricheff, I. I.: The usefulness of computed tomography during and after radiation therapy in patients with brain tumors. Radiology, *121*, 79–83, 1976.

Pollock, J. A. and Newton, T. H.: The anterior falx artery: Normal and pathologic anatomy. Radiology, *91*, 1089–1095, 1968.

Rosenbaum, A. E. and Stein, R. L.: Abnormal supratentorial deep cerebral veins. In Newton, H. and Potts, D. G. Eds.: Radiology of the Skull and Brain, Vol. 2. St. Louis: C. V. Mosby, 1974.

Sansregret, A. and Ledoux, R.: Lesser wing meningiomas: A few unfamiliar differential diagnoses. Neuroradiology, *2*, 9–14, 1971.

Sauer, J., Fiebach, O. Otto, H., Löhr, E. Strötges, M. W. and Bettag, W.: Comparative studies of cerebral scintigraphy. Angiography and encephalography for detection of meningiomas. Neuroradiology, *2*, 102–106, 1971.

Schall, G. L., Heffner, R. R. and Handmaker, H.: Brain scanning in oligodendrogliomas. Radiology, *116*, 367–372, 1975.

Sellwood, R. 'B.: The radiological approach to metastatic cancer of the brain and spine. British Journal of Radiology, *45*, 647–651, 1972.

Silverberg, G. D. and Hanberry, J. W.: Meningeal invasion by gliomas. Journal of Neurosurgery, *34*, 549–554, 1971.

Stannard, M. W.: Cerebral scintigraphy in the diagnosis of meningioma. European Neurology, *13*, 85–91, 1975.

Stattin, S.: Meningeal vessels of the internal carotid artery and their angiographic significance. Acta Radiologica, *55*, 329–336, 1961.

Stattin, S.: Significance of some angiographic signs of intracranial meningiomas. Acta Radiologica Diagnosis, *5*, 530–535, 1966.

Steinhoff, H., Lanksch, W., Kazner, E., Grumme, T., Meese, W., Lange, S., Aulich, A., Schindler, E. and Wende, S.: Computed tomography in the diagnosis and differential diagnosis of glioblastomas. A qualitative study of 295 cases. Neuroradiology, *14*, 193–200, 1977.

Steven, J. L.: Some pitfalls in the angiographic diagnosis of intracranial tumor pathology. Clinical Radiology, *12*, 194–198, 1961.

Tadmor, R., Davis, K., Roberson, G. and Kleinman, G.: Computed tomography in primary malignant lymphoma of the brain. Journal of Computed Assisted Tomography, *2*, 135–140, 1978.

Tarcan, Y. A., Farjman, W., Marc, J. and Berg, D.: "Doughnut" sign in brain scanning. American Journal of Roentgenology, *126*, 842–852, 1976.

Taveras, J. M. and Wood, E. H.: Diagnostic Neuroradiology. Baltimore: Williams and Wilkins, 1976.

Thomson, J. L. G.: Computerised axial tomography and the diagnosis of glioma: a study of 100 consecutive histologically proven cases. Clinical Radiology, *27*, 431–444, 1976-A. 431–441, 1976a.

Thomson, J. L. G.: The computed axial tomograph in acute herpes simplex encephalitis. British Journal of Radiology, *49*, 86–87, 1976b.

Trevisian, C. and Dettori, P.: Diagnostic problems of cerebral metastases. Neuroradiology, *3*, 216–222, 1972.

Vassiloathis, J. and Ambrose, J.: Computerized tomography scanning appearances of intracranial meningiomas. Journal of Neurosurgery, *50*, 320–327, 1979.

White, E. and Greitz, T.: Subependymal venous filling sequence at cerebral angiography. Influence of grey and white matter distribution. Acta Radiologica Diagnosis, *13*, 272–285, 1972.

Wickbom, I.: Angiographic determination of tumour pathology. Acta Radiologica, *40*, 529–546, 1953.

Williams, J. L. and Beiler, D. D.: Brain scanning in nontumourous conditions. Neurology, *16*, 1159–1166, 1966.

Willis, R. A.: Pathology of Tumours. London: Butterworth, 1967.

Yock, D. H. and Marshall, W. H.: Recent ischemic brain infarcts at computed tomography: Appearances pre- and postcontrast infusion. Radiology, *117*, 559–608, 1975.

Zimmerman, R. D., Leeds, N. E. and Naidich, T. P.: Ring blush associated with intracerebral hematoma. Radiology, *122*, 707–711, 1977.

7 Supratentorial Deep Lesions

INTRODUCTION

Lesions situated deeply in the cerebral hemisphere, especially those within the thalamus and lateral ventricle, may present clinically as a hyperpressure syndrome or organic dementia without localizing neurological signs. Computed tomography has simplified diagnosis and management of these patients, because it effectively outlines the site and size of the lesion and demonstrates its effect on the brain. It has superceded pneumography. Angiography with magnification and subtraction techniques is the logical complementary examination to computed tomography because it portrays the vascular anatomy and may suggest possible histology of the lesion. This information is essential in planning management, which may include attempted surgical removal, needle biopsy and/or irradiation. Consequently angiographic diagnosis is especially emphasized in this chapter. Radioisotope imaging, because of the increased distance of the camera from the lesion, frequently gives false-negative or only weakly positive results in tumors of the ventricles, basal ganglia and corpus callosum (Fig. 7–1).

VENTRICULAR AND PARAVENTRICULAR LESIONS

These lesions include:
  Intraventricular: meningioma, choroid plexus papilloma, arteriovenous malformation, hematoma.
  Paraventricular: plaques of multiple sclerosis, tuberous sclerosis, astrocytoma, ependymoma.

Computed Tomography

Axial computed tomography is particularly useful in deep lesions which are difficult and often dangerous to investigate by other neuroradiological techniques. Intraventricular masses such as meningioma (Fig. 7–1), blood clot (Fig. 7–2) and the glomus bodies of the choroid plexus (Fig. 7–3) are demonstrated to best advantage, their effects on adjacent parts of the brain being clearly shown (Claveria et al., 1977). Ventricular epidermoids — tumors showing characteristic pneumographic features, described as resembling "cottage cheese" or "a cauliflower" (Dyke and Davidoff, 1937; Tytus and Pennybacker, 1956) — are also well visualized, and computed tomography is usually adequate in differentiating intraventricular glioblastomas which rarely may simulate this appearance (Shapiro, 1950). It is even more reliable in the diagnosis of diseases producing focal paraventricular lesions such as tuberous sclerosis (Fig. 7–4), multiple sclerosis (see Ch. 10) and subependymal astrocytoma (Fig. 7–9).

Angiography

Supratentorial Hydrocephalus. Symmetrical enlargement of both lateral ventricles is usually caused by an obstructive lesion situated either within the brain, e.g., vermis metastasis, aqueduct stenosis, or extraventricularly, e.g., convexity adhesions (see Ch. 10). An enlarged lateral ventricle simulates — and, indeed, is — an avascular space-occupying lesion situated in the depths of the cerebral hemisphere (Fig. 7–5). Unilateral carotid angiography presents a typical appearance, due to the particular displacements of arteries and veins around

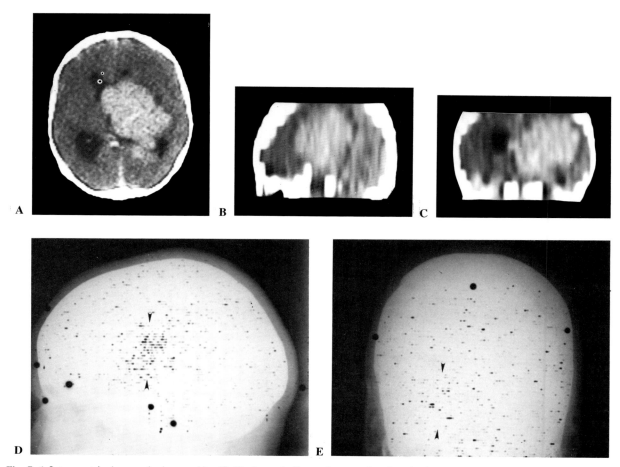

Fig. 7–1 Intraventricular meningiomas. (A–C) Horizontal slice and coronal and sagittal reconstructions of an enhanced computed tomogram in a 29-year-old man. The nodular tumor has well-defined margins and blushes vividly; it fills the cavity of the right lateral ventricle and produces minimal displacement relative to its size. Hydrocephalus is caused by outflow obstruction at the level of the 3rd ventricle. (D and E) Scintigram in a middle-aged woman with a recurrent intraventricular meningioma (*arrowheads*).

the sausage-shaped mass in each hemisphere, from which a diagnosis of supratentorial hydrocephalus can be made. These angiographic signs, which are illustrated in Figures 7–6 and 7–7, consist of tethering of the midline vessels between the two ventricles, and of appreciable straightening and stretching of hemispherical arteries and veins around each ventricle. Therefore, in summary:

1. The pericallosal artery and internal cerebral vein are in the midline.

2. The pericallosal artery follows a wideswept and geometric course between the dilated anterior horns, and the sylvian vessels are slightly elevated and stretched laterally by the dilated temporal horns. The lenticulostriate arteries are flattened outward beneath the dilated ventricular body, and the gap between them and the sylvian vessels is narrowed (Andersen, 1958; Leeds and Goldberg, 1970).

3. The thalamostriate vein is displaced downward and outward with the thalamus, and the internal cerebral vein is flattened (Shah and Kendall, 1971).

The subependymal veins of the roof of the lateral ventricle elongate, and this sign is more reliable evidence of ventricular enlargement than an increased sweep of the pericallosal artery (Galligioni et al., 1969; Azar-Kia et al., 1974).

4. The lateral posterior choroidal artery and branches of the posterior pericallosal artery separate, which is seen in the lateral arterial view of the vertebral angiogram (Fig. 7–8; see Widened Atrium, below).

5. If the third ventricle is dilated, the anterior thalamoperforator arteries are elongated and stretched, especially the hypothalamic segment (Fig. 7–17; George et al. 1975b).

Solitary Enlarged Lateral Ventricle. Obstruction to the outflow of cerebrospinal fluid at a foramen of Monro, as shown in Figure 7–5, is uncommon (Thompson et al., 1973; Segall et al., 1974). Carotid angiography reveals the signs of ventricular enlargement listed above, except that the pericallosal artery has a round shift and the internal cerebral artery is contralaterally displaced, in correspon-

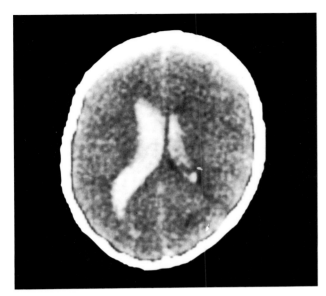

Fig. 7–2 Intraventricular hematoma. Ventricular slice of an unenhanced computed tomogram in a 32-year-old woman with subarachnoid hemorrage. Angiography showed a ruptured aneurysm of the anterior communicating artery.

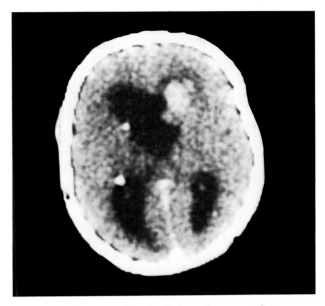

Fig. 7–4 Tuberous sclerosis. Enhanced computed tomogram showing calcified tubers, bilateral and paraventricular in distribution, in an 11-year-old girl from a family with the disease. Right frontal astrocytoma, two calcified paraventricular tubers and hydrocephalus are present—a pathognomonic picture.

dence with the degree of ventricular enlargement. Local lesions at the foramen of Monro may be revealed in the lateral venous phase through deformity of the venous angle. The angle may be closed by obstruction or rendered obtuse by an adjacent neoplasm (Rosa and Viale, 1971).

Widened Atrium. Solid intraventricular tumors or a mass in the adjacent subependymal floor of this part of the lateral ventricle, or hydrocephalus, show a characteristic displacement on vertebral and ca-

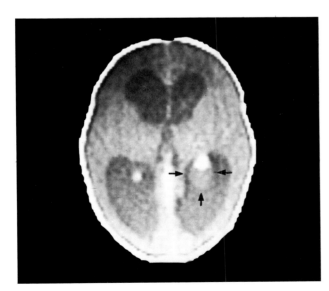

Fig. 7–3 Asymmetrical glomus bodies in an infant with hydrocephalus. The enhanced ventricular slice shows the right glomus *(arrows)* to be considerably larger than the left one.

rotid angiography (Galloway et al., 1964). Vertebral injection in such cases reveals an increase in the normal gap between the lateral posterior choroidal artery and branches of the posterior pericallosal artery (Fig. 7–8). This sign indicates merely atrial involvement, and a more precise angiographic diagnosis is possible only if a "tumor blush" or hypertrophied feeding arteries are present (Fig. 7–9).

Carotid angiography reflects atrial involvement, i.e., a retrosylvian or posterior temporoparietal mass, through forward and upward dislocation of the sylvian triangle, combined with spreading of the distal sylvian arteries (Figs. 6–35 and 7–9). In the lateral venous phase, deformity of the medial atrial vein and its tributaries may be a more accurate guide to the presence of an atrial mass (Hooshmand et al., 1974).

Enlarged Temporal Horn. Neoplasms in the temporal lobe may enlarge the horn by growth or by isolating fluid in the tip. The temporal horn participates in the uniform ventricular enlargement of hydrocephalus, producing an avascular temporal mass which gives rise to arterial displacements that may be misinterpreted as a neoplasm. If the temporal horn is sufficiently large, as in Figures 7–5 and 7–11, the sylvian arteries will show the typical hydrocephalic deformity, i.e., upward and outward displacement. Isolated massive enlargement of the temporal horn may in addition elevate the anterior choroidal artery while depressing the posterior cerebral artery (Fig. 7–10; Chase and Taveras, 1963; LeMay and Ojemann, 1973). The sylvian vein may be elevated.

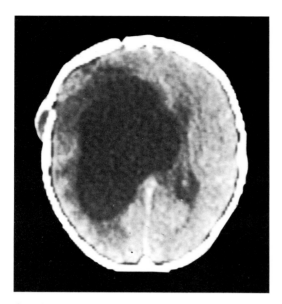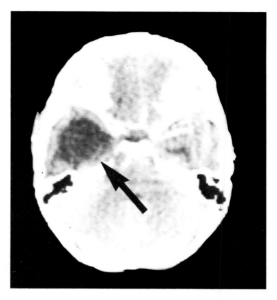

Fig. 7–5 Dilatation of a single lateral ventricle due to obstruction at the foramen of Monro, a postoperative complication in a 15-year-old boy with a pyogenic brain abscess. The arrow points to the dilated temporal horn. For the original appearance of the brain abscess, see Figure 6–21.

Blood Supply of Intraventricular Neoplasms. Tumors of the cavity of the lateral ventricle, such as meningiomas or papillomas of the choroid plexus, usually derive their blood supply from the anterior choroidal, medial and/or lateral posterior choroidal arteries and these vessels become enlarged and tortuous (Fig. 7–11; Stanley, 1968; Banna and Appleby, 1969; Banna, 1971; Thompson et al., 1973). The lenticulostriate arteries supply ganglionic neoplasms, including those that encroach upon the cavity of the ventricle.

Lesions of the Third Ventricle

Tumors within the third ventricle regularly produce obstructive hydrocephalus (Stein et al., 1969). Colloid cysts and initially solid neoplasms obstruct the foramina of Monro. As a result, the lateral ventricles and sometimes the anterior end of the third ventricle dilate, and the third ventricle behind the tumor collapses. Computed tomography reveals all except the smallest of these lesions, through a pattern of deformity or obliteration of the third ventricle associated with tumor enhancement. Pneumography with tomography remains the "last-resort" technique for demonstrating small lesions. Suprasellar masses that impinge on the anterior end of the third ventricle are discussed in Chapter 5. Tumors that deform the posterior end of the third ventricle are discussed below; see Pineal-Region and Incisural Lesions.

Colloid Cyst of the Third Ventricle. A firm diagnosis of colloid or paraphyseal cyst of the third ventricle is impossible on clinical grounds, yet radiological methods will accurately demonstrate it. Correct diagnosis is important since the tumor is benign and amenable to successful surgical removal. Colloid cysts form in the lower attachment of the septum pellucidum and protrude into the roof of the third ventricle as a smooth filling defect immediately behind the foramina of Monro. They manifest by producing obstructive hydrocephalus, and this is the key to the radiological diagnosis: gross dilatation of the lateral ventricles is always present. Initially the cyst causes intermittent obstruction through a ball-valve action at the foramina of Monro; therefore, it need be no larger than 1 cm. in diameter. More usually, however, the cyst is larger. If it is sufficiently large to obstruct the middle of the body of the third ventricle, the optic and infundibular recesses dilate as well as the lateral ventricles. The majority of such patients are demented (Sage et al., 1975).

Plain Radiographs: In about half of the patients the skull radiographs are normal. In the remainder, enlargement of the pituitary fossa or erosion of the dorsum sellae reflects the presence of obstructive hydrocephalus. Colloid cysts do not calcify: according to Taveras and Wood (1976), the presence of suprasellar calcification rules out this diagnosis.

Computed Tomography: Unless the dedicated technique described in Chapter 5 is applied, a small cyst may be missed and the only clue to its presence will be grossly dilated lateral ventricles and a normal-sized third ventricle. When imaged without enhancement, colloid cysts exhibit a high density and smooth outline (Isherwood et al., 1977), and vertebral and bilateral carotid angiography is necessary to rule out a giant midline aneurysm (Fig. 7–12).

Pneumography: This is the original diagnostic

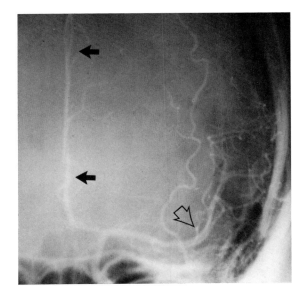

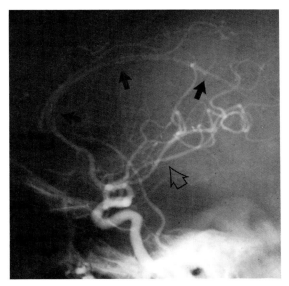

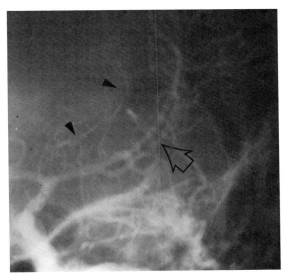

Fig. 7–6 Angiographic appearances of supratentorial hydroce-phalus—arterial signs. Symmetrical dilatation of the frontal horns of the lateral ventricles tethers the wideswept pericallosal artery in the midline *(black arrows)* and dilatation of the tempo-ral horn displaces the sylvian vessels upward and outward *(open arrow)*. The lenticulostriate arteries *(arrowheads)* are also dis-placed outwards and depressed, and they approximate to the sylvian vessels.

method and probably remains the definitive exami-nation for excluding a colloid cyst. Bull and Sutton (1949) described the "hanging-head" lateral and anteroposterior views which, when combined with tomography, will never fail to demonstrate the smallest colloid cyst. Without these special projec-tions, that is, by using only "routine" encephalogra-phic views, the diagnosis is easily missed (Fig. 7–13). Giant basilar aneurysms can be excluded if the floor of the third ventricle is shown to be intact. This is done by manipulating gas around the cystic lesion, to demonstrate its origin from the roof of the ventricle.

Angiography: In addition to the features of ob-structive hydrocephalus which are constantly pres-ent, about 50 percent of patients will show signs upon carotid and vertebral angiography which point to the diagnosis of colloid cyst. These are: (1) In the carotid venous phase, lateral view: local elevation of the internal cerebral vein in the vicinity of the foramen of Monro in large cysts, and an opening out of the venous angle due to draping ("humping") of the internal cerebral vein over the lesion (Fig. 7–14). (2) Carotid venous phase, anteroposterior view: the medial half of each thalamostriate vein is elevated and may be everted, i.e., it assumes a superolateral convexity (Batnitzky et al., 1974). (3) Vertebral arterial phase, lateral view: the medial posterior choroidal artery loses its distal hairpin configuration and shows circumferential draping over the posterior aspect of the mass (Sackett et al., 1975; Rothman et al., 1976).

Glioma of the Third Ventricle. Computed tomog-raphy will reveal such lesions unfailingly. It pro-vides information on paraventricular spread and the degree of accompanying hydrocephalus. Exception-

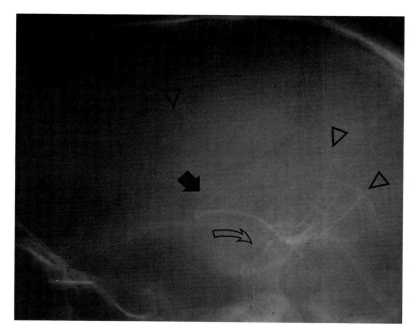
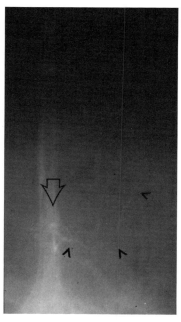

Fig. 7—7 Angiographic appearances of supratentorial hydrocephalus (continued) — venous signs. The symmetrically dilated bodies of the lateral ventricles tether the internal cerebral vein *(open curved arrow)* to the midline and flatten it. Each dilated ventricle is outlined by displaced veins — inferiorly and laterally by the thalamostriate vein *(open arrowheads, frontal view)*, and above by subependymal veins *(open arrowheads, lateral view)*. The black arrow points to a closed venous angle. In the anterior posterior projection the thalamostriate vein is displaced laterally around the margins of the lateral ventricle *(arrows)*.

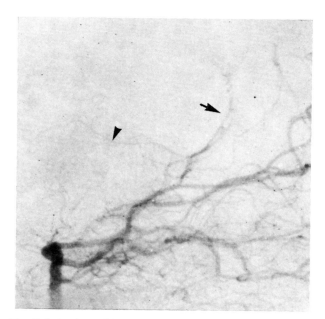

Fig. 7—8 Angiographic appearances of supratentorial hydrocephalus (continued). Enlargement of the lateral ventricles is visible on the lateral arterial view of the vertebral angiogram, manifested by forward displacement of branches of the lateral posterior choroidal artery *(arrowhead)* and backward displacement of the posterior callosal artery *(arrow)*. Widening of the space between these arteries indicates enlargement of the atrium of the lateral ventricle. Diagnosis: astrocytoma of the third ventricle causing obstructive hydrocephalus.

ally, conventional pneumography and angiography are useful in providing additional information in the sagittal and coronal planes, which axial tomographic slicing fails to reveal.

Pneumography remains the reliable alternative to computed tomography for fulfilling neurosurgical diagnostic requirements (Fig. 7–15). The arterial phase of carotid angiography may demonstrate the presence only of obstructive hydrocephalus in small tumors of the third ventricle. Specific angiographic abnormalities caused by such tumors may be confined to the carotid venous phase and the small perforating arteries of the vertebrobasilar system. They are, if present:

1. Upward and backward displacement of the internal cerebral vein by the intraventricular mass; the venous angle may be obliterated and the proximal part of the vein corrugated or deformed (Fig. 7–16).

2. Stretching and elongation of the anterior thalamoperforating branches of the posterior communicating artery (Fig. 7–17). In a dilated third ventricle due to obstructive hydrocephalus, the hypothalamic (paraventricular) segment of the artery is most severely stretched, and in tumors of the third ventricle the arteries tend to be bowed (George et al., 1975a and 1975b).

3. Occasionally a tumor of the third ventricle causes detectable stretching and upward displacement of the medial posterior choroidal arteries (Fig. 7–17; Galloway et al., 1964).

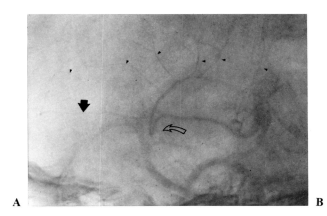

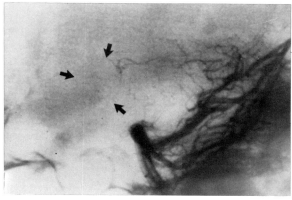

A

B

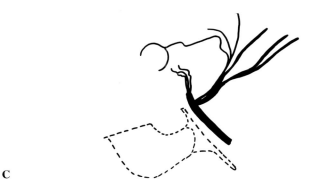

C

Fig. 7–14 Colloid cyst of the 3rd ventricle (continued). Specific angiographic signs. (A) Carotid venous phase, lateral projection. The venous angle is rendered more acute because the part of the internal cerebral vein just posterior to it is wrapped over the top of the cyst ("beaking" — *curved open arrow*). The remainder of the internal cerebral vein is flattened by hydrocephalus. A reliable sign of enlargement of the lateral ventricles is elongation of the septal vein *(large arrow)* and the subependymal veins *(arrowheads)*. (B) Another patient. Vertebral angiogram, lateral arterial phase, demonstrates downward displacement of the medial posterior choroidal artery and bowing of two terminal branches around the cyst *(arrows)*. (C) Line drawing of radiograph. This case was described and illustrated by S. L. G. Rothman, W. E. Allen, III and J. F. Simeone in *Neuroradiology, 11*, 123–129, 1976.

and position of the third ventricle. The large bag of fluid in the midline of the brain produces ipsilateral displacement of the pericallosal artery and internal cerebral vein, as these structures curve around it on either side. The internal cerebral vein is also elevated by the third ventricle (Fig. 7–24; Holman and MaCCarty, 1959; Morris, 1962; Probst, 1974; Osborn and Poole, 1975).

Neoplasms

Lipoma of the corpus callosum, a benign tumor sometimes implicated as the cause of clinical deficit, shows characteristic radiological signs (Fig. 7–25; Sutton, 1949; Mullan and Hannan, 1950).

Malignant gliomas or metastatic deposits arising within the corpus callosum or spreading into it from an adjacent hemisphere distort the normal anatomy. Tumors that cross the commissure from one hemisphere to the other assume a "butterfly" configuration on radioisotope or computed-tomographic imaging. Noninvasive imaging techniques are more reliable in detecting the extent of callosal tumors than angiography or pneumography.

Tumors of the caput or anterior half of the body of the corpus callosum can be shown by computed tomography to encroach upon and distort the lateral ventricles (Fig. 7–26). The area of attenuation produced by contrast enhancement in such cases

serves to confirm the diagnosis. Carotid angiography may be helpful, provided the quality of the examination is adequate, viz., including rapid-serial, magnification and subtraction techniques. The following signs may be present: (1) Elevation of the pericallosal artery, which may supply the tumor via penetrating cortical branches arising from its undersurface (Fig. 7–27; Osborn and Poole, 1975). "Shaggy" cortical branches may also provide a clue to the presence of a neoplasm (Leeds, Rosenblatt and Zimmerman, 1971). If widesweeping of the pericallosal artery is the only sign present, a differential diagnosis may be impossible from hydrocephalus, which is a commoner cause of this configuration. (2) The pial vessels deforming the roof of the corpus callosum (callosal "blush" or "moustache") may be elevated by a tumor or hydrocephalus; therefore an increase in the distance between these vessels and the roof veins of the lateral ventricles must be present before a mass can be suspected (Fig. 7–27; Huang and Wolf, 1964). (3) Displacement of the anterior cerebral artery from the midline. (4) "Tumor blush."

Tumors arising from or invading the splenium of the corpus callosum (Fig. 7–28) are supplied from the posterior cerebral arteries, and angiographic evidence of the presence of a neoplasm may have to be sought by vertebral angiography (Zatz et al., 1967). (1) An increase in the sweep or elevation of

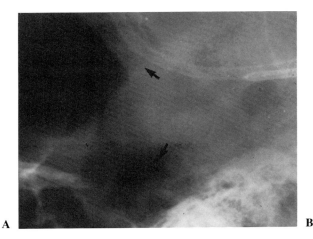
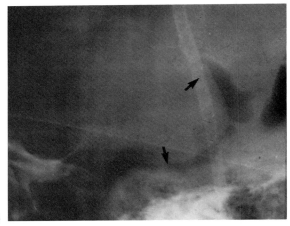
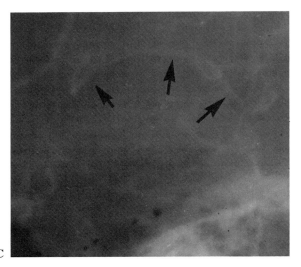

Fig. 7—15 Recurrent glioma of the 3rd ventricle. (A and B) Air ventriculography in the brow-up and brow-down positions reveals a circular mass *(arrows)* filling the 3rd ventricle and dilating its anterior recesses as well as the lateral ventricles. (C) Carotid venous phase, lateral view. The arrows point to an elevated internal cerebral vein with an accentuated convexity; the venous angle is abnormally acute. These observations point to localized enlargement of the third ventricle usually caused by an intraventricular mass.

the posterior pericallosal artery indicates swelling of the splenium (Fig. 7–29). This artery arises from the occipital branch of the posterior cerebral artery in the cistern of the quadrigeminal plate, and becomes visible at the posterior-inferior border of the splenium behind the lateral posterior choroidal artery. From this origin it ascends around the splenium to enter the cistern of the corpus callosum running forward to join the pericallosal artery (Galloway et al., 1964; Osborn and Poole, 1975). (2) Drainage through medullary and early draining veins. (3) Enlargement of the splenium may be confirmed by identifying the vein of the splenium and observing displacement relative to the internal cerebral vein (Fig. 7–29; Zatz et al., 1967). (4) The medial atrial vein may be enlarged and displaced (Fig. 7–29; Hooshmand et al., 1974).

GANGLIONIC MASSES

These lesions distort the caudate nucleus, lentiform nucleus (putamen and globus pallidus) or thalamus.

Computed tomography is the examination of choice for studying their extent and space-taking effects including ventricular enlargement. Angiography remains valuable for identifying causal lesions such as aneurysms and also for anatomical diagnosis because the small, deep-seated arteries and veins which are usually displaced. The most important of these are the following.

(1) *Lenticulostriate Arteries* (Fig. 7–30). The *lateral branches* which arise from the trunk of the middle cerebral artery run parallel to each other as they traverse the lentiform nucleus. Usually four to eight in number, they are seen in frontal view to follow an S-shaped course on the right and a reversed-S on the left. In lateral view they fan out, although in most normal subjects they are usually not recognized, being obscured by the overlying sylvian branches of the middle cerebral artery (Andersen, 1958). Useful measurements in the frontal projection are (Leeds and Goldberg, 1970):

Most lateral branch to middle cerebral artery = 11–14 mm.

Most medial branch to midline = 25 mm.

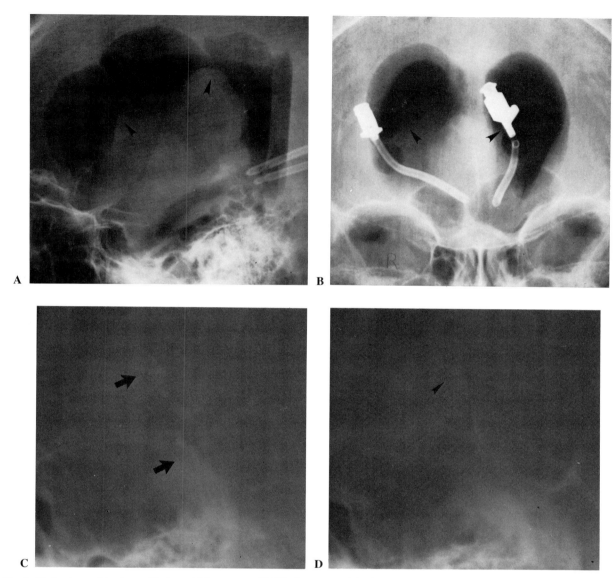

Fig. 7–16 Angiographic signs of 3rd-ventricle tumors: (1) Displacement of the internal cerebral vein. (A-D) A patient with an ependymoma obliterating the 3rd ventricle and splaying the lateral ventricles, as shown by gas ventriculography (A and B, *arrowheads*). The *right* internal cerebral vein (*arrows*, C) has a corrugated appearance, being elevated and displaced backward and sideways — the typical deformity caused by a midline mass arising from the floor of the 3rd ventricle. The *left* internal cerebral vein *(arrowhead*,D) is distorted in the same way.

The *medial branches* are usually not seen unless pathologically hypertrophied. They run a straight course and pass into the medial ganglionic substance from the proximal part of the anterior or middle cerebral artery (Fig. 7 – 30).

(2) *Thalamostriate Vein and Tributaries, the Venous Angle and the Internal Cerebral Vein.* These venous structures drain the subependymal region of each lateral ventricle in the vicinity of the septum pellucidum, caudate nucleus and thalamus. Minor pathological variations in their course may sometimes be confirmed by comparison with the opposite side (Probst, 1970a and 1970b).

(3) *Medial and Lateral Posterior Choroidal Arteries* (Galloway and Greitz, 1959; Pachtman et al., 1974). The *medial posterior choroidal artery* arises proximally from the posterior cerebral artery within the interpeduncular or crural cistern, then runs parallel to the posterior cerebral artery in close proximity to the brainstem and turns superiorly to enter the quadrigeminal plate cistern, assuming the shape of the figure 3, with the pineal gland at the middle. The superior portion of the 3 turns anteriorly and runs forward in the tela choroidea, in the roof of the third ventricle. The artery may be identified in lateral view from this typical configuration, but it

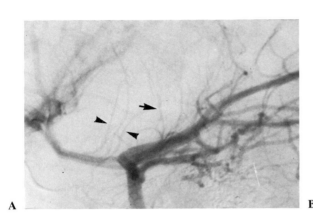

A

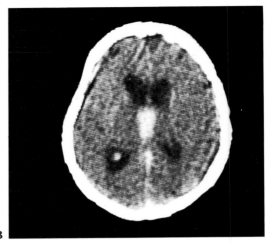

B

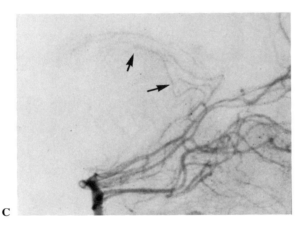

C

Fig. 7–17 Angiographic signs of 3rd-ventricle tumors (continued): (2) Stretched thalamoperforator arteries. (A) A patient with an astrocytoma. The vertebral angiogram shows elongation, stretching and bowing of the anterior thalamoperforator arteries *(arrowheads)*. The posterior thalamoperforator arteries *(arrow)* are slightly compressed. (3) Elevated medial posterior choroidal artery. (B and C) A patient with a low-grade glioma of the 3rd ventricle. The computed tomogram shows an enhancing mass occupying the 3rd ventricle, causing obstructive hydrocephalus. The lateral vertebral angiogram demonstrates an increased superior curve of the medial posterior choroidal artery *(arrows)*, due to enlargement of the posterior part of the 3rd ventricle.

is obscured by the posterior cerebral artery in frontal view.

(4) The *lateral posterior choroidal artery* takes origin from the posterior cerebral artery more distally, i.e., more posteriorly, than the medial posterior choroidal artery. It follows an arcuate course as it lies on the posterior aspect of the pulvinar of the thalamus in the retrothalamic (ambient-wing) cistern and then enters the choroidal fissure to anastomose with the anterior choroi-

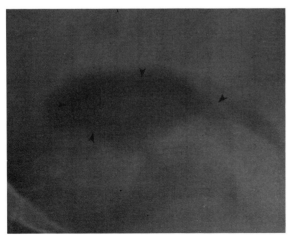

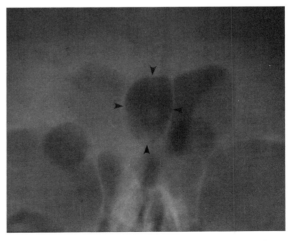

Fig. 7–18 Pellucidal cyst. Brow-up lateral and frontal ventriculograms demonstrate a pellucidal cyst *(arrowheads)* flanked by lateral ventricles of normal shape and size. Two burrholes are present.

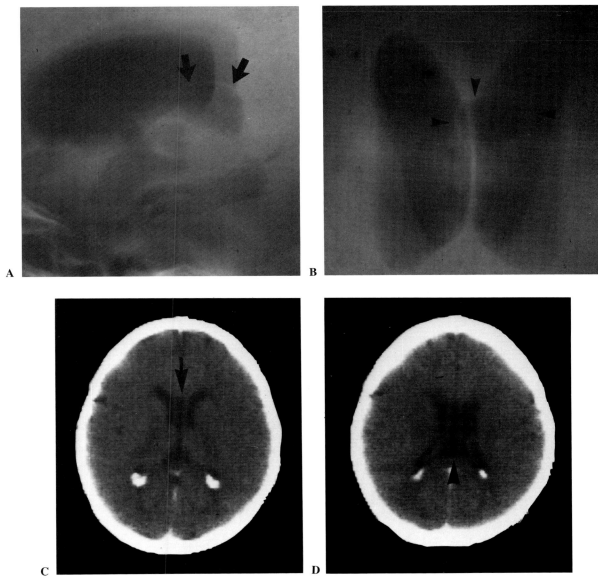

Fig. 7–19 Cavum vergae. (A and B) Brow-up lateral and frontal ventriculogram of a patient with obstructive hydrocephalus. Arrows point to the air-filled cavum vergae above the tela choroidea of the 3rd ventricle. (C and D) Computed tomogram of another patient with a pellucidal cyst *(arrow)* and a cavum vergae *(arrowhead)*.

dal artery. The lateral artery may be identified in lateral view from its arcuate course and its posterior position to the medial artery. It can sometimes be recognized in frontal view in normal subjects (Galloway and Greitz, 1959).

(5) *The Anterior and Posterior Thalamoperforator Arteries* (Fig. 7–31; George et al., 1975a and 1975b). The *anterior arteries* arise from the posterior communicating artery and are related to the third ventricle, optic tract, hypothalamus and thalamus. The course forms an acute angle posteriorly to the posterior communicating artery. George and his colleagues (1975b) subdivided these arteries into interpeduncular, paraventricular

or hypothalamic and thalamic segments. The interpeduncular segment consists of a posterior convex loop around the optic tract, then the artery runs parallel to the third ventricle within the hypothalamus, and finally it turns abruptly laterally opposite the massa intermedia to ramify within the thalamus.

The *posterior thalamoperforating arteries* arise from the termination of the basilar artery or from the proximal part of the posterior cerebral artery. They may be subdivided into interpeduncular, mesencephalic and thalamic segments. These arteries also form an acute angle similar to the anterior thalamoperforating arteries and follow a short undulating course across the interpeduncular cistern. The

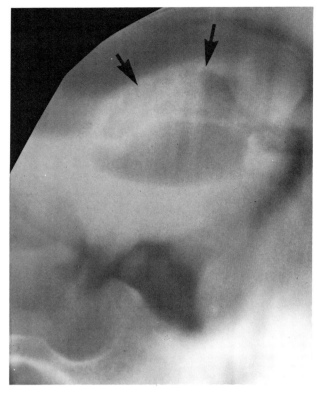

Fig. 7–20 Cavum velum interpositum. The dilated cavum velum interpositum *(arrows)* is visible above the 3rd ventricle. It is seen while the patient is erect during filling of the ventricles.

main segment, the mesencephalic portion, is straight as it penetrates and traverses the midbrain to reach the floor of the third ventricle. Then it curves laterally to ramify within the thalamus.

Tumors of the Caudate Nucleus
Any growth within the caudate nucleus will compress or obliterate the ipsilateral lateral ventricle (Fig. 7–32). However, selective growth may obstruct the foramen of Monro and produce ventricular dilatation. Evidence of the tumor on computed tomography and angiography is then overshadowed by the signs of unilateral ventricular enlargement (Fig. 7–33). Without hydrocephalus, tumors of the caudate nucleus and its vicinity show minimal angiographic changes. Signs when present may be limited to distortion of veins, notably those around the venous angle, e.g., enlargement, stretching or displacement of the caudate or subependymal veins, stretching of the septal veins, opening out or flattening of the venous angle, and/or midline shift of the anterior part of the internal cerebral vein (Johanson, 1954; Probst, 1970a; Salomon and Lazorthes, 1971; Azar-Kia et al., 1974).

Intraganglionic Masses
Space-occupying lesions in the vicinity of the internal capsule are most often hematomas, less fre-

quently gliomas or neoplastic metastases. Intracerebral hematomas in this location tend to complicate systemic arterial hypertension, as discussed in Chapter 3; Figure 3–3 illustrates the typical computed-tomographic and angiographic appearances: "the mass without a shift" (Andersen, 1958; Westberg, 1966; Huckman et al., 1970; Terbrugge et al., 1977).

Carotid angiography permits lateral ganglionic masses to be distinguished from medial masses, by displacement of the lenticulostriate arteries (Fig. 7–34). Lateral masses, which include hematomas complicating aneurysms of the middle cerebral artery as well as neoplasms, displace these arteries medially and widen the gap between the lateral branches and the insular segment of the middle cerebral artery (Fig. 7–35). Medial ganglionic masses, which include a dilated lateral ventricle as well as neoplasms and intracapsular hematomas, displace the arteries laterally and narrow the gap. Mass lesions tend also to *spread* and *straighten* them, while a dilated lateral ventricle produces only lateral deviation and crowding (see Fig. 7–34; compare B and C). Large ganglionic masses produce a square shift of the angiographic U-loop, usually elevating the proximal part of the internal cerebral vein and closing the venous angle (Probst, 1970b; Salomon and Lazorthes, 1971).

Thalamic Tumors
Computed tomography usually provides an adequate diagnosis. Displacement of the lateral and third ventricle and distortion of the tissue planes suffices to indicate the extent of the mass, and contrast enhancement may provide additional clues to its histology (Fig. 7–36). Pneumography may be helpful in demonstrating further displacements, e.g., elevation of the floor of the lateral ventricle, compression of the lateral margin of the body of the lateral ventricle, and displacement or bowing of the third ventricle (Fig. 7–38). Demonstration of a thalamic neoplasm by computed tomography or pneumoencephalography may indicate the need for angiographic examination, especially injection of the vertebral artery in order to study its ganglionic branches.

Vertebral angiography with magnification and subtraction techniques may reveal abnormalities of the thalamoperforating arteries and the posterior choroidal and other branches of the posterior cerebral artery (Galloway and Greitz, 1959). Angiographic signs include stretching or distortion, hypertrophy or neovascularity (Figs. 7–37 and 7–38). Comparisons between the same vessels on each side may reveal subtle but important diagnostic differences. Tumor circulation may be present. The lateral thalamoperforating (geniculate) branches of the posterior cerebral artery may increase in caliber and length to supply a thalamic

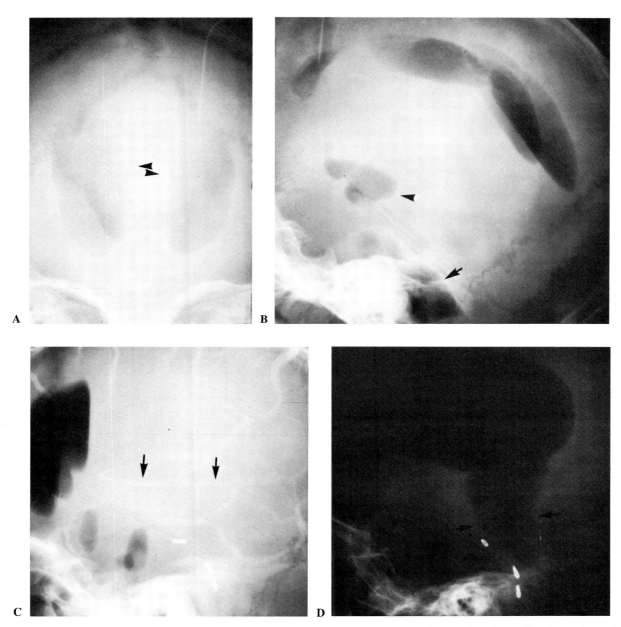

Fig. 7–21 Cavum vergae acting as a mass. (A and B) Preoperative ventriculography. The frontal view shows dilated lateral ventricles and suture diastasis, with a midline cyst *(arrowheads)*. The lateral view shows forward displacement of the 3rd ventricle *(arrowhead)* and 4th ventricle *(arrow)*. (C) Postoperative carotid angiogram, lateral venous phase, shows flattening and convex-downward depression of the internal cerebral vein. (D) Postoperative ventriculogram after surgical opening of the cyst. The air-filled cyst extends through the incisura *(arrows)*. Comparison with (B) shows how the cyst displaces the 3rd ventricle, aqueduct and 4th ventricle forward to produce severe obstructive hydrocephalus.

neoplasm (Fig. 7–38). In the same way, the lateral posterior choroidal artery may hypertrophy and its arcuate course around the pulvinar be wideswept (Fig. 7–38; Margolis et al., 1972); the asymmetry between the two branches in the frontal view will confirm lateral deviation on the affected side. In tumors extending to the midline, the medial posterior choroidal artery may be displaced backward and its sweep increased (Fig. 7–37).

Carotid angiography in the investigation of thalamic masses frequently reveals only a midline displacement of the internal cerebral vein (Taveras and Wood, 1976). In the frontal venous view, the thalamostriate vein may be elevated and compressed. In the lateral venous view, the venous angle may be opened and the internal cerebral vein elevated and its normal anterior curve accentuated, separating it from the basal vein of Rosenthal (Fig.

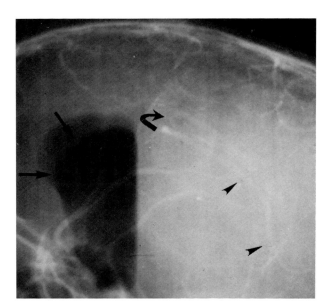

Fig. 7–22 Cyst of the velum interpositum acting as a mass. Lateral carotid angiogram, venous phase, demonstrates marked elevation of the internal cerebral vein *(arrowheads)* and closure of the venous angle *(curved arrow)*. The large arrows indicate the anterior and superior limits of the cyst.

7–38; Guidicelli and Salamon, 1970; Probst, 1970b). Arterial signs include widening of the angiographic U-loop, lateral crowding of the lenticulostriate arteries in frontal view and elevation of the axis of the middle cerebral artery on lateral view (Margolis et al., 1972). According to Potts and Taveras (1963), this effect on the middle cerebral artery is the result of upward and outward rotation of the sylvian fissure by the thalamic tumor.

PINEAL REGION AND INCISURAL LESIONS

Lesions of the posterior end of the third ventricle arise from a variety of structures—pineal gland, thalamus, vein of Galen, posterior third ventricle, quadrigeminal plate, incisural edge (CFT: confluence of falx and tentorium), and adjacent infratentorial structures such as the pons and superior vermis. Poppen and Marino's (1968) series of 20 posterior third ventricle tumors comprised 15 pinealomas and 1 each of the following: medulloblastoma, glioblastoma multiforme, astrocytoma, spongioblastoma and metastasis from the gastrointestinal tract. A feature of most lesions in this region is gross supratentorial hydrocephalus, but specific signs may also be visible in the computed tomogram, pneumogram or angiogram which enable a precise diagnosis to be made (Olson and Abell, 1969; Greitz, 1972). Non-tumoral aqueduct

obstruction is discussed in Chapter 10. Aneurysm of the vein of Galen is described in Chapter 3.

"Pinealoma"

This term includes various histological growths of the pineal gland such as teratoma, pinealoblastoma, pinealocytoma and germinoma, which it is not possible to separate radiologically. "Pineal region tumor" is probably the better term for the radiologist to use when describing these lesions, since he is unable to say that a mass in this region arises from the pineal gland (Papo and Salvolini, 1974; Tod et al., 1974; Messina et al., 1976).

Calcification. As stated in Chapter 1, visible deposits of physiological calcification in the pineal gland are unusual before adulthood. Secondly, the physiological pineal calcification rarely exceeds 1 cm. in diameter. If dense calcification is observed in the pineal region before the age of 20 years, pinealoma should be suspected; also, it should be suspected at any age if the deposits are large (Fig. 7–39; Harwood-Nash and Fitz, 1976). About 25 percent of pinealomas, and all histological varieties, calcify. The deposits of calcification may be speckled, curvilinear or conglomerate in type.

Computed Tomography. Unenhanced slices will reveal pathological pineal calcification, deformity of obstructive hydrocephalus (Figs. 7–39 and 7–40). Enhancement is common and may be discrete or irregular, and reveal subependymal seeding or extension. Computed tomography is the ideal means of monitoring the efficacy of radiotherapy or surgical treatment including ventriculoatrial shunting (Fig. 7–41).

Pneumography. Although superceded by computed tomography in diagnosis, pneumoencephalography may be required in the anatomical delineation of a mass prior to direct surgical attack. Distortion of the posterior end of the third ventricle is a hallmark of pineal tumors (Fig. 7–42). The pineal recesses are effaced and the aqueduct may be flattened if the neoplasm extends through the incisura, and eventually the aqueduct will be occluded (Tod et al., 1974).

Angiography. Over three-quarters of pineal-region tumors are accompanied by dilated supratentorial ventricles, and signs of hydrocephalus usually dominate the angiographic picture. In tumors that are sufficiently large, however, local signs may enable a diagnosis of pineal-region neoplasm to be made. A midline "tumor blush" may be present which is usually irrigated by branches of the posterior choroidal or thalamoperforator arteries. (Fig. 7–43 and 7–44; Tamaki et al., 1973).

Important displacements of branches of the posterior choroidal arteries may be detected by means of magnification and subtraction techniques. Pinealomas displace the medial posterior choroidal artery,

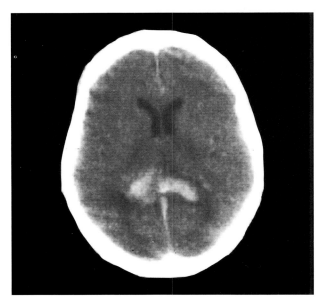

Fig. 7–28 Lymphoma of the splenium of the corpus callosum. Enhanced computed tomogram in a 28-year-old girl with disseminated Hodgkin's disease, showing a mass with a butterfly distribution distorting the normal anatomy of the splenium.

pontomesencephalic vein backwards, separating these vessels from the clivus. If the brainstem is significantly affected, secondary retrodisplacement of the precentral cerebellar vein and choroidal point of the posterior inferior cerebellar artery will also occur. Lesions in this situation may derive a blood supply from the tentorial or dorsal meningeal branches of the meningohypophyseal trunk of the cavernous part of the internal carotid artery: a vivid "tumor blush" may be present (Fig. 7–53; Cortes et al., 1964; Wallace et al., 1967; El Gammal et al., 1974; Palacios et al., 1975). Pneumography remains useful and may be essential to distinguish between intra-axial and extra-axial tumors. This is achieved by opacifying the prepontine cistern. Lateral pneumopolytomography of the clivus may outline the tumor and also reveal bone destruction. Posterior displacement of the aqueduct reflects the degree of brainstem dislocation (Fig. 7–54).

Anterolateral Masses. These lesions are usually solitary or saddle (dumbbell) meningiomas or neurofibromas. Asymmetrical displacement is a hallmark of these tumors. If *solely supratentorial* in location, the following displacements may be present: (1) Indentation of the posterior end of the third ventricle on lateral view, and flattening of one side on frontal view (e.g., Fig. 7–55; Taveras, 1960). (2) Medial displacement of the ipsilateral posterior cerebral artery (Fig. 7–55). (3) The middle cerebral artery and basal vein of Rosenthal may be elevated. If *solely infratentorial*, the tumor may displace only the superior cerebellar artery and precentral cerebellar vein (Fig. 7–56). If both *supratentorial* and

infratentorial (Fig. 7–57), the displacements may affect the arteries and veins of both compartments, Saddle lesions are usually neurofibromas or meningiomas and show similar appearances, but neurofibromas more commonly have a vascular supply from the external carotid artery, while meningiomas tend to be avascular (Levine et al., 1973). Both neoplasms may receive blood supply from the tentorial artery (Wallace et al., 1967).

Incisural (Tentorial) Herniation. The brain may herniate through the incisura if the pressure in one intracranial compartment exceeds the pressure in the other. This situation is usually the consequence of a space-occupying lesion or obstructive hydrocephalus (Liliequist, 1960).

Anterior incisural herniation occurs when the uncus is displaced medially and compressed by the tentorium (Fig. 7–58). This type of hemispherical distortion is reflected in carotid angiography as a downward and medial displacement of the anterior choroidal and posterior communicating arteries. The causal lesion, e.g., massive extracerebral hematoma or glioma, is usually obvious. Enhanced computed tomography shows deformity of the lateral aspect of the suprasellar cistern. With progressive herniation the ipsilateral cerebral peduncle becomes compressed (Naidich et al., 1976; Leeds and Naidich, 1977).

Complete transtentorial herniation occurs when the medial part of the temporal lobe is displaced downward through the incisura, compressing the brainstem (Fig. 7–59; Stovring, 1977). Carotid angiography now reveals, in addition to anterior incisural herniation, a tentorial step in lateral view. The posterior cerebral artery is carried downward and medially by the temporal lobe but at the posterior margin of the incisura the posterior temporal and occipital branch are forced to curve upward. This posterior tentorial step is an important clue to the presence of complete transtentorial herniation.

The enhanced computed-tomographic findings include flattening and/or rotation of the suprasellar "star" and perimesencephalic cistern, which is produced as the tentorium compresses the contralateral side of the brainstem; displacement and rotation of the brainstem; and displacement of the ipsilateral posterior communicating or posterior cerebral artery. With more severe downward herniation, progressive obliteration of the suprasellar "star" and perimesencephalic cistern occurs (Fig. 7–59; Osborn, 1977b).

Bilateral brainstem compression by both temporal lobes, e.g., complicating supratentorial obstructive hydrocephalus, produces a pear-shaped deformity of the brainstem (Fig. 7–60; Liliequist, 1960). Each posterior cerebral artery is compressed between the temporal lobe and tentorial edge, and both arteries become occluded if bilateral herniation occurs (Komaki and Handel, 1974).

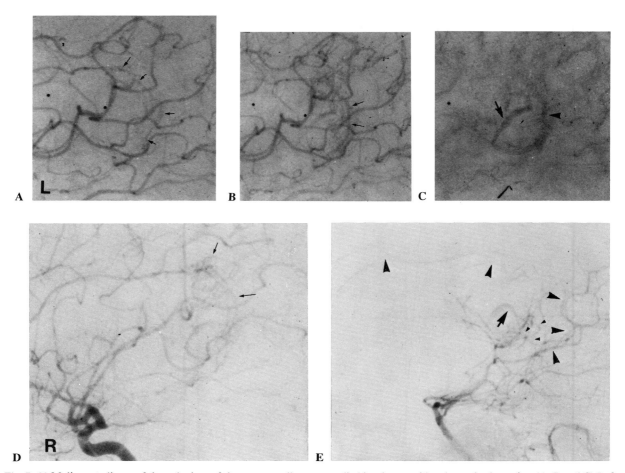

Fig. 7–29 Malignant glioma of the splenium of the corpus callosum supplied by the carotid and vertebral arteries. (A, B and C) Left carotid angiogram, lateral series. In the arterial phase (A) the arrows point to a widened sweep of the posterior pericallosal artery, which is prominent. A half-second later, a "tumor blush" commences (B, *arrows*). The intermediate phase (C) shows hypertrophy of the draining veins: the arrowhead points to an enlarged vein of the splenium and the arrow to an engorged medial atrial vein. (D) Injection of the *right* carotid artery reveals a "tumor blush" in the vicinity of the splenium *(arrows)*. (E) Vertebral angiogram, arterial phase: the large arrowheads indicate the wideswept posterior pericallosal artery. The small arrowheads point to numerous penetrating tumor vessels arising from its inferior aspect. The arrow denotes an early filling vein.

"Brain Death." Compression of the intracranial contents accompanying mass disorders such as tentorial herniation leads to a terminal and irreversible hyperpressure state known as "brain death." Blood flow ceases beyond the level at which the cerebral vessels penetrate the skull, and the demonstration of angiographic stasis possesses clinical value in the diagnosis of death. This picture must not be confused with clinical disease processes which occlude arteries, e.g., traumatic carotid occlusion, or artifactual occlusion produced during direct puncture of the carotid artery (Pribram, 1961). To avoid confusion, Greitz and his colleagues (1973) recommended aortocranial studies with prolonged filming. In order to verify circulatory stasis, the serial angiograms should cover an interval of 30 seconds. Then, after waiting for 30 minutes, another 30-second run should be made.

Several angiographic patterns of "brain death"

are recognized: (Bradac and Simon, 1974): (1) Occlusion of the internal carotid artery above the bifurcation in the neck, with a tapered configuration (Fig. 7–61). (2) The contrast column terminates intracranially at the carotid siphon (Fig. 7–62). Only rarely are the anterior and middle cerebral arteries opacified; the veins never fill, and the 30-second seriogram confirms the impression of circulatory arrest. Although Pribram (1961) reported that emergency surgical measures can lead to a resumption of normal arterial flow demonstrable by angiography, carotid pseudo-occlusion is usually a terminal event and the patient is always unrousable when the angiogram is commenced. This terminal clinical picture may be a decisive point in the radiological differentiation of carotid occlusion: a diagnosis of "brain death" is untenable in a conscious patient.

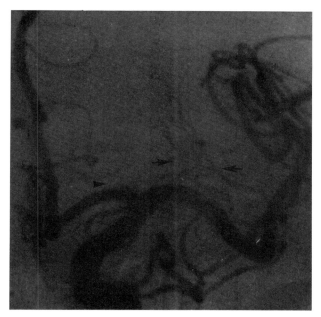

Fig. 7–30 Normal lenticulostriate arteries. Four lateral branches are visible, following a parallel course in the ganglionic substance *(arrows)*. Note their relationship to the insular segment of the middle cerebral artery. The medial lenticulostriate branches arise from the proximal segment of the anterior cerebral artery and ascend vertically in the ganglionic substance *(arrowhead)*.

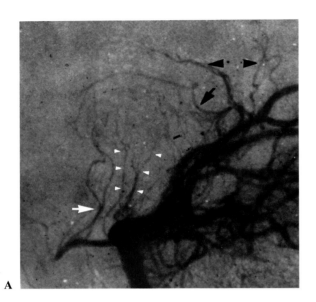

A

Fig. 7–31 Normal vertebral anatomy. (A) Vertebral angiogram, lateral arterial phase. *(Anterior large black arrow)* Anterior thalamoperforator arteries arising from the posterior communicating arteries and looping around the optic tract. *(Small white arrowheads)* Posterior thalamoperforator arteries arising from the basilar tip and penetrating the midbrain to ramify within the thalamus. *(Parallel black bars)* Lateral thalamoperforator arteries. *(Large posterior black arrow)* Medial posterior choroidal artery. *(Anterior large posterior black arrowhead)* Lateral posterior choroidal artery. *(Posterior large black arrowhead)* Posterior pericallosal artery. The large black arrowheads define the atrium of the lateral ventricle. (B and C) Diagrams of arteries and veins in the pineal region. 1. Posterior cerebral artery. 2. Posterior pericallosal artery. 3. Medial posterior choroidal artery. 4. Lateral posterior choroidal artery. 5. Thalamoperforating arteries. 6. Superior cerebellar artery. a. Great vein of Galen. b. Superior vermian vein. c. Precentral cerebellar vein. d. Internal cerebral vein. e. Posterior mesencephalic vein. f. Basal vein of Rosenthal. (After Sones and Hoffman, 1975.)

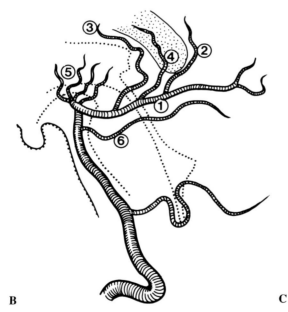

B

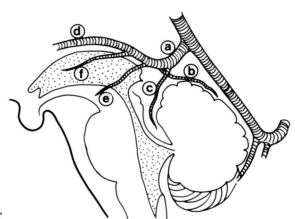

C

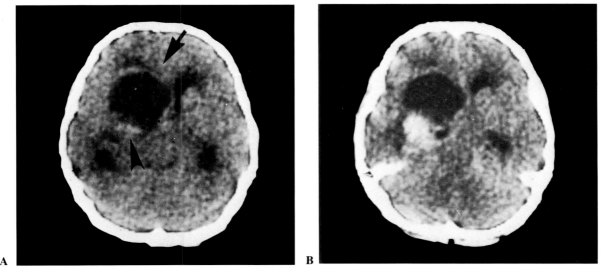

Fig. 7–32 Cystic astrocytoma of the caudate nucleus. (A) Unenhanced computed tomogram shows a large cyst in the left caudate nucleus, compressing the left lateral ventricle *(arrow)*. The posterior margin of the cyst is irregular and the adjacent tissue shows increased density *(arrowhead)*. (B) Post-contrast slice at a slightly lower level shows the vividly enhancing solid part of the astrocytoma.

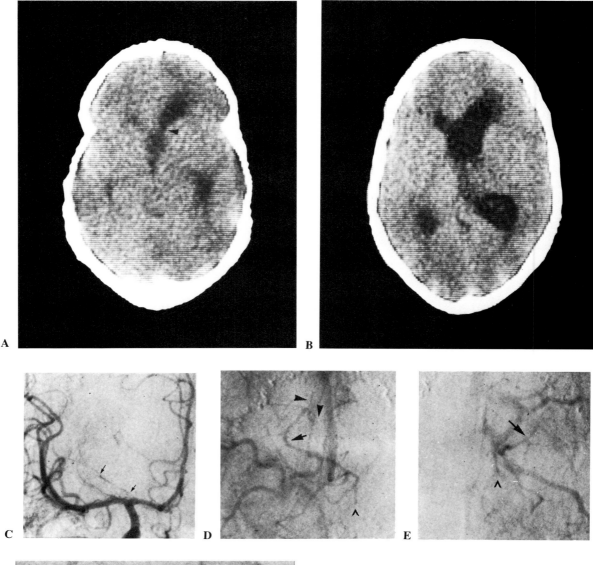

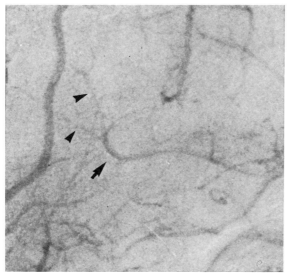

Fig. 7–33 Astrocytoma of the caudate nucleus. (A and B) Enhanced computed tomogram. The arrowhead points to a mass in the right caudate nucleus. A slice 2.5 cm. higher shows midline displacement, caused mainly by the enlarged right lateral ventricle, which is obstructed at the foramen of Munro. (C) Right carotid angiogram, frontal arterial view. Slight contralateral displacement of the anterior cerebral artery is present. The lateral lenticulostriate branches and the insular segment of the middle cerebral artery are deviated laterally. The arrows point to the anterior choroidal artery, also deviated laterally — an appearance compatible with a medially situated mass — tumor or hydrocephalus — or a dilated temporal horn. (D and E) Bilateral carotid angiograms, frontal venous views. Both internal cerebral veins are displaced to the left side *(open arrowheads)*. The right thalamostriate vein (D, *arrow*) is deviated around the caudate nucleus and the caudate veins (D, *arrowheads*) are stretched. Compare the normal course of the *left* thalamostriate vein (E, *arrow*). (F) Right carotid angiogram, lateral venous view, shows deformity of the venous angle (F, *arrow*) and stretching of caudate veins (F, *arrowheads*).

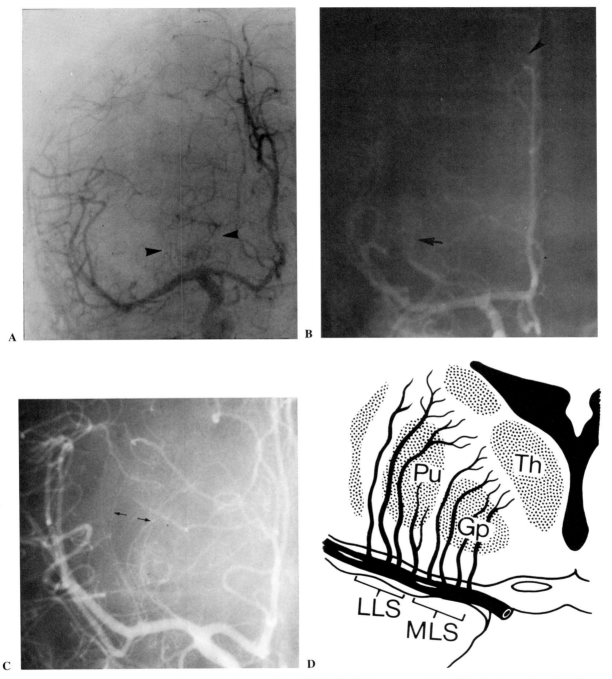

Fig. 7–34 Displacements of the lateral lenticulostriate arteries. (A) Medial displacement and straightening *(arrowheads)* with separation from the insular segment of the middle cerebral artery, caused by a hemorrhage into the external capsule. Note the presence of a square shift and falcine herniation of the anterior cerebral artery. (B) Lateral displacement and flattening *(arrow)* accompanied by lateral displacement of the insular segment of the middle cerebral artery and narrowing of the intervening gap, due to obstructive hydrocephalus. Additional signs of hydrocephalus: straightened pericallosal artery which is taut, and acute angulation of a branch of the pericallosal artery over the corpus callosum. *(arrowhead)*. (C) Spreading, elongation and bowing *(arrows)*, due to an intraganglionic mass. Bowing of the medial lenticulostriate branches *(medial arrow)* suggests extension of the lesion towards the midline. Diagnosis: ganglionic glioblastoma multiforme extending into the corpus callosum. (D) Ganglionic distribution of the normal lateral (LLS) and medial (MLS) arteries. (Gp) globus pallidus. (Pu) putamen. (Th) thalamus.

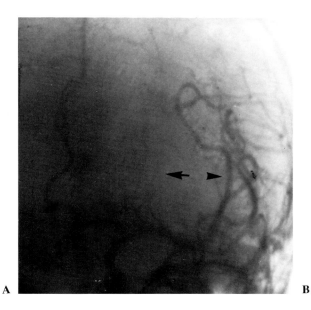

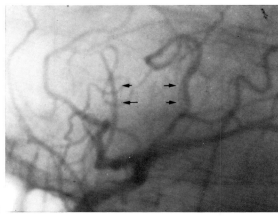

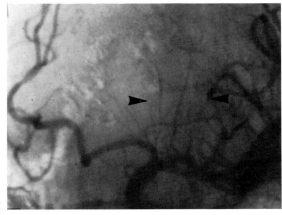

Fig. 7–35 Ganglionic astrocytoma spreading into the island of Reil—a diagnosis made by displacement of arteries. (A) Frontal arterial view shows a square shift, lateral displacement of the insular segment *(arrowhead)* and medial dislocation of the lenticulostriate arteries *(arrow).* (B) Lateral arterial view shows spreading of the intrasylvian branches of the middle cerebral artery *(arrows)*—a reliable indication that the intrasylvian mass involves the island of Reil. (C) Oblique arterial view: the arrowheads show that the displaced lenticulostriate arteries are spread *(arrowheads),* indicating that the mass has an intraganglionic component.

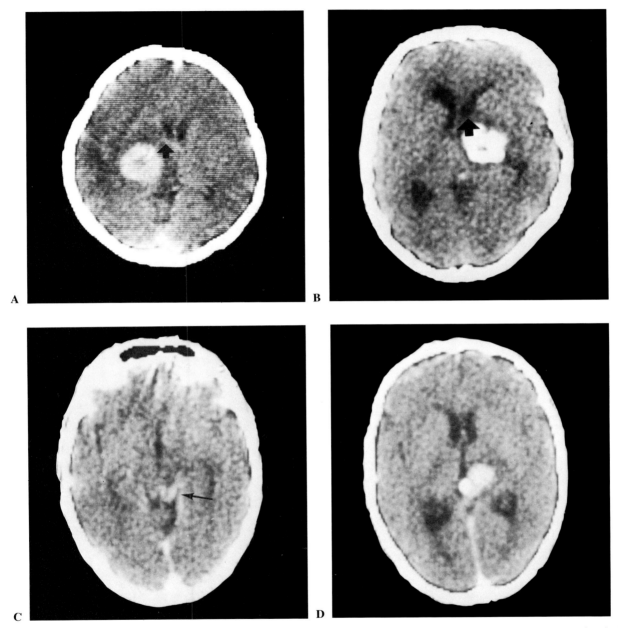

Fig. 7–36 Thalamic masses shown by computed tomography. (A) Malignant glioma. A well-defined enhancing mass occupies the left thalamus, producing only minimal elevation of the floor of the lateral ventricle *(arrow)* and a slight tilt of the septum pellucidum. (B) Ependymoma. A calcified neoplasm of the right thalamus is shown, elevating the floor of the lateral ventricle *(arrow)*. (C and D) Malignant astrocytoma of the thalamus and midbrain. The arrow points to an enhancing lesion to the right of the midbrain and the quadrigeminal plate. A slice made 2 cm. higher shows extension into the pulvinar of the thalamus. In all three patients, note the absence of pineal displacement and significant supratentorial hydrocephalus.

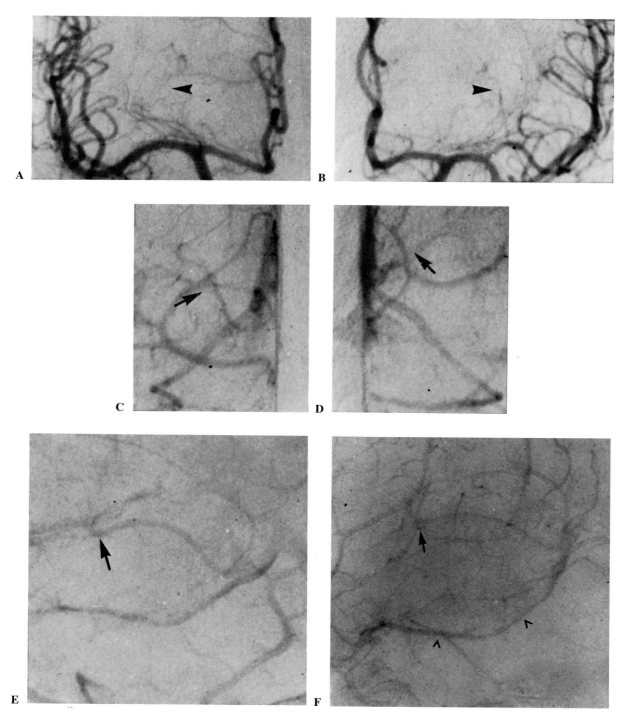

Fig. 7—37 Angiographic signs of a tumor of the left thalamus. Some vessel displacements are subtle, and they may be confirmed by comparison with the normal configuration of the opposite side. (A and B) Bilateral carotid angiograms, frontal arterial views: Arrowheads indicate the lenticulostriate arteries, which are stretched and displaced outwards on the left side. (C and D) Frontal venous views: the arrows indicate the thalamostriate veins, of which the left is compressed and elevated by the mass. (E and F) Lateral venous views; the arrows point to the venous angle. Compared with the normal right angle, the left internal cerebral vein is blunted and elevated with the internal cerebral vein. The left basal vein *(open arrows)* is depressed and stretched.

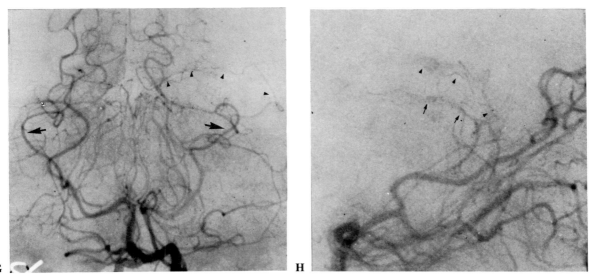

Fig. 7–37 continued (G and H) Left vertebral angiogram. In frontal arterial view, the arrows point to the lateral posterior choroidal arteries and the arrowheads indicate stretching and lateral displacement of the left one and its branches. In lateral arterial view (H), the course of this artery is wideswept on the left *(arrowheads)*, compared to the normal configuration on the right *(arrows)*.

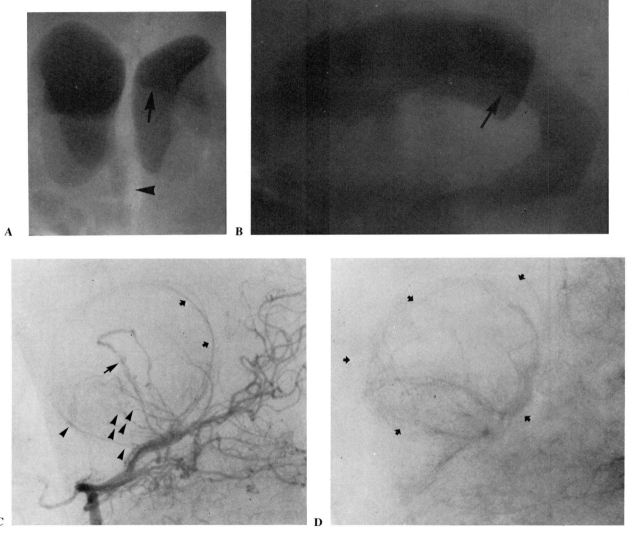

Fig. 7–38 Glioblastoma multiforme of the thalamus. (A and B) Ventriculogram, brow-up views. The floor of the left lateral ventricle in the region of the pulvinar is elevated *(arrow)*, and the 3rd ventricle is displaced to the right side *(arrowhead)*. (C and D) Vertebral angiogram, lateral views of arterial and early venous phases. In the arterial phase, the small arrows point to the lateral posterior choroidal artery which is bowed and wideswept by the large mass in the pulvinar. Large arrow indicates a hypertrophied medial posterior choroidal artery: the superior loop is elevated and stretched with an irregular contous, suggesting neoplastic encasement. The arrowheads point to hypertrophied lateral thalamoperforating arteries which supply blood to the tumor; the most anterior branch is bowed to make almost a complete circle with the displaced lateral posterior choroidal artery. In the venous phase, a ring-blush *(arrows)* is visible in the vicinity of the thalamus.

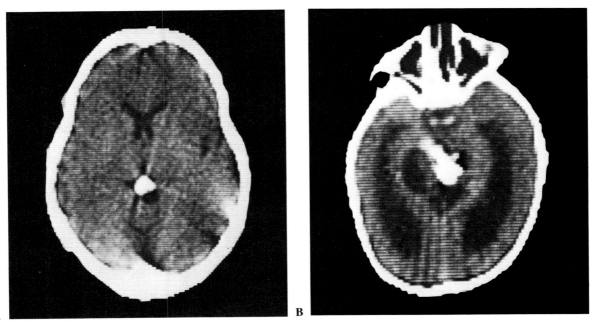

Fig. 7–39 Calcified pineal tumors shown by unenhanced computed tomography. (A) Pinealoma. The extent of the calcification exceeds 1 cm. in diameter, but the tumor has not yet produced obstructive hydrocephalus. (B) Pineal teratoma causing supratentorial hydrocephalus in a baby. Subsequent enhancement revealed a larger tumor surrounding the dense, lobulated deposits of calcification shown here.

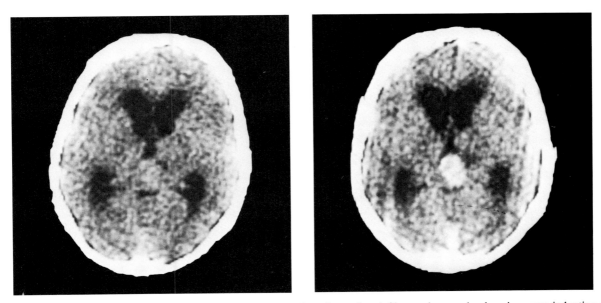

Fig. 7–40 Pinealoma in a 22-year-old girl. Computed tomograms (unenhanced on left) reveal an oval enhancing mass indenting and widening the posterior part of the 3rd ventricle, and producing obstructive hydrocephalus.

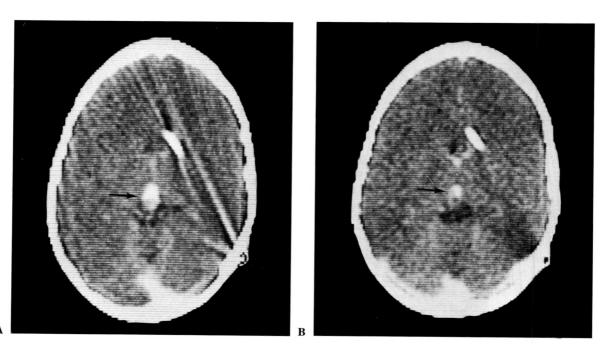

Fig. 7–41 Pinealoma response to radiotherapy monitored by enhanced computed tomography. The arrow points to the tumor. (A) Initial examination after ventriculo-atrial shunting and immediately prior to radiotherapy. (B) Same slice, 45 days later, showing considerable shrinkage of the tumor.

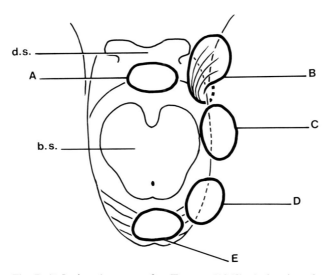

Fig. 7–47 Incisural masses after Taveras (1960). A drawing of the incisura viewed from above shows the position of extraneural tumors. Anterior midline masses (A) lie between the dorsum sellae (d.s.) and the brainstem (b.s.). Anterolateral tumors (B) may be saddleshaped. Other locations are lateral (C), postero-lateral (D) and posterior midline (E).

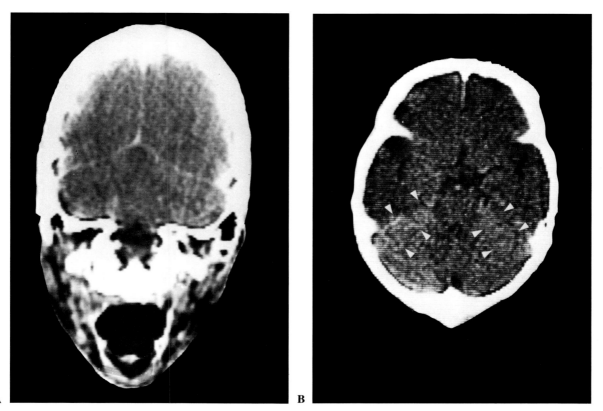

Fig. 7–48 The normal tentorium cerebelli shown by enhanced computed tomography in 5 patients. (A) Coronal slice, depicting the sloping configuration of the tentorium. (B, C, D, E) Horizontal slices made at different angles below the level of the torcular Herophili (B) Broad bands of the tentorium can be identified laterally, as they form its lateral margin *(white arrowheads)*.

(Fig. continues on next page.)

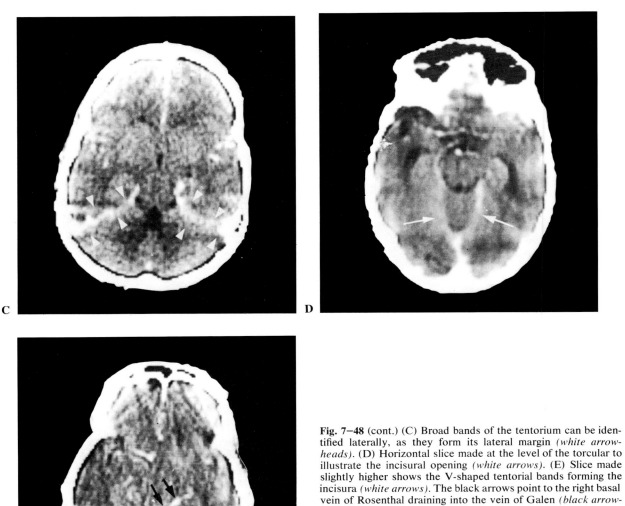

C

D

E

Fig. 7–48 (cont.) (C) Broad bands of the tentorium can be identified laterally, as they form its lateral margin *(white arrowheads)*. (D) Horizontal slice made at the level of the torcular to illustrate the incisural opening *(white arrows)*. (E) Slice made slightly higher shows the V-shaped tentorial bands forming the incisura *(white arrows)*. The black arrows point to the right basal vein of Rosenthal draining into the vein of Galen *(black arrowhead)*.

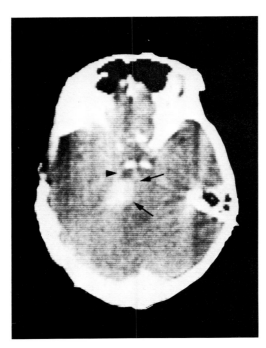

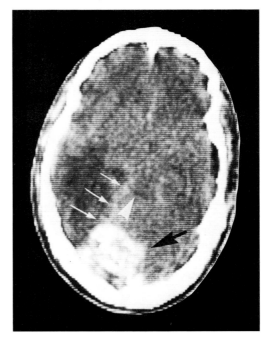

Fig. 7–49 Incisural breast metastasis. The enhancing mass has a well-rounded medial border *(arrows)*. The arrowhead indicates a dilated prepontine cistern.

Fig. 7–50 Meningeal chondrosarcoma above and below the tentorium. Tentorial slice shows the lateral tentorial bands *(white arrows)* forming the medial border of the low-density supratentorial component. The irregular enhancing mass indicated by the black arrow lies at the incisura, distorting and compressing the quadrigeminal-plate cistern *(white arrowhead)*.

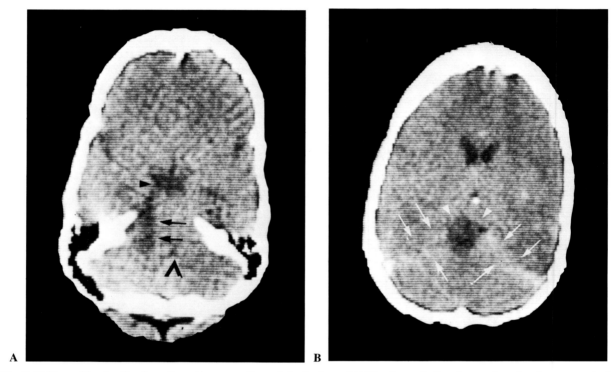

Fig. 7–51 Dermoid extending from the petrous apex through the incisura. (A) Unenhanced slice shows a low-density mass at the level of the left petrous tip *(arrows)*, compressing and displacing the 4th ventricle *(open arrowhead)*. The mass extends forward to the incisura and deforms the posterolateral aspect of the suprasellar cistern *(arrowhead)*. (B) Enhanced slice made 10 cm. higher at the level of the lateral tentorial bands *(arrows)*. The mass within the incisura *(arrowheads)* has a rhomboid shape.

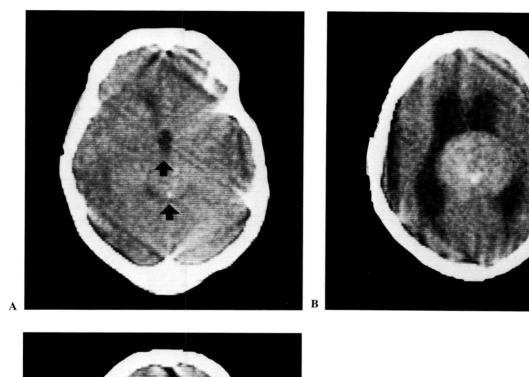

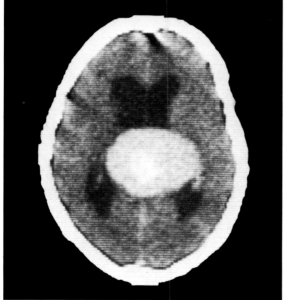

Fig. 7–52 Falx-tentorial junction meningioma shown by computed tomography. (A) Unenhanced slice made at the level of the pineal shows a mass indenting the posterior end of the 3rd ventricle *(upper arrow)* and compressing the midbrain, the quadrigeminal-plate cistern is splayed and displaced posteriorly *(lower arrow)*. (B) Unenhanced slice 13 mm. higher shows dilatation of the lateral ventricles and a large central mass containing calcified deposits. (C) Postinjection slice at the same level shows the mass to have well-defined borders and to enhance densely.

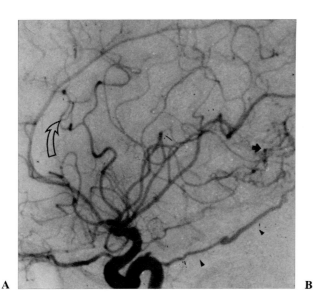

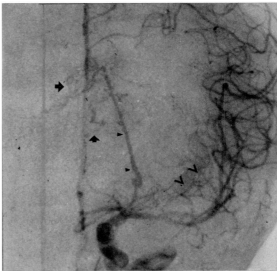

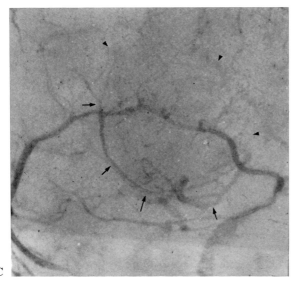

Fig. 7–53 Tentorial meningioma (same patient as Fig. 7–52) demonstrated by angiography. (A and B) Frontal and lateral arterial-phase views of the left carotid angiogram show: a hypertrophied tentorial branch of the meningohypophyseal artery *(arrowheads)* with an extensive "tumor blush" at the incisura *(arrow)*. Ventricular dilatation is manifested by the increased sweep of the pericallosal artery *(open curved arrow on lateral)* and lateral displacement of the lenticulostriate arteries *(open arrowheads on frontal)*. (C) Lateral venous phase of the same examination: the arrows point to the internal cerebral vein with a reversed curve caused by the supratentorial mass effect. The arrowheads outline a "tumor blush."

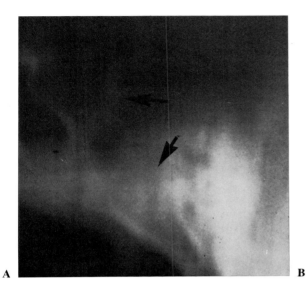

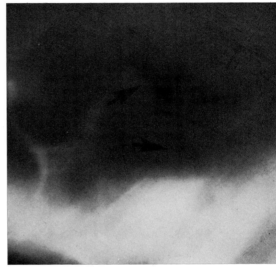

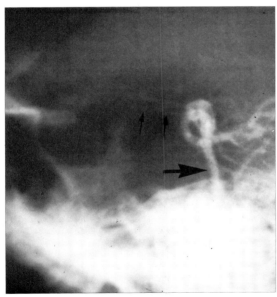

Fig. 7–54 Chordoma of the clivus. (A) Lateral midline tomogram shows extensive destruction of the clivus and dorsum sellae *(arrows)*. (B) Lateral pneumoencephalogram showing a soft-tissue mass filling the prepontine cistern and spreading into the interpeduncular cistern *(arrows)*. The ventricular system fails to fill. (C) Lateral arterial phase of vertebral angiogram. The basilar artery is retrodisplaced by the prepontine mass *(large arrow)*. The posterior communicating arteries are stretched and bowed superiorly, defining the cephalic extent of the lesion *(small arrows)*.

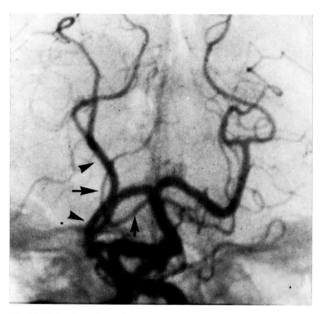

Fig. 7–55 Incisural meningioma – supratentorial growth. Frontal arterial phase of vertebral angiogram shows medial displacement of the right posterior cerebral artery *(arrowheads),* as compared with the left. The right superior cerebellar artery, being infratentorial, is not displaced *(arrows).*

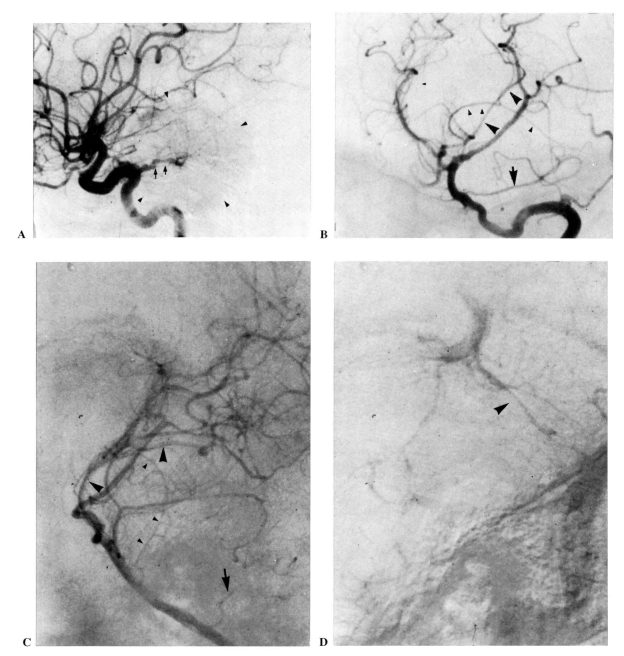

Fig. 7–56 Incisural meningioma (continued) — infratentorial growth. (A) Left carotid angiogram. The arrows point to a hypertrophied tentorial branch of the meningohypothyseal artery entering the tumor. The arrowheads outline the "tumor blush." (B and C) Frontal and lateral phases of left vertebral angiogram. Large arrowheads outline the elevated and stretched course of the left superior cerebellar artery: its marginal branch *(small arrowheads)* is stretched and arched over the tumor. The large arrow points to the left anterior inferior cerebellar artery, which is depressed. (D) Lateral venous phase of the same angiogram. The arrowhead points to a retrodisplaced precentral cerebellar vein.

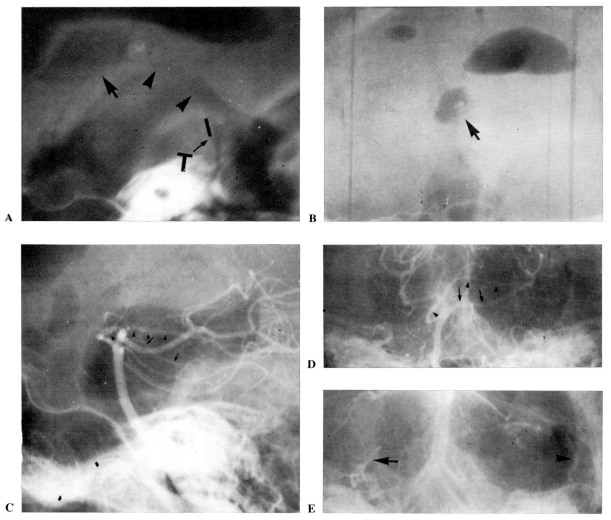

Fig. 7–57 Incisural meningioma (continued) — supratentorial plus infratentorial growth. (A and B) Frontal and lateral pneumoenceph-alograms made with the patient erect. The supratentorial component of the mass elevates and indents the floor of the 3rd ventricle *(arrow)* and aqeduct *(arrowheads)*. According to Taveras (1960), the angled defect of the 3rd ventricle seen in frontal view is character-istic of indisural masses. (T) mid-point of Twining's line, indicating retrodisplacement of the 4th ventricle. (C and D) Frontal and lateral arterial phases of the left vertebral angiogram. The trunk of the basilar artery is displaced to the right of midline. The arrows point to a stretched, elongated and slightly depressed left posterior cerebral artery, and the arrowheads show elevation and medial displacement of the left superior cerebellar artery — signs that the incisural mass is saddle-shaped, i.e., above and below the tentorium. (E) Frontal venous phase of the same angiogram. The left petrosal vein *(arrowhead)* is bowed and displaced outward, compared with the normal right *(arrow)*.

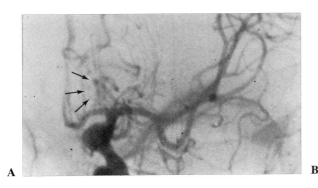

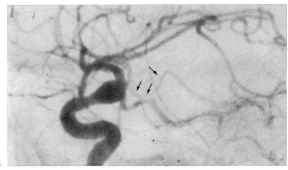

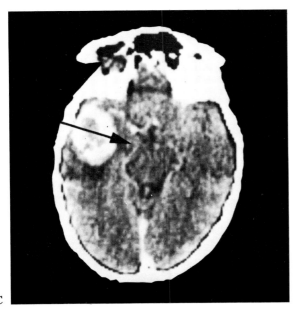

Fig. 7–58 Anterior incisural herniation. (A and B) Left carotid angiogram of a patient with a fatal hemorrhage of the external capsule, which was confirmed in frontal view by medial displacement and straightening of the lenticulostriate arteries. The angiogram also shows evidence of anterior incisural herniation, viz., localized displacement of the anterior choroidal artery as it curves around the uncus *(arrows)*. The direction of displacement is downward in the lateral view and medial in frontal view. (C) Enhanced computed tomogram of another patient, with a left temporal hematoma. The arrow points to medial dislocation of the posterior cerebral artery and compression of the proximal segment of the left cerebral peduncle.

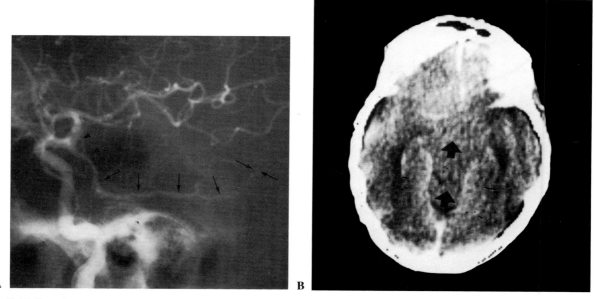

Fig. 7–59 Complete transtentorial herniations. (A) Left carotid angiogram in a patient with a massive subdural hematoma. Marked downward displacement is present of the anterior choroidal artery *(arrowheads)* and posterior communicating and posterior cerebral arteries *(arrows)*. A tentorial step is shown posteriorly *(apposing arrows)*. (B) Enhanced computed tomogram made at a level just above the torcular Herophili in a patient with a large parasagittal meningioma. The outlines of the suprasellar cistern are defined posteriorly by opacified branches of the circle of Willis *(upper arrow),* but obliteration of the suprasellar "star" is evident. The tentorial incisura is outlined by the contrast medium and within it the rotated and distorted cistern of the quadrigeminal plate is visible *(lower arrow).*

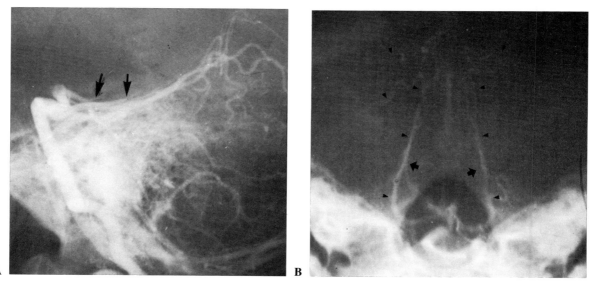

Fig. 7–60 Brain death in a patient with diffuse cerebral contusion and complete transtentorial herniation, shown by vertebral angiography. (A) Lateral arterial view. Both posterior cerebral arteries are occluded *(large black arrows);* only the superior cerebellar arteries are opacified. (B) Frontal projection. The arrows point to the proximal occlusion of the posterior cerebral arteries. The arrowheads indicate the superior cerebellar arteries outlining the brainstem, which has a pear-shaped configuration due to the complete transtentorial herniation.

8 Posterior Fossa Lesions

INTRODUCTION

The posterior cranial fossa is a separate chamber within the skull, which houses the pons, medulla and cerebellum and the blood vessels and covering membranes. These structures communicate above via the midbrain through the tentorial opening with the supratentorial brain, and below through the foramen magnum with the spinal cord.

Lesions of the posterior fossa are classified into one of three compartments or areas, viz., anterior, posterior or cerebellopontine angle. This classification is based on the topographical relationship of the lesion to certain anatomical structures in the midline which are identifiable angiographically and pneumographically.

1. Anterior Compartment Lesions. These lesions lie anterior to the precentral cerebellar vein (vertebral angiography) and to the aqueduct of Sylvius and fastigium of the 4th ventricle (pneumography). They may arise from the clivus, fourth ventricle or brainstem, the latter including tumors arising in or spreading into the midbrain, pons and medulla.

2. Posterior Compartment Lesions. These lesions lie posterior to the precentral cerebellar vein and the aqueduct and fourth ventricle. They are situated in the cerebellar vermis or hemispheres or their coverings or in the retrocerebellar space.

3. Cerebellopontine Angle Masses. These lesions comprise typical angle lesions, such as acoustic neuromas, but also those which extend through the incisural opening into the middle cranial fossa or into the remainder of the posterior fossa, or both.

The lesions most frequently encountered in the posterior fossa are listed in Table 8–1. In adults they include metastatic deposits of cancer (usually in the vermis), acoustic neuroma, meningioma and glioma; and non-neoplastic processes such as infarction, hematoma and atrophy. In children, about 50 percent of intracranial neoplasms arise below the tentorium. The majority are of three varieties, each of which accounts for about 30 percent of infratentorial childhood tumors, viz., brainstem glioma, medulloblastoma and cerebellar astrocytoma.

Incisural masses are excluded from this discussion, having been described in Chapter 7. Craniovertebral angle and foramen magnum lesions are treated in Chapter 9.

PLAIN RADIOGRAPHY

Plain radiographs of the skull are less often useful in posterior fossa lesions than in supratentorial masses—with the exception of acoustic neuromas, of which the plain-film and tomographic changes may be distinctive. Apart from these site-specific changes, abnormalities of the skull are uncommon in infratentorial lesions. They include deformity of the occipital bone associated with a dermoid or other hindbrain anomaly; thinning of the vault (Fig. 8–1), sometimes also adjacent calcification in a slow-growing astrocytoma; destruction of the clivus and adjacent calcification of a chordoma. Most patients with posterior fossa masses, if they survive long enough, will exhibit calvarial changes of raised intracranial pressure—either the acute or the chronic pattern, as outlined in Chapter 1.

Table 8-1 Lesions Most Frequently Encountered in the Three Compartments within the Posterior Fossa

1. ANTERIOR COMPARTMENT LESIONS
Clivus
  – Meningioma (most common)
  – Chordoma
  – Aneurysm of the basilar artery
  – Epidermoid
  – Exophytic pontine glioma
  – Giant-cell tumor
  – Metastatic tumor
  – Meningeal deposits
  – Plasmacytoma
  – Supratentorial lesions extending inferiorly along the clivus, e.g., meningioma, chromophobe adenoma, optic nerve glioma, nasopharyngeal carcinoma
Brainstem
  – Glioma (most common)
  – Arteriovenous malformation
  – Hematoma
  – Infarct
  – Metastasis
  – Infection (tuberculosis and encephalitis)
  – Syringobulbia
  – Demyelinating disease
Fourth Ventricle
  – Ependymoma (most frequent)
  – Exophytic glioma from the brainstem
  – Epidermoid
  – Choroid plexus papilloma
  – Hematoma
  – Outlet obstruction (post-meningitic, post-cysticercosis)
  – Porencephaly (postoperative or post-traumatic)
2. POSTERIOR COMPARTMENT LESIONS
Extracerebellar
  – Meningioma
  – Hematoma
  – Metastasis
  – Abscess
  – Dural arteriovenous malformation
  – Dermoid
  – Lymphoma
  – Arachnoid cyst
Intracerebellar
  – Metastasis (in adults, most common)
  – Medulloblastoma and astrocytomas (in children, most common)
  – Hematoma
  – Capillary hemangioblastoma
  – Arteriovenous malformation
3. CEREBELLOPONTINE-ANGLE LESIONS
  – Acoustic neuroma (most common, adults)
  – Meningioma
  – Epidermoid
  – Metastasis
  – Aneurysm of the basilar artery
  – Arteriovenous malformation
  – Arachnoid cyst
  – Adhesions ("arachnoiditis")
  – Rare: exophytic glioma from the brainstem or fourth ventricle, choroid plexus papilloma, plasmacytoma and glomus jugulare tumor

Calcification: Deposits of pathological calcification are frequently missed, especially in patients with generously pneumatized mastoid cells in whom radiographic examination of the skull is inadequate. Camp in 1930 pointed out the historical fact that the accepted incidence of infratentorial calcification doubled after Towne introduced the radi-ographic projection that bears his name and which reveals the posterior fossa. It may be noted that probably the first calcified brain tumor demonstrated radiologically was a calcified glioma of the posterior fossa, described by Fittig in 1902 (Burrows 1971).

Cerebellar astrocytomas, being more benign, are more likely to calcify than supratentorial ones — 20 percent, according to Kalan and Burrows (1962). The histological deposits found in medulloblastomas, on the other hand, are microscopical in extent, and such tumors seldom exhibit radiological calcification (Martin and Lemmen, 1952; McRae and Elliot, 1958). Therefore, infratentorial deposits when visible in the plain radiographs of infants or children possess differential diagnostic importance. This statement conflicts with the diagnostic significance of calcified deposits demonstrable in computed tomograms, see below. In adults, infratentorial meningiomas, ependymomas and choroid-plexus papillomas may calcify. Calcification in the cerebellopontine angle may represent atheromatous deposits in the walls of a tortuous basilar artery or a meningioma. One-fifth of angle meningiomas calcify (Gold et al., 1969), and a larger proportion additionally show adjacent bone changes (Fig. 8–2).

ANTERIOR AND POSTERIOR COMPARTMENT LESIONS

It is convenient to separate those lesions of the posterior fossa which occupy the cerebellopontine angle and to consider them as a separate group, since they form a distinct entity clinically and radiologically (see p. 385). Other posterior-fossa lesions, viz., those in either anterior or posterior compartment, will be considered together when computed tomography and pneumography are discussed, but separately when vertebral angiography is considered.

Computed Tomography
Complete examination of all anatomical structures of the posterior fossa is possible only if a satisfactory technique is followed and if the slices are carefully analyzed. On account of the partial-volume effect and frequent artifactual densities produced by density variations associated with the petrous pyramids, multiple thin slices are required to demonstrate displacement or deformity of one or more of the following structures:

Posterior end of the 3rd ventricle — deformed or displaced by lesions of the thalamus, pineal, midbrain, tentorium, superior vermis and vein of Galen.

Fourth ventricle — displaced forward or backward or sideways, its contour being deformed by an adjacent or intraventricular mass; enlarged by outlet obstruction.

Cerebellopontine-angle   cisterns — compressed,

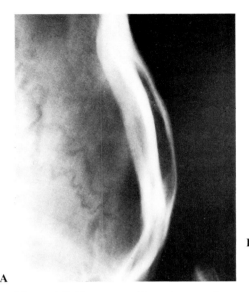

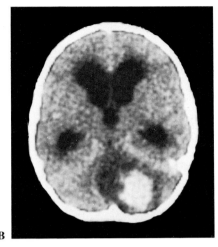

B

A

Fig. 8–1 Thinning of the occipital bone caused by a slow-growing cerebellar astrocytoma in a 12-year-old boy. (A) Asymmetrical thinning and slight bulging of the occipital squame. (B) Enhanced computed tomogram showing a cystic lesion of the right cerebellar hemisphere, producing supratentorial obstructive hydrocephalus.

obliterated, dilated or enlarged by a mass arising within or growing into it.

Parenchymal abnormalities shown before and after contrast enhancement—calcification, bone destruction and changes in normal tissue density.

A high proportion of posterior fossa tumors produce supratentorial obstructive hydrocephalus—up to 90 percent in children, and about half of these show associated periventricular lucencies due to transependymal extravasation (see Fig. 8 – 12). The presence of hydrocephalus should always prompt a careful search for a posterior fossa lesion.

Coronal slices or coronal and lateral reconstructions may contribute significantly to the diagnosis by defining the relationship of the mass to the tentorium and 4th ventricle (see Fig. 8 – 72; Wolf et al., 1976).

The value of computed tomography in the diagnosis of posterior fossa lesions has been reviewed by Bilaniuk et al. (1980), Gado et al. (1977), Naidich et al. (1977) and Thomson (1978).

Brainstem Glioma: These tumors vary greatly in computed-tomographic appearances. The diagnosis depends on demonstrating abnormal density changes and enlargement or deformity of the brainstem; tumor enhancement through the injection of contrast medium frequently occurs with minimal opacification in about 50% of cases (Figs. 8 – 4 and 8 – 6; Bilaniuk et al., 1980).

In about 80 percent of gliomas the unenhanced brainstem shows increased attenuation (Fig. 8 – 3); the remainder show a low- or mixed-density pattern (Fig. 8 – 4). The commonest site of occurrence is the pons, but extension to involve adjacent intraaxial structures can often be demonstrated, e.g., 4th ventricle, cerebellar peduncles or the midbrain and thalamus (Fig. 8 – 5). Exophytic growth from the brainstem into the prepontine cistern produces a tumor picture that may be difficult to interpret (Fig. 8 – 6).

Enlargement of the brainstem occurs at the expense of its circumferential cisterns, which are

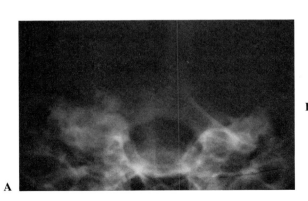

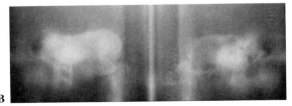

B

A

Fig. 8–2 Calcified meningioma of the cerebellopontine-angle. (A) Nodular deposits are present opposite the mouth of the right internal auditory canal. (B) Petrous tomography shows focal sclerosis of the right petrous pyramid, indicating a diagnosis of meningioma. The calcified nodule has been blurred out in the tomogram.

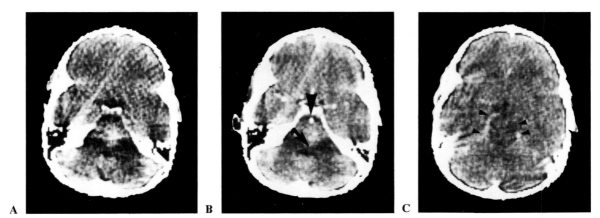

Fig. 8–3 Brainstem glioma. (A) Unenhanced slice shows a patchy high-density lesion within the brainstem. (B and C) Enhanced slices. The expanded brainstem has displaced the basilar artery forward and reduced the prepontine cistern to a slit-like crescent *(large arrowhead)*. It also compresses the apex of the 4th ventricle *(large arrow)*. On the higher slice (C) the brainstem appears less dense than normal *(arrowheads),* due to the overall increase in density of the brain produced by the contrast medium.

compressed or obliterated. The prepontine cistern, which is the cistern most readily studied in the horizontal plane, can be consistently shown to be narrow (Figs. 8–3 and 8–4) or absent (Fig. 8–6). The perimesencephalic cistern may be displaced laterally and the quadrigeminal-plate cistern posteriorly; and the cerebral peduncle may be enlarged (see Figs. 8–3 and 8–4). The 4th ventricle is displaced backward, and its anterior angles may be blunted. If the growth extends into a cerebellar peduncle, the 4th ventricle will be displaced sideways.

Other brainstem lesions may be misdiagnosed as tumor. A fresh hematoma will appear on unenhanced slices as a well-defined, high-density patch within the brainstem (Fig. 8–7), but within weeks the lesion alters in appearance, becoming isodense and then hypodense. Infarcts appear hypodense from the beginning, and they are usually more focal and homogeneous than gliomas (Fig. 8–8). Prepon-

tine masses such as meningioma or chordoma of the clivus or a giant aneurysm of the basilar artery are important in the differential diagnosis of brainstem masses, especially if the prepontine cistern is obliterated and the 4th ventricle is displaced backward (Fig. 8–9).

Medulloblastoma: Most medulloblastomas present a characteristic appearance, viz., a central mass on the floor of the posterior fossa obliterating or deforming the 4th ventricle and producing obstructive hydrocephalus (Figs. 8–10 and 8–11). In the unenhanced scan, the tumor commonly shows the following features: increased or isodense tissue attenuation, a sharply circumscribed outline which is oval, round or loculated, a circumferential halo which probably represents pooling of cerebrospinal fluid rather than edema. Stippled deposits of calcium, although rare, may be visible. Hydrocephalus is usually present. After the in-

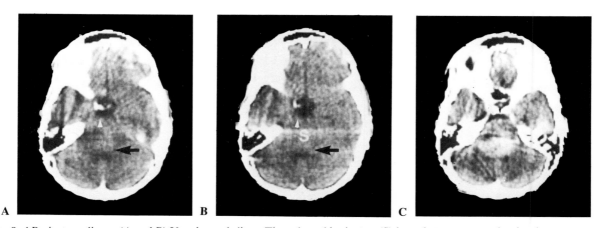

Fig. 8–4 Brainstem glioma. (A and B) Unenhanced slices. The enlarged brainstem (S) has a heterogeneous density; it compresses the prepontine cistern asymmetrically on the left *(white arrowhead)* more than the right side, and flattens and retrodisplaces the 4th ventricle *(arrow).* (C) Enhanced slice reveals a densely blushing brainstem lesion.

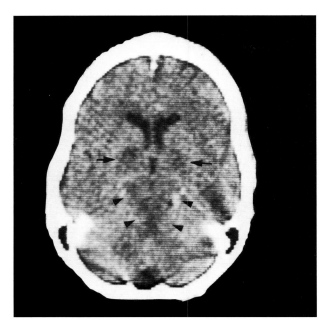

Fig. 8–5 Brainstem glioma extending into both thalamic regions. The low-density brainstem lesion *(arrowheads)* is continuous with like-density lesions in each thalamus *(arrows).*

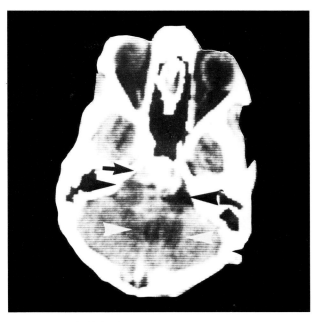

Fig. 8–6 Exophytic brainstem glioma occupying the prepontine cistern. Postenhancement slice shows a dense blushing mass obliterating the prepōntine cistern *(arrow)* and extending into the right cerebellopontine-angle cistern *(black arrowhead).* The 4th ventricle *(white arrowhead)* is deformed from a previous exploratory craniotomy.

jection of contrast medium, the tumor blushes vividly and homogeneously, confirming the presence of well-defined margins and presenting appearances unlike a brainstem glioma.

Computed tomography is the ideal method of demonstrating medulloblastoma dissemination. Follow-up studies may reveal further spread or regrowth of tumor (Fig. 8–12). Medulloblastoma is one of the few primary intracranial neoplasms likely to spread to bone, and the picture of sclerotic de-

posits in a skeleton with ununited epiphyses is quite characteristic (Banna et al., 1970).

Ependymoma: This tumor, slightly less frequent than brainstem glioma or medulloblastoma, is found within or in the vicinity of the 4th ventricle. Not infrequently it extends through a lateral recess and thence into a cerebellopontine angle or the brainstem (Fig. 8–13), or downward through the fora-

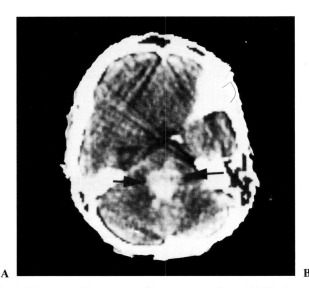

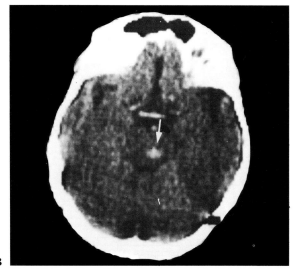

A   B

Fig. 8–7 Intra-axial hematomas. Non-contrast slices. (A) The increased density *(arrows)* indicates hemorrhage extending into the 4th ventricle from the brain stem. (B) Another patient. The small hematoma *(white arrow)* occupies the right side of the tegmentum.

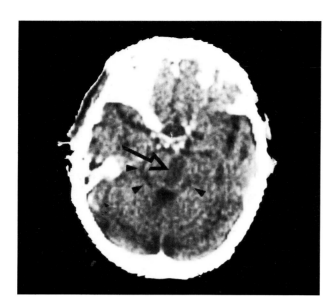

Fig. 8–8 Pontine infarction. The outline of the pons *(arrowheads)* is deformed. A sharply defined, low-density lesion occupies the right half of the pons *(open arrow)*.

men of Magendie into the cisterna magna or the cervical subarachnoid space. Other cases show an irregular ring of growth along the margins of the 4th ventricle, exhibiting an oval or irregular outline with fronds or pseudopods (Fig. 8 – 14).

In the unenhanced scan ependymomas usually show increased or isodense tissue attenuation; Naidich and his colleagues (1977) could find no ependymoma with a reduced attenuation. About 50 percent calcify. Contrast injection usually results in total tumor enhancement if a ring pattern does not occur.

Astrocytoma: The majority of astrocytomas are located in a cerebellar hemisphere and extend toward the midline or into the vermis (Fig. 8 – 15). Less frequently they are located centrally within the vermis (Fig. 8 – 15). About 50 percent are cystic: low-density lesions with defined borders are usually cystic, but "solid" tumors may show a reduced density due to the presence of cysts, edematous tissue or necrosis (Latchaw et al., 1977). Compare the appearances of the solid astrocytoma illustrated in Figure 8 – 15 with the two cystic cases in Figure 8 – 16.

The diagnosis of cerebellar astrocytoma depends upon demonstrating an enhancing lesion and a space-occupying effect, e.g., displacement of the 4th ventricle. In the majority of cases, a portion at least of the tumor enhances, but some low-grade astrocytomas fail to do so at all (Gado et al., 1977). The portion of the cystic tumor to enhance corresponds to the mural nodule(s). These nodules vary in appearance: ring-like, round or crescentic (Fig. 8 – 16).

Differential diagnostic features favoring astrocytoma are: low-density or isodense appearances before enhancement (unlike ependymoma and medulloblastoma); chunky calcified deposits in 20 percent (unlike the stippled calcification seen in 12 percent of medulloblastomas); a circumferential halo (unlike medulloblastoma); and nodular crescentic or ring enhancement (unlike the homogeneous opacification of medulloblastoma).

Capillary Hemangioblastoma: These uncommon tumors possess no features which enable the diagnosis to be made by computed tomography; only vertebral angiography reveals a distinctive appearance (see p. 384). Most hemangioblastomas are solitary, cystic and situated in a cerebellar hemisphere, but some are multifocal, solid and vermian in situation. They are most often misdiagnosed as metastatic deposits, having the same well-defined borders, except that peritumoral edema is unusual (Fig. 8 – 17).

Malignant Metastases: Cancer deposits, which are the commonest posterior-fossa tumors of adults, present no uniform picture. They may be solitary (Fig. 8 – 18) or multiple (see Fig. 8 – 21) and show ring-like or homogeneous enhancement after injection of contrast medium. In the unenhanced scan the low-density pattern of brain edema is usually present, with a circular or solitary zone of increased density within it. Enhancement produces a ring lesion in about 70 percent of cases (Gado et al., 1977).

Non-Neoplastic Lesions: *Hematomas* are imaged reliably and characteristically as high-density masses with well-defined margins (Fig. 8 – 19); on the unenhanced scan, no other pathological entity produces a similar picture. Cerebellar hematomas are usually a spontaneous event for which contrast enhancement fails to demonstrate a cause, while subdural and extradural infratentorial collections are almost invariably associated with trauma.

Infarcts usually affect the brainstem (Fig. 8 – 8) or a cerebellar hemisphere (Fig. 8 – 20). Initial hyperfusion with contrast enhancement and obstructive hydrocephalus due to edema may occasionally cause diagnostic confusion, but the usual picture presents no difficulty in diagnosis, viz., a low-density lesion exerting no mass effect upon the brain.

Otogenic cerebellar abscess possesses the same characteristics as supratentorial abscesses (see p. 252).

Multiple Lesions: Multiple or multifocal enhancing foci present similar diagnostic possibilities as in the supratentorial compartment, although no specific vascular territories can be usefully defined in the posterior fossa. Most multiple lesions are metastatic cancer (Fig. 8 – 21), but it is important always to consider other causes. Extensive primary tumor growth may result in an appearance of multiplicity (Fig. 8 – 22). Similarly, vascular lesions may be mul-

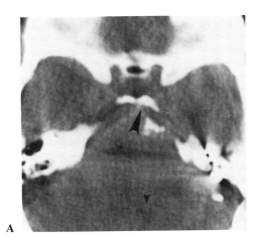

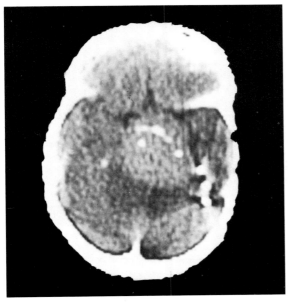

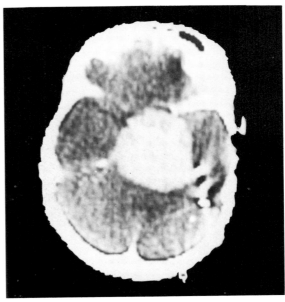

Fig. 8–9 Clivus meningioma. (A and B) Unenhanced slices reveal a central mass with surrounding edema *(arrowheads)*, containing deposits of calcium. The posterior aspect of the dorsum sellae is eroded *(large arrowhead)*. The 4th ventricle is deformed and retrodisplaced *(small arrowhead)*. (C) Post-enhancement slice confirms the well-defined margins of a vividly blushing tumor.

tifocal—either cerebellar hemorrhage (see Fig. 3–37) or giant arteriovenous malformation (Fig. 8–23).

Scintigraphy

The disappointing results of scintigraphic imaging of masses on the floor of the skull contrast with the high accuracy of this technique in detecting supratentorial hemispherical and convexity lesions. This marked difference appears to be caused by the scintigraphically unfavorable topography of the infratentorial chamber (Fig. 8–24; Burrows 1976). However, certain tumors appear to be exceptions, notably large acoustic neurofibromas (Baum et al., 1972; Burrows, 1975) and their ease of diagnosis justifies the continued use of scintigraphy to investi-

gate cases of unilateral sensorineural deafness if computed tomography is not available.

The three scintigraphic patterns found by De-Land et al. (1970) in their series of posterior-fossa lesions correspond closely, although not completely, to the three topographical territories defined in this Chapter, viz., (1) cerebellopontine angle (see p. 385); (2) axial region, i.e., anterior compartment; and (3) cerebellar hemisphere, i.e., posterior compartment.

Anterior Compartment: The area of increased density must lie in the midline on the posterior-tilted view. Only about 25 percent of lesions in this compartment give positive results. Medulloblastomas are usually not demonstrated: "in a child with clinical signs of a cerebellar lesion and a normal

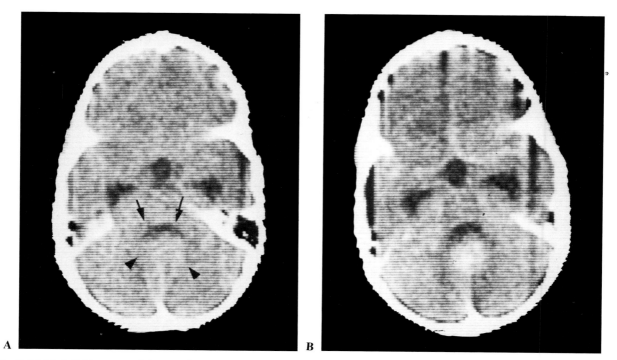

Fig. 8–10 Medulloblastoma of the vermis in a 5-year-old boy. A. Noncontrast slice shows a dense lesion in the superior vermis *(arrowheads)* indenting the 4th ventricle, splaying its floor and displacing it forward *(arrows)*. (B) Same slice after enhancement with contrast medium. The 3rd ventricle and both temporal horns are enlarged due to supratentorial hydrocephalus.

radioisotope scan, a medulloblastoma is more likely than a cerebellar astrocytoma or an ependymoma" (Mealey, 1966). Apart from the high false-negative yield, the results may be misinterpreted: in the posterior-tilted scintigram, normal torcular activity may

be misread as a tumor; in the lateral scintigram, abnormal activity if anterior and low resembles a cerebellopontine-angle tumor and if more posterior, a hemispherical tumor.

Posterior Compartment: Cerebellar hemisphere

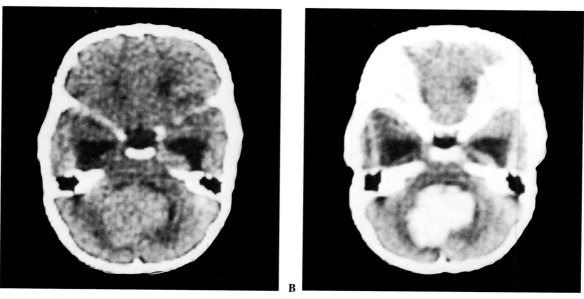

Fig. 8–11 Medulloblastoma—typical appearances. (A) Noncontrast slice reveals a dense mass with circumferential edema situated in the middle of the posterior fossa. (B) Contrast injection causes vivid enhancement of the mass. Both temporal horns are dilated due to hydrocephalus.

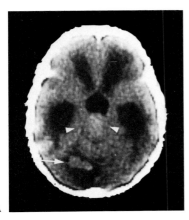
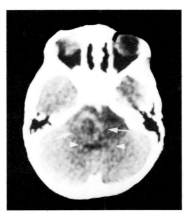
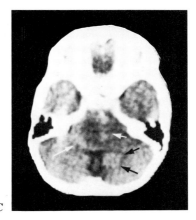

Fig. 8–12 Medulloblastoma spread. (A) An unenhanced slice in a 7-year-old girl with a surgically verified tumor. Two masses are visible, producing supratentorial hydrocephalus—left cerebellar hemisphere *(white arrow)* and pineal region *(white arrowheads)*. Low-density areas surrounding the dilated frontal and temporal horns indicate transependymal resorption, a frequent sign in obstructive hydrocephalus. (B and C) Seeding in a 4-year-old girl with medulloblastoma, slice C made 45 days after slice B. The blushing "doughnut" lesion in the brainstem *(white arrows)* shows interval growth, and a second lesion has appeared in the right cerebellar hemisphere *(black arrows)*. Although a presumptive diagnosis of brainstem glioma was made, histological sections revealed medulloblastoma.

activity may lie high or low, usually surrounded by a clear area separating it from the physiological basal and torcular activity (Fig. 8–25). Only about 50 percent of lesions in this situation can be identified scintigraphically.

Excluding cerebellopontine-angle lesions, therefore, the diagnostic yield of scintigraphy in posterior-fossa lesions is low. Burrows (1976) in his series of proven tumors found false-negative results in 16 neoplastic metastases out of 37, in both meningio-mas, and in 5 capillary hemangioblastomas out of 8. Neurosurgeons complain of two additional deficiencies of the scintigraphic method, viz., (1) lack of specificity: an area of abnormal activity may not represent a space-occupying lesion (Fig. 8–26); and (2) failure to image the ventricular system and demonstrate hydrocephalus. As a consequence, other contrast studies are usually required before posterior-fossa craniotomy can be undertaken.

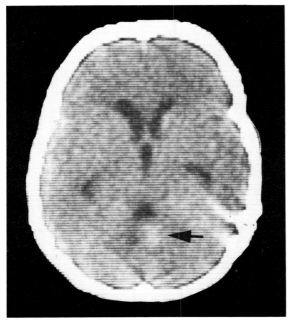
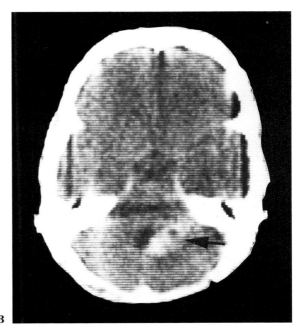

Fig. 8–13 Ependymoma of the 4th ventricle. (A) Enhanced slice shows a blushing lesion with ill-defined margins encroaching on the 4th ventricle *(arrow)*. (B) 11 months later, scan following craniotomy shows a recurrence of the tumor which is extending into the right cerebellopontine angle *(arrow)*.

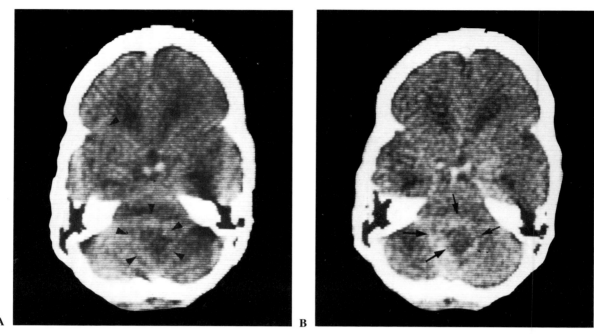

Fig. 8–14 Ependymoma of the 4th ventricle. (A) Unenhanced scan shows a "doughnut" lesion *(arrowheads)*, surrounded by a halo of edema and itself enveloping a 4th ventricle with an irregular contour. (B) Same slice, after contrast injection: the irregular contour of the 4th ventricle enhances *(arrows)*, but the halo is abolished by the increased tissue density produced by the contrast medium.

Vertebral Angiography

Applied Vascular Anatomy of the Posterior Fossa
Correct angiographic interpretation depends on a knowledge of the normal vascular anatomy, and the great detail of the posterior-fossa structures justifies a preliminary description of those of its arteries and veins which are relevant clinical diagnosis (Fig. 8–27; Savoiardo and LeMay, 1970).

Vertebral Artery Trunk: Each artery penetrates

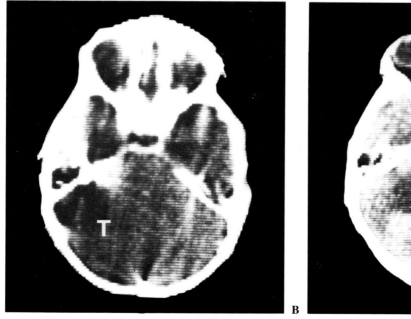
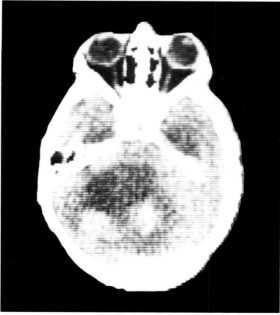

Fig. 8–15 Cerebellar astrocytoma. (A) Unenhanced slice shows an extensive low-density lesion occupying the entire left cerebellar hemisphere and crossing the midline (T). (B) After an injection of contrast medium, two tumor nodules enhance within the low-density lesion.

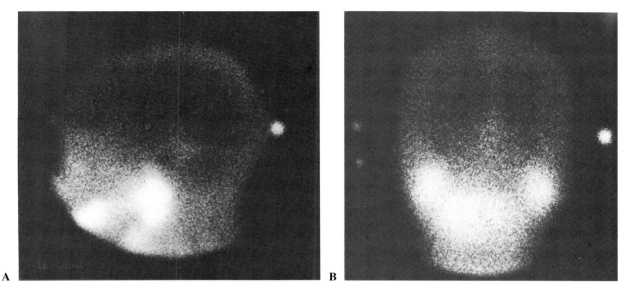

Fig. 8–24 Capillary hemangioblastoma extending through the tentorial hiatus. Lateral and posterior-tilted scintigrams show increased activity in the axial midline of the posterior fossa.

anterior inferior cerebellar artery is usually present (Naidich et al., 1976b). The right and left posterior inferior cerebellar arteries or the ipsilateral anterior inferior and posterior inferior cerebellar arteries may arise from a common trunk. This variation, if not recognized, may lead to the aberrant combination of arterial loops being mistaken for a neoplasm of the brainstem or 4th ventricle.

Anterior Inferior Cerebellar Artery: This is a paired artery which arises from the middle third of the basilar artery, and provides blood to the anterior aspect of the inferior surface of the cerebellum and lateral two-thirds of the pons and upper medulla. There are two major branches, viz., the rostrolateral and caudomedial arteries. The rostrolateral branch runs upward and laterally, close to the 7th and 8th cranial nerves, and describes a double arterial loop called the M segment (Fig. 8–29; Naidich et al., 1976b). Sometimes a single loop is present. In 70 percent of cases, the proximal loop of the M (or a single loop) is related to the porus acousticus. The loop lies anterior to the flocculus, and beyond it the rostrolateral branch passes into the great horizontal fissure. The other branch, the

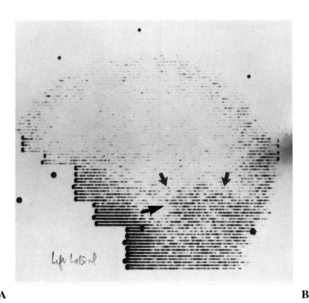

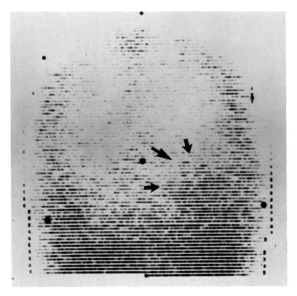

Fig. 8–25 Metastatic deposits in the right cerebellar hemisphere from breast cancer. A clear zone surrounds the area of increased activity *(arrows)*.

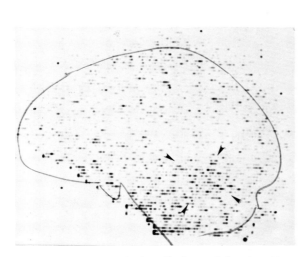

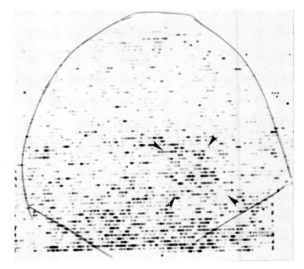

Fig. 8−26 Brainstem infarct in a 66-year-old man *(arrows)*, confirmed at autopsy.

caudomedial artery, varies in size and passes downward in relation to the 9th and 10th cranial nerves to supply the lateral aspect of the floccular and biventral lobules. The anatomical significance of the anterior inferior cerebellar artery, as pointed out by Naidich and his colleagues, is its association with the lower cranial nerves, as well as the flocculus, brachium pontis, great horizontal fissure and biventral lobule.

Pontine Arteries: Paired transverse pontine arteries arise from the distal half of the basilar artery. According to Gerald and Wieder (1975), 2 to 5 branches are present on each side, which extend circumferentially over a distance of 5 to 10 mm. from the basilar artery. These arteries outline the ventral surface and belly of the pons.

Superior Cerebellar Artery: The superior cerebellar arteries arise from the distal trunk of the basilar artery opposite the superior margin of the pons within the interpeduncular cistern. Each runs posterolaterally within the perimesencephalic cistern, circumscribing and then passing over the superior surface of the pons to the quadrigeminal-plate cistern, where they terminate as the superior vermian arteries (Mani and Newton, 1969). The largest proximal branch is the marginal artery, which ramifies on the anterior surface of the cerebellar hemisphere, defining the superior and lateral aspect of the cerebellum. Several small hemispherical branches arise from the perimesencephalic segment. The superior vermian segments define the undersurface of the medial margin of the tentorium above and superior vermis below. The superior vermian branches pass downward and medially and then approximate each other posterior to the quadrigeminal-plate cistern. These arteries form the inferior margin of the incisura.

Posterior Cerebral Artery: These arteries also

arise from the distal end of the basilar artery and have a similar appearance to the superior cerebellar arteries, except that they have a course above the tentorium. After passing around the midbrain they extend posteromedially and laterally as calcarine and parieto-occipital branches (Margolis and New-

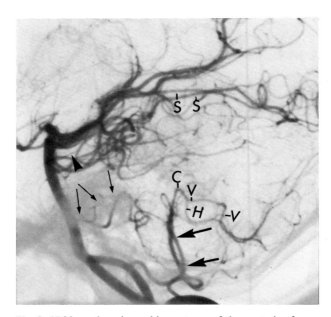

Fig. 8−27 Normal angiographic anatomy of the posterior fossa: lateral vertebral arteriogram. *(Arrowhead)* Pontine arteries; *(small arrows)* anterior inferior cerebellar artery; *(large arrows)* posterior medullary segment of posterior inferior cerebellar artery; (C) choroidal point; (H) hemispheric branches of posterior inferior cerebellar artery; (S) superior cerebellar artery; (V) vermian branches of posterior inferior cerebellar artery. Thus, the following segments of the posterior inferior cerebellar artery can be defined: posterior medullary segment, choroidal point and hemispheric and vermian branches.

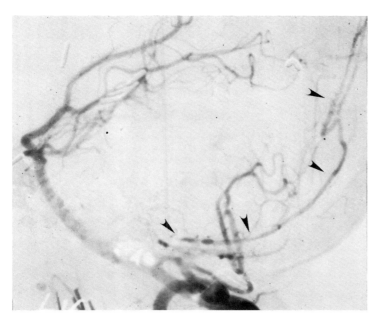
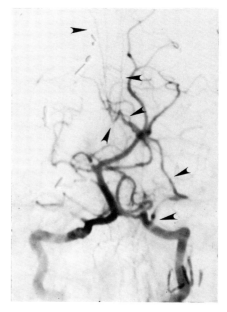

Fig. 8–28 Hypertrophied posterior meningeal artery *(arrowheads)* arising from the intradural part of the left vertebral artery. The patient was a young girl with a choroid plexus papilloma of the right temporal lobe, and the right posterior cerebral artery was clipped during attempted removal of the tumor. Postoperative vertebral angiography reveals that the tentorium and the tumor bed receive a meningeal blood supply.

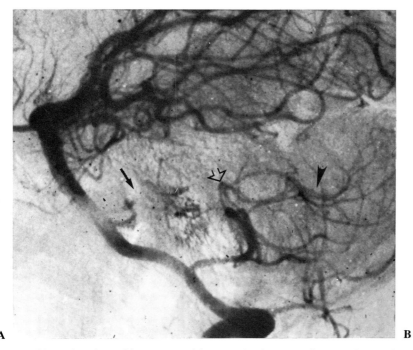
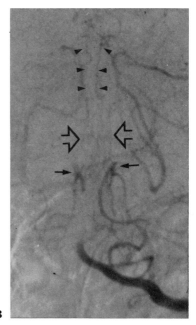

A   **B**

Fig. 8–29 Normal angiographic anatomy of the posterior fossa (continued): The anterior and posterior inferior cerebellar arteries. (A) The **M** segment of the anterior inferior cerebellar artery is visible above the segment of the 7th and 8th cranial-nerve complexes *(black arrow)*. The posterior inferior cerebellar artery wraps itself around the medulla and then ascends behind it (posterior medullary segment) to loop over the top of the tonsil—the caudal loop or choroidal arch *(open arrow)*. Then the artery winds itself around the tonsil to produce an acute hook at the copular point *(arrowhead)*, finally branching into vermian and tonsillohemispherical branches. (B) The choroidal points of both posterior inferior cerebellar arteries are well shown *(small arrows)*. The inferior vermian arteries *(open arrows)* have courses parallel to the midline. The superior vermian veins *(arrowheads)* are visible in the midline.

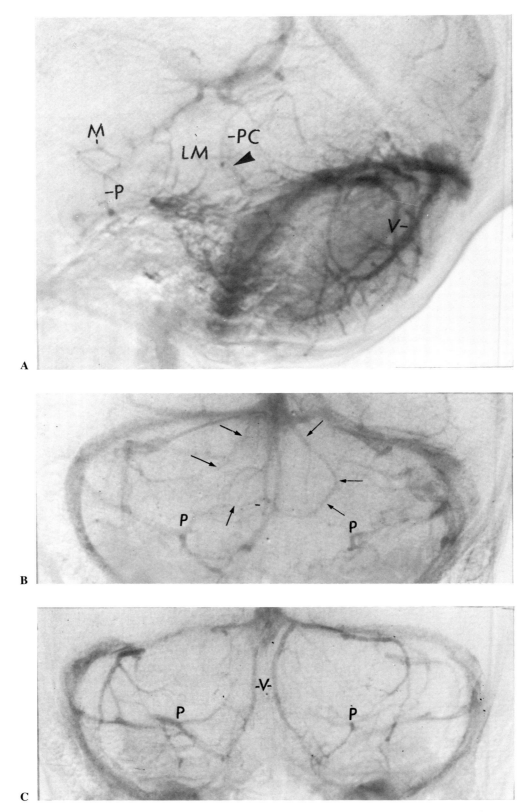

Fig. 8–30 Normal angiographic anatomy of the posterior fossa (continued): veins. (A) Lateral view. (LM) Lateral mesencephalic vein; (M and P) pontomesencephalic vein; (PC) precentral cerebellar vein; (V) inferior vermian veins; *(arrowhead)* colliculocentral point. (B and C) Frontal view. (P) petrosal veins; (V) inferior veins; *(arrows)* veins outlining the midbrain.

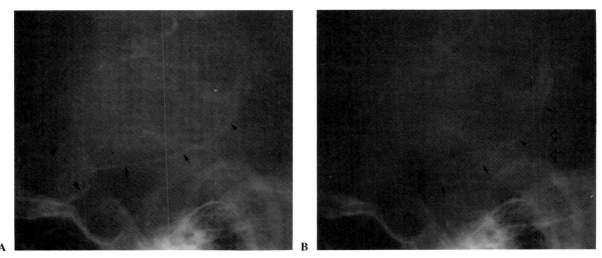

Fig. 8–31 Normal angiographic anatomy of the posterior fossa (continued): the basal and posterior mesencephalic veins. These veins may be confused, due to their similar configuration and course. (A) The vein identified by the arrows is the basal vein, because it opacifies from the deep middle cerebral veins *(arrowhead)*. It drains into the vein of Galen in this patient. (B) Two seconds later: the vein identified by the arrows is the posterior mesencephalic vein, because the anterior mesencephalic vein *(proximal arrow)* drains into it, and the precentral cerebellar vein is visible *(open arrows)*. No supratentorial veins drain into the posterior mesencephalic vein, which in this patient also empties into the vein of Galen. For diagrammatic representation after Sones and Hoffman (1975), see Figure 7–31, p. 320.

ton, 1972). The arterial branches of the posterior cerebral artery which are pertinent to a discussion of posterior-fossa lesions are: the posterior thalamoperforating and posterior choroidal arteries (see Ch. 7, p. 308). The posterior thalamoperforator arteries are important in demonstrating tumor extension into the thalamus or midbrain. The medial and lateral posterior choroidal arteries, in conjunction with the posterior callosal arteries, reveal the size of the lateral ventricles (Galloway and Greitz, 1959).

Veins: The posterior-fossa veins which are important in diagnosis have been described by Huang and Wolf and their colleagues. Veins which can be identified angiographically include the following, in lateral view: pontomesencephalic veins, posterior and lateral mesencephalic veins, precentral cerebellar veins, inferior vermian veins, tonsillar veins, and the superior and inferior retrotonsillar veins. In frontal view: the petrosal veins, inferior vermian veins, veins of the lateral recesses of the 4th ven-

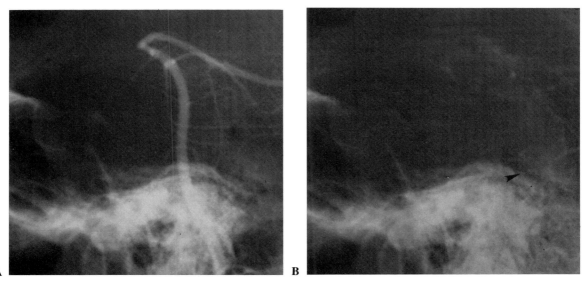

Fig. 8–32 Meningioma of the clivus shown by vertebral angiography. (A) Lateral view, arterial phase: the basilar artery is displaced backwards by an avascular mass. (B) Venous phase, the anterior pontomesencephalic vein is displaced backward and deformed *(arrow)*.

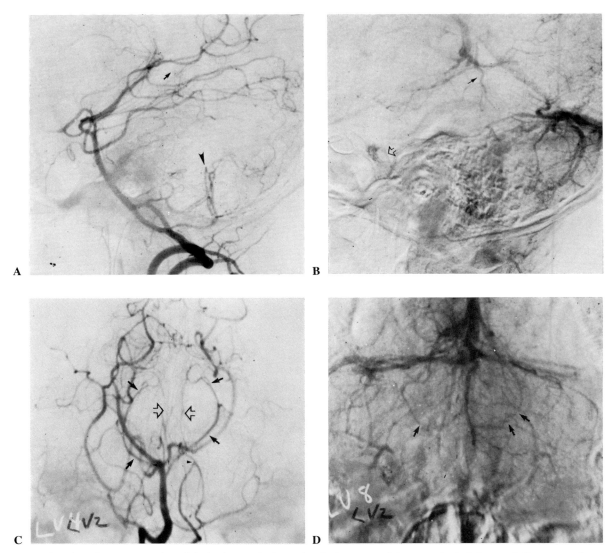

Fig. 8–33 Pontine glioma. Expansion of the brainstem is shown by displacement of the posterior inferior cerebellar artery, the precentral cerebellar vein and the circumferential stem vessels. (A) Lateral view of vertebral angiogram, arterial phase. The basilar artery is compressed against the clivus. *(Arrowhead)* Choroidal point, displaced backward. *(Arrow)* Precentral branches of the superior cerebellar arteries displaced backward. (B) Venous phase. *(Open arrow)* Pontine part of anterior pontomesencephalic vein, displaced forward against the clivus. *(Arrow)* Precentral cerebellar vein, displaced backward. (C) Frontal view of vertebral angiogram, arterial phase showing expansion of the brainstem to the left side. *(Arrowheads)* Choroidal points, separated from each other, each being displaced laterally and the left more than the right. *(Arrows)* superior cerebellar arteries which, with the posterior cerebral arteries, outline the asymmetrical brainstem. *(Open arrows)* Inferior vermian arteries in normal position. (D) Frontal view of vertebral angiogram, venous phase. *(Double arrows)* Lateral mesencephalic veins displaced laterally, indicating enlargement of the brainstem to the left, as compared to the right *(one arrow)*.

tricle, and peduncular veins arising from the ponto-mesencephalic veins.

These veins have been classified into three groups by Huang and Wolf and by George (1974), viz., superior, anterior and posterior (Fig. 8–30). (1) The *superior or Galenic group* represent those veins that drain into the vein of Galen and include, according to Huang and Wolf (1965), the precentral cerebellar vein, posterior mesencephalic vein and superior vermian veins (Fig. 8–30). The precentral cerebellar vein is formed by the junction of

the two brachial veins in a fissure defined anteriorly by the margins of the inferior part of the aqueduct and the upper part of the 4th ventricle, and posteriorly by the central lobule of the vermis. It then ascends between the central lobule and the aqueduct to drain into the vein of Galen (Fig. 8–30; Huang and Wolf, 1966; Hopkins and Bakay, 1975). The precentral cerebellar vein has a gentle curve convex forward. In frontal view it has an inverted **Y** configuration in the midline between the two inferior vermian veins, the short arms of the **Y** being formed by the brachial veins. However, the vein may not be seen in frontal view as it may be obscured by the paired inferior vermian veins. The posterior mesencephalic vein parallels the course of the basal vein of Rosenthal but lies beneath the tentorium. It may be distinguished from the basal vein because it possesses no sylvian or temporal branches (Fig. 8–31) and follows a course around the peduncles and brainstem to drain into the vein of Galen. The superior vermian or culminate veins define the superior surface of the vermis. The superior cerebellar cistern lies between these veins and the straight sinus. (2) The *anterior group,* i.e., those veins which drain into the petrosal sinus, include the anterior pontomesencephalic, the vein of the lateral recess of the 4th ventricle and the petrosal vein (Huang et al., 1968a).

The anterior pontomesencephalic vein has a characteristic notch between the mesencephalic and pontine segments of the interpeduncular fossa (Fig. 8–30). The pontine segment descends along the anterior surface of the pons. It lies on the belly of the pons and defines the anterior extent of the pons more accurately than the basilar artery. The petrosal vein is best seen in frontal projection. It lies in the cerebellopontine angle just above the porus acousticus at a 45-degree angle (Bull and Kozlowski, 1970). The brachial veins lie on the brachium pontis and course anterolaterally to drain into each petrosal vein. The vein of the lateral recess of the 4th ventricle courses medially and inferiorly and then turns upwards to lie in close proximity to the lateral recess of the 4th ventricle (Huang and Wolf, 1967). These veins are not usually well seen in lateral projection. (3) The *posterior or tentorial group* of veins drain into the straight sinus. The veins of importance in this group are the inferior vermian veins (Huang et al., 1969). They occupy a paracentral location in the frontal projection and are formed by junction of tonsillar tributaries (predominantly superior and inferior retrotonsillar veins; see Fig. 8–30). In lateral view the inferior vermian veins have a gentle curve convex posteriorly and lie several centimeters from the occipital bone. The point of junction of the vermian veins with the tonsillar veins occurs just below the copula pyramidis, and this junction is called the *copular point.* The copular point may be recognized by the characteristic loop beneath the copula pyramidis which is similar to that of the vermian artery.

Lesions of the Anterior Compartment: Displacements

1. Clivus and Adjacent Masses: The commonest of these are chordoma and meningioma, and also aneurysm of the basilar artery (Table 8–1). The trunk of the basilar artery and the anterior pontomesencephalic vein are displaced backward from the clivus: Kendall and Lee (1977) found that the extent to which these vessels were dislocated corresponded to the size of the mass in 95 percent of cases of chordoma. Characteristically meningiomas receive a portion of their blood supply from hypertrophied meningeal arteries and show a homogeneous stain, but occasionally they may be avascular (Fig. 8–32). Conversely, chordomas—although traditionally avascular—may exhibit a profuse blood supply including staining and hypertrophied feeding vessels (Kendall and Lee, 1977; Smink et al., 1977).

2. Brainstem Masses: The commonest intrinsic lesion deforming the brainstem both in adults and children is a glioma (Table 8–1). The tumor may be confined to the pontomedullary axis, producing symmetrical swelling of the stem; or it may grow excentrically and invade the midbrain, 4th ventricle or a cerebellar hemisphere via the peduncle. Finally, a small proportion of brainstem gliomas spread exophytically, usually invading the prepontine cistern.

The following angiographic signs of a brainstem mass are encountered:

(A) Posterior Inferior Cerebellar Artery: Displacement of the medullary segments, particularly the posterior one, so that the choroidal point is displaced backward and the gap between the basilar artery and the medullary segments is widened. The posterior inferior cerebellar artery may be flattened, losing its normal caudal and cranial loops, and assuming the configuration on lateral view of an open accordion (Fig. 8–33 and 8–34; Huang and Wolf, 1969; George, 1974). In frontal view, each lateral medullary segment is displaced laterally and the choroidal points therefore separate if the tumor grows into the vallecula or 4th ventricle (Fig. 8–33).

(B) Anterior Inferior Cerebellar Artery: Displacement downward, particularly unilateral flattening of the brachial and floccular parts of the artery, serve as a guide to growth into the brachium pontis and cerebellar peduncle (Figs. 8–36 and 8–37; Naidich et al., 1976b).

(C) Basilar Artery and Pontine Branches: The trunk of the basilar artery is usually flattened forward against the clivus by the enlarged brainstem (Figs. 8–33 and 8–37), but occasionally it may retain a normal position. Exophytic growth may, paradoxically, cause posterior displacement of the basilar trunk, as shown in Fig. 8–38, and this possibility emphasizes the importance of identifying the transverse pontine arteries and the anterior pontomesencephalic vein, which are more reliable indicators of the position of the belly of the pons (Sarwar et al., 1977). According to Gerald and Wieder (1975), the transverse pontine arteries are rarely traced for more than 10 mm. behind the basilar artery in lateral view of the vertebral angiogram. In

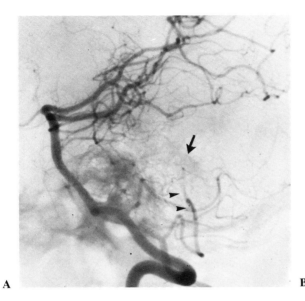

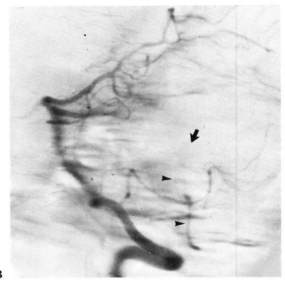

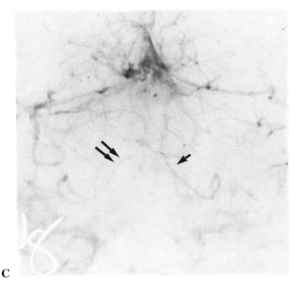

A

B

C

Fig. 8–34 Brainstem glioma spreading into the right cerebellar peduncle. (A and B) Lateral view of vertebral angiogram with tomography. *(Arrowheads)* Retrodisplaced posterior medullary segment. *(Arrow)* Choroidal blush. (C) Frontal view of vertebral angiogram, venous phase. *(Double arrows)* Vein of the right lateral recess of the 4th ventricle, with abnormal convex-lateral curve, compared to the normal vein of the left side *(single arrow)*. This deformity indicates a mass lesion situated adjacent to the 4th ventricle and in the peduncle.

brainstem gliomas they may be stretched, displaced and enlarged, and lie anterior to the basilar trunk (Figs. 8–37 and 8–38).

(D) *Superior Cerebellar and Posterior Cerebral Arteries:* In frontal view these arteries follow a wideswept course around an enlarged brainstem and they may be taut (Fig. 8–33). In lateral view, the quadrigeminal and precentral branches of the superior cerebellar artery are displaced backward (Fig. 8–33).

(E) *Displacement of Veins:* These vessels frequently show changes in brainstem tumors, e.g., enlargement of the outline of the midbrain in the frontal view, manifested by outward displacement of the lateral mesencephalic veins and inferior and lateral displacement of the peduncular veins (Fig. 8–33 and 8–37). The anterior pontomesencephalic vein, because of its close relationship to the belly of the pons, is the most sensitive indication of an enlarged brainstem (Figs. 8–33 and 8–35; Bradac, 1970; Bradac et al., 1971). The precentral cerebellar vein is regularly displaced backward (Figs. 8–33, 8–35 and 8–38; Huang and Wolf 1966). According to Savoiardo and Vaghi (1974), the brainstem is abnormally large if the gap between the anterior pontomesencephalic vein and the precentral cerebellar vein exceeds 23 mm. The position of the lateral mesencephalic vein may aid in differentiating anterior midbrain masses from posterior midbrain or tegmental masses: in anterior masses, this vein is displaced backward and in tegmental masses forward (Fig 8–35). Tegmental tumors also cause localized arcuate deformity of the precentral cerebellar vein and reversal of the normal convex-

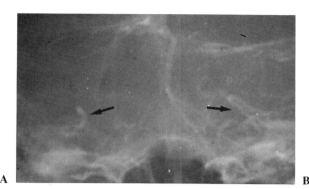
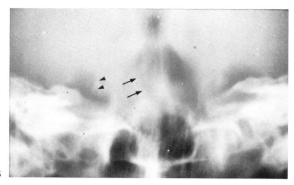

A   B

Fig. 8–52 Trigeminal neuroma in Meckel's cave, deforming the petrosal vein. (A) Vertebral angiogram, venous phase, frontal view. The petrosal veins *(arrows)* are asymmetrical, due to lateral displacement of the right vein. (B) Pneumotomogram with the patient erect. *(Arrowheads)* Lateral outline of mass. *(Arrows)* Defect in the right lateral recess of the 4th ventricle.

recess, malleus and incus ossicles, canal for the facial nerve ("cat's eyes"), cochlea and carotid canal. The *vestibular plane* lies approximately 4 mm. behind the cochlear plane. The structures visualized, in addition to some seen in the cochlear plane, are: mastoid antrum and Koerner's septum, the semicircular canals, vestibule, oval window, jugular foramen, internal auditory canal, jugular tubercle and hypoglossal canal.

The *internal auditory canal* comprises the porus, or mouth, and the canal proper (Fig. 8–61; Valvassori and Pierce, 1964). The porus is defined by the medial margin of the posterior wall. The canal extends from the porus to a point 2 mm. medial to the vestibule—an average distance of 8 mm. The vertical diameter of the canal averages 5 mm., but wide variations in size are found. The hallmark is symmetry between the two canals, and diagnostic evaluation rests largely upon accurate comparison. According to Valvassori (1969), the canal is definitely abnormal in the presence of: (1) a difference in width greater than 2 mm. between comparable parts of each canal (Fig. 8–62); (2) erosion of the cortical margin of the canal; (3) a posterior wall more than 3 mm. shorter than the other side; and (4) the falciform crest closer to the inferior than to the superior wall of the canal. On rare occasions the canal may be extremely wide and yet be a normal variant, and both canals may be affected (Fig. 8–63; Fraser and Carter, 1975). Bilateral abnormal funnelling is virtually confined to patients with generalized neurofibromatosis who harbor two acoustic neuromas (see Fig. 8–71), although Hill and his colleagues (1977) reported a case of non-tumor widening of the canal in this disease.

Pericanalicular erosion of the superior surface of the petrous pyramid may be the manifestation of extensive extrameatal growth of an acoustic neuroma. However, lesions such as epidermoids and meningiomas also erode the pyramid extensively, and the porus and internal auditory canal may be destroyed in this process (Fig. 8–64; Phelps et al.,

1970). Angle calcification is more likely to represent meningioma (Fig. 8–2) or arteriosclerosis than acoustic neuroma.

Computed Tomography

The computed tomographic technique, discussed earlier in this chapter, should be adequate to demonstrate some or all of the following signs of a cerebellopontine-angle mass: (1) altered density of the tumor tissue, including cystic change (Figs. 8–70 and 8–75). (2) Tumor calcification, usually indicating meningioma (Fig. 8–72). (3) The distinctive pattern of tumor enhancement following contrast injection—compare Figures 8–66 and 8–69. (4) Bone erosion, which might produce only funnelling of the internal auditory canal or extend to amputation of the petrous tip (Figs. 8–65 and 8–69), also bilateral changes (Figs. 8–71). (5) Deformity of the cerebellopontine-angle cistern: cutoff and widening to a trumpet-shape with the mouth of the trumpet capping the anterior margin of the

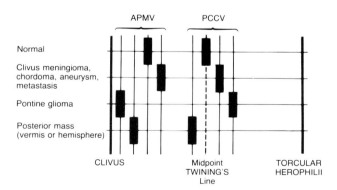

Fig. 8–53 Topographical diagnosis in the venous phase of lateral vertebral angiography. Displacement of the anterior pontomesencephalic vein (APMV) and precentral cerebellar vein (PCCV) lesions of the clivus and of the anterior and posterior compartments. The top horizontal line indicates the positions of these veins in normal subjects, relative to the clivus, the midpoint of Twining's line and torcular Herophili.

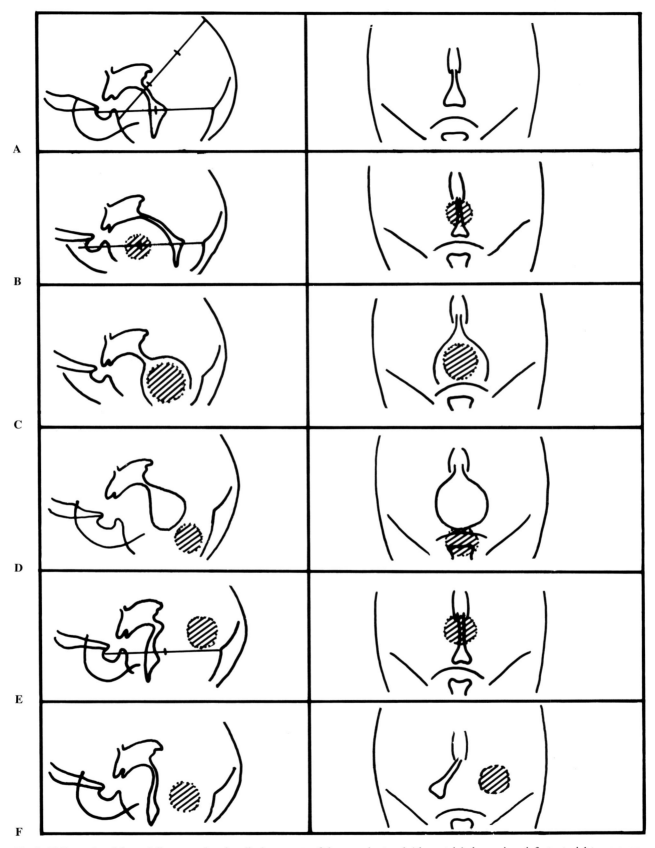

Fig. 8–54 Lateral and frontal diagrams showing displacements of the aqueduct and 4th ventricle by various infratentorial tumors, according to Sutton (1950). (A) Normal. The middle of Twining's line and one-third segments of the Stockholm line are marked. (B) Brainstem and clivus mass. (C) Intra-fourth-ventricular tumor. (D) Outlet obstruction. (E) Vermian tumor. (F) Cerebellar-hemispherical tumor.

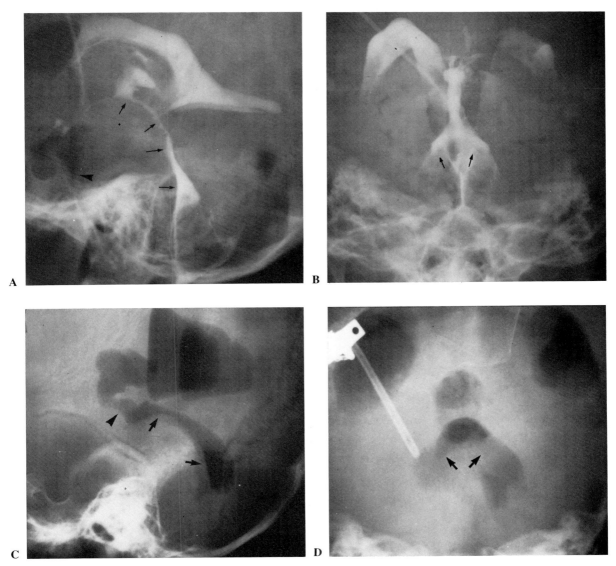

Fig. 8–55 Brainstem tumors shown by pneumography. (A and B) A 15-year-old girl with a pontine glioma. In lateral view, positive contrast medium outlines an irregular aqueduct and a compressed 4th ventricle, which is displaced backward (A, *arrows*). The swollen brainstem is confirmed by partial obliteration of the prepontine cistern (A, *arrowhead*). Note the absence of supratentorial hydrocephalus. In frontal view the 4th ventricle is shown to be widened, with the tumor encroaching upon it *(arrows)*. (C and D) Medulloblastoma in a 6-year-old boy. In lateral view, the aqueduct is foreshortened (C, *arrowhead*) and the 4th ventricle is splayed, displaced and deformed (C, *arrows*) over a mass arising from the midline of the floor of the posterior fossa. In the frontal view, the arrows point to the tumor invading the 4th ventricle. Suture diastasis and supratentorial hydrocephalus are present.

mass (Figs. 8–65 and 8–66); or obliteration due to adhesions. (6) Contralateral displacement of the 4th ventricle which may be slit-like and rotated away from the affected angle (Fig. 8–70). (8) Supratentorial hydrocephalus, although this is an inconstant feature.

Several authors have reviewed the value and described the appearances of computed tomography in lesions of the cerebellopontine-angle, notably Naidich et al. (1976a) Gyldensted et al. (1976); Kendall and Symon (1977); and Dubois et al. (1978).

Acoustic Neuroma: The majority of these tumors have an isodense or low-density appearance, without contrast enhancement, and a peritumoral halo of edema is unusual. Thus, unenhanced neuromas which are too small to displace the 4th ventricle are easily overlooked. Contrast injection produces a blush in almost all tumors, although small neuromas may remain undetected. The typical acoustic neuroma is a uniformly enhancing round or oval mass with well-defined margins (Figs. 8–65 and 8–66). Cystic changes or a ring-like lesion are only occasionally seen (Figs. 8–69 and 8–70). Tumor calcification is uncommon. Bilateral tumors usually

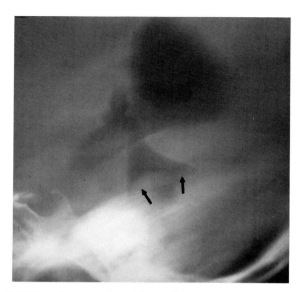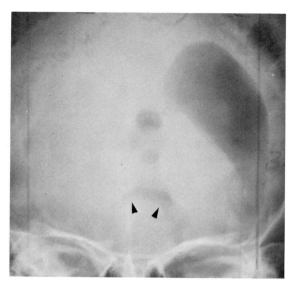

Fig. 8–56 Ependymoma of the 4th ventricle revealed by ventriculography. The lateral view outlines the upper surface of the tumor obstructing the 4th ventricle *(arrows)*, exerting a ball-valve action on the ventricular system. The 4th ventricle is displaced upward, above Twining's line, and forward; and the aqueduct has been assimilated. Supratentorial hydrocephalus is present. The frontal view also outlines the upper surface of the tumor *(arrowheads)*, and the distorted 4th ventricle caps it.

indicate generalized neurofibromatosis (Fig. 8–71).

The structural effects of an acoustic neuroma on the brain and adjacent petrous pyramid depend on the size of its extrameatal components. These space-occupying signs shown on computed tomography, which have been described above, concern cerebellopontine angle masses in general, and they may be produced by meningiomas and epidermoids as well as acoustic neuromas. The majority of these signs were described many years ago in respect of plain radiographs and pneumoencephalography (Liliequist, 1959). These other features include unilateral dilatation of the cerebellopontine angle or circumsencephalic cistern (ambient) (Figs. 8–65 to 8–67), rotation and displacement of the fourth ventricle (Figs. 8–65 to 8–67) rotation and compression of the brainstem (Fig. 8–67) and a thin radiolucent collection circumscribing the tumor due to pooling of cerebrospinal fluid or cerebellar atrophy (Figs. 8–67 to 8–72).

False-negative computed tomographic results may be obtained in small acoustic neuromas. The smallest tumor identified by Gyldensted et al. (1976) was 0.7 cm. in diameter, but one of the authors (E. H. B.) has failed to demonstrate three cases of acoustic neuroma, all of which were subsequently proved by oil cisternography or operation to be larger than 1 cm. in diameter. Opacification of the cerebellopontine angle and brainstem cisterns may permit visualization of even these small neoplasms and obviate the need for pneumoencephalography and pantopaque cisternography (Dubois et al., 1978). Computed tomography after intro-

duction of small amounts of air has been found to be extremely helpful (Kricheff et al., 1980 and Sortland, 1979).

Meningioma: Meningioma, one of the two angle tumors that may erode or deform the petrous bone, exhibits the same space-occupying effects upon the angle cistern and 4th ventricle as acoustic neuroma. The computed tomographic signs that distinguish it are psammomatous calcification of the same pattern as in the supratentorial compartment, and a tissue density significantly higher than normal brain, so that it can usually be distinguished on unenhanced slices (Figs. 8–72 and 8–73). The causes of this higher density are believed to be a combination of increased blood content and psammoma-body calcification. Contrast injection produces more vivid and homogeneous tumor enhancement than occurs even in acoustic neurofibromas: the margins of the mass are sharply outlined and usually smooth (Fig. 8–72 and 8–73). A circumferential collar of edema may be present (Figs. 8–72 and 8–73).

Meningiomas may extend beyond the confines of the cerebellopontine angle, in one of several directions: (1) inferiorly to the foramen magnum; (2) laterally to displace the cerebellar hemisphere medially from its subtentorial position (Fig. 8–73); (3) superiorly through the tentorial incisura to deform the midbrain (see Fig. 8–73).

Epidermoid (Cholesteatoma): These curious lesions evoke great interest (Tytus and Pennybacker, 1956; Long et al., 1973; Norman and Newton, 1975; Fawcitt and Isherwood, 1976). Cerebellopontine-angle epidermoids may erode and destroy

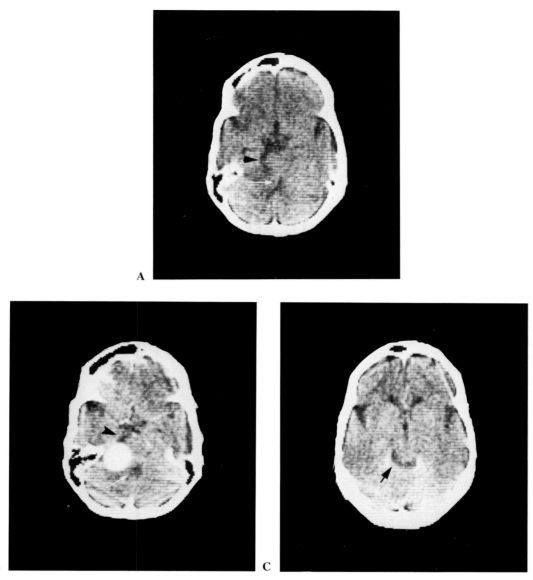

Fig. 8–67 Incisural extension of left acoustic neuroma. (A) Unenhanced slice shows lateral displacement and deformity of the 4th ventricle *(white arrow)*. The left side of the perimesencephalic cistern *(black arrowhead)* is dilated. (B and C) Enhanced slices show a sharply defined spherical mass arising from the left cerebellopontine angle. It indents the dilated left side of the perimesencephalic cistern *(arrowhead)*, and displaces the 4th ventricle *(white arrow)*. Incisural involvement is shown by deformity of the left side of the quadrigeminal-plate cistern *(black arrow)*.

and Lüdecke, 1971; Gold and Kieffer, 1972; Novy and Jensen, 1975). The patient's head is positioned obliquely on the fluoroscopic table so that the cistern to be examined is horizontal and its porus and internal auditory canal are in a vertical position. Then the cistern is slowly filled by tilting the table head-downward, and overhead and cross-table spot-films are made (Fig. 8–82). An angle lesion is excluded if contrast medium enters the internal auditory canal, which is best demonstrated in the cross-table view. Very small extrameatal lesions can be demonstrated in this way, e.g., angle adhe-

sions or tumors of the 8th nerve which are the size of a matchhead (Fig. 8–83). Larger angle tumors characteristically obliterate the apex of the contrast triangle in the overhead view, in addition to resulting in failure of the auditory canal to fill (Fig. 8–84). Still larger tumors, by raising the pressure in the posterior fossa, seal off the cisterns at the level of the foramen magnum and prevent the passage of oily contrast medium into the head. Fortunately most such patients exhibit papilledema, which, through contraindicating lumbar puncture, prevents cisternographic examination. Other causes of non-

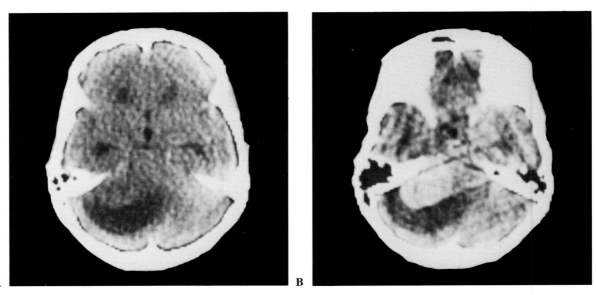

Fig. 8—68 Acoustic neuroma trapping cerebrospinal fluid. (A) Unenchanced slice shows a crescent of edema partly outlining the tumor. (B) Enhanced slice.

filling are: arachnoid scarring from previous infection, hemorrhage or surgery; exophytic cerebellar or brainstem tumors; and an ectatic basilar artery (Baker, 1963; Long et al., 1972).

Gas Cisternography (Meatography): Air or gas introduced by lumbar or suboccipital injection was used for many years to outline small angle masses. The technique of fractional pneumoencephalography developed by Lindgren (1950) and others was described and critically evaluated by Liliequist (1959). Tomography became an integral part of the examination (Morris and Wylie, 1973).

Small extrameatal masses deform the cistern into which they protrude without displacing or distorting the 4th ventricle. Success of the examination depends upon demonstrating this deformity. The standard Scandinavian technique of fractional pneumoencephalography possesses the advantage of enabling constant comparison between the two cerebellopontine-angle cisterns. Figure 8–85A shows the characteristic widening and foreshortening of such a cistern deformed by a tumor. Special techniques employing small volumes of gas and oblique tomographic projections, as described by

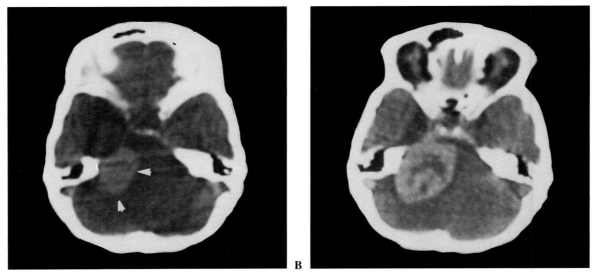

Fig. 8—69 Acoustic neuroma doubling in size. (A) Initial examination: Enhanced slice shows a vividly blushing, well-defined mass *(arrowheads)* adjacent to an eroded petrous pyramid. (B) Repeat examination 18 months later: the tumor has doubled in size. The lucencies within the mass may represent necrosis or old hemorrhage.

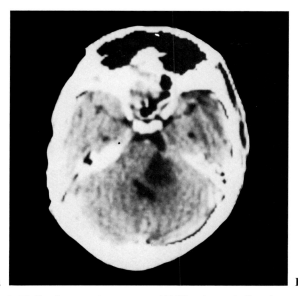 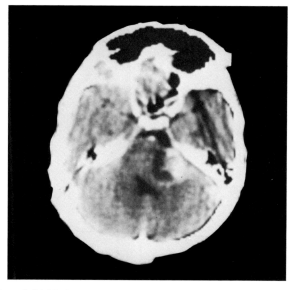

A   B

Fig. 8–70 Cystic acoustic neuroma. (A) Unenhanced slice shows three fluid-filled structures. These are, from front to back: the widened right cerebellopontine-angle cistern, the cystic medial half of the neuroma, and an angled 4th ventricle. (B) Enhanced slice made at the same level shows the enhancing capsular ring and the solid part of the tumor, which lies in the cerebellopontine angle. Funnelling of the right internal auditory canal confirmed the diagnosis of acoustic neuroma.

Ziedses des Plantes (1968) and Isherwood (1972), refined the accuracy of the method in experienced hands.

Large angle tumors, in addition to obliterating the cistern, cause a characteristic deformity of the 4th ventricle (Fig. 8–85B; see Ventriculography below).

Metrizamide Cisternography: See Sortland et al.

(1977) and Rosenbaum and Drayer (1977).

Radioisotope Cisternography: See Mamo and Houdart (1972).

Ventriculography

Ventricular opacification has no place in the diagnosis of small cerebellopontine-angle tumors. However, large tumors deform the 4th ventricle in a

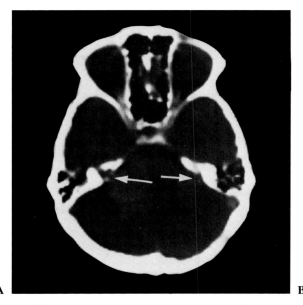 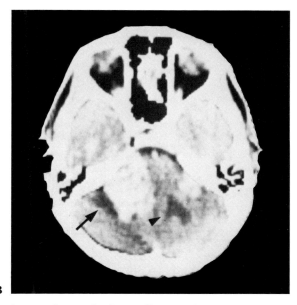

A   B

Fig. 8–71 Bilateral acoustic neuromas in a patient with cutaneous stigmata of generalized neurofibromatosis. (A) Unenhanced slice shows erosion of both internal auditory canals *(white arrows)*. (B) Enhanced slice made at the same level shows a large tumor in the left cerebellopontine angle, displacing the 4th ventricle *(arrowhead)* and trapping of pool of cerebrospinal fluid *(arrow)*. A small tumor is present in the right cerebellopontine angle.

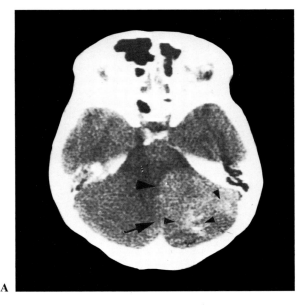

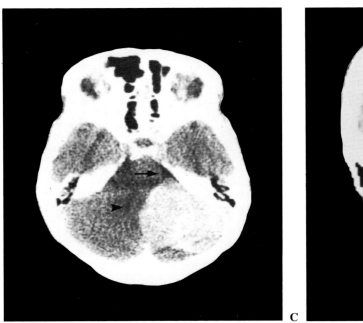

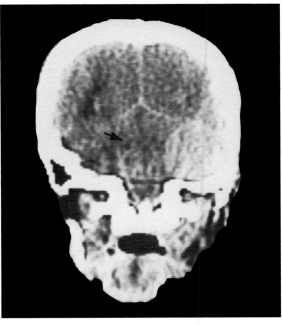

Fig. 8–72 Meningioma. (A) Unenhanced slice shows a well-circumscribed mass of increased density in the right cerebellopontine angle, extending to the cerebellar convexity *(black arrows)*. Speckled deposits of calcium are present within the tumor *(arrowheads)*. (B) Enhanced slice: the tumor blushes intensely. The arrow points to a widened cerebellopontine-angle cistern capping the anterior aspect of the tumor. The rotated displaced ventricle is also seen *(arrow head)*. (C) Enhanced coronal slice: the displaced 4th ventricle *(arrow)* and the position of the tentorium are definable in relation to the tumor. See Wolf et al. (1976).

characteristic way and ventriculography remained a standard preoperative diagnostic procedure in many neurological centers, until replaced by vertebral angiography or computed tomography.

Figure 8–85B illustrates the deformity of the 4th ventricle produced by large tumors, viz., contralateral and posterior dislocation, with flattening and a rotational deformity which has been likened to the blade of an airplane propellor, a paddle (Greitz, 1974) or a bananna shape (Taveras and Wood,

1976). Supratentorial hydrocephalus is a frequent but not invariable accompaniment. For 50 years the combination of enlarged lateral ventricles, a paddle-shaped and displaced 4th ventricle and erosion of the contralateral petrous pyramid represented the traditional appearance to the neurosurgeon of a mass in the corner of the posterior fossa which Harvey Cushing once described as the "bloody angle" of brain surgery.

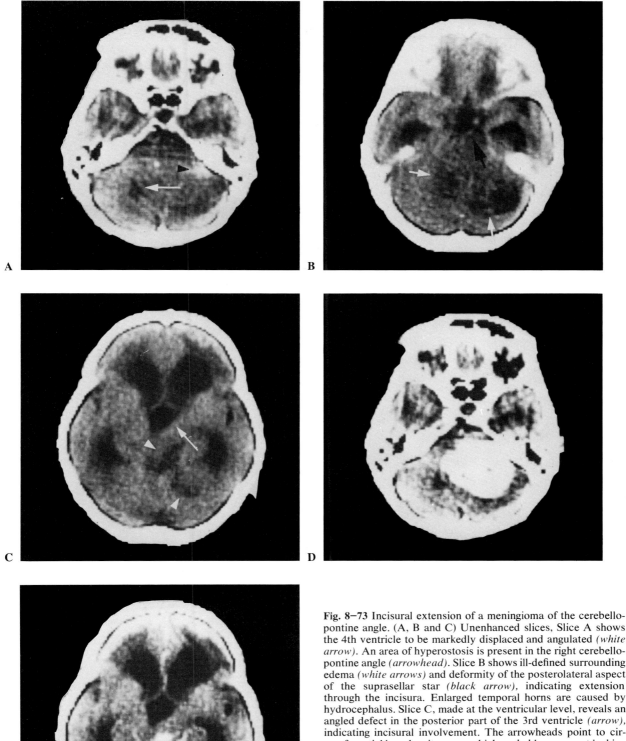

Fig. 8–73 Incisural extension of a meningioma of the cerebellopontine angle. (A, B and C) Unenhanced slices, Slice A shows the 4th ventricle to be markedly displaced and angulated *(white arrow)*. An area of hyperostosis is present in the right cerebellopontine angle *(arrowhead)*. Slice B shows ill-defined surrounding edema *(white arrows)* and deformity of the posterolateral aspect of the suprasellar star *(black arrow)*, indicating extension through the incisura. Enlarged temporal horns are caused by hydrocephalus. Slice C, made at the ventricular level, reveals an angled defect in the posterior part of the 3rd ventricle *(arrow)*, indicating incisural involvement. The arrowheads point to circumferential low-density areas which probably represent leaking of cerebrospinal fluid around the tumor. Marked hydrocephalus with transependymal extravasation is present. (D and E) Enhanced slices confirm the tumor. Slice D shows the intensely blushing mass with sharply defined margins in the right cerebellopontine angle. Slice E, made at the ventricular level, shows cephalic extension of the tumor through the incisura to deform the third ventricle.

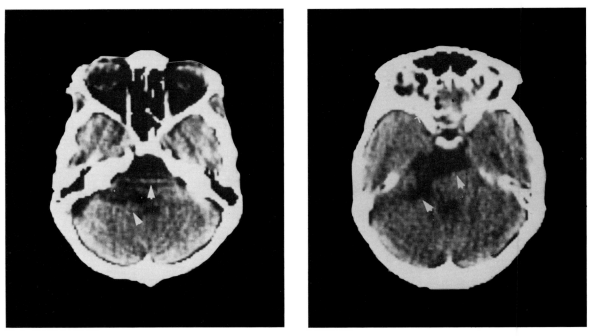

Fig. 8–74 Epidermoid of the left cerebellopontine angle and clivus. A low-density lesion occupying the left cerebellopontine angle and retroclival region is visible, which failed to enhance upon contrast infusion *(arrowheads)*.

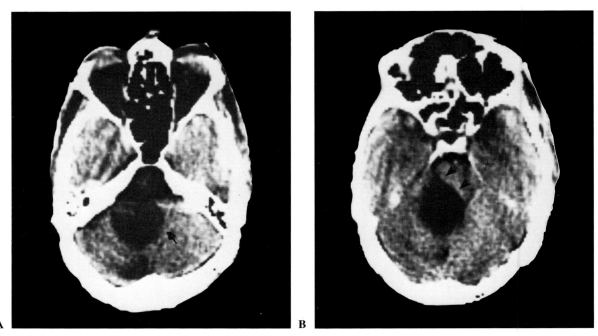

Fig. 8–75 Epidermoid of the left cerebellopontine angle. A cystic lesion of unusually low tissue attenuation is present, which fails to show contrast enhancement. (A) Posterior fossa slice shows a displaced and slit-like 4th ventricle *(arrow)*. Despite the large size of the mass, no petrous erosion was visible. (B) Slice 10 mm. higher shows distortion of the brainstem *(arrowheads)* by upward extension of the cystic mass.

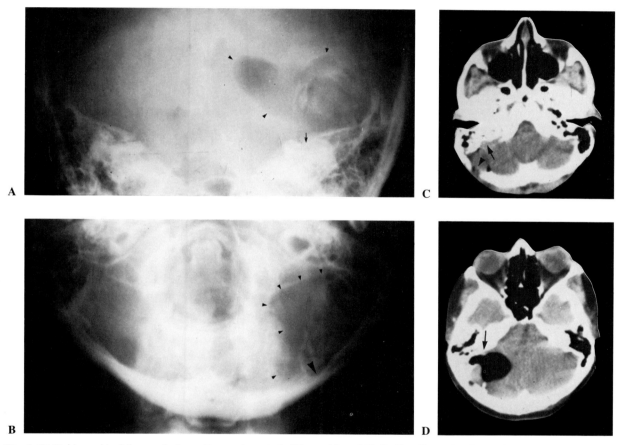

Fig. 8–76 Epidermoid of the cerebellopontine angle and skull base. (A and B) Skull radiographs show a lucency with a well-defined margin *(arrowheads)*, contiguous with a defect in the petrous bone in proximity to Meckel's cave *(arrow)*. Thinning of the inner table is present *(large arrowhead)*. Vague density within the lucency may represent debris. (C and D) Computed tomography confirms that the lesion has replaced the inner and outer tables of the occipital bone *(arrowhead)*. The cystic mass in the cerebellopontine angle shows the typical low attenuation of an epidermoid *(arrows)*. (Reproduced by courtesy of Dr. H. Oestreich, White Plains Hospital, White Plains, New York.)

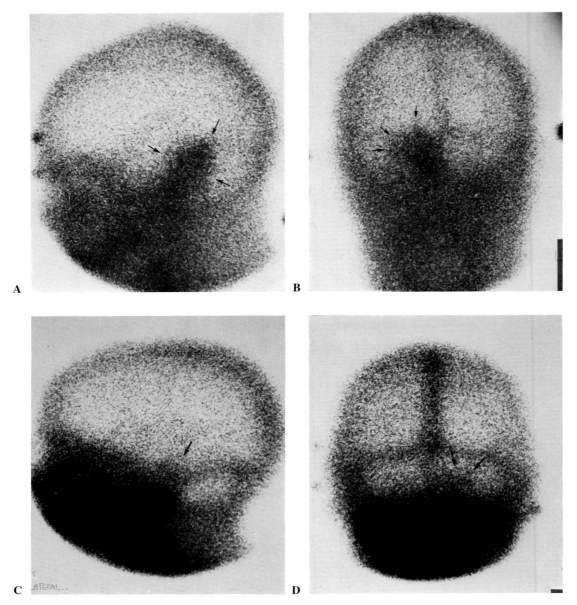

Fig. 8–77 Scintigraphic appearances of acoustic neuromas. (A and B) Diagrammatic representation of a large tumor in the right cerebellopontine angle *(arrows):* it rises up from the normal basal activity associated with the neck muscles and parotid gland. (C and D) Small left tumor, projecting into the infratentorial "window" on the posterior-tilted view *(arrows).*

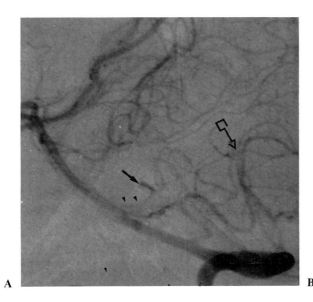

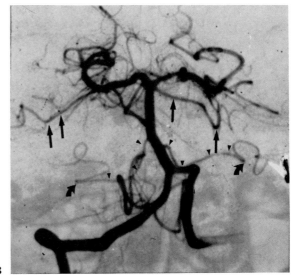

A

B

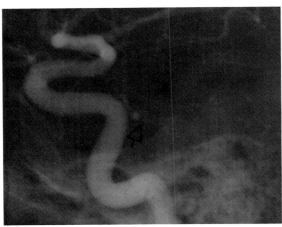

C

Fig. 8–78 Angiography of cerebellopontine-angle masses—meningioma. (A) Vertebral arteriogram, lateral view. The anterior inferior cerebellar artery is depressed *(arrowheads)* and the proximal part of the **M** segment (which is related to the 7th and 8th nerves at the porus acousticus) is closed and compressed by the neoplasm *(arrow)*. The open arrow points to the choroidal point of the posterior inferior cerebellar artery, which is displaced downward. No "tumor blush" is visible. (B) Vertebral arteriogram, straight frontal view. The arrows point to the superior cerebellar arteries, the left one being elevated and its proximal course hidden by the posterior cerebral artery. The arrowheads indicate the anterior inferior cerebellar arteries, the left one being stretched and displaced downward. Curved arrows indicate the meatal loop of each artery, the left loop being depressed and compressed. (C) Left carotid angiogram, lateral view, showing a vascular supply to the tumor from the tentorial branch of the meningohypophyseal artery *(open arrow)*.

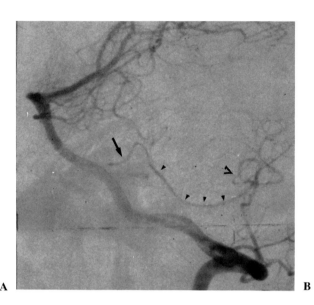

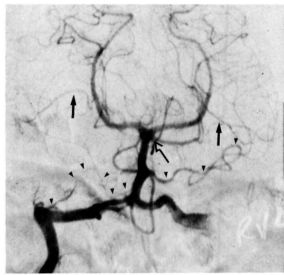

A

B

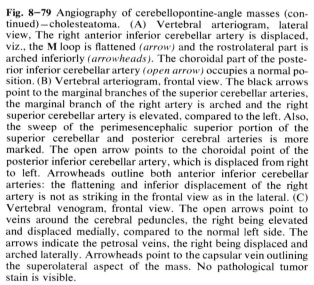

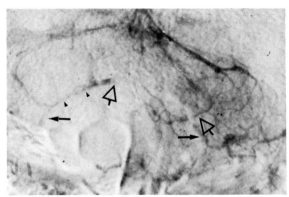

C

Fig. 8–79 Angiography of cerebellopontine-angle masses (continued)—cholesteatoma. (A) Vertebral arteriogram, lateral view, The right anterior inferior cerebellar artery is displaced, viz., the **M** loop is flattened *(arrow)* and the rostrolateral part is arched inferiorly *(arrowheads)*. The choroidal part of the posterior inferior cerebellar artery *(open arrow)* occupies a normal position. (B) Vertebral arteriogram, frontal view. The black arrows point to the marginal branches of the superior cerebellar arteries, the marginal branch of the right artery is arched and the right superior cerebellar artery is elevated, compared to the left. Also, the sweep of the perimesencephalic superior portion of the superior cerebellar and posterior cerebral arteries is more marked. The open arrow points to the choroidal point of the posterior inferior cerebellar artery, which is displaced from right to left. Arrowheads outline both anterior inferior cerebellar arteries: the flattening and inferior displacement of the right artery is not as striking in the frontal view as in the lateral. (C) Vertebral venogram, frontal view. The open arrows point to veins around the cerebral peduncles, the right being elevated and displaced medially, compared to the normal left side. The arrows indicate the petrosal veins, the right being displaced and arched laterally. Arrowheads point to the capsular vein outlining the superolateral aspect of the mass. No pathological tumor stain is visible.

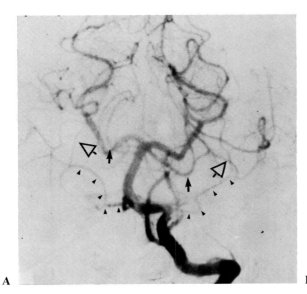
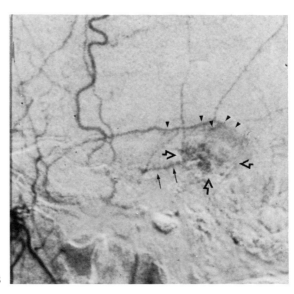

A B

Fig. 8–80 Angiography of cerebellopontine-angle masses (continued)—acoustic neuroma. (A) Vertebral arteriogram, frontal view. The arrows point to the superior cerebellar arteries, the right artery being elevated and displaced medially, compared to the normal left side. The open arrows are the marginal branches, the right one being elevated, displaced laterally and stretched. Arrowheads indicate the anterior inferior cerebellar arteries, the right artery being elevated, stretched and arched medially. B. Right external carotid angiogram, lateral view. The open arrows point to a tangle of vessels representing a tumor stain. The vascular supply to the tumor arises from the posterior branch of the middle meningeal artery *(arrowheads)* and a branch of the ascending pharyngeal artery *(arrows)*.

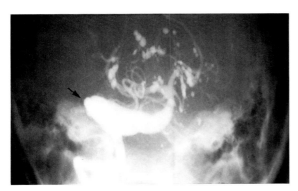
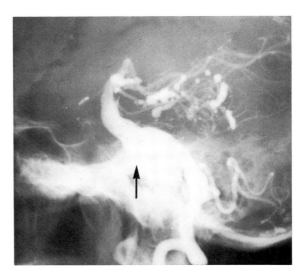

Fig. 8–81 Ectasia of the basilar artery: an atherosclerotic fusiform aneurysm of the trunk simulating a cerebellopontine-angle lesion *(arrow)* is present, surrounded by residues of an oil myelogram.

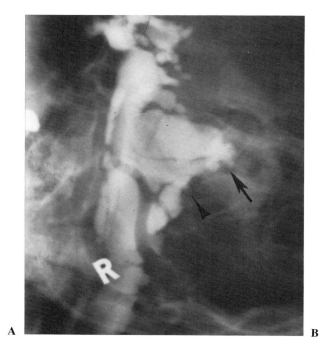

A

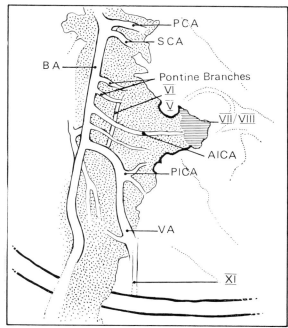

B

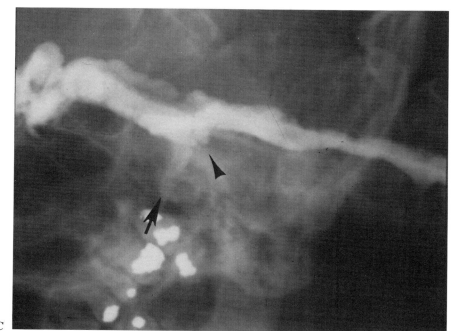

C

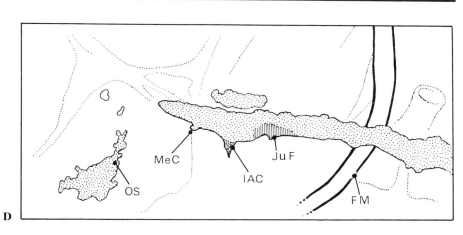

D

Fig. 8–82 Normal oil cisternogram. (A and B) Anteroposterior spot-film and line drawing. (C and D) Lateral ("cross-table") spot-film and line drawing. *(Arrow)* Internal auditory canal—a fingerlike projection on lateral view, a denser contrast shadow on anteroposterior view. *(Arrowhead)* jugular foramen. (AICA) Anterior inferior cerebellar artery. (BA) Basilar artery. (FM) Foramen magnum. (IAC) Internal auditory canal. (JuF) Jugular foramen. (MeC) Meckel's cave. (OS) Overspill. (PCA) Posterior cerebral artery. (PICA) Posterior inferior cerebellar artery. (SCA) Superior cerebellar artery. (VA) Vertebral artery. (V) Trigeminal nerve. (VI) Abducent nerve. (VII/VIII) Facial and auditory nerves. (IX) Accessory nerve. (This case was described and illustrated by E. H. Burrows in the British Journal of Radiology, *42*, 902–913, 1969.)

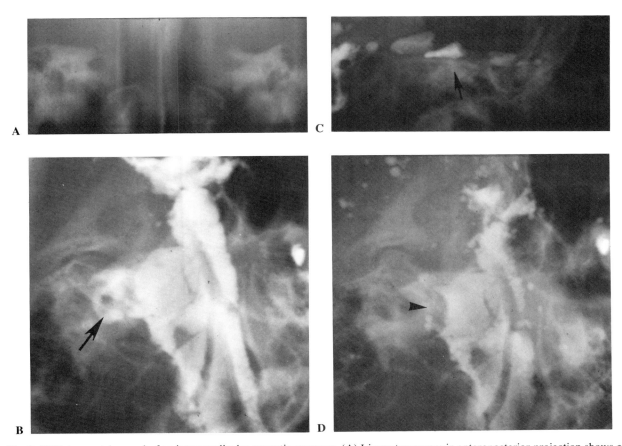

Fig. 8–83 Extrameatal spread of an intracanalicular acoustic neuroma. (A) Linear tomogram in anteroposterior projection shows erosion of the posterior wall and slight flaring of the left porus acousticus, compared to the normal right. (B and C) Initial oil examination of the left cerebellopontine angle. In the lateral view, the porus fails to fill *(arrow)*. In the anteroposterior view, the apex of the triangle is irregular—compared with normal angle filling in Figure 8–82A. This appearance indicates the presence of a lesion, and the eroded porus points to the diagnosis of an 8th nerve tumor. (D) Repeat oil examination 14 months later. The apex of the triangle has now been obliterated by extrameatal spread of the tumor *(arrowhead)*. An acoustic neuroma was removed at operation.

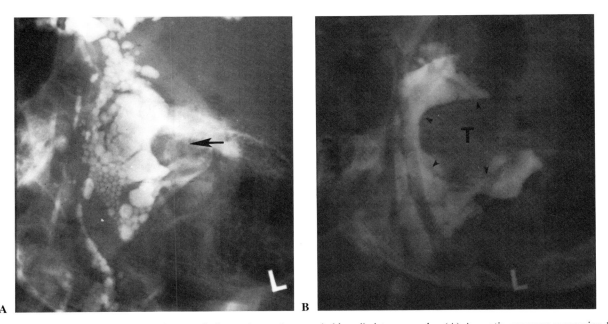

Fig. 8–84 Small and large neuromas in a cerebellopontine angle, revealed by oil cisternography. (A) Acoustic neuroma measuring 1.3 cm. in diameter *(arrow)* when removed at operation, which could not be demonstrated by enhanced computed tomography. Abnormal otological tests and an eroded left porus acousticus indicated that the computed-tomographic result was false-negative. (B) Trigeminal neuroma measuring 3.2 cm. in diameter (T, *arrowheads*), obliterating the cistern of the left cerebellopontine angle and abutting on the left vertebral and basilar arteries. The left porus acousticus was normal.

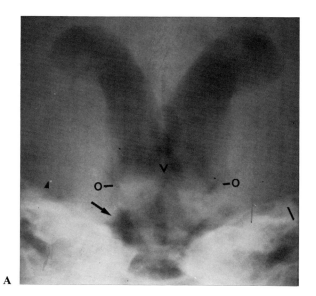

Fig. 8–85 Extrameatal acoustic neuromas outlined by gas cisternography. (A) Small neuroma, i.e., 1.5 cm. in diameter. *(Arrow)* Gas in right cistern which is widened and foreshortened and outlines the inferomedial surface of the tumor. (O) Crural cisterns, which are symmetrical and unrelated to the angle mass. (V) Fourth ventricle which shows no deformity or displacement, due to the small size of the tumor. (B and C) Larger neuroma, i.e., 2.6 cm. in diameter, deforming the angle as well as the 4th ventricle. The lateral view shows retrodisplacement of the aqueduct and 4th ventricle *(arrowhead)*. In frontal tomography, *(black arrow)* widened and foreshortened left cistern, revealing part of the tumor. The adjacent porus acousticus is eroded. In this case, the crural cisterns were not filled and the oblique gas shadow *(open arrowhead)* outlines the superior surface of the angle tumor. *(Black arrowheads)* 4th ventricle, displaced and deformed into the shape of a propellor blade or banana—see Figure 8–86.

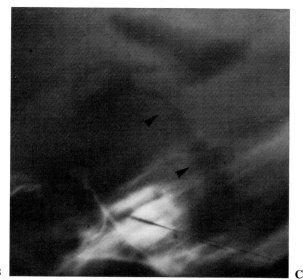

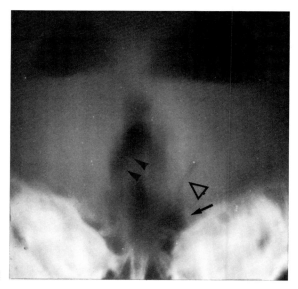

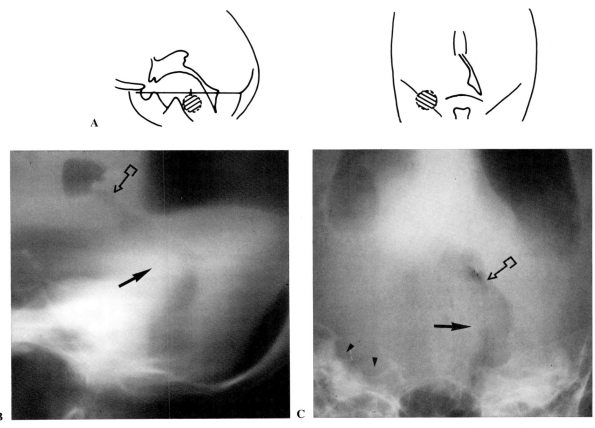

Fig. 8–86 The 4th ventricle in tumors of the cerebellopontine angle. (A) Diagram showing displacement backward and laterally of the aqueduct and 4th ventricle which is flattened and rotated. (For normal configuration and relationship to Twining's line, see Fig. 8 – 54A). (B and C) Characteristic propellor-blade or banana shaped deformity of a displaced 4th ventricle *(arrows),* caused by a large acoustic neuroma eroding the superior surface of the petrous bone *(arrowheads).* The aqueduct *(open arrows)* is retrodisplaced and tilted sideways.

REFERENCES

Azar-Kia, N., Palacios, E. and Spak, M.: The megadolichobasilar artery anomaly and expansion of the internal auditory meatus. Neuroradiology, *11,* 109 – 111, 1976.

Baker, H. L.: Myelographic examination of the posterior fossa with positive contrast medium. Radiology, *81,* 791 – 801, 1963.

Banna, M., Lassman, L. P. and Pearce, G. W.: Radiological study of skeletal metastases from cerebellar medulloblastoma. British Journal of Radiology, *43,* 173 – 179, 1970.

Baum, S., Rothballer, A. B., Shiffman, F. and Girolamo, R. F.: Brain scanning in the diagnosis of acoustic neuromas. Journal of Neurosurgery, *36,* 141 – 147, 1972.

Bilaniuk, L. T., Zimmerman, R. A., Littman, P., Gallo, E., Rorke, L. B., Bruce, D. A. and Schut, L.: Computed tomography of brain stem gliomas in children. Radiology, *134:* 89 – 96, 1980.

Bradac, G. B.: The ponto-mesencephalic veins (radio-anatomical study). Neuroradiology, *1,* 52 – 57, 1970.

Bradac, G. B., Holdorff, B. and Simon, R. S.: Aspects of the venous drainage of the pons and the mesencephalon. Neuroradiology, *3,* 102 – 108, 1971.

Braun, I. F., Naidich, T. P., Leeds, N. E., Koslow, M., Zimmerman, H. and Chase, N. E. Dense intracranial epidermoid tumors. Radiology, *122,* 717 – 719, 1977.

Bull, J.: Difficulty in differentiating between fourth ventricle and brain stem masses. Acta Radiologica Diagnosis, *1,* 814 – 820, 1963.

Bull, J. W. D.: Massive aneurysm at the base of the brain. Brain, *92,* 535 – 570, 1969.

Bull, J. W. D. and Kozlowski, P.: The angiographic pattern of the petrosal veins in the normal and pathological. Neuroradiology, *1,* 20 – 26, 1970.

Burns, J. B., Hoffman, J. C. and Brylski, J. R.: The posterior inferior cerebellar artery in fourth ventricular dilatation. Acta Radiologica Diagnosis, *13,* 58 – 65, 1972.

Burrows, E. H.: Positive contrast examination (cerebellopontine cisternography) in extrameatal acoustic neurofibromas. British Journal of Radiology, *42,* 902 – 913, 1969.

Burrows, E. H.: Intracranial calcification. In Newton, T. H. and Potts, D. G., Eds., Radiology of the Skull and Brain, Vol. 1, book 2. St. Louis: C. V. Mosby, 1971.

Burrows, E. H.: Scintigraphic diagnosis of acoustic neurofibromas. British Journal of Radiology, *48,* 1000 – 1006, 1975.

Burrows, E. H.: Clinical reliability of posterior fossa scintigraphy. Clinical Radiology, *27,* 473 – 481, 1976.

Camp, J. D.: Intracranial calcification and its roentgenologic significance. American Journal of Roentgenology, *23,* 615 – 624, 1930.

Davis, K. R., Roberson, G. H., Taveras, J. M., New, P. F. J. and Trevor, R.: Diagnosis of epidermoid tumor by computed tomography. Radiology, *119,* 347 – 353, 1976.

De Land, F. H., James, A. E., Jr. and Wagner, H. N.: Patterns for differentiation of posterior fossa neoplasms as detected by brainscans. Nuklearmedizin (Stuttgart), *9,* 303 – 316, 1970.

Dowding, D. V. and Whall, M.: The value of lead shields in

reducing radiation dosage to the eye during neuroradiological procedures. Radiography (London), *42*, 181–184, 1976.

Dubois, P. J., Drayer, B. P., Bank, W. O., Deeb, Z. L. and Rosenbaum, A. E.: An evaluation of current diagnostic radiologic modalities in the investigation of acoustic neurilemmomas. Radiology, *126*, 173–179, 1978.

Fawcitt, R. A. and Isherwood, I.: Radiodiagnosis of intracranial pearly tumors with particular reference to the value of computer tomography. Neuroradiology, *11*, 235–242, 1976.

Fraser, R. A. R. and Carter, B. L.: Unilateral dilatation of the internal auditory canal. Neuroradiology, *9*, 227–229, 1975.

Gabrielsen T. O., Seeger, J. F. and Amundsen, P.: Some new angiographic observations in patients with Chiari Type I and II malformations. Radiology, *115*, 627–634, 1975.

Gado, M., Huete, I. and Mikhael, M.: Computerized tomography of infratentorial tumors. Seminars in Roentgenology, *12*, 109–120, 1977.

Galloway, J. R. and Greitz, T.: The medial and lateral choroid arteries. An anatomic and roentgenographic study. Acta Radiologica, *53*, 353–366, 1959.

George, A. E.: A systematic approach to the interpretation of posterior fossa angiography. Radiologic Clinics of North America, *12*, 371–400, 1974.

Gerald, B. and Wieder, S.: Displacement of pontine arteries by fungating pontine astrocytomas. American Journal of Roentgenology, *125*, 833–838, 1975.

Gold, L. H. A., Kieffer, S. A. and Peterson, H. P.: Intracranial meningiomas; a retrospective analysis of the diagnostic value of plain skull films. Neurology, *19*, 873–878, 1969.

Gold, L. H. A. and Kieffer, S. A.: Positive contrast evaluation of the posterior cranial fossa. Radiology, *102*, 63–70, 1972.

Goodbody, R. A. and Gamlen, R. R.: Cerebellar hemangioblastoma and genitourinary tumors. Journal of Neurology, Neurosurgery and Psychiatry, *37*, 606–609, 1974.

Greitz, T.: Technical aspects of the pneumoencephalographic and ventriculographic examination of the fourth ventricle. Neuroradiology, *6*, 259–269, 1974.

Greitz, T. and Laurén, T.: Anterior meningeal branch of the vertebral artery. Acta Radiologica Diagnosis, *7*, 219–224, 1968.

Greitz, T. and Sjögren, S. E.: The posterior inferior cerebellar artery. Acta Radiologica Diagnosis, *1*, 284–297, 1963.

Gyldensted, C., Lester, J. and Thomsen, J.: Computer tomography in the diagnosis of cerebellopontine angle tumors. Neuroradiology, *11*, 191–197, 1976.

Hill, M. C., Oh, K. S. and Hodges, F. J.: Internal auditory canal enlargement in neurofibromatosis without acoustic neuroma. Radiology, *122*, 730, 1977.

Hitselberger, W. E. and House, W. F.: Acoustic neuroma: The adaptation of polytomography and iophendylate to the early diagnosis of acoustic tumors. The American Surgeon, *33*, 791–796, 1967.

Hodes, P. J.: Cerebello-pontine angle tumors: their roentgenologic manifestations. Radiology, *57*, 395–406, 1951.

Hopkins, L. N. and Bakay, L.: Precentral cerebellar vein in cystic astrocytomas of the vermis. Journal of Neurology, Neurosurgery and Psychiatry, *38*, 816–818, 1975.

Huang, Y. P. and Wolf, B. S.: Veins of posterior fossa–superior or Galenic draining group. American Journal of Roentgenology, *95*, 808–821, 1965.

Huang, Y. P. and Wolf, B. S.: Precentral cerebellar vein in angiography. Acta Radiologica, *5*, 250–262, 1966.

Huang, Y. P. and Wolf, B. S.: The vein of the lateral recess of the fourth ventricle and its tributaries. Roentgen appearance and anatomic relationships. American Journal of Roentgenology, *101*, 1–21, 1967.

Huang, Y. P. and Wolf B. S.: Angiographic features of fourth ventricle tumors with special reference to the posterior inferior cerebellar artery. American Journal of Roentgenology, *107*, 543–564, 1969.

Huang, Y. P. and Wolf, B. S.: Differential diagnosis of fourth ventricle tumors from brain stem tumors in angiography. Neuroradiology, *1*, 4–19, 1970.

Huang, Y. P., Wolf, B. S., Antin, S. P. and Okudera, T.: Veins of posterior fossa - anterior or petrosal draining group. American Journal of Roentgenology, *104*, 36–56, 1968.

Huang, Y. P., Wolf, B. S. and Okudera, T.: Angiographic anatomy of the inferior vermian vein of the cerebellum. Acta Radiologica Diagnosis, *9*, 327–344, 1969.

Isherwood, I.: Air meatography. Clinical Radiology, *23*, 65–77, 1972.

Kalan, C. and Burrows, E. H.: Calcification in intracranial gliomata. British Journal of Radiology, *35*, 589–602, 1962.

Kendall, B. E. and Lee, B. C. L.: Cranial chordomas. British Journal of Radiology, *50*, 687–698, 1977.

Kendall, B. and Shah, S.: Investigation of meningiomas of cerebellar convexities. Neuroradiology, *4*, 162–170, 1972.

Kendall, B. and Symon, L.: Investigation of patients presenting with cerebellopontine angle syndromes. Neuroradiology, *13*, 65–84, 1977.

Kerber, C. W., Margolis, M. T. and Newton, T. H.: Tortuous vertebrobasilar system: A cause of cranial nerve signs. Neuroradiology, *4*, 74–77, 1972.

Kieffer, S. A., Binet, E. F. and Gold, L. H. A.: Angiographic diagnosis of intra- and extra-axial tumors in the cerebellopontine angle. American Journal of Roentgenology, *124*, 297–309, 1975.

Kricheff, I. I., Pinto, R. S., Bergeron, R. T., and Cohen, W.: Air-CT cisternography and canalography for small acoustic neuromas. American Journal of Neuroradiology, *1*:57–63, 1980.

Latchaw, R. E., Gold, L. H. A., Moore, Jr., J. S. and Payne, J. T.: The nonspecificity of absorption coefficients in differentiation of solid tumors and cystic lesions. Radiology, *125*, 141–144, 1977.

LeMay, M. and Rubens, A. B.: The neuroanatomical changes associated with dilated corpus callosal and distended ambient cisterns. British Journal of Radiology, *44*, 14–20, 1971.

Levine, H. L., Ferris, E. J. and Spatz, E. L.: External carotid bloody supply to acoustic neurinomas. Report of two cases. Journal of Neurosurgery, *38*, 516–520, 1973.

Liliequist, B.: The subarachnoid cisterns. An anatomic and roentgenologic study. Acta Radiologica Supplementum, *185*, 1959.

Lindgren, E.: Encephalographic examination of tumors of the posterior fossa. Acta Radiologica, *34*, 331–338, 1950.

Long, J. M., Kier, E. L. and Hilding, D. A.: Pitfalls of posterior fossa cisternography using 2 ml of iophendylate (Pantopaque). Radiology, *102*, 71–75, 1972.

Long, J. M, Kier, E. L. and Schechter, M. M.: The radiology of epidermoid tumors of the cerebellopontine angle. Neuroradiology, *6*, 188–192, 1973.

McRae, D. L. and Elliot, A. W.: Radiological aspects of cerebellar astrocytomas and medulloblastomas. Acta Radiologica, *50*, 52–66, 1958.

Mamo, L. and Houdart, R.: Radioisotopic cisternography: contribution to the diagnosis of cerebellopontine angle tumors. Journal of Neurosurgery, *37*, 325–331, 1972.

Mani, R. L. and Newton, T. H.: The superior cerebellar artery: arteriographic changes in the diagnosis of posterior fossa lesions. Radiology, *92*, 1281–1287, 1969.

Margolis, M. T., Newton, T. H. and Hoyt, W. F.: Cortical branches of the posterior cerebral artery. Anatomic-radiologic correlation. Neuroradiology, *2*, 127–135, 1971.

Margolis, M. T. and Newton, T. H.: Borderlands of the normal and abnormal posterior inferior cerebellar artery. Acta Radiologica Diagnosis, *13*, 163–176, 1972.

Margolis, M. T. and Newton, T. H.: The posterior inferior cerebellar artery. In Newton, T. H. and Potts, D. G., Eds., Radiology of the Skull and Brain. Vol. 2. St. Louis: C. V. Mosby, 1974.

Martin, F. and Lemmen, L. J.: Calcification in intracranial

neoplasms. American Journal of Pathology, 28, 1107–1131, 1952.

Mealey, J. Jr.: Brain scanning in childhood. Journal of Pediatrics, 69, 399–403, 1966.

Megret, M.: A landmark for the choroidal arteries of the fourth ventricle - branches of the posterior inferior cerebellar artery. Neuroradiology, 5, 85–90, 1973.

Michael, W. F.: Posterior fossa aneurysms simulating tumors, Journal of Neurology, Neurosurgery and Psychiatry, 37, 218–223, 1974.

Morris, L. and Wylie, I. G.: Tomography in cerebral pneumoencephalography. Clinical Radiology, 24, 221–230, 1973.

Naidich, T. P., Lin, J. P., Leeds, N. E., Kricheff, I. I., George, A. J., Chase, N. E., Pudlowski, R. M. and Passalaqua, A.: Computed tomography in the diagnosis of extra-axial posterior fossa masses. Radiology, 120, 333–339, 1976-A.

Naidich, T. P., Kricheff, I. I., George, A. E. and Lin, J. P.: The normal anterior inferior cerebellar artery. Radiology, 119, 355–373, 1976-B.

Naidich, T. P., Kricheff, I. I., George, A. E. and Lin, J. P.: The anterior inferior cerebellar artery in mass lesions. Radiology, 119, 375–383, 1976-C.

Naidich, T. P., Lin, J. P., Leeds, N. E., Pudlowski, R. M., and Naidich, J. B.: Primary tumors and other masses of the cerebellum and fourth ventricle. Differential diagnosis by computed tomography. Neuroradiology, 14, 153–174, 1977.

Newton, T. H.: The anterior and posterior meningeal branches of the vertebral artery. Radiology, 91, 271–279, 1968.

Norman, D. and Newton, T. H.: Ceruminous tumors of the cerebellopontine angle. Neuroradiology, 10, 1–4, 1975.

Novy, S. and Jensen, K. M.: Filling defects and nonfilling defects of the internal auditory canal in posterior fossa myelography. American Journal of Roentgenology, 124, 265–270, 1975.

Okawara, S. H.: Solid cerebellar hemangioblastoma. Journal of Neurosurgery, 39, 514–518, 1973.

Osborn, J. D.: A comparative study of special petrous views and tomography in the diagnosis of acoustic neuromas. British Journal of Radiology, 48, 996–999, 1975.

Peeters, F. L. M.: The vertebral angiogram in patients with tumors in or near the midline. Neuroradiology, 5, 53–58, 1973.

Phelps, P. D., Toland, J. A., and Sheldon, P. W. E.: Erosions of the petrous temporal bone. Journal of Laryngology and Otology, 84, 1205–1230, 1970.

Pribram, H. F. W., Hudson, J. D. and Joynt, R. J.: Posterior fossa aneurysms presenting as mass lesions. American Journal of Roentgenology, 105, 334–340, 1969.

Reidy, J., De Lacey, G. J., Wignall, B. K. and Uttley, D.: The accuracy of plain radiographs in the diagnosis of acoustic neuromas. Neuroradiology, 10, 31–34, 1975.

Rosenbaum, A. E. and Drayer, B. P.: CT cisternography with metrizamide. Acta Radiologica Supplementum, 355, 1977.

Ross, P., Du Boulay, G. and Keller, B.: Normal measurements in angiography of the posterior fossa. Radiology, 116, 335–340, 1975.

Salamon, G. M., Combalbert, A., Raybaud, C. and Gonzalez, J.: An angiographic study of meningiomas of the posterior fossa. Journal of Neurosurgery, 35, 731–741, 1971.

Sarwar, M., Batnitzky, S. and Schechter, M. M.: Tumorous aneurysms. Neuroradiology, 12, 79–97, 1976.

Sarwar, M., Batnitzky, S. and Schechter, M. M.: Anterior pontomesencephalic vein and basilar artery in exophytic brain-stem glioma. Radiology, 124, 403–408, 1977.

Savoiardo, M., and LeMay, M.: Diagnosis of posterior fossa lesions by angiography. British Journal of Radiology, 43, 291–302, 1970.

Savoiardo, M. and Vaghi, M. A.: Angiography in brain stem tumors. Neuroradiology, 8, 99–112, 1974.

Scanlan, R. L.: Positive contrast medium (iophendylate) in diagnosis of acoustic neuromas. Archives of Otolaryngology, 80, 698–707, 1964.

Schechter, M. M., Bull, J. W. D. and Carey, P.: Two new encephalographic signs of pressure hydrocephalus. British Journal of Radiology, 31, 317–325, 1958.

Schechter, M. M. and Zingesser, L. H.: The spinal arteries. Acta Radiologica Diagnosis, 5, 1124–1131, 1966.

Seeger, J. F. and Gabrielsen, T. O.: Angiography of eccentric brain stem tumors. Radiology, 105, 343–351, 1972.

Shiffman, E., Dancer, J., Rothballer, A. B., Berrett, A. and Baum, S.: The diagnosis and evaluation of acoustic neurofibromas. Otolaryngologic Clinics of North America, 6, 189–228, 1973.

Smaltino, F., Bernini, F. P. and Elefante, R.: Normal and pathologic findings of the angiographic examination of the internal auditory artery. Neuroradiology, 2, 216–222, 1971.

Smink, K. W. F., Hekster, R. E. M. and Bots, G. T. A. M.: Clivus chordoma with distinct vascularity demonstrated by angiography. Neuroradiology, 13, 273–277, 1977.

Sones, P. J. and Hoffman, J. C.: Angiography of tumors involving the posterior third ventricle. American Journal of Roentgenology, 124, 241–249, 1975.

Sortland, O.: Computed tomography combined with gas cisternography for the diagnosis of expanding lesions in the cerebellopontine angle. Neuroradiology, 18, 19–22, 1979.

Sortland, O., Nornes, H. and Djupesland, G.: Cisternography with metrizamide in cerebellopontine angle tumors. Acta Radiologica Supplementum, 355, 1977.

Sutton, D.: The radiological assessment of the normal aqueduct and 4th ventricle. British Journal of Radiology, 23, 208–218, 1950.

Takahashi, M., Okudera, T., Tomanaga, M. and Kitamura, K.: Angiographic diagnosis of acoustic neurinomas: Analysis of 30 lesions. Neuroradiology, 2, 191–200, 1971.

Takahashi, M., Wilson, G. and Hanafee, W.: The significance of the petrosal vein in the diagnosis of cerebellopontine angle tumors. Radiology, 89, 834–840, 1967.

Takahashi, M., Wilson, G. and Hanafee, W.: The anterior inferior cerebellar artery: Its radiographic anatomy and significance in the diagnosis of extra-axial tumors of the posterior fossa. Radiology, 90, 281–287, 1968.

Théron, J. and Lasjaunais, P.: Participation of the external and internal carotid arteries in the blood supply of acoustic neurinomas. Radiology, 118, 83–88, 1976.

Thijssen, H. O. M., Marres, E. H. M. and Slooff, J. L.: Arachnoid cyst simulating intrameatal acoustic neuroma. Neuroradiology, 11, 205–207, 1976.

Thomson, J. L. G.: Computerised axial tomography in posterior fossa lesions. Clinical Radiology, 29, 233–250, 1978.

Twining, E. W.: Radiology of the third and fourth ventricle, Part II. British Journal of Radiology, 12, 569–598, 1939.

Tytus, J. S. and Pennybacker, J.: Pearly tumors in relation to the central nervous system. Journal of Neurology, Neurosurgery and Psychiatry, 19, 241–259, 1956.

Valvassori, G. E.: The abnormal internal auditory canal: The diagnosis of acoustic neuroma. Radiology, 92, 449–459, 1969.

Valvassori, G. E. and Pierce, R. H.: The normal internal auditory canal. American Journal of Roentgenology, 92, 1232–1241, 1964.

Van Damme, W., Reolon, M., Pereira, N. and Wackenheim, A.: Arterial and venous signs of tumors within the fourth ventricle. Neuroradiology, 13, 209–214, 1977.

Wallace, S., Goldberg, H. I., Leeds, N. E. and Mishkin, M. M.: The cavernous branches of the internal carotid artery. American Journal of Roentgenology, 101, 34–46, 1967.

Wastie, M. L.: The significance of the failed pneumoencephalogram. Journal of the Neurological Sciences, 17, 309–321, 1972.

Wende, S. and Lüdecke, B.: Technique and value of gas and

Pantopaque cisternography in the diagnosis of cerebellopontine angle tumors. Neuroradiology, *2*, 24 – 29, 1971.

Wolf, B. S., Nakagawa, H. and Staulcup, P. H.: Feasibility of coronal views in computed scanning of the head. Radiology, *120*, 217 – 218, 1976.

Wolf, B. S., Newman, C. M. and Khilnani, M. T.: The posterior inferior cerebellar artery on vertebral angiography. American Journal of Roentgenology, *87*, 322 – 337, 1962.

Wolpert, S. M.: The neuroradiology of hemangioblastomas of the cerebellum. American Journal of Roentgenology, *110*, 56 – 66, 1970.

Wolpert, S. M.: Angiography of posterior fossa tumors. New York: Grune and Stratton, 1976.

Ziedses Des Plantes, B. G.: X-ray examination in cerebellopontine angle tumors. Psychiatria, Neurologia, Neurochirurgia, *71*, 133 – 139, 1968.

9 Skull Base Including Cranio-Vertebral Junction

INTRODUCTION

The skull base and craniovertebral junction are anatomical areas often overlooked in clinical and radiological diagnosis. The delicate upper cervical vertebrae together with the occiput and their interconnecting ligaments and muscles form a rigid yet flexible funnel-shaped tube which supports the head and houses the brainstem and upper spinal cord. In front lie the nasopharynx and the floors of the temporal fossae, structures that can only be seen properly in the full-axial projection.

Bony abnormalities around the foramen magnum are not uncommon findings but not all are symptomatic. It is necessary to formulate radiological criteria for deciding which abnormalities are relevant—that is, likely to produce clinical signs and symptoms—and which may be dismissed as insignificant. Clinical localization to the upper cervical region is imprecise, and complaints such as limb weakness, neck pain and ataxia are common features of certain neurological diseases, e.g., multiple sclerosis, amyotrophic lateral sclerosis and subacute combined degeneration. McRae (1960), in a study of 68 patients with bony abnormalities of the craniovertebral angle, found that 21 had been diagnosed as multiple sclerosis and a further 17 as cases of cervical disc prolapse or posterior fossa tumor.

RADIOLOGICAL EXAMINATION AND MEASUREMENTS

Projections

The most useful view for evaluating the craniovertebral junction is a lateral projection of the skull—provided that it is made with a central ray that is horizontal, and preferably with the patient supine. Adequate study of the relationship of the occiput and its foramen magnum to the atlas and axis is possible on the routine lateral view of the skull, since the craniovertebral angle is not usually excluded by optimal coning of the beam. The radiographic centering for this projection is far more appropriate for studying this area than the routine lateral projection of the cervical spine.

Lateral midline tomograms (Fig. 9–1) may be necessary, especially if the mastoid air cells are well pneumatized, to show the anterior and posterior rims of the foramen magnum, the clivus and its relation to the tip of the odontoid process (apical ligament), the atlas and the axis. The horizontal-ray lateral view, when made with the patient supine, serves as a dynamic test of the integrity of the atlantoaxial joint: it reveals the full extent of any abnormal slippage due to laxity or rupture of the transverse ligament, because the weight of the neck muscles will force the odontoid process to separate from the anterior arch of the atlas when the patient is placed in this position.

Further lateral tomograms made 1 cm. apart on each side of the midline will demonstrate the integrity of the laminae and apophyseal joints of the atlas and axis.

The anteroposterior ("through-mouth") projec-

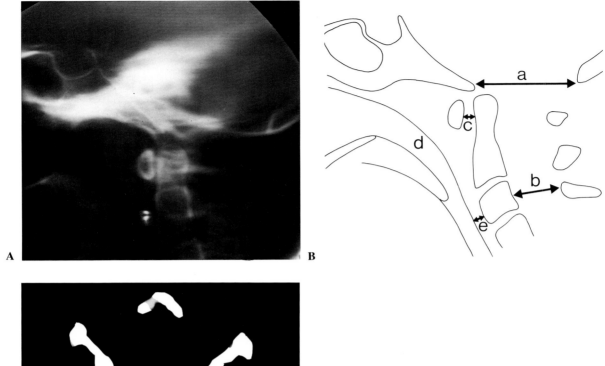

Fig. 9–1 (A and B) The craniovertebral angle. a. Foramen magnum. b. Sagittal diameter of the cervical spine at C3. c. Atlantoodontoid gap. d. Nasopharyngeal soft-tissue space. e. Retropharyngeal (prevertebral) space. (C) Computed tomogram of base. The dimensions of the foramen magnum can be measured accurately and its symmetry verified.

tion of the odontoid process is an amplifying view which is essential in congenital skeletal anomalies and destructive lesions of the upper cervical spine, in order to gauge their full extent, and particularly the side-side functional asymmetry of the neck. Tomograms or zonograms in this plane are useful to show the occipital condyles and lateral borders of the foramen magnum which may be selectively distorted by basilar impression.

Boogaard's Basal Angle and Platybasia

The basal angle, as measured by anthropologists using an inclinometer, is the angle between the floor of the anterior cranial fossa and the clivus. Boogaard, a Dutch scientist, described it in 1865, 32 years before his countryman W. C. Roentgen discovered x-rays. Anthropologists point out that man has the smallest basal angle (usually 120–140°), that primates have angles greater than 150 degrees and most subprimate mammals angles approximating 180 degrees. Measured on a lateral radiograph, Boogaard's measurement is the angle at the middle of the pituitary fossa between lines drawn to the nasion and the anterior rim of the foramen magnum.

An extremely wide range of normal values is found in humans (Fig. 9–2). A skull with a basal angle of over 140 degrees is said to be platybasic, but this description possesses no clinical relevance. Although underdevelopment of the skull base, e.g., in achondroplasia (Fig. 1–64), produces a characteristically small angle, there is no scientific evidence to indicate that the basal angle reflects developmental patterns or particular defects. A wide basal angle may be present in mongolism, and in bone-softening states that cause basilar impression (Burwood, Gordon and Taft, 1973).

A second anthropological measurement is the angle between the clivus and odontoid process

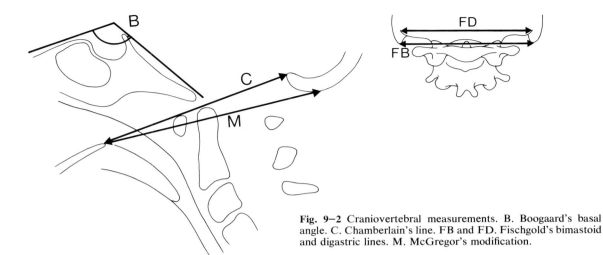

Fig. 9–2 Craniovertebral measurements. B. Boogaard's basal angle. C. Chamberlain's line. FB and FD. Fischgold's bimastoid and digastric lines. M. McGregor's modification.

which, like the basal angle, approaches 180 degrees in lower mammals and reptiles. This angle is rendered more acute in cases of basilar impression that cause stenosis by deforming the bones and compressing the medulla and cervical spinal cord, and it is more useful to the neuroradiologist than some conventional measurements described elsewhere (Wackenheim, 1974).

Foramen Magnum and Upper Cervical Spinal Canal

Although the dural sheath of the craniovertebral junction is usually described as funnel-shaped, only the foramen magnum is round: the cervical spinal canal is triangular in cross-section. Throughout its length the interpedicular (side-side) diameter is nearly twice as great as the sagittal (front-back) diameter. Therefore the spinal cord, which is suspended within the canal like a loose-fitting round peg in a triangular hole, can expand sideways but there is less room for anteroposterior movement. Lindgren (1937) and Boijsen (1954) first drew attention to the importance of measuring the sagittal diameter of the cervical canal. Of Boijsen's seven cases of cervical intraspinal tumor with bone changes, five showed increased sagittal diameters and only two widened interpedicular diameters, and in both of these the sagittal diameters were increased. Narrowing as well as widening is important. Stenosis of the craniovertebral canal may result from congenital underdevelopment or deformity of the skull base, or from severe hypertrophic osteophytosis of degenerative joint disease.

Evaluation of the shape and dimensions of the craniovertebral funnel is important in neuroradiological interpretation, because focal neurological disorders of the foramen magnum are usually caused by neural compression. Cervical myelography is always necessary to demonstrate the level and extent of compression, but local narrowing or widening of the bony canal should be positively excluded before contrast investigations. A range of normal values is available, based on the measurement of about 800 normal adults reported by various authors (Boijsen, 1954; Wolf, Khilnani and Malis, 1956; Payne and Spillane, 1957; Burrows, 1963). The following are the mean sagittal diameters:

Foramen magnum: 34 (26 – 40 mm.)
Atlas: 22 (13 – 16 mm.)
Axis: 19 (15 – 27 mm.)
C3: 18 (12 – 25 mm.)

Atlanto-Odontoid Gap

If a neuroradiologist is accustomed to viewing lateral skull radiographs made with a horizontal ray of a supine patient, his eye will be adjusted to the maximum gap allowable. If the patient is examined erect or prone, this gap narrows and the anterior arch is displaced upward. The odontoid usually lies within 2 mm. of the anterior arch of the atlas in adults, and this relationship is so constant that any degree of widening is significant (Wholey, Bruwer and Baker, 1958). However, in children the transverse ligament is less rigid, and a slightly wider gap need not be abnormal (Caffey, 1973). In traumatic, inflammatory and neoplastic processes, widening may point to more extensive involvement of the adjacent cervical vertebrae and the contents of the dural tube.

Retropharyngeal Space

The average width of this layer of soft tissues at the lower level of the axis is 3.5 mm. in adults and children, according to Wholey et al. (1958), who evaluated the lateral cervical spine radiographs of 600 normal subjects. They found a wide range of normal variation, but expressed the view that a space wider than 7 mm. is always suspicious and merits further investigation.

Measurements for Basilar Impression (Fig. 9–2)

Chamberlain's Line and McGregor's Modification: Chamberlain's (1939) line joins the posterior end of the hard palate to the posterior lip of the foramen magnum. Because of the difficulty in identifying the posterior lip without tomography in some cases of basilar impression, McGregor (1948) drew his line to the lowest point of the occipital squame. The diagnosis of basilar impression is made by relating the position of the odontoid process to these lines. In normal subjects, the tip should lie below Chamberlain's line and not more than 6 mm. above McGregor's line. Exceptions to this rule are commonly found, and the diagnosis of basilar impression should never rest solely on measurement. These lines may be criticized, in addition to being subject to the limitation of all biological measurements, in that a facial reference point is utilized to draw conclusions on the craniovertebral junction. Certain normal or asymptomatic deformities may give rise to a high odontoid process: platybasia, occipitalization of the atlas, a congenitally short clivus, or combinations of these.

Digastric and Bimastoid Lines (Fischgold et al., 1952): The bimastoid line joins the tips of the two mastoid processes and bisects the atlanto-occipital joints at the very tip of the odontoid process. The digastric line joins the two digastric notches and lies about 1 cm. above the atlanto-occipital joints. These measurements, although less convenient to make than Chamberlain's or McGregor's lines, are more reliable. Basilar impression is almost certainly present if the atlanto-occipital joint lies at the level of the digastric line.

INDIVIDUAL PATHOLOGICAL ENTITIES

Congenital and Developmental Dysplasias

A large number of skeletal anomalies involve the craniovertebral angle, but the majority do not give rise to symptoms. The importance of the latter to the radiologist depends on his ability to be able to dismiss them as chance findings of no significance (List, 1941; McRae, 1960).

Asymptomatic anomalies include: (1) Defects in the arch of the atlas—spina bifida is common; other defects such as a sagittally split atlas are rare. (2) Ponticuli: osseous bridging of the grooves for the vertebral arteries as they cross the lateral masses of the atlas (ponticulus lateralis) or its posterior aspect (ponticulus posticus). (3) Asymmetry of the atlanto-occipital and atlantoaxial joints. Wackenheim (1970) has drawn attention to the facial asymmetry accompanying such anomalies, as depicted in the portraits of Modigliani and certain other artists.

Symptom-producing anomalies include the following three mechanical lesions:

Basilar impression
Occipitalization of the atlas
Atlantoaxial dislocation
Each is usually a congenital abnormality, although the same deformity may result from acquired disease. Congenital hindbrain descent, which may be symptomatic, is sometimes accompanied by skeletal anomalies. Congenital fusion of the cervical vertebrae (Klippel-Feil's syndrome) is symptomatic only if associated with another defect at the craniovertebral junction.

Basilar Impression

Basilar impression is defined as an invagination or upturning into the skull of the margins of the foramen magnum. The entire occiput may be deformed in this way, or only a particular segment of the rim of the foramen magnum (Fig. 9–3). It is difficult to set radiological criteria for the diagnosis of minor degrees of basilar impression. No single line of measurement is entirely reliable, since each may give different results, depending on the pattern of deformity present. For example: in anterior impression the odontoid process will rise above both Chamberlain's and McGregor's lines, but in posterior impression it will transgress only McGregor's line, and Chamberlain's measurement may remain normal. Apart from measurements, there are three radiological features to confirm: (1) The high-lying odontoid process may lie within the foramen magnum, and its tip maintains a normal relationship to the basiocciput (which, if hypoplastic, is tilted upward). (2) The clivus-odontoid angle is narrowed nearly to 90 degrees. (3) The medial parts of the petrous pyramids are tilted upward, above the horizontal plane.

Tonsillar herniation may be a feature of severe basilar impression, but this deformity is not a true ectopia of the Chiari type, as proven by the fact that the upper cervical nerve roots retain their normal horizontal or slightly downward path outward toward the intervertebral foramina. Rather, the herniation reflects a "normal brain-abnormal skull" situation. The caudal loop of the posterior inferior cerebellar artery is depressed and both vertebral arteries and the proximal basilar show unusual looping, due to the concertina effect (Klaus, 1969).

Basilar impression is either a congenital (primary) affection, when it is usually an isolated asymptomatic deformity which may be familial (Bull, Nixon, and Pratt, 1955), or a complication of the following: (1) Bone-softening diseases, e.g., osteogenesis imperfecta (Hurwitz and MacSwiney, 1960; Dirheimer and Babin, 1971), Paget's disease (Bull, Nixon, Pratt and Robinson, 1959), disordered bone metabolism in celiac disease and after gastric surgery (Hurwitz and Shepherd, 1966; Hurwitz and Banerji, 1972). (2) Severe fracture or a process that deforms by destruction, e.g., osteomyelitis or neoplastic metastases. (3) Mongolism (Burwood and Watt, 1974).

Occipitalization of the Atlas (Atlanto-Occipital Assimilation)

This congenital abnormality consists of fusion of the atlas to the occipital bone, and fusion of C2 – 3 is a common accompaniment (Fig. 9 – 4). About 25 percent of cases have an associated Chiari malformation (McRae and Standen, 1966). An identical morbid-anatomical situation may be produced by collapse of the craniovertebral junction due to inflammatory or neoplastic destruction, e.g., tuberculous osteomyelitis. Surprisingly little limitation of head movement occurs. About half of the patients present with medullary or upper cervical symptoms and signs. It is significant that a similar proportion of cases studied at autopsy have shown secondary atrophic changes on the anterior surface of the medulla oblongata and upper spinal cord due to odontoid compression. Tomography reveals that the odontoid process forms the anterior rim of the foramen magnum. McRae and Barnum (1953) found that symptoms due to pressure on the medulla oblongata are likely to be present if the effective anteroposterior diameter of the foramen magnum is reduced to less than 19 mm. In four of their 25 patients, an associated dural band was found at operation to be pressing against the posterior surface of the medulla. They believe this band, which cannot be identified by radiological methods, to play a significant part in causing symptoms and signs.

Atlantoaxial Dislocation

About 50 percent of patients with this anomaly present with related symptoms. The radiological feature essential for the diagnosis is widening of the atlanto-odontoid gap (Measurements, see above). There are two types of atlantoaxial dislocation: (1) odontoid process intact, i.e., attached to the body of the axis; and (2) separate odontoid process. If an intact axis vertebra is present, atlantoaxial instability is the result of softening or rupture of the transverse ligament. Apart from trauma, the most frequent cause in acute cases is infection—pyogenic or tuberculous osteomyelitis. Most chronic cases occur in rheumatiod patients (Fig. 9 – 5; Sharp and Purser, 1961). In younger subjects this type of atlantoaxial instability is seen in mongols (Tishler and Martel, 1965). McRae (1960) described six cases which he believed to be congenital in origin. Atlantoaxial dislocation is also encountered in osteogenesis imperfecta.

If the odontoid is detached from the body of the axis so that it moves with the atlas, the descriptive term "separate odontoid process" is preferable, since fractures may be difficult or impossible to differentiate from congenital defects. According to Greenberg (1968), the line of separation in fractures usually lies below the level of the superior articular facets of the atlantoaxial articulations, and in congenital anomaly the line is above them. Three congenital anomalies of the odontoid exist: agenesis, separate apical segment only (ossiculum terminale), and separate complete odontoid (os odontoideum — Minderhoud, Braakman and Penning, 1969). Odontoid hypoplasia is a feature of mucopolysaccharidosis IV (Morquio-Brailsford's disease).

Functional radiological and ciné studies in patients with separate odontoid process show that considerable alterations in position occur during movement between the odontoid and the body of the axis: the odontoid, being attached by the apical ligament to the tip of the clivus, moves with the atlas *en bloc*. This abnormal movement disrupts normal anatomical alignments and threatens to compress the spinal cord and vertebral arteries. The cross-sectional diameter of the spinal canal may be considerably reduced during flexion, as shown by measuring the distance between the posterior aspect of the odontoid process and the posterior rim of the foramen magnum or the anterior aspect of the posterior arch of the atlas. Vertebrobasilar ischemia is more difficult to demonstrate, but occlusion of the vertebral arteries leads to drop attacks (Barton and Margolis, 1975). Vulnerability of the spinal cord in atlantoaxial instability is well demonstrated in Figure 9 – 6, which explains why dislocation alone is more serious than dislocation with separate odontoid process. Mongols and patients with os odontoideum are an anesthetic hazard, especially during intubation and the use of muscle relaxants.

Other Stenotic Lesions

Apart from the secondary stenosis produced by the above three deformities (Fig. 9 – 7), several other conditions may narrow the neural tube. They are (1) Achondroplasia. (2) Occipital dysplasia, in which the foramen magnum is small and deformed as a result of premature fusion of one or more occipital synchondroses (Kruyff, 1965). (3) Chronic fluorine intoxication, in which thickening of the skull base, ligamentous calcification and protruding osteophytes may compress the medulla and spinal cord and produce a severe myelopathy (Møller and Gudjonsson, 1932). Singh, Jolly, Bansal and Mathur (1963) illustrated their important report of this disease in India with an autopsy specimen in which the osteophytic overgrowth obliterated half of the spinal canal. (4) Paget's disease and other bone-softening conditions in which stenosis of the foramen magnum is a complication of the gross deformity of the skull base. (5) Spondylosis of the atlantoaxial joint (Fig. 9 – 8). (6) Congenital spinal stenosis (see Chap. 11).

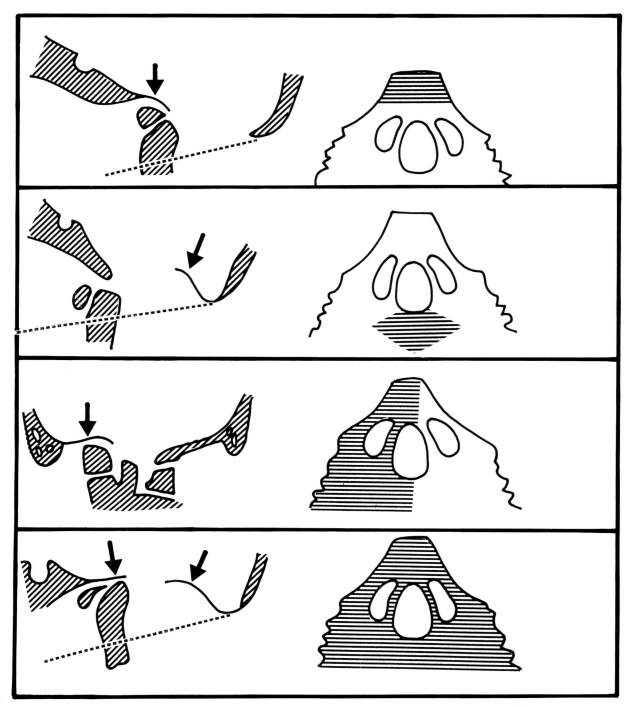

Fig. 9–3 Basilar impression. (A) Various types, drawn after Wackenheim (1974). Broken line is McGregor's modification. *(Top)* Anterior impression. *(Middle, above)* Posterior impression. *(Middle, below)* Asymmetric unilateral impression. *(Bottom)* Generalized impression.

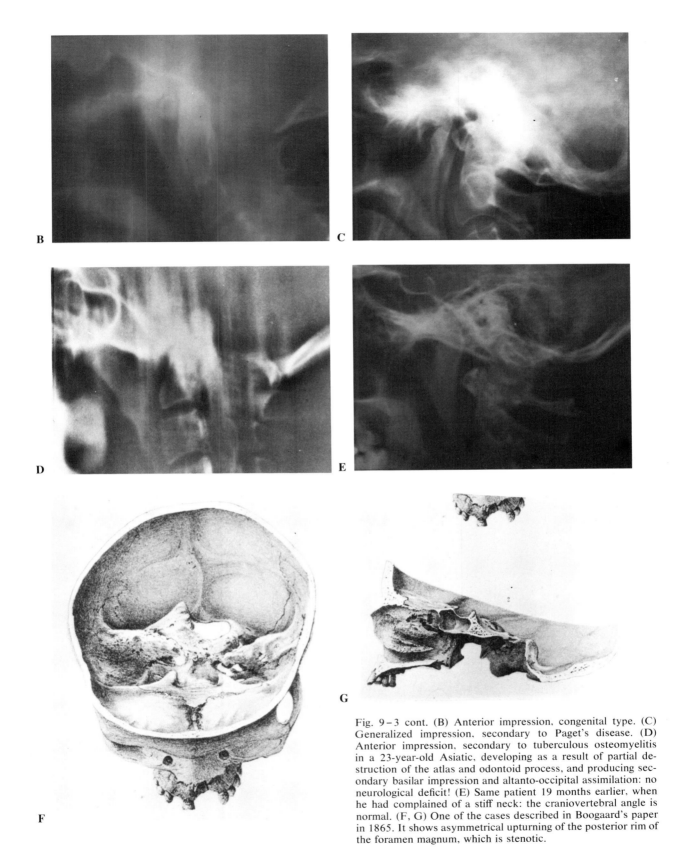

Fig. 9–3 cont. (B) Anterior impression, congenital type. (C) Generalized impression, secondary to Paget's disease. (D) Anterior impression, secondary to tuberculous osteomyelitis in a 23-year-old Asiatic, developing as a result of partial destruction of the atlas and odontoid process, and producing secondary basilar impression and altanto-occipital assimilation: no neurological deficit! (E) Same patient 19 months earlier, when he had complained of a stiff neck: the craniovertebral angle is normal. (F, G) One of the cases described in Boogaard's paper in 1865. It shows asymmetrical upturning of the posterior rim of the foramen magnum, which is stenotic.

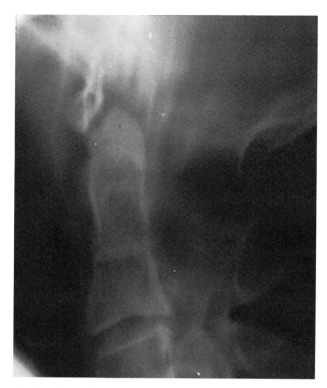

Fig. 9−4 Congenital atlanto-occipital assimilation and C2−3 fusion, asymptomatic patient.

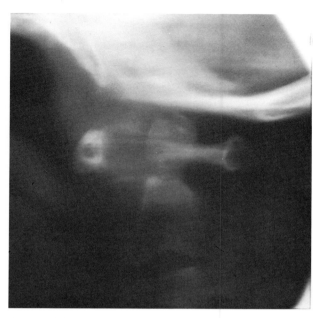

Fig. 9−5 Atlanto-axial dislocation, caused by laxity of the transverse ligament in a patient with rheumatoid arthritis. Note the widened atlanto-odontoid gap, and the groove on the anterior surface of odontoid process caused by the transverse ligament.

Hindbrain Anomalies

In 1891 Chiari described hindbrain ectopia in a group of patients with congenital hydrocephalus, and classified them as follows:

Type 1: Ectopic tonsils, which are elongated and narrow and closely applied to the posterior aspect of the upper cervical cord, reaching the C1−2 level. No other part of the hindbrain is misplaced; and in particular, the fourth ventricle occupies a normal position.

Type 2: Tonsillar ectopia combined with ectopia of the inferior cerebellar vermis and caudal location of the pons and medulla. Thus the entire brainstem lies at a lower level than normal—the fourth ventricle is at or below the foramen magnum, and the tonsils are often considerably lower. Meningocele or myelomeningocele and/or syringomyelia may be associated findings. All the patients are hydrocephalic, probably due to outlet obstruction. This type of Chiari anomaly is sometimes called the Arnold-Chiari malformation.

Type 3: Total hindbrain ectopia, with the cerebellum located in a high cervical meningocele (rare).

Type 4: Hypoplasia of the cerebellum (rare).

Radiological Findings: The tonsillar ectopia that comprises the type 1 Chiari anomaly may be impossible to distinguish from secondary brain descent, i.e., tonsillar herniation caused by an expanding intracranial lesion. Gas myelography will reveal a soft-tissue mass on the posterior surface of the upper cervical cord and sometimes a compromised cisterna magna (Liliequist, 1960). Oil myelography made with the patient supine (Baker, 1963; Davies, 1967) shows two almond-shaped filling defects, often with pointed tips (Fig. 9−9). Metrizamide cervical myelography with or without computerized tomography will sometimes demonstrate the findings to advantage (Fig. 9−9). The diagnosis of the type 1 Chiari anomaly can be made if the first pair of cervical nerve roots is shown to pass upward to reach the intervertebral foramina, rather than horizontally, as is the normal arrangement; and if contrast filling reveals a fourth ventricle that is normal in size, shape and position (Fig. 9−9). The extracranial position of the cerebellar tonsils can be demonstrated by vertebral angiography (Fig. 9−10). The unusually wide range of normal variation in the appearances of the tonsils has been stressed by Bloch, Van Rensburg and Danziger (1974). Low-lying tonsils are not uncommon in otherwise normal individuals, and their presence below the level of the foramen magnum may occasionally be an isolated myelographic finding.

The Chiari type 2 anomaly tends to exhibit longer, flatter tonsils which may reach to below the level of the axis, but the diagnosis depends on demonstrating the ectopic position of the fourth ventricle. Computed tomography or ventriculography is required for this purpose, since the fourth ventri-

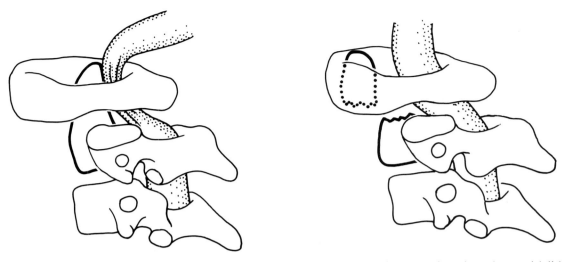

Fig. 9–6 Atlanto-axial dislocation. Diagram showing why atlanto-axial dislocation alone is more serious than atlanto-axial dislocation with separation of the odontoid process (after Watson-Jones, 1952).

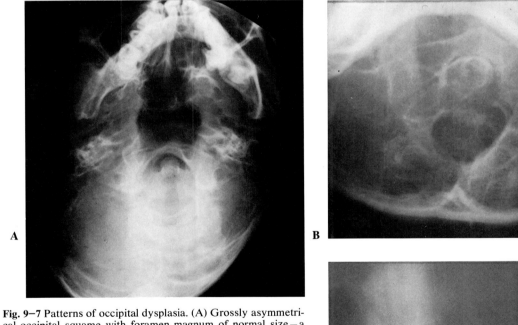

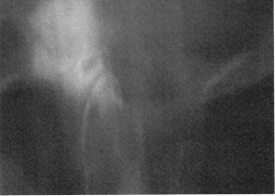

Fig. 9–7 Patterns of occipital dysplasia. (A) Grossly asymmetrical occipital squame with foramen magnum of normal size – a chance finding in a young male. (B and C) Severe stenosis of the foramen magnum complicating congenital basilar impression, the patient was a 50-year-old woman with long-tract signs, in whom the initial diagnosis was multiple sclerosis. The foramen magnum has a "figure-of-eight" outline and the odontoid process occupies the anterior half, as a result of incomplete development of its anterior rim.

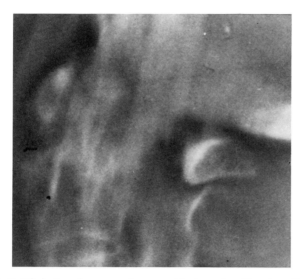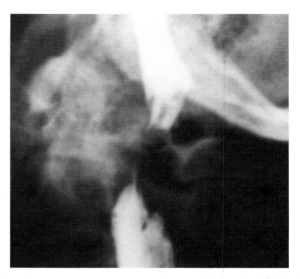

Fig. 9–8 Spinal cord compression caused by hypertrophic osteoarthritis of the atlanto-axial joint, in an 82-year-old man. Relief followed decompression laminectomy.

cle usually does not fill from a lumbar contrast injection. Obstructive hydrocephalus is invariably seen (Fig. 9–11). Vertebral angiography may reveal unexpected arterial anomalies (Lasjaunia et al., 1977).

Skeletal abnormalities are present in no more than about 50 percent of patients (Davies, 1967; Appleby, Foster, Hankinson and Hudgson, 1968). They include all or some of the following features: chronic hydrocephalus, including a depressed pineal gland; deformities of the craniovertebral angle, of which only accentuation of its funnelled shape is characteristic; and an abnormally wide lower cervical canal if syringomyelia is an additional complication.

Klippel-Feil and Associated Anomalies

The clinical syndrome described by Klippel and Feil in 1912 was *une homme sans cou,* "a man without a neck." The syndrome consists of a short neck, low hair line and an absence of individually formed cervical vertebrae. Although cervical fusion leads to limitation of neck movements, neurological deficit is rare since the cervical spinal canal is not stenotic. Patients with the Klippel-Feil syndrome alone have a full life expectancy. However, children with an associated occipital or cervical meningocele usually do not survive to adulthood (Fig. 9–12).

Acquired Masses Around the Foramen Magnum

Abnormal masses within or around the foramen magnum comprise the following groups:

1. Local masses such as aneurysm, primary neoplasm (neurofibroma or meningioma) or metastasis.
2. Invasive neoplasms spreading by contiguity from the fourth ventricle (choroid plexus papilloma, ependymoma), cerebellopontine angle (chol-

esteatoma), brainstem (glioma) cerebellar hemisphere (astrocytoma, metastasis), or the clivus (chordoma, myeloma).

3. Brain descent causing tonsillar herniation secondary to distant intracranial neoplasms or posterior-fossa arachnoiditis (outlet obstruction) (see Fig. 9–13). About one-third of foramen magnum lesions are benign and thus curable. The most important of these is meningioma (Marc and Schechter, 1975).

Plain radiography including tomography of the foramen magnum is essential, not only to reveal destruction but also to exclude a congenital anomaly of the craniovertebral junction. Calcified deposits although rare, may be specific: curvilinear calcification indicates a giant aneurysm of the vertebral artery, tightly-packed granular deposits point to a meningioma or a fourth ventricle tumor such as an ependymoma.

Gas myelography, if supplemented by tomography, and oil myelography made with the patient supine, will show a soft-tissue mass emerging from the foramen magnum behind the spinal cord. This mass, depending upon its size and position, will narrow or obliterate the cisterna magna, displace the spinal cord laterally or completely plug the upper cervical spinal canal. Slowly growing tumors causing brain descent will exhibit tonsillar herniation that is indistinguishable from the congenitally ectopic tonsils of the Chiari types 1 and 2 anomalies (Wickbom and Hanafee, 1963). In other cases of tumor or outlet obstruction due to arachnoiditis, the retromedullary space may be plugged or obliterated by herniated tonsil (Fig. 9–14) (Stein, Leeds, Taveras, and Pool, 1963). Obstructive hydrocephalus is invariably present in the acquired lesions. If such patients are submitted to pneumoencephalography, air fails to enter the ventricular system. Instead, it passes

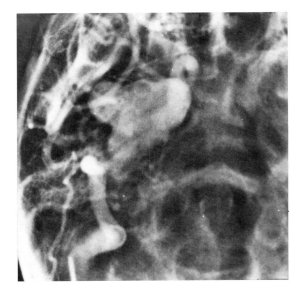

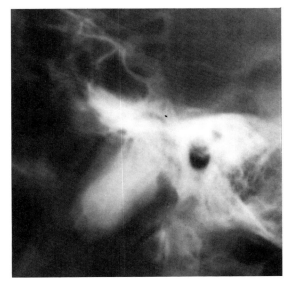

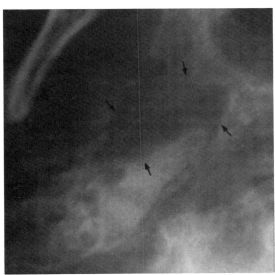

Fig. 9-19 Aneurysm of the internal carotid artery eroding the floor of the middle cranial fossa *(arrows),* and presenting as a soft-tissue mass on the right side of the nasopharynx. Preangiographic diagnosis: nasopharyngeal carcinoma!

seous midline defect of the body of the sphenoid bone is characteristic of this type of congenital brain herniation. The defect, which involves the floor of the anterior cranial fossa and may extend from the cribriform plate to the pituitary fossa, is difficult to recognize without tomography and full axial views. The extent of brain descent can be shown by pneumography, viz., herniation of the anterior end of the third ventricle through the defect, or by carotid angiography which shows downward displacement of the proximal part of the anterior cerebral artery (Pollock, Newton and Hoyt, 1968).

Petrous Pyramid
Destruction of the upper (i.e., intracranial) surface of the petrous bone is discussed in Chapter 8; see

Table 9-1. A wide variety of lesions erode the undersurface of the pyramid around the jugular foramen. The most important is the glomus jugulare tumor, but the following have been reported: neuroma of the 9th, 10th and 11th cranial nerves, chordoma, giant-cell tumor of bone, cholesteatoma and carcinoma—either hematogenous in origin or due to direct spread from the nasopharynx, salivary glands or external auditory meatus.

Chemodectoma (Glomus Jugulare and Carotid Body Tumors). Chemodectomas are the tumors of the chemoreceptor tissue of the body, located along blood vessels and nerves. Most often they occur in the microscopic glomus bodies in the adventitia of the jugular bulb (glomus jugulare) or the middle ear (glomus tympanum), or at bifurcation of the common carotid artery (carotid body tumor). They also

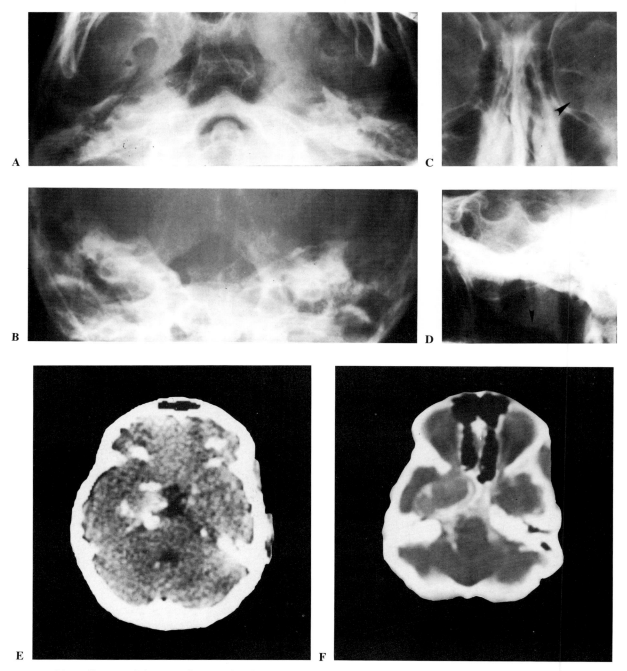

Fig. 9–20 Neurofibroma of the gasserian ganglion in a young man with cutaneous stigmata of generalized neurofibromotosis. Skull radiographs showing destruction of the floor of the left middle cranial fossa (A), petrous apex (B) and superior orbital fissure *(arrowhead, C)*, with a soft-tissue nasopharyngeal mass *(arrowhead, D)*. (E and F) Computed tomograms showing a parasellar mass with a well-defined outline which has destroyed the following structures: anterior clinoid process, lateral saddle of the pituitary fossa (encroaching upon the suprasellar "star" from the left side) and the petrous apex, extending into the left cerebellopontine angle.

occur on the 9th and 10th cranial nerves, aortic body, lung and in the retroperitoneum and larynx. The tendency to multicentric and bilateral involvement is so strong that bilateral angiography has been advised (Berk, 1961; Cook, 1977).

Radiological signs depend on the site of origin

and route of spread of the tumor (Rice and Holman, 1963; Hawkins, 1966; Miller et al., 1969). Glomus tumors arising from the tympanum are smaller, and destroy the inner and middle ear structures, presenting with otic signs rather than lower cranial nerve palsies — typically, a shiny, blue polyp on the

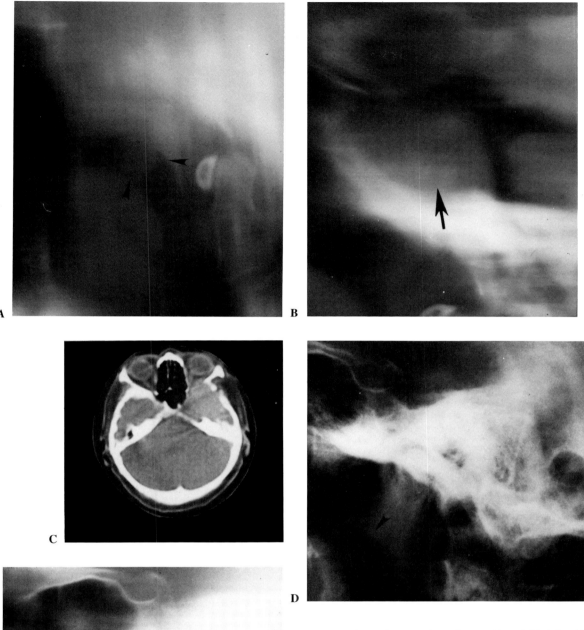

Fig. 9–21 Nasopharyngeal carcinoma. (A and B) Adenoid cystic carcinoma (cylindroma) of the nasopharynx in a middle-aged woman with an abducent palsy and a pedunculated nasopharyngeal swelling. Extensive destruction of the clivus and sphenoid body is present. The pedunculated mass is visible in the nasopharynx (A, *arrowheads*). (B) Midline tomopneumogram, showing the tumor mass replacing the destroyed clivus and sphenoid body. Calcified deposits *(arrow)* led to an erroneous pre-biopsy diagnosis of chordoma. (C) Nasopharyngeal carcinoma causing unilateral proptosis due to invasion of a spheroid ring. Computed tomogram shows destructive parasellar mass. (D and E) Sclerosing nasopharyngeal carcinoma. No destruction accompanies the large soft-tissue mass (D, *arrowhead*), but tomography confirmed the basal sclerosis (E). This case was published and illustrated by M. L. Wastie in the *British Journal of Radiology, 45,* 570–574, 1972.

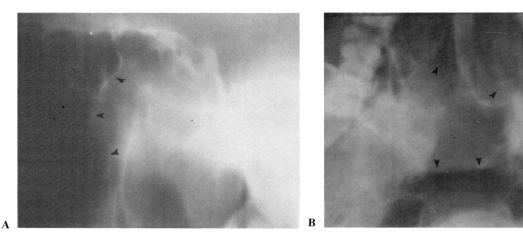

A   B

Fig. 9–22 Juvenile angiofibroma of the nasopharynx. A 14-year-old boy with nosebleeds and nasopharyngeal obstruction. (A) Median sagittal tomogram outlining a well-defined soft-tissue mass extending upward into the sphenoidal sinus and forward, to produce a characteristic concave indentation of the posterior wall of the maxillary sinus *(arrowheads)*. (B) The full-axial view shows the mass encroaching upon the right maxillary sinus, destroying the pterygoid plates on both sides and penetrating the sphenoidal sinus *(arrowheads)*.

eardrum and ipsilateral deafness. Glomus jugulare tumors erode the rim of the jugular foramen (Fig. 9–25), then enlarge and destroy the undersurface of the petrous pyramid. From there they extend

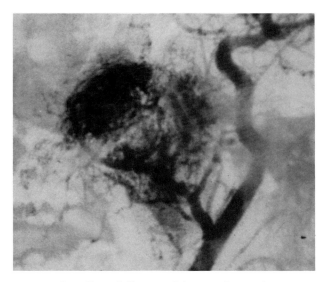

Fig. 9–23 Juvenile angiofibroma of the nasopharynx (same case as Fig. 9–22). Common carotid angiogram: well-circumscribed tumor with coarse hypervascularity, supplied chiefly by the internal maxillary branch of the external carotid artery.

forward and erode the floor of the ipsilateral temporal fossa; backward toward the foramen magnum and hypoglossal canal; and medially to amputate the petrous tip (Fig. 9–26). The erosion is infiltrative and possesses no corticated margin. Occasionally glomus tumors calcify (Moody, Ghatak and Kelly, 1976).

Angiographic investigation, which is essential for management, should be complete in three respects: (1) selective study of the external carotid artery amplified by internal carotid and vertebral arteriograms, because all three vessels may supply blood to the tumor (El Gammal, 1971). The typical picture is shown in Figure 9–27; (2) the subtraction technique, preferably combined with magnification is desirable for jugular tumors and essential for demonstrating tympanic tumors (Ziedses Des Plantes, 1971); and (3) venography may reveal an obstructed jugular vein, indicating unsuspected downward growth of the tumor (Cornell, 1969). Absence of the characteristic angiographic stain excludes a glomus tumor as the cause of any basal erosion—an important diagnostic point, in view of the wide asymmetry of the normal jugular foramina (Fig. 9–25B).

Sclerosis of the Base
See Table 9–2 and Figure 9–28.

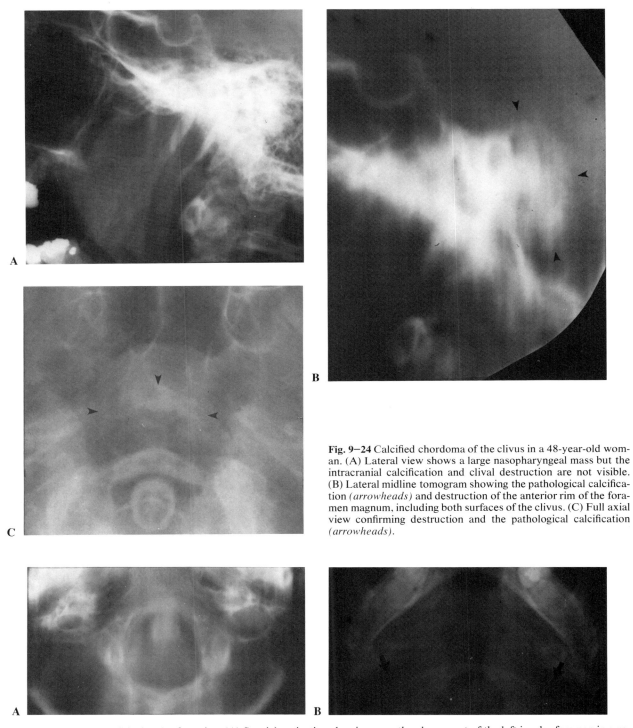

Fig. 9–24 Calcified chordoma of the clivus in a 48-year-old woman. (A) Lateral view shows a large nasopharyngeal mass but the intracranial calcification and clival destruction are not visible. (B) Lateral midline tomogram showing the pathological calcification *(arrowheads)* and destruction of the anterior rim of the foramen magnum, including both surfaces of the clivus. (C) Full axial view confirming destruction and the pathological calcification *(arrowheads)*.

Fig. 9–25 Asymmetry of the jugular foramina. (A) Special projection showing smooth enlargement of the left jugular foramen in a patient with a proven chemodectoma of the glomus jugulare. (B) A boy with blood-stained discharge from the left ear and a coincidental large jugular bulb—a normal variant. Jugular asymmetry may require angiography to rule out a tumor.

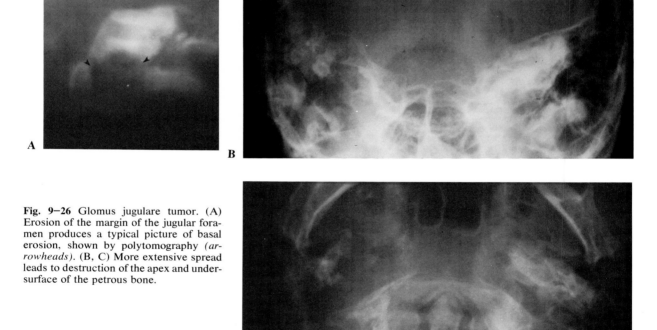

Fig. 9–26 Glomus jugulare tumor. (A) Erosion of the margin of the jugular foramen produces a typical picture of basal erosion, shown by polytomography *(arrowheads)*. (B, C) More extensive spread leads to destruction of the apex and undersurface of the petrous bone.

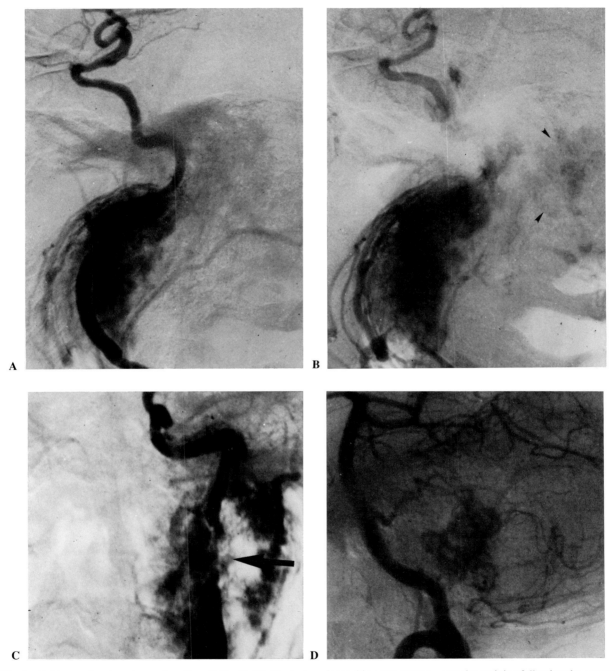

Fig. 9–27 Glomus jugulare tumor (continued) (A, B, C): Typical angiographic appearances — streaky staining following the course of the blood vessels from the carotid bifurcation to the skull base. Note displacement of large vessels and stenosis of a segment of the internal carotid artery through involvement of its wall *(arrow)*. Blotchy posterior-fossa staining [*arrowheads in* (B)] was confirmed by selective vertebral angiography (D).

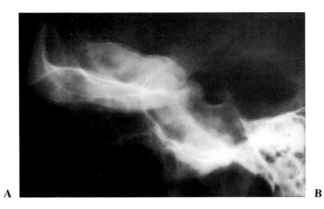

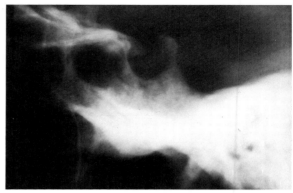

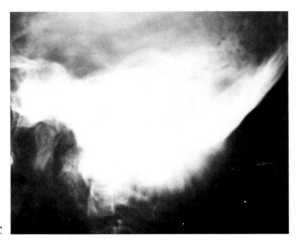

Fig. 9–28 Sclerosis of the base. (A) Fibrous dysplasia of bone, involving the sphenoid and ethmoid bones in an 18-year-old youth. (B) Sphenoid metastasis from breast cancer in a 56-year-old woman. (C) Osteogenic sarcoma involving the occipital squame and basiocciput, clivus and sphenoid body in a 21-year-old man.

REFERENCES

Appleby, A., Bradley, W. G., Foster, J. B., Hankinson, J. and Hudgson, P.: Syringomyelia due to chronic arachnoiditis at the foramen magnum. Journal of the Neurological Sciences, 8, 451–464, 1969.

Appleby, A., Foster, J. B., Hankinson, J. and Hudgson, P.: The diagnosis and management of the Chiari anomalies in adult life. Brain, 91, 131–140, 1968.

Baker, H. L., Jr.: Myelographic examination of the posterior fossa with positive contrast medium. Radiology, 81, 791–801, 1963.

Balériaux-Waha, D., Mortelmans, L. L., Dupont, M. G. and Jeanmart, L.: Computed tomography for lesions of the craniovertebral angle. Neuroradiology, 13, 59–61, 1977.

Barton, J. W. and Margolis, M. T.: Rotational obstruction of the vertebral artery at the atlanto-axial joint. Neuroradiology, 9, 117–120, 1975.

Berk, M. E.: Chemodectoma of glomus intravagale: a case report and review. Journal of the Faculty of Radiologists, 12, 219–226, 1961.

Bloch, S., Van Rensburg, M. J. and Danziger, J.: The Arnold-Chiari malformation. Clinical Radiology, 25, 335–341, 1974.

Boijsen, E.: The cervical spinal canal in intraspinal expansive processes. Acta Radiologica, 42, 101–115, 1954.

Boogaard, J. A.: De indrukking der grondvlakte van den schedel door de wervelkolom, hare oorzaken en gevolgen. Nederlands Tijdschrift voor Geneeskunde, 2, 81–108, 1865.

Bull, J. W. D., Nixon, W. L. B. and Pratt, R. T. C.: The radiological criteria and familial occurrence of primary basilar impression. Brain, 78, 229–247, 1955.

Bull, J. W. D., Nixon, W. L. B., Pratt, R. T. C. and Robinson, P. K.: Paget's disease of the skull and secondary basilar impression. Brain, 82, 10–22, 1959.

Burwood, R. J., Gordon, I. R. S. and Taft, R. D.: The skull in mongolism. Clinical Radiology, 24, 475–480, 1973.

Burwood, R. J. and Watt, I.: Assimilation of the atlas and basilar impression. A review of 1500 skull and cervical spine radiographs. Clinical Radiology, 25, 327–333, 1974.

Burrows, E. H.: The sagittal diameter of the spinal canal in cervical spondylosis. Clinical Radiology, 14, 77–86, 1963.

Caffey, J.: Pediatric X-ray Diagnosis. 6th Ed. Chicago: Year Book Medical Publishers, 1973.

Chamberlain, W. B.: Basilar impression (platybasia): a bizarre developmental anomaly of the occipital bone and upper cervical spine with striking and misleading neurologic manifestations. Yale Journal of Biology and Medicine, 11, 487–496, 1939.

Chiari, H.: Ueber Veraenderungen des Kleinhirns infolge von Hydrocephalie des Grosshirns. Deutsche Medizinische Wochenshrift, 17, 1172, 1891.

Cook, P. L.: Bilateral chemodectoma in the neck. Journal of Laryngology, 91, 611–618, 1977.

Cornell, S. H.: Jugular venography. American Journal of Roentgenology, 106, 303–307, 1969.

Danziger, J., Lewer Allen, K. and Bloch, S.: Intracranial chordomas. Clinical Radiology, 25, 309–316, 1974.

Davies, H. W.: Radiological changes associated with Arnold-Chiari malformation. British Journal of Radiology, 40, 262–269, 1967.

Di Chiro, G. and Anderson, W. B.: The clivus. Clinical Radiology, 16, 211–223, 1965.

Dirheimer, Y. and Babin, E.: Basilar impression and hereditary fragility of the bones. Neuroradiology, 3, 41–43, 1971.

El Gammal, T.: The blood supply of chemodectomas of the head and neck; report of two cases. British Journal of Radiology, 47, 515–518, 1971.

Fischgold, H., David, M. and Bregeat, P. R.: La tomographie de la base du crâne en neuro-chirurgie et neuro-ophtalmologie. Paris: Masson et Cie, 1952.

Greenberg, A. D.: Atlanto-axial dislocations. Brain, 91, 655–684, 1968.

Hawkins, T. D.: Radiological investigation of glomus jugulare tumors. Acta Radiologica, 5, 201–210, 1966.

Holman, C. B. and Miller, W. E.: Juvenile nasopharyngeal fibroma: roentgenologic characteristics. American Journal of Roentgenology, 94, 292–298, 1965.

Holman, C. B., Olive, I. and Svien, H. J.: Roentgenologic features of neurofibromas involving the gasserian ganglion. American Journal of Roentgenology, 86, 148–153, 1961.

Hurwitz, L. J. and Banerji, N. K.: Basilar impression of the skull in patients with adult coeliac disease and after gastric surgery. Journal of Neurology, Neurosurgery and Psychiatry, 35, 92–96, 1972.

Hurwitz, L. J. and MacSwiney, R. R.: Basilar impression and osteogenesis imperfecta in a family. Brain, 83, 138–149, 1960.

Hurwitz, L. J. and Shepherd, W. H. T.: Basilar impression and disordered metabolism of bone. Brain, 89, 223–234, 1966.

Kendall, B.: Invasion of the facial bones by basal meningiomas. British Journal of Radiology, 46, 237–244, 1973.

Kendall, B. E. and Lee, B. C. P.: Cranial chordomas. British Journal of Radiology, 50, 687–698, 1977.

Klaus, E.: Vertebralisbefunde bei der basilären Impression. Der Radiologe, 9, 293–299, 1969.

Klippel, M. and Feil, A.: Un cas d'absence des vertebres cervicales avec cage thoracique remontant jusqu'à la base du crâne (cage thoracique-cervicale). Nouvelle Iconographie de la Salpêtrière, 25, 223, 1912.

Kruyff, E.: Occipital dysplasia in infancy. Radiology, 85, 501–506, 1965.

Lasjaunias, P., Moret, J., Manelfe, C., Théron, J., Hasso, T. and Seeger, J.: Arterial anomalies at the base of the skull. Neuroradiology, 13, 267–272, 1977.

Liliequist, B.: Encephalography in the Arnold-Chiari malformation. Acta Radiologica, 53, 17–32, 1960.

Lindgren, E.: Ueber Skeletveraenderungen bei Ruckenmarkstumoren. Nervenarzt, 10, 240–248, 1937.

List, C. F.: Neurologic syndromes accompanying developmental anomalies of occipital bone, atlas and axis. Archives of Neurology and Psychiatry, 45, 577–616, 1941.

McGregor, M.: The significance of certain measurements of the skull in the diagnosis of basilar impression. British Journal of Radiology, 21, 171–181, 1948.

McRae, D. L.: The significance of abnormalities of the cervical spine. American Journal of Roentgenology, 84, 1–25, 1960.

McRae, D. L. and Barnum, A. S.: Occipitalization of atlas. American Journal of Roentgenology, 70, 23–46, 1953.

McRae, D. L. and Standen, J.: Roentgenologic findings in syringomyelia and hydromyelia. American Journal of Roentgenology, 98, 695–703, 1966.

Marc, J. A. and Schechter, M. M.: Radiological diagnosis of mass lesions within and adjacent to the foramen magnum. Radiology, 114, 351–365, 1975.

Margolis, M. T. and Newton, T. H.: An angiographic sign of cerebellar tonsillar herniation. Neuroradiology, 2, 3–8, 1971.

Miller, W. E., Holman, C. B., Dockerty, M. B. and Devine, K. D.: Roentgenologic manifestations of malignant tumors of the nasopharynx. American Journal of Roentgenology, 106, 813–823, 1969.

Minderhoud, J. M., Braakman, R. and Penning, L.: Os odontoideum. Clinical, radiological and therapeutic aspects. Journal of Neurological Sciences, 8, 521–544, 1969.

Møller, P. F. and Gudjonsson, S. V.: Massive fluorosis of bones and ligaments. Acta Radiologica, 13, 269–304, 1932.

Moody, D. M., Ghatak, N. R. and Kelly, D. L.: Extensive calcification in a tumor of the glomus jugulare. Neuroradiology, 12, 131–135, 1976.

Moscow, N. P. and Newton, T. H.: Angiographic features of hypervascular neuromas of the head and neck. Radiology, 114, 635–640, 1975.

Payne, E. E. and Spillane, J. D.: The cervical spine. An anatomico-pathological study of 70 specimens (using a special technique) with particular reference to the problem of cervical spondylosis. Brain, 80, 571–596, 1957.

Pollock, J. A., Newton, T. H. and Hoyt, W. T.: Transsphenoidal and transethmoidal encephaloceles; a review of clinical and roentgen features in eight cases. Radiology, 90, 442–453, 1968.

Potter, G.: Sclerosis of the base of the skull as a manifestation of nasopharyngeal carcinoma. Radiology, 94, 35–38, 1970.

Rice, R. P. and Holman, C. B.: Roentgenographic manifestations of tumors of glomus jugulare (chemodectoma). American Journal of Roentgenology, 89, 1201–1208, 1963.

Schechter, M. M., Liebeskind, A. L. and Azar-Kia, B.: Intracranial chordoma. Neuroradiology, 8, 67–82, 1974.

Schindler, E. and Jung, H.: A juvenile nasopharyngeal angiofibroma with an unusual vascular supply. Neuroradiology, 10, 49–54, 1975.

Sharp, J. and Purser, D. W.: Spontaneous atlanto-axial dislocation in ankylosing spondylitis and rheumatoid arthritis. Annals of the Rheumatic Diseases, 20, 47–77, 1961.

Singh, A., Jolly, S. S., Bansal, B. C. and Mathur, C. C.: Epidemic fluorosis: epidemiological, clinical and biochemical study of chronic fluorine intoxication in Panjab (India). Medicine, 42, 229–246, 1963.

Smith, P. H., Benn, R. T. and Sharp, J.: Natural history of rheumatoid cervical luxations. Annals of the Rheumatic Diseases, 31, 431–439, 1972.

Stein, B. M., Leeds, N. E., Taveras, J. M., and Pool, J. L.: Meningiomas of the foramen magnum. Journal of Neurosurgery, 20, 740–751, 1963.

Swinson, D. R., Hamilton, E. B., Mathews, J. A. and Yates, D. A. H.: Vertical subluxation of the axis in rheumatoid arthritis. Annals of the Rheumatic Diseases, 31, 359–363, 1972.

Tishler, J. and Martel, W.: Dislocation of the atlas in mongolism. Radiology, 84, 904–906, 1965.

Tsai, F. Y., Lisella, R. S., Lee, K. F. and Roach, J. F.: Osteosclerosis of base of skull as a manifestation of tumor invasion. American Journal of Roentgenology, 124, 256–264, 1975.

Wackenheim, A.: Facial asymmetry and transverse dislocation of the cervico-occipital joint. Neuroradiology, 1, 112–116, 1970.

Wackenheim, A.: Roentgen Diagnosis of the Craniovertebral Angle. Heidelberg: Springer, 1974.

Wastie, M. L.: The significance of the failed pneumoencephalogram. Journal of the Neurological Sciences, 17, 309–321, 1972a.

Wastie, M. L.: The value of tomography in carcinoma of the nasopharynx. British Journal of Radiology, 45, 570–574, 1972b.

Watson-Jones, R.: Spontaneous hyperaemic dislocation of the atlas. Proceedings of the Royal Society of Medicine, 25, 586–590, 1932.

Watson-Jones, R.: Fractures and Joint Injuries. 4th Ed. Edinburgh: E. and S. Livingstone, 1952.

Weinstein, M. and Newton, T. H.: Caudal dislocation of the pons in adult Arnold-Chiari malformation: an angiographic evaluation. American Journal of Roentgenology, 126, 798–801, 1976.

Westberg, G.: Angiographic changes in neurinoma of the trigeminal nerve. Acta Radiologica Diagnosis, 1, 513–520, 1963.

Wholey, M. H., Bruwer, A. J. and Baker, H. L.: The lateral roentgenogram of the neck (with comments on the atlanto-odontoid-basion relationship). Radiology, *71*, 350–356, 1958.

Wickbom, I. and Hanafee, W.: Soft tissue masses immediately below the foramen magnum. Acta Radiologica Diagnosis, *1*, 647–658, 1963.

Wilson, G. H. and Hanafee, W. N.: Angiographic findings in 16 patients with juvenile nasopharyngeal angiofibroma. Radiology, *92*, 279–284, 1969.

Wolf, B. S., Khilnani, M. and Malis, L.: The sagittal diameter of the bony cervical spinal canal and its significance in cervical spondylosis. Journal of the Mount Sinai Hospital, *23*, 283–292, 1956.

Wood, E. H. and Himadi, G. M.: Chordomas: roentgenologic study of 16 cases previously unreported. Radiology, *54*, 706–716, 1950.

Ziedses des Plantes, B. G.: L'angiographie de la tumeur glomique. Journal Belge de Radiologie, *54*, 287–291, 1971.

Zingesser, L. H. and Schechter, M. M.: The radiology of masses lying within and adjacent to the tentorial hiatus. British Journal of Radiology, *37*, 486–510, 1964.

10 Hydrocephalus, Brain Atrophy, Neonatal Lesions, and Degenerative Lesions

INTRODUCTION

A variety of lesions of diverse causes and affecting mainly neonates and elderly individuals are considered in this Chapter. Several of the entities discussed, including hydrocephalus and brain atrophy, are radiological symptoms, of which the etiology is frequently not demonstrable and the clinical correlation and relevance may not be clear. In preparing this material the authors have relied upon their experience as practicing neuroradiologists to select for description familiar entities and recurring situations, some of which remain difficult to classify clinically or etiologically.

HYDROCEPHALUS

Hydrocephalus is a symptom, not a disease. Russell (1966) defined hydrocephalus as an excessive accumulation of cerebrospinal fluid within the skull, due to a disturbance of its secretion, its flow or its absorption. The term describes only an increased fluid volume—it is not concerned with the intracranial pressure, which in a hydrocephalic may be high, low or normal. Frequently the cause of hydrocephalus is impossible to determine. Once an obstructing lesion has been ruled out by computed tomography or pneumography, the contribution of radiology to the etiological classification of hydrocephalus is limited. Surgical management of the condition is empirical, aimed at restoring patency of the cerebrospinal fluid pathway.

Conventional classifications of hydrocephalus require revision, as a result of Adams's concept of normal-pressure hydrocephalus (see below), as well as the introduction of more searching diagnostic methods. For example, the concept of hydrocephalus with raised pressure or hydrocephalus without raised pressure has been invalidated by Adams's work. Even more important, dynamic studies have shown that a division of hydrocephalus into "communicating" and "obstructive" types is false, since many cases of so-called communicating hydrocephalus have an extraventricular obstructive cause. Brain's (Brain and Walton, 1969) definition of hydrocephalus, viz., an increase in the volume of the cerebrospinal fluid within the brain, might be interpreted to exclude extracerebral accumulations of excess fluid—the so-called "hydrocephalus *ex-vacuo*" following trauma or disease. On account of these doubts, radiologists are wise to use the word "hydrocephalus" as a descriptive term and to be cautious of affixing etiological labels to it, if an obstructive cause cannot be demonstrated.

Etiology

Tumors. The commonest cause of hydrocephalus except in infants is an intracranial mass, which is most often neoplastic. Three mechanisms are responsible, viz., (1) Oversecretion of cerebrospinal fluid by a tumor of the choroid plexus, about 50 percent of which produce hydrocephalus—a rare cause. (2) Direct obstruction of a narrow part of the ventricular system, e.g., pineal neoplasm or even a convexity subdural hematoma obliterating the aqueduct by compression. (3) Obstruction of the cerebrospinal fluid in the leptomeningeal pathways

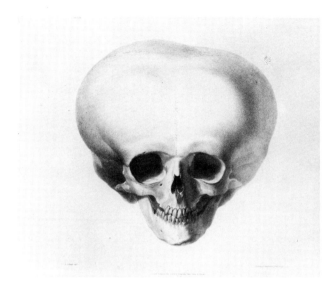

Fig. 10-1 The skull of James Cardinal (1795–1825), the patient in whom the London physician, Richard Bright, made a diagnosis of chronic hydrocephalus. Lithography by George Scharfe, taken from Richard Bright's *Reports of Medical Cases,* plate 36, London: Longman, 1827–1831. Reproduced by courtesy of the Wellcome Trustees, London.

by neoplastic or hemorrhagic exudate, e.g., medulloblastoma. A rare cause is obstruction of the third ventricle by an ectatic basilar artery (Greitz et al., 1969).

Congenital Malformations. Such lesions, a frequent cause of infantile hydrocephalus, affect two levels: the outlet of the fourth ventricle and the aqueduct of Sylvius, sometimes simultaneously. Hindbrain ectopia, which is frequently associated with a myelocele (see below), is a common cause of outlet obstruction in infants. Atresia of the foramina of Luschka and Magendie (Dandy-Walker's syndrome), on the other hand, is very rare.

Congenital atresia or stenosis of the aqueduct of Sylvius cannot be differentiated radiologically from other forms of non-tumor aqueductal obstructions. According to Russell (1966), the most frequent congenital malformations are forking of the aqueduct with one channel a dead end, and an aqueduct obstructed at its distal end by a paper-thin membrane. Congenital stenosis of a foramen of Monro is a doubtful entity.

Infection. Coccal or coliform organisms are probably the most frequently isolated, producing a ventriculitis or pyocephalus. The thick exudate and granulation tissue is most likely to obstruct the aqueduct of Sylvius or produce a collar of fibrin around the tentorial hiatus. Antituberculous medication is said to provoke leptomeningeal adhesions and, eventually, calcification. Northfield (1973), in a study of 100 hydrocephalic infants, found that the majority were caused by a combination of factors, viz., malformation complicated by infection, or infection complicated by trauma; only four had neoplasms.

Trauma. Dilatation of the ventricles is a recognized sequel of intracranial hemorrhage. The hemorrhage may be spontaneous due to rupture of an aneurysm, accidental after head injury or iatrogenic following craniotomy (Hawkins et al., 1976). Other rare traumatic events with a similar potential complication include: surgical spillage of cholesteatomatous fluid during evacuation of an epidermoid or of lipoid during shunting procedures in cases of dysostosis multiplex (Hurler's syndrome); and the adhesive reaction of foreign substances still sometimes used in diagnosis and therapy, e.g., talc, kaolin, sterile barium preparations, thorotrast and iodophendylate (Pantopaque).

Compensatory. Hydrocephalus *ex vacuo* or compensatory hydrocephalus describes the accumulation of cerebrospinal fluid within or around the brain that accompanies shrinkage of brain substance in the normal ageing process. Such accumulations may also complicate events producing focal brain damage – birth, ischemia, trauma, craniotomy.

"Normal-Pressure Hydrocephalus" (Treatable Dementia). In 1965 Adams and his colleagues reported the dramatic benefit of ventriculoatrial drainage in a group of patients with dementia combined with hydrocephalus. Clinical features of this treatable syndrome, apart from the dementia, are gait disturbance and incontinence and an absence of clinical or mechanical signs of raised intracranial pressure. Scientific confusion continues to shroud the causative mechanism in those cases which are unassociated with tentorial or convexity blockage (Benson et al., 1970). Greitz (1969) implied that the mechanism is a mechanical one, in which the passage of cerebrospinal fluid over the hemispherical convexities is prevented by "brain distension."

Radiological Contrast Diagnosis
The radiological diagnosis of hydrocephalus rests upon demonstrating enlargement of the cerebrospinal fluid pathway, i.e., ventricles, cisterns and convexity channels. Computed tomography has largely replaced pneumography for this purpose, and especially in neonates and infants the resulting decline in morbidity has been dramatic (Naidich et al., 1976; El Gammal et al., 1976; Palmieri et al., 1978). Dynamic studies of the movement of cerebrospinal fluid, which are useful in the differential diagnosis of hydrocephalus, are performed by monitoring the passage of substances introduced into the lumbar or suboccipital spinal canal – radioisotope (Bannister et al., 1967; James et al., 1970) or metrizamide cisternography (Hindmarsh and Greitz,

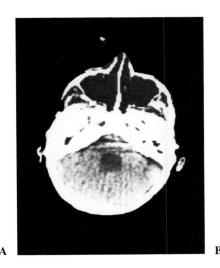
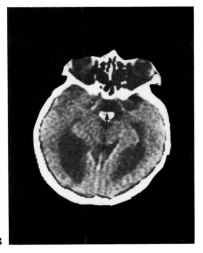
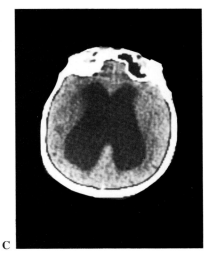

A   B   C

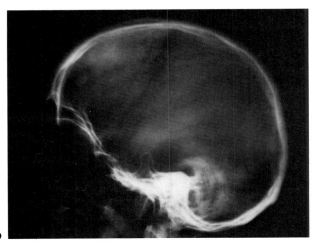

D

Fig. 10–7 Post-hemorrhagic adhesions of the basal cisterns, causing obstructive hydrocephalus. (A, B and C) Computed tomogram, slices made respectively at the level of the fourth ventricle, pituitary fossa and lateral ventricles. The anterior end of the third ventricle *(middle slice)* herniates into the fossa over the dorsum sellae *(arrow)*. (D) Lateral skull radiograph, showing a vault of normal size and a large pituitary fossa with an unusually high dorsum sellae.

1963; Marions and Lying-Tunell, 1977). Therefore, non-filling is never more than a suggestive sign of brain distension or of tentorial- or convexity-block hydrocephalus.

Computed tomography, in replacing pneumoencephalography as the technique for static evaluation of the cerebrospinal pathway, provides no greater certainty in the diagnosis of treatable dementia. (1) An absolute increase in ventricular size documented by serial examinations is a more reliable indication than any particular sign such as enlarged temporal horns or a dilated third or fourth ventricle. (2) Demonstration of widened convexity sulci or interhemispherical or sylvian fissures does not exclude the diagnosis of normal-pressure hydrocephalus, because their presence does not imply that a patent and functioning cerebrospinal-fluid pathway exists (Fig. 10–12). (3) Ventriculoatrial shunting usually fails to reduce the size of the enlarged ventricles, although it may have cured the patient of his dementia (Shenkin et al., 1975).

Cisternography is the definitive diagnostic test for treatable dementia because it documents the diversion of cerebrospinal fluid from its normal pathways. The test requires a lumbar puncture to introduce a radionuclide such as iodinated human serum albumen (RIHSA) or indium-DTPA, or the water-soluble contrast medium metrizamide into the spinal fluid. Diffusion of the radionuclide through the cerebrospinal fluid pathways is monitored during the next 24 to 48 hours by means of a scintillation camera or in the case of metrizamide by a computed-tomographic scanner.

If normal diffusion occurs, the radioactivity (or the contrast medium) can be demonstrated over the cerebral hemispheres and in the parasagittal regions within 12 to 24 hours; the ventricular area is free of all activity (or contrast medium). In patients with normal-pressure hydrocephalus, by contrast, the ventricular activity (or filling) is early and persistent—up to 72 hours, and its intensity contrasts with the lack of radioactivity (or sulcal contrast filling) over the surfaces of the hemisphere (Fig. 10–13 and 10–14; Di Chiro et al., 1964; Benson et

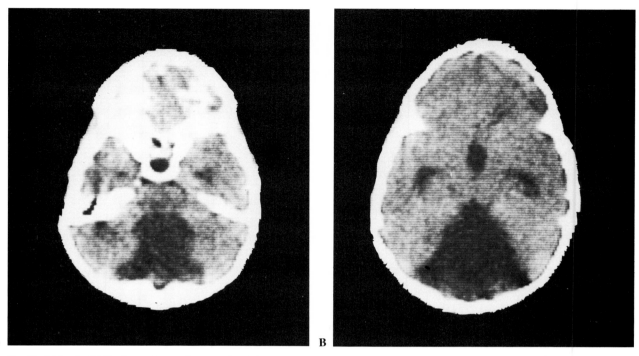

A   B

Fig. 10–8 Dandy-Walker's syndrome, i.e., atresia of the foramina of Luschka and Magendie resulting in distension of the fourth ventricle and obstructive hydrocephalus. Computed tomograms of the posterior fossa. (A) Hypoplastic cerebellar hemispheres separated by a giant fourth ventricle. (B) Higher slice, showing that the bag of cerebrospinal fluid extends up to the tentorium.

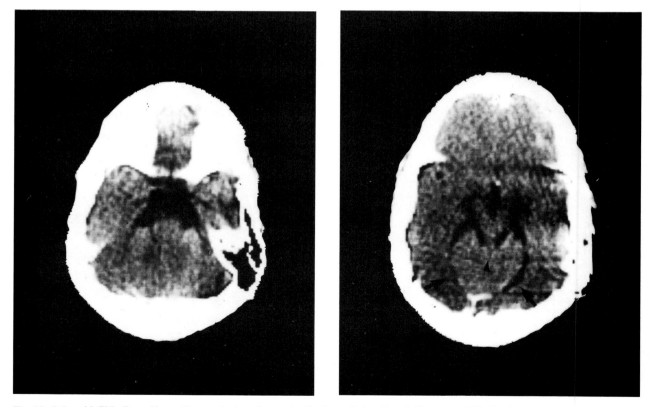

Fig. 10–9 Arnold-Chiari's malformation producing obstructive hydrocephalus. Basal slices reveal hindbrain descent; the fourth ventricle is not visible. Breaking of the tectum *(arrowhead)* is present. Heart shaped pseudotumor appearance of the cerebellum *(arrows)*.

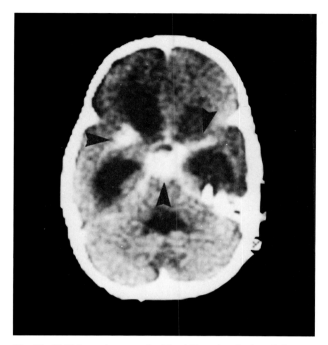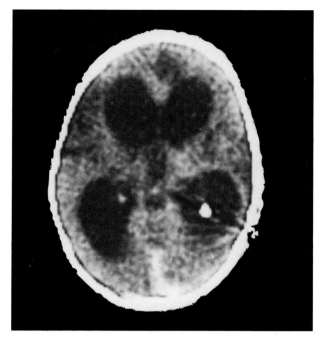

Fig. 10–10 Tuberculous meningitis obliterating the basal cisterns and causing gross hydrocephalus. Enhanced slices show blushing basal exudate *(arrows)* and extensive bilateral cortical infarction. See Enzmann et al. (1976).

al., 1970; Hindmarsh, 1977). Computed cisternography with metrizamide will probably replace the radionuclide method, since it provides more information about the morphological state of the patient's brain at the cost of less radiation.

Plain Radiographs of the Skull
About one-third of patients with hydrocephalus have symmetrically enlarged heads (Fig. 10–1) (Kingsley and Kendall, 1978). Macrocrania is a sign of chronicity; therefore it is a feature of the syndrome of non-neoplastic hydrocephalus. The second characteristic radiological feature of hydrocephalus is an enlarged pituitary fossa with an amputated dorsum sellae. The possibility of a neoplasm being responsible for the case illustrated in Figure 10–6, can be dismissed: macrocrania caused by a tumor, although it does occur (page 27) is rare without suture diastasis.

The reader should now consult the section in Chapter 1, Generalized Deformity, page 27. The following illustrations and their captions are relevant:

Suture diastasis due to tumor hydrocephalus: Fig. 1–19.

Macrocrania due to hydrocephalus of aqueduct stenosis: Fig. 1–21.

Macrocrania, before and after ventriculoatrial drainage: Fig. 1–22.

Thickened vault of successful drainage: Fig. 1–50.

Deformed pituitary fossa due to non-tumor hydrocephalus: Fig. 5–43.

Macrocrania due to cerebellar astrocytoma: Chapter 1, page 27.

Deformed pituitary fossa due to non-tumor hydrocephalus: Fig. 10–7.

Craniolacunia, Myelomeningocele and Hydrocephalus. Craniolacunia, lacunar skull or *Lückenschädel* is a neonatal cranial dysplasia of no importance, except that children with this deformity are very likely to have severe and/or multiple lesions of the central nervous system (Fig. 10–15; McRae, 1966). These lesions frequently include hydrocephalus due to aqueductal stenosis and/or the Arnold-Chiari malformation. The cranial dysplasia is thought to represent a developmental defect of the membrane bone, because it never involves the base of the skull. Although the characteristic lacunae affect the inner table, they are not caused by raised intracranial pressure—they may develop *in utero* and disappear by the third month of life, before brain markings appear. Nearly 50 percent of children with encephaloceles or myelomeningocele have craniolacunia.

Complications
These are spontaneous or iatrogenic. Spontaneous complications include the following: (1) Transependymal extravasation of cerebrospinal fluid. An alternative pathway of absorption of cerebrospinal fluid is believed to exist—or to be accentuated—in

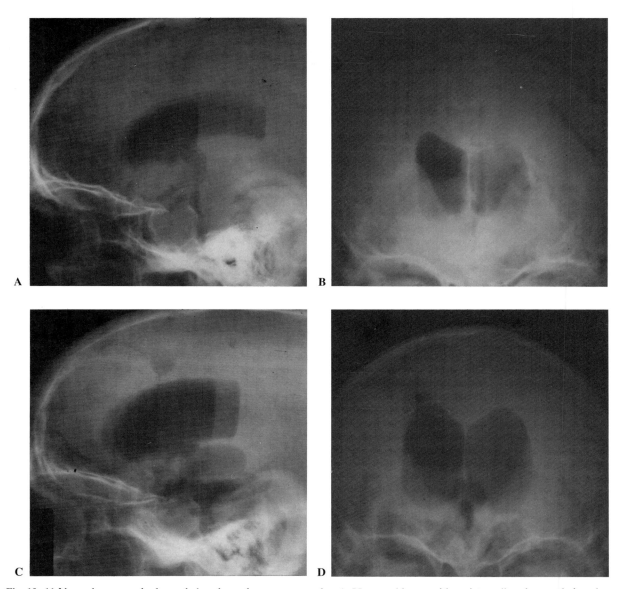

Fig. 10–11 Normal-pressure hydrocephalus shown by pneumography. A 55-year-old man with an intrasellar chromophobe adenoma. (A and B) Preoperative pneumogram: brow-up views show no suprasellar tumor growth, and frontal horns of normal size and shape. (C and D) Pneumoencephalogram made two years later, following frontal craniotomy for the pituitary tumor and the subsequent onset of dementia. Striking ventricular enlargement and widening of the basal cisterns is now present, with non-filling of the convexity sulci.

hydrocephalus, viz., passage across the ependymal membrane (Lux et al., 1970; James et al., 1974). Computed tomography reveals this activity as periventricular low attenuation (Fig. 10–16). The greater frequency of this phenomenon in tumor cases suggests that it occurs when hydrocephalus is of relatively rapid and recent onset and that it may not persist if the hydrocephalus becomes chronic (Kingsley and Kendall, 1978). (2) Ventricular diverticula. Secondary diverticula may form in infantile hydrocephalus from the walls of the lateral ventricles, which may be symptomatic (Granholm and Rådberg, 1963). The mechanism of formation is not

clear, and the resulting appearances may be incorrectly interpreted as arachnoid cyst, porencephalic cyst or ventricular-puncture cyst (Lorber and Grainger, 1963). The diagnosis of hydrocephalic diverticulum in the case illustrated in Figure 10–17 was suggested by the clinical circumstances.

Iatrogenic complications are concerned less nowadays with the performance of ventriculography and more directly with the insertion of ventriculoatrial shunts. (3) Accidental rupture of cortical veins. This accident is not an infrequent cause of extracerebral collections in hydrocephalics, both subdural (Fig. 10–18) and extradural (Sengupta

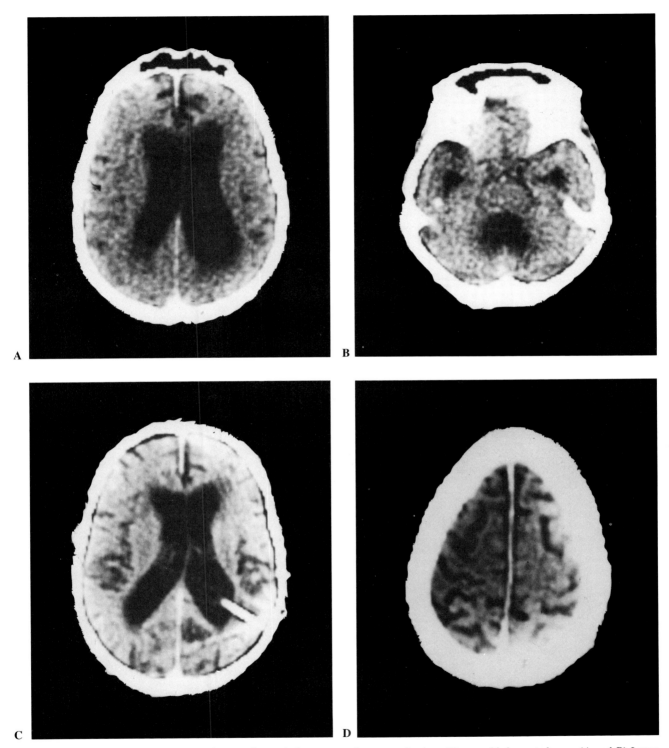

Fig. 10–12 Normal-pressure hydrocephalus—diagnosis by computed tomography in a 66-year-old demented man. (A and B) Large lateral ventricles and fourth ventricle. Prominent hemispheric sulci are visible. (C and D) Repeat examination 17 months later, 1 year after ventricular drainage which successfully reversed the patient's dementia. Despite shunting and clinical cure, the lateral ventricles are not significantly smaller, and the cortical sulci remain abnormally wide.

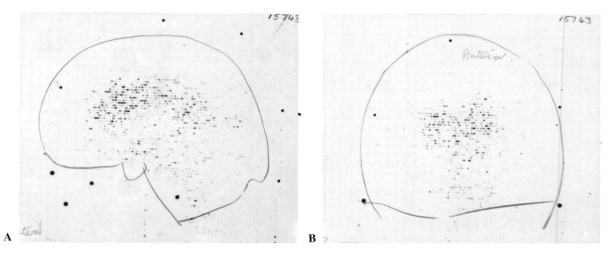

Fig. 10–13 Normal-pressure hydrocephalus—diagnosis by radioisotope cisternography with RIHSA (radio-iodinated human serum albumen). (A and B) Lateral and frontal views made 48 hours after intrathecal injection, showing persistence of radionuclide in the ventricles and absence of sagittal or cortical activity.

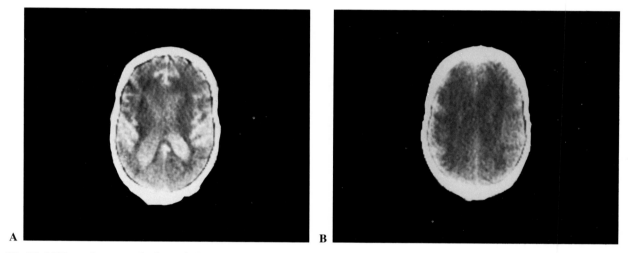

Fig. 10–14 Normal-pressure hydrocephalus—diagnosis by computed tomography with intrathecal metrizamide. (A) 6 hours after injection, showing prompt (and abnormal) filling of the lateral ventricles as well as the lower convexity sulci. (B) 24 hours after injection, with no apparent filling of the convexity sulci.

and Hankinson, 1972). These collections may calcify and present years later as a calcified envelope surrounding the hemisphere beneath the valve—see Figure 1–13). (4) Shunt dependency (Fig. 10–18). This condition is defined as the presence of small ventricles after a shunt procedure. This appearance may present a diagnostic problem, because if the shunt becomes obstructed the intracranial pressure may rise acutely. This situation is difficult to treat because of the small size of the ventricles. Therefore, small ventricles, rather than being the goal of shunt procedures, are to be avoided because of potential risks (Naidich et al., 1976). Another sign of shunt dependence is progressive ventricular enlargement, as may be demonstrated by repeated computed tomography. This type of

enlargement is caused either by malfunction or dependence. If the shunt is functioning, the ventricles enlarge because more fluid is being produced than can be diverted by the shunt. (5) Extracranial complications. These are connected with the intrathoracic end of the drain—see Starer (1973).

BRAIN ATROPHY

The radiological diagnosis of degenerative diseases of the brain depends on demonstrating an abnormal shrinkage of brain substance. This is achieved by means of computed tomography or pneumoencephalography, which yields evidence of widened lateral ventricles and/or cortical sulci, interhemispheric

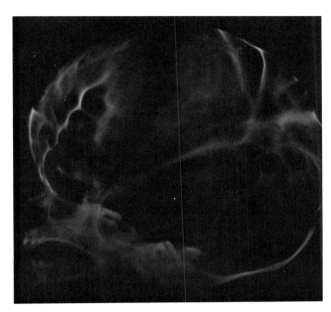

Fig. 10–15 Craniolacunia in a 3-month-old baby with hydrocephalus associated with a fatal myelomeningocele (postmortem radiograph).

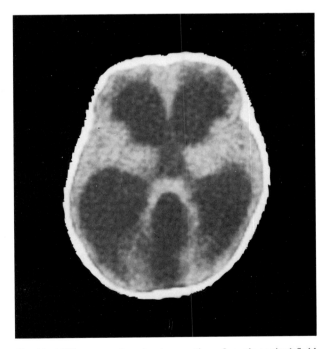

Fig. 10–16 Transependymal extravasation of cerebrospinal fluid in a baby with severe hydrocephalus due to outlet obstruction. The dilated ventricles have an irregular low-density perimeter.

or sylvian fissures, and basal cisterns. Etiological diagnosis rests partly on the pattern of distribution, i.e., a generalized or focal process, whether the process is limited to the gray matter or appears to single out specific parts of the white matter.

The radiological evaluation of brain degeneration is complicated by two facts: (1) *The human brain alters with ageing,* tending to atrophy as the subject grows older. Postmortem cutting of an aged brain reveals deepened sulci, widened fissures and enlarged ventricles, due to the physiological process of neuronal loss. Using computed tomography in 170 patients aged up to 75 years, Haug (1977) documented statistically the increase that occurs in four parameters with ageing, viz., cellae mediae and anterior horns of the lateral ventricles, the width of the third ventricle and the width of the interhemispherical fissure. The picture of the ageing process, as documented by computed tomography or pneumography, is no different to that revealed at necropsy (Huckman et al., 1977). (2) *No correlation exists between mental function and morphological appearance:* a demented patient may show no atrophy, conversely a grossly atrophic brain does not rule out the preservation of normal cognitive function (Gosling, 1955; Huckman et al., 1975; Claveria et al., 1977).

The first aim of radiological investigation in demented subjects or others suspected of cerebral degenerative disease, is to identify treatable lesions, e.g., normal-pressure hydrocephalus or a frontal-lobe meningioma. A secondary aim is to show a pattern of shrinkage out of keeping with the patient's age which could explain the clinical picture, e.g., gross generalized atrophy in a young subject, or a unilateral or more focal atrophic process.

Measurements
Brain atrophy is associated with enlarged ventricles and wide surface spaces for cerebrospinal fluid. Therefore, the diagnosis of atrophy, and particularly of minor degrees, requires a familiarity with the variations in size and shape of these structures which are accepted as normal. A large literature dealing with planimetric measurements of ventricular size is available, based initially on pneumography and since 1975 on computed tomography of the brain. See Davidoff and Epstein (1958) and Gyldensted (1977).

Pneumography. Although pneumoencephalography is now an obsolete examination, Figure 10–19 is included as an introduction to computed-tomographic planimetry, and to illustrate the most important ratios, lines and measurements used to assess ventricular size. Historically, the search for a single indicator of ventricular enlargement produced the following:

1. Evans's ratio. Evans (1942) described a ratio, the maximum width of the frontal horns of the lateral ventricles divided by the maximum width of the *inner* tables of the skull, with a normal value of 0.2 to 0.25. He believed that values exceeding 0.3 indicate ventricles that are definitely enlarged.

2. Schiersmann's ratio. Schiersmann (1952) related the maximum width of the *outer* tables of the

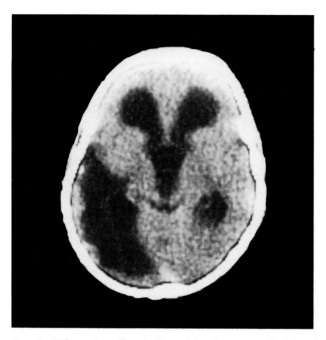
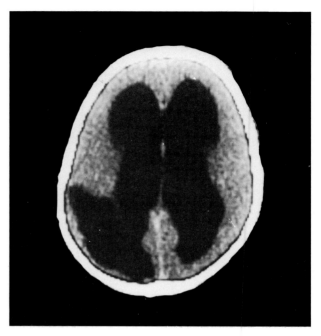

Fig. 10—17 Secondary diverticulum arising from the wall of the left lateral ventricle in infantile hydrocephalus. The patient was an adolescent with a right hemiplegia of gradual onset, without any history of trauma or surgery.

skull to the combined maximum width of the cella media of each lateral ventricle, thus inverting Evans's ratio. A result of 4 or over is normal, and 3 or under is abnormal.

3. Bruijn (1959) believed that the maximum width of the cellae mediae—"the most reliable single indicator"—should not exceed 4 cm.

4. Burhenne and Davies (1963) claimed that a ventricular span, i.e., maximum width of the frontal horns of both lateral ventricles, exceeding 5 cm. indicates brain atrophy.

5. Engeset and Skraastad (1964) introduced the septum-caudate distance (Fig. 10-19,B), which provides a sensitive indication of shrinkage of the head of the caudate nucleus. Upon evaluating and comparing all these measurements in a series of patients, Engeset and Skraastad found that a satisfactorily close correlation exists between them, and

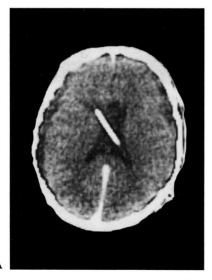
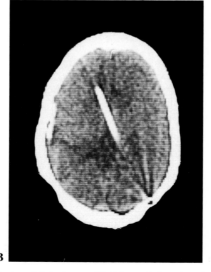
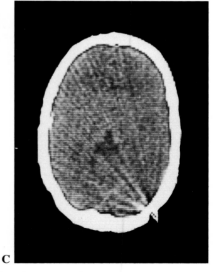

A   B   C

Fig. 10—18 Iatrogenic complications of ventriculoatrial drainage. (A) Bilateral chronic subdural hematomas in a patient with aqueductal stenosis, found three months after the insertion of a ventricular drain. (B and C) Ventricular obliteration due to shunt dependency.

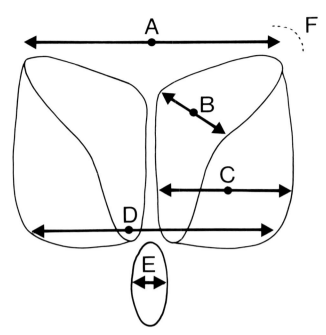

Fig. 10–19 Measurements of ventricular size based on pneumography. (A) Maximum width of cellae mediae. Normal = 50 mm. (B) Septum–caudate distance, i.e., angle of septum pellucidum and corpus callosum to the most medial point of the inferolateral wall of the lateral ventricle. Normal = 15 mm. (C) Maximum width of frontal horn. Normal = 25 mm. (D) Transventricular diameter, i.e., maximum width of both frontal horns. Normal = 50 mm. (E) Maximum width of posterior part of the third ventricle. Normal = 5–10 mm. (F) Superolateral angle of the lateral ventricle.

concluded that each was adequate on its own as a "single-indicator" parameter. Since ventricular size must be interpreted in the context of the age of the patient, diagnostic evaluation of minor grades of enlargement calls for caution. The technique of lumbar pneumography itself may provoke ventricular enlargement, although usually of insignificant degree according to Moseley and Sondheimer (1975).

Computed Tomography. Planimetric criteria of the normality of ventricles and sulci are based on measuring the size of these structures in miniature photographs of radiographs of the tomographic slices (Huckman et al., 1975; Gyldensted and Kosteljanetz, 1975 and 1976; Gyldensted, 1977). However, the variation in viewing systems of the various commercial scanners reduces the value of absolute measurements and suggests that ventricular size is best related to the width of the skull, and expressed as a ratio. Hahn and Rim (1976) recommended two ratios, the first being the maximum bifrontal diameter related to brain width at this level and the second the maximum bicaudate diameter to brain width at its level. They reported that the first (bifrontal) ratio averaged 31 percent, and the second (bicaudate) ratio 15 percent in 200 normal subjects.

Widened sulci are caused by cortical shrinkage. Absolute measurements are as vulnerable to misinterpretation as is the assessment of ventricular size, being as likely to be influenced by physiological ageing as by cerebral degeneration. Hemispheric sulci are easily deformed by pathological processes, and may be obliterated by edema, compression or adhesions (Fig. 10–20).

Huckman and his colleagues (1975) observed that actual measurements of ventricular size and cortical sulci seldom modify the classification of brain atrophy provided by subjective assessment of these parameters on computed tomography. Roberts et al. (1976) found a clear and significant correlation between ventricular size and the ventricular span shown by pneumography and ventricular area measured by computed tomography. However, they found that the relationship between sulcal width and the presence of cortical atrophy was less clear, especially in computed tomography.

Degenerative Syndromes

The Aging Brain ("Cerebral Atrophy")
This brain is small and greatly reduced in weight. The convolutions are thin and separated by wide sulci, especially the frontal lobes, as a result of cortical atrophy. Brain slices reveal that the supratentorial ventricles are dilated, having lost their anatomical shape due to periventricular or central atrophy (Nielsen et al., 1966a and 1966b). These features may be well documented by pneumography or computed tomography (Fig. 10–21).

Roberts and his colleagues (1977), in evaluating the relationship between cortical atrophy and dementia in elderly subjects, concluded the following: (1) Slight but definite ventricular enlargement is usually present in the normal elderly. (2) In the elderly patient without clinically obvious cerebrovascular disease or infarction, there is a broad correlation between the degree of ventricular dilatation and the degree of intellectual impairment. Therefore, if only slight ventricular enlargement is encountered in a grossly demented patient, an alternative diagnosis to degenerative atrophy should be considered. Conversely, if ventricular dilatation is greater than expected from the degree of intellectual impairment, obstructive or normal-pressure hydrocephalus must be excluded. (3) No correlation can be shown between mental state and evidence of cortical atrophy in elderly subjects, as assessed by sulcal widening on computed tomography.

Alzheimer's Disease. Although this condition, a slowly progressive presenile disturbance of memory in which the patient's cognitive and intellectual capabilities are significantly impaired and the process leads finally to dementia, has a specific histo-

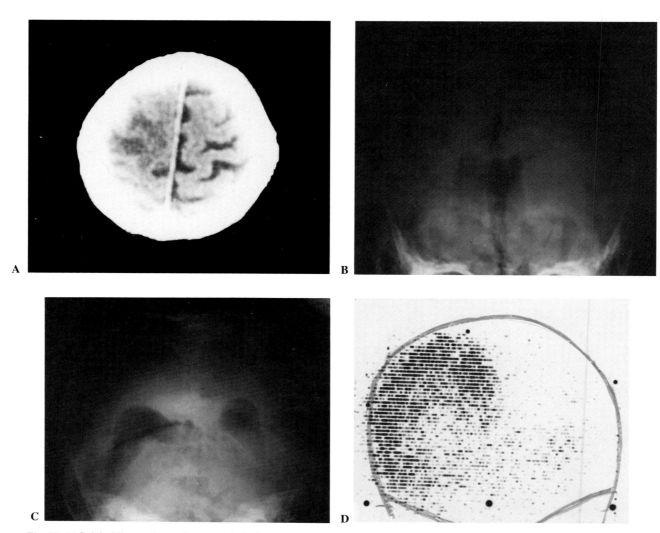

Fig. 10—20 Sulci obliterated by adjacent pathological processes. (A) Left cortical edema due to an underlying glioblastoma multiforme. (B) Cortical non-filling (and hemispherical shift) due to acute subdural hematoma. (C and D) Blockage of the convexity sulci of the right hemisphere, shown by pneumoencephalography and confirmed by radioisotope cisternography. A middle-aged man with a history of severe head injury.

logical pattern, the radiological appearances are identical to those of the physiological ageing brain. If the "cracked walnut" appearance of the brain surface, shown by computed tomography and indicating severe cortical atrophy, is associated with large ventricles in an adult, the underlying process may be Alzheimer's disease. However, no specific diagnosis is possible radiologically (Huckman et al., 1977).

Pick's disease is an atrophic process of the brain of younger individuals, affecting the frontal and parietal lobes, which show selective cortical atrophy.

Jakob-Creuzfeldt's syndrome, a disease probably with a slow-virus etiology, is another cause of progressive dementia of young persons (Fig. 10-22). Profound brain atrophy may be present, with occasional cerebellar dysfunction (Rao et al., 1977), but there is no specific pattern which enables the diag-

nosis to be made radiologically (Schechter, 1970). Transmission has been observed from affected individuals in the course of handling pathological specimens or making biopsies, therefore strict precautions must be adopted when dealing with suspected cases.

Multi-Infarct Dementia. Hachinski et al. (1974) pointed out the important fact that the typical case of slowly progressive dementia of old age does not have an atherosclerotic etiology. Most such cases show Alzheimer-like degeneration of the brain histologically, and there is no relation between these changes and arterial disease. Instead, Hachinski and his colleagues postulated that the dementia caused by chronic cerebrovascular insufficiency in elderly individuals is attributable to the summation effect of multiple small cerebral infarcts, rather than to a gradual process of neuronal loss. Experience

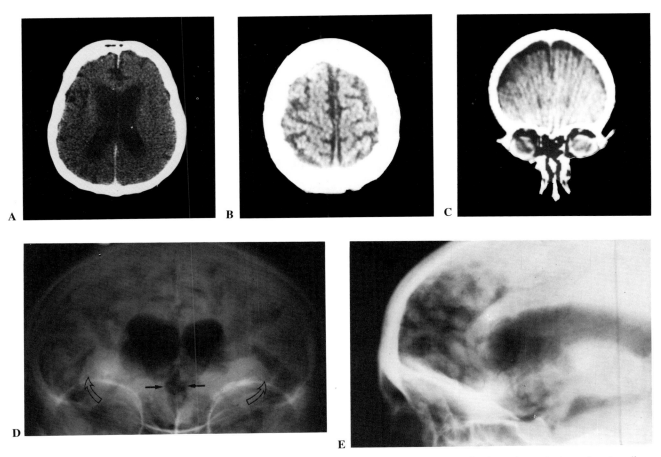

Fig. 10–21 The aging brain of a severely demented woman. (A, B and C) Computed tomogram, horizontal ventricular and vertex slices and coronal slice. (D and E) Pneumoencephalogram, brow-up lateral and frontal views. Both techniques reveal a generalized pattern of wide cortical sulci, including those on the medial surfaces of the hemispheres outlining the falx cerebri. The ventricles are large and the lateral ventricles have round superolateral angles. The third ventricle is wide *(black arrows)*, and gas has accumulated in the sylvian fissures *(open arrows)* indicating atrophy in the region of the island of Reil.

with computed tomography confirms the existence of the entity they proposed, viz., multi-infarct dementia (Fig. 10–23).

Degeneration in Focal Neurological Syndromes

Cerebellar Atrophy. Certain congenital, neoplastic and metaneoplastic, and degenerative conditions are characterized by selective atrophy of the brainstem, vermis and cerebellar hemispheres which may sometimes manifest clinically as ataxia, vertigo and other neurological signs. Pneumographic and computed-tomographic refinements in the past decade have revealed the existence of more cerebellar atrophy than previously—occurring also in patients in whom no clinical suspicion of cerebellar disease exists. The relation between clinical and radiologically-demonstrable cerebellar atrophy, and also the clinical significance of the latter, was studied by LeMay and Abramowicz (1966), Thiébaut et al. (1966) and Kennedy et al. (1976). Of these, LeMay and Abramowicz described measurements for use

as an index of cerebellar atrophy, viz., two or more sulci in the cerebellar vermis each exceeding 4 mm. in width, and measured on a posterior-fossa pneumotomogram made in the sagittal midline. Computed tomography has revealed further signs which may be used as evidence of cerebellar atrophy, including enlargement of the fourth ventricle and dilatation of the subarachnoid spaces lateral to the cerebellum and the cerebellopontine angles (Fig. 10–24; Allen et al., 1979). Kennedy and his colleagues, using the criterion of sulcal width to compare clinical and pneumographic findings in a large series of patients, concluded that vermian atrophy, if shown radiologically to be severe, is usually associated with clinical signs of cerebellar disease. There is a good correlation between clinical severity and radiological severity in such cases.

No etiological conclusion is justified from the radiological appearances, but the well-established association of cerebellar atrophy with chronic alcoholism and metastatic disease should prompt an appropriate search.

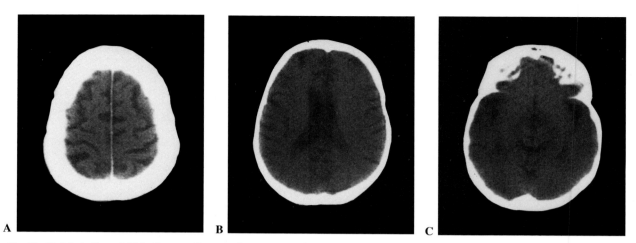

Fig. 10–22 Jakob-Creuzfeldt's disease. Computed tomogram of a 35-year-old woman with progressive dementia and extrapyramidal deficit, in whom a histopathological diagnosis of the disease was subsequently made. (A) Vertex slice showing wide cortical sulci. (B) Ventricular slice: the ventricles show moderate abnormal width. (C) Tentorial slice showing atrophy of the vermis and sylvian fissures.

Huntington's Chorea. In this familial and fatal disease, the pathological lesion affects the caudate and lenticular nuclei which atrophy severely in the advanced stages. Computed tomography and pneumography may reveal a flat thalamic impression or even a rounded lateral ventricle, due to decrease in size of the basal ganglia (Fig. 10–25).

Experience with pneumoencephalography in patients with Huntington's chorea demonstrated a good correlation between the radiological appear-ances and the neuropathological features, e.g., increased width of the bodies of the lateral ventricles due to atrophy of the caudate nucleus, and cortical atrophy—features often found in other forms of atrophy or with ventricular dilatation from any cause. No single feature can be regarded as specific of the diagnosis; nor does a normal pneumoenceph-alogram rule out the disease (Gath and Vinje, 1968). Computed tomography reveals the atrophic fea-tures of the disease and may be more specific diag-

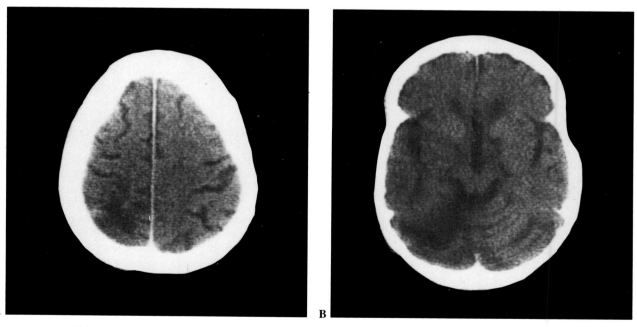

Fig. 10–23 Multi-infarct dementia in a 72-year-old woman. The patient, who was grossly demented, had experienced several step-like illnesses and a bruit was audible over the sternum and neck. Computed tomography revealed four separate low-density lesions, of which two are illustrated. (A) Convexity slice, showing an infarct of the left parietal lobe. Grossly widened hemispherical sulci are also present. (B) Tentorial slice, showing an infarct of the left cerebellar hemisphere, with atrophy of the cerebellar folia and sylvian fis-sures.

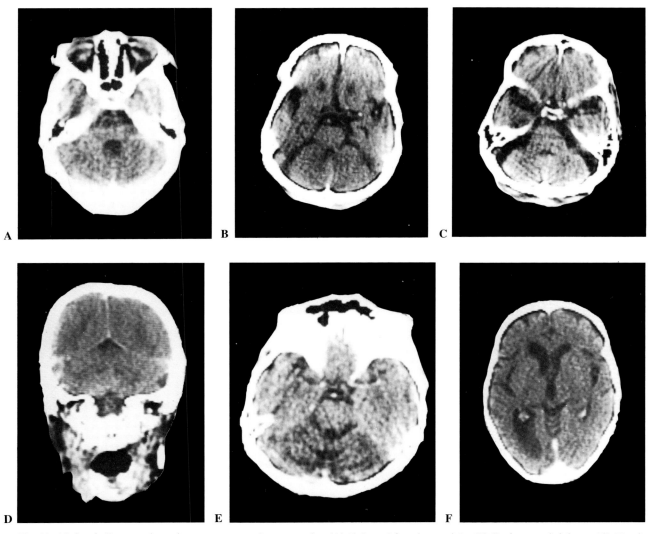

Fig. 10–24 Cerebellar atrophy—signs on computed tomography. (A) Enlarged fourth ventricle. (B) Brainstem shrinkage. (C) Hemispheric shrinkage. (D, E) Widened folia and subtentorial pooling of cerebrospinal fluid. (F) Vermian atrophy.

nostically when supplemented by measurements (Terrence et al., 1977).

Parkinsonism. Generalized cortical and ventricular atrophy is a frequent finding in parkinsonian brains at autopsy. Gath et al. (1975) studied the pneumoencephalograms of 45 parkinsonian patients. They found cortical atrophy to be present in 78 percent and cortical atrophy in 47 percent; the septum-caudate distance (Fig. 10–19) was increased in 75 percent. However, there was no definite correlation between the severity or duration of the clinical symptoms and the degree of atrophy. Experience of computed tomography confirms the nonspecific nature of the atrophic process in this disease (Huckman et al., 1977). Cavitation of the lentiform nucleus was reported in a case of postencephalitic parkinsonism by Kendall and his colleagues (1977).

Degeneration Associated with External Factors

Trauma. Traumatic atrophy, if interpreted in the wider sense, includes the sequelae of cerebral infarction, hemorrhage, abscess, irradiation and craniotomy, apart from acute head injury. These effects are discussed and illustrated in Chapter 4; see page 164. They include the loss of brain tissue and the formation of cysts. Post-traumatic destruction of brain substance if extensive involves the white matter as well as the cortex, and causes localized expansion of a ventricle, shift of the midline structures and cortical atrophy (Fig. 10–26). Porencephalic cysts are discussed in the next section, Neonatal Lesions, although it should be stressed that they may be revealed for the first time only late in life (see Fig. 4–29, B–C). Less frequently, shrinkage or cyst formation follows arterial occlusion (Fig.

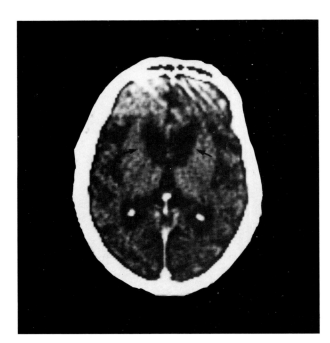

Fig. 10–25 Huntington's chorea. Computed tomogram, enhanced ventricular slice, showing the rounded anterior horns of the lateral ventricles *(arrows)* caused by selective atrophy of the heads of the caudate nuclei. Gross generalized atrophy is present, shown by the large third and lateral ventricles, and wide sylvian fissures.

10–27; Hunter et al., 1962; Schechter, 1970).

Infection. The sequelae of encephalitis are radiologically similar to those of trauma, viz., shrinkage of brain tissue and occasionally cyst formation. Figure 10–28 illustrates the evolution of a unilateral focus of herpes-simplex encephalitis. Infective atrophic lesions possess no specific morphological features although computed tomography has shown the lesions of herpes-simplex encephalitis frequently to be bilateral and symmetrical (see Fig. 10–38).

Chronic Alcoholism. Several studies have revealed the prevalence of wide ventricles in patients suffering from alcohol abuse or Korsakoff's syndrome (Fig. 10–29; Lynch, 1960; Fox et al., 1976; Kennedy et al., 1976; Van Gall et al., 1978). Fox and his colleagues found that one-third of alcoholics without dementia showed signs of cerebral atrophy on computed tomography. Severe and selective vermian and cerebellar atrophy is a particular indication of chronic alcoholism.

Drug Abuse, Including Cannabis. Campbell and his colleagues (1971) claimed to have demonstrated brain atrophy in young men smoking cannabis, but other workers using computed tomography have failed to confirm this finding in chronic cannabis users and heavy marijuana smokers (Co et al., 1977; Kuehnle et al., 1977).

Demyelination
Computed tomography and to some extent scintigraphy have brought demyelinating diseases such as multiple sclerosis for the first time within the diagnostic province of the neuroradiologist.

Multiple Sclerosis. This, the commonest of the primary demyelinating diseases, is characterized by periods of exacerbation and remission. The pathological lesion consists of focal patches of myelin destruction disseminated throughout the brain and spinal cord. During remission the destroyed myelin is removed by macrophages and the astrocytes proliferate, resulting in the gray or sclerotic plaques that give the disease its name.

During the acute stage or exacerbations of the disease, plaques larger than 2 cm. in diameter may be revealed by scintigraphy (Fig. 10–30; Antunes et al., 1974; Cohan et al., 1975). However, since most plaques are smaller and since many patients are not examined during attacks of the disease, positive results are exceptional.

Descriptions of the findings in two large series of patients, in whom a clinical diagnosis of multiple sclerosis had been made, suggests that computed tomography has a more definite part to play. Gyldensted (1976) reported the results in 110 patients of whom 90 percent showed generalized brain atrophy and 36 percent low-density periventricular plaques; less than 20 percent had normal scans. Almost all the patients with plaques showed atrophy; there were 82 plaques in 40 patients, situated adjacent to the frontal or occipital horns or the trigones of the lateral ventricles. These findings were confirmed by Cala and her colleagues (1978) in a series of 100 patients which included serial studies in sixteen. Figure 10–30 illustrates the regressive nature of the plaques of demyelination which should not be mistaken on the initial examination for multiple infarcts or virus encephalitis. Similar findings of nodules or ring lesions, usually in a periventricular situation, have been reported by others (Lebow et al., 1978; Sears et al., 1978; Weinstein et al., 1978). The reason why contrast medium accumulates is probably a breakdown of the blood-brain barrier. Crocker et al. (1976) pointed out that steroid therapy re-establishes the integrity of this barrier. As a consequence, lesions that blush after contrast injection during computed tomography may be found to diminish markedly in size, or disappear altogether, after steroid administration. Weinstein et al. (1978) pointed out that contrast enhancement disappears in time, even without steroid therapy, and that the area of affected brain becomes isodense or of low density. Weinstein and his colleagues also observed that the distribution of lesions seen on computed tomography frequently does not conform to the areas of clinical involvement. The presence of single or multiple foci of increased density in the white

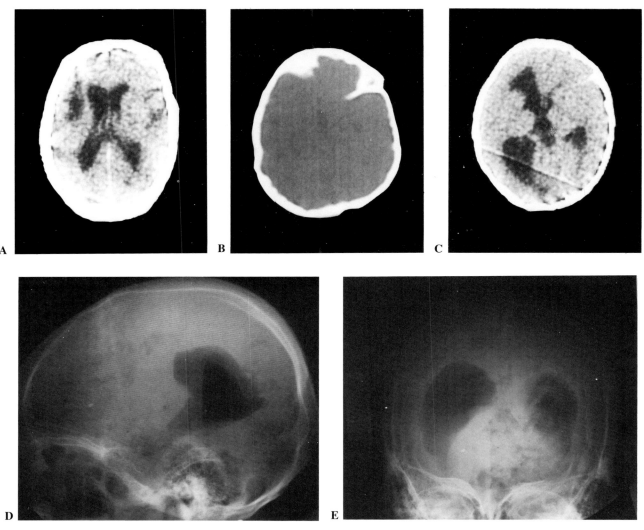

Fig. 10–26 Post-traumatic brain damage. (A) Computed tomogram, ventricular slice, of a patient two years after left temporal craniotomy for aneurysm. The anterior half of the left lateral ventricle is wide and an adjacent "brain scar" indicates the site of the surgeon's approach. (B and C) Computed tomograms of a 25-year-old woman with late-onset epilepsy, showing cerebral hemiatrophy and cranial asymmetry. The only relevant history was a forceps delivery. (D and E) Pneumoencephalogram of an 8-year-old mentally backward boy who sustained a non-accidental head injury at the age of 2 years, with evacuation of a subdural hematoma. The vault is uniformly thick and slightly asymmetrical, corresponding to the unilateral ventricular enlargement, and the cortical sulci over the damaged right hemisphere failed to fill due to adhesions.

matter or periventricular situation in the absence of a mass effect should prompt consideration of the diagnosis of acute multiple sclerosis.

The introduction of the newer scanners with improved discrimination between gray and white matter permits greater diagnostic capability, particularly of lesions affecting the white matter (Arimitsu et al., 1977 and Weinstein et al., 1977).

Schilder's Disease. Diffuse sclerosis is a demyelinating disorder of childhood in which the white matter of the occipital lobes and corpus callosum are affected. The computed-tomographic appearances in several cases have been described (Huckman et al., 1977).

Congenital demyelinating diseases (leukodystrophies) are described in the next section, Neonatal Lesions.

Other Lesions

Disseminated Necrotizing Leukoencephalopathy. Cases of this condition have been described, in which the computed tomogram has revealed extensive low-density areas throughout both cerebral hemispheres, wide lateral ventricles and symmetrical deposits of calcification in the white matter and basal ganglia (Flament-Durand et al., 1975; Kendall et al., 1977). Diffuse white-matter degeneration

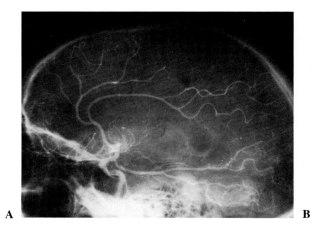

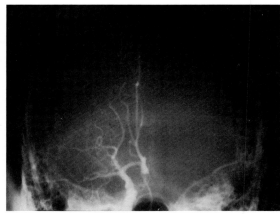

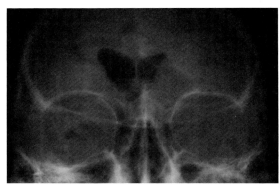

Fig. 10–27 Focal atrophy resulting from traumatic occlusion of the middle cerebral artery. During World War II, the patient while fleeing from the Japanese in Burma, suddenly developed a left hemiplegia, from which he had partially recovered. (A and B) Right carotid angiogram 25 years later, showing occlusion of the trunk of the middle cerebral artery with profuse collateral circulation from the cortical branches of the anterior and posterior cerebral arteries, and ipsilateral hemispherical displacement. (C) Pneumoencephalogram confirms that the ipsilateral hemispherical displacement is due to shrinkage of the right cerebral hemisphere.

may occur in such patients, who have been subjected to radiotherapy and prolonged courses of antimetabolite drugs, including intrathecal methotrexate for malignant meningitis following lymphosarcoma and leukemia (Fig. 10–31).

Epilepsy, Schizophrenia and Infantile Autism. Radiological abnormalities in these conditions have been described and their clinical implications discussed by Brett and Hoare (1969), Newcombe et al. (1975); Johnstone et al. (1976); and Hauser et al. (1975).

NEONATAL LESIONS

A wide variety of brain lesions may be identified by radiological means in the neonatal period. Computed tomography illuminates these lesions and it has largely replaced other methods of investigation (Harwood-Nash, 1977; Kendall and Kingsley, 1978).

Malformations
Table 10–1 lists major cerebral malformations according to the stages of development of the human fetus. This section deals with those conditions not mentioned and illustrated in previous chapters.

Cranioschisis. Figure 10–32 illustrates a large congenital defect of the parietal vault, with brain herniation. See Chapter 1, Meningoencephalocele.

Dysgenesis of the Commissural Plate. Cessation of or aberrant intrauterine development of the corpus callosum causes the pattern of midline deformities discussed in Chapter 7 (p. 304), viz., agenesis or lipoma. Callosal lipoma is usually a solitary lesion, agenesis is frequently associated with porencephaly (Fig. 10–33).

Hindbrain Anomalies. The Arnold-Chiari malformation is discussed and illustrated in Chapter 9 (p. 422). The Dandy-Walker syndrome is described earlier in this Chapter under Hydrocephalus (p. 446, Fig. 10–9).

Holoprosencephaly. Development of the prosencephalic single ventricle is controlled by the mesodermal analogue of the medial facial structures. Aberrant or stunted growth leads to a common frontal horn, lobar holoprosencephaly and/or features of the medial cleft syndrome (Fig. 10–34; Kurlander et al., 1966).

Hydranencephaly is a congenital anomaly consisting of complete or near-complete absence of the cerebral hemispheres. The brain resembles a bag of fluid, and the cortical mantle may be paper-thin (Fig. 10–35). Angiography may be necessary to

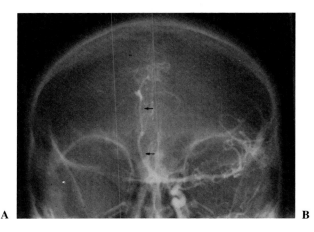

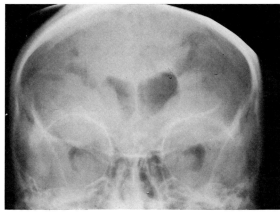

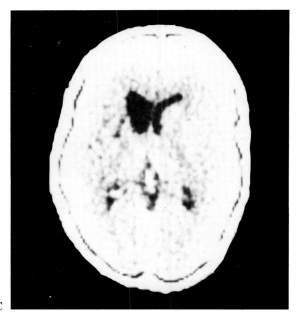

Fig. 10-28 Hemispheric atrophy due to herpes simplex encephalitis. A 25-year-old woman was admitted with an acute febrile illness and left hemispherical signs. (A) Left carotid angiogram on admission revealed considerable swelling of the left frontal lobe. *(Arrows)* Pericallosal artery displaced from the midline. (B) Pneumoencephalogram 6 months later, after the patient had developed considerable intellectual deficit. Selective enlargement of the left lateral ventricle including its temporal horn is present, as well as bilaterally wide cortical channels. (C) Computed tomogram.

differentiate hydranencephaly from gross hydrocephalus or bilateral congenital subdural collections (Poser et al., 1955; La Torre and Occhipinti, 1969).

Porencephaly. Cavities within the brain or on its surface that contain cerebrospinal fluid may be produced by many factors (Table 10-2). These cavities, irrespective of their cause, may communicate with the ventricular system (Fig. 10-36) or they may be closed and then frequently appear as avascular space-occupying lesions. In about one-third of cases of porencephaly, ventricular distortion and midline shift is present (Ramsey and Huckman, 1977). In neonates examined by computed tomography, a grossly disorganized brain with multiple fluid-filled clefts represents congenital porencephaly, or schizencephaly, a disorder of sulcation and migration, the result of intrauterine cerebral infarction and subsequent cystic formation

(Yakovlev and Wadsworth, 1946; Harwood-Nash, 1977).

Anoxic and Hypoxic States. Prolonged anoxia of the brain such as a complicated childbirth or respiratory distress may produce a characteristic clinical picture of "decerebration" or "decortication." Modern methods of resuscitation can bring patients to the stage of *coma dépassé,* i.e., cerebral death with intact cardiac function, although respiration is no longer spontaneous. Cerebral damage in such patients may be revealed by computed tomography (Fig. 10-37).

Viral and Other Infections. Herpes and other viral encephalitides as well as pyogenic microorganisms produce a variety of intracranial lesions which are best visualized by computed tomography. Cerebral abscess has been described in Chapter 6 (p. 252). Meningitis was discussed earlier in this Chapter

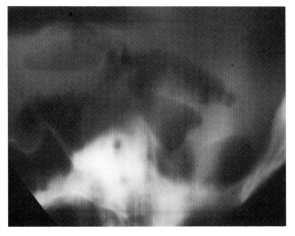 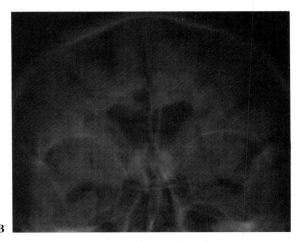

A   B

Fig. 10–29 Brain atrophy associated with chronic alcoholism in a severely demented 56-year-old man, shown by pneumoencephalography. (A) Median sagittal tomogram of the posterior fossa, showing a shrunken vermis and cerebellar hemispheres. The fourth ventricle, as well as the cisterna magna, vermian sulci and prepontine cistern are all widened. (B) Brow-up perorbital view, showing wide dilatation of the cortical sulci and sylvian fissures of both hemispheres. Normal lateral ventricles.

Table 10–1 Malformations (After DeMyer, 1971, and Harwood-Nash, 1977)

1. Disorders of Organogenesis
A. Disorders of Closure
   – Cranioschisis (meningocele, encephalocele: Fig. 1 – 40)
   – Callosal (agenesis: Fig. 7 – 25, lipoma: Fig. 7 – 25)
   – Teratoma
   – Arnold-Chiari malformation: Fig. 9 – 12
   – Dandy-Walker's syndrome: Fig. 10 – 9
B. Disorders of Diverticulation
   – Septo-optic dysplasia
   – Holoprosencephaly (Fig. 10 – 34)
C. Disorders of Sulcus Formation and Migration
   – Lissencephaly
   – Polymicrogyria
   – Schizencephaly
   – Heterotopias
D. Disorders of Size
   – Microcephaly: Fig. 1 – 24
   – Macrocephaly (megalancephaly obstructive hydrocephalus, e.g., aqueduct stenosis: Fig. 10 – 4)
E. Destructive Lesions
   – Hydraencephaly (Fig. 10 – 35)
   – Porencephaly: Fig. 4 – 29
   – Hypoxia
   – Inflammatory (rubella, cytomegalic inclusion, toxoplasmosis, herpes simplex, etc.)
2. Disorders of Histogenesis
   – Tuberous sclerosis: Fig. 1 – 16
   – Encephalotrigeminal angiomatosis: Fig. 1 – 17
   – Generalized neurofibromatosis
   – Vascular lesions, e.g., Galenic aneurysm: Fig. 3 – 27
   – Neonatal neoplasia

Table 10–2 Causes of Porencephaly (After Ramsey and Huckman, 1977)

1. Present at Birth
   – Germ plasm defect, e.g., schizencephaly
   – Intrauterine vascular accident (Fig. 10 – 36)
2. Acquired Defects
   – Birth trauma
   – Head injury later in life
   – Postinflammatory, e.g., meningitis
   – Vascular-mediated, e.g., embolism, thrombosis, spasm
   – Intracerebral hematoma, spontaneous or traumatic
   – Surgical
   – Hydrocephalus

tions, viz., tuberous sclerosis (p. 20), encephalotrigeminal angiomatosis or Sturge-Weber's syndrome (p. 22), generalized neurofibromatosis or Von Recklinghausen's disease (p. 68). Von Hippel-Lindau's syndrome (p. 377) and ataxia teleangiectasia. Computed tomography has revolutionized the diagnosis and management of the intracranial and intraorbital manifestations of these conditions (Kingsley, 1977).

Congenital Demyelinating Diseases (Leukodystrophies)
Conventional neuroradiology has played a negligible part in the diagnosis of the diseases grouped under the generic term *leukodystrophy,* its usefulness being confined to the demonstration of cerebral atrophy in established cases. Experience with computed tomography has altered this situation considerably, and this method may now in some instances represent an alternative to brain biopsy in diagnosis (Table 10 – 3; Erdohazi, 1975; Kendall et al., 1977; Robertson et al., 1977; Lane et al., 1978). The leukodystrophies include a heterogeneous group of progressive degenerative neurological disorders characterized by a diffuse demyelination of

under Hydrocephalus (Fig. 10 – 10). The symmetrical distribution of the low-attenuation lesions in the atrophic brain shown in Figure 10 – 38 suggests a viral etiology.

Phakomatoses. The phakomatoses, or neuroectodermal dysplasias, are hereditary conditions characterized by the development of tumors in the skin or central nervous system. They comprise 5 condi-

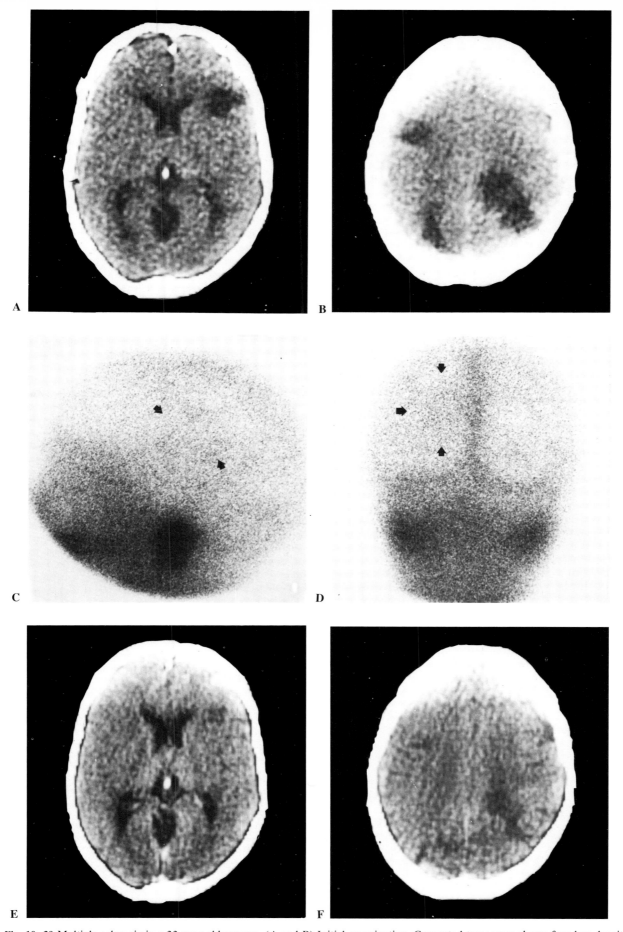

Fig. 10–30 Multiple sclerosis in a 33-year-old woman. (A and B) Initial examination. Computed tomogram shows four low-density, non-enhancing lesions in the cerebral hemispheres. (C and D) Scintigram made at the same time: right lateral and posterior scans show ill-defined activity in the parieto-occipital region, corresponding to the larger lesion *(arrows)*. (D and F) Repeat examination 16 months later, showing considerable regression of the plaques.

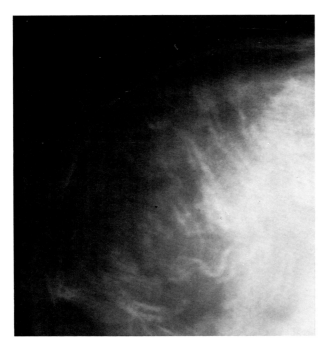

Fig. 10–31 Calcification following methotrexate therapy in an 18-year-old man with a reticulum-cell sarcoma. Progressive cortical calcification developed after treatment with intrathecal methotrexate.

Table 10–3 Leukodystrophies

A. Sudanophilic leukodystrophy
   1. Adrenoleukodystrophy
B. Spongiform leukodystrophy
   1. Canavan's diffuse sclerosis
   2. Alexander's disease
C. Sphingolipidosis
   1. Metachromatic leukodystrophy
   2. Globoid cell leukodystrophy (Krabbe's disease)
D. Lysosomal disease

white matter. Most are hereditary sex-linked recessive disorders. According to Eiben and Di Chiro (1977), the computed-tomographic characteristics of a leukoencephalopathy other than adrenoleukodystrophy include: (1) multiple noncoalescent areas of reduced density, (2) absence of periventricular involvement, (3) early frontal-lobe involvement, and (4) relative sparing of the occipital lobes, even though each centrum ovale may be affected.

Adrenal Leukodystrophy. The biochemical lesion is a breakdown of normal myelin which is replaced by sudanophilic material, and the brain lesion is accompanied by atrophy of the adrenal cortex. Typically, the patient is a 5-year-old boy with cortical blindness and computed tomography reveals bilateral though not necessarily symmetrical occipital and parietal lesions, with sparing of the frontal and temporal lobes. In the patient reported by Duda and Huttenlocher (1976), the lesions were imaged by cerebral scintigraphy and computed tomography although they failed to enhance upon contrast injection (Fig. 10–39; Greenberg et al., 1977). Since adrenal insufficiency occurs late and neurological symptoms are protean, biopsy may be required for diagnosis.

Spongiform Leukodystrophy (Canavan's Diffuse Sclerosis). The feature of this variety of leukodystrophy is an almost complete demyelination of white matter in the brain. The white matter is replaced by a loose glial network which appears to be edematous. In the cases so far described, an important feature of the computed-tomographic picture is sparing of the internal capsules in a hemisphere of which the white matter is extensively replaced. A less specific finding is widening of the interhemispherical fissure indicating atrophy (Fig. 10–40; Boltshauser and Isler, 1976; Kendall et al., 1977).

Globoid-Cell Leukodystrophy (Krabbe's Disease).

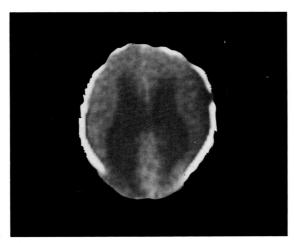

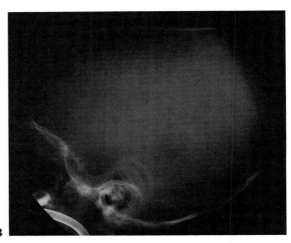

A   B

Fig. 10–32 Parietal meningoencephalocele. (A) Computed tomogram made soon after birth, showing herniation of the left lateral ventricle through a midline parietal defect. (B) Lateral skull radiograph made at the age of 27 months. The vault has been deformed by the herniating brain; the edges of the defect are everted.

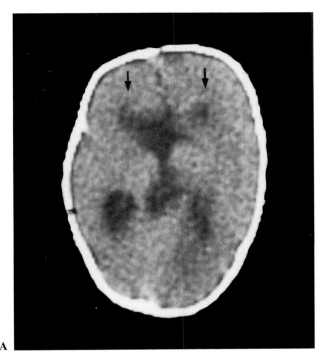 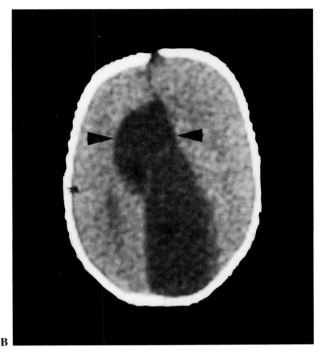

A   B

Fig. 10–33 Agenesis of the corpus callosum in a 4-month-old boy with seizures. (A) The ventricular slice shows widely displaced, pointed frontal horns *(arrows)*. (B) Higher slice showing a wide third ventricle *(arrowheads)* communicating with a giant porencephalic cyst.

In this disease of infants which is usually fatal before the age of 2 years, abnormal cerebrosides accumulate in the central nervous system, especially in multinucleated globoid cells in the demyelinated area. Although a generalized pattern of white matter involvement might be expected, the histologically proven case illustrated in Figure 10–41 exhibited only cortical atrophy.

Metachromatic Leukodystrophy. Sulphatides are deposited in cells of the central and peripheral nervous system and abdominal viscera. The patients, in addition to the leukodystrophy, may have a peripheral neuropathy (Fig. 10–42).

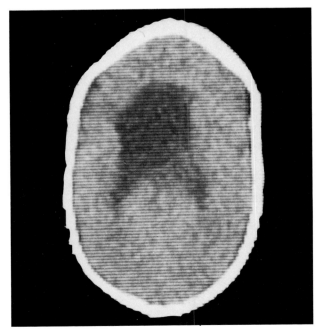 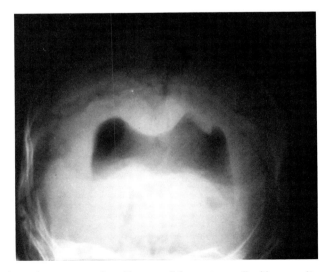

Fig. 10–34 Lobar holoprosencephaly shown by computed tomography and pneumography. Absence of the septum pellucidum results in a flat anterior aspect of the frontal horns.

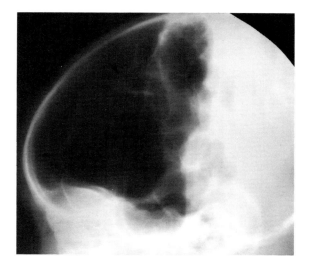

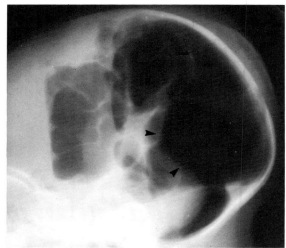

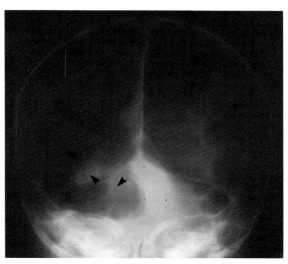

Fig. 10–35 Hydranencephaly. Both cerebral hemispheres are thin-walled bags of fluid surrounding the basal ganglia. Pneumoencephalogram showing partial invagination of the cortical mantle (arrows) in the brow-up and brow-down positions.

Kendall and his colleagues advanced several criteria for the diagnosis of leukodystrophy by computed tomography, viz.: (1) an appropriate clinical picture must be present; (2) the low-density lesions of the white matter are bilateral; (3) they tend to be symmetrical; (4) the gray matter is unaffected; and (5) the disease runs a progressive course, leading to atrophy and death—therefore, serial examination is essential to exclude reversible or static lesions of similar appearance.

Differential Diagnosis. (1) Demyelination associated with systemic illnesses, e.g., meningo-encephalomyelitis. (2) Spinal muscular atrophy. Radiological and microscopical studies in various types of muscular dystrophy and atrophy have revealed white-matter changes and wide lateral ventricles (Fig. 10–43; Hovstad et al., 1976). (3) Vascular lesions, e.g., multiple infarction. (4) Disseminated necrotizing leukoencephalopathy: see page 463.

Birth Trauma
Neuroradiologists are familar with the difficulty of investigating neonates and infants who fail to thrive or who exhibit neurological symptoms or signs such as seizures, hemiparesis, an enlarging head or a floppy state. The pattern of intracranial changes found in such infants is frequently attributed to abnormal birth trauma, and sometimes a relevant history can be elicited. In the majority, however, no etiological relationship can be established, and the question of whether the lesion dates from the fetal, birth or postnatal period remains unanswerable.

Congenital porencephaly (Fig. 10–44) is a frequent finding in patients with seizures or a hemisyndrome.

Cerebral "no-growth" (Fig. 10–45) is found in backward infants and neonates who fail to thrive. A diffusely shrunken brain—indicating an atrophic process, and not merely a failure of growth—may

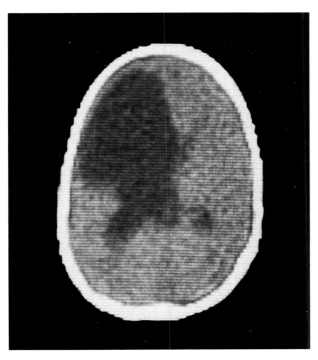

Fig. 10—36 Porencephaly. Computed tomogram of a 5-year-old boy with seizures, showing left frontal porencephaly communicating with the ventricular system.

be encountered, accompanied by an excess of cerebrospinal fluid around the brain and a microcranium.

Outlet obstruction (Fig. 10–46) and stenosis at the level of the aqueduct are the main cause of an enlarging head, due to obstructive hydrocephalus. Another cause is subdural collections (Fig. 10–47).

Cortical infarction (Fig. 10–48) is an important cause of infantile hemisyndromes or paralysis. Some of these cases are caused by traumatic occlusion of the carotid artery in the neck. Lesions occurring in early life deform the ipsilateral half of the skull as well as the brain (see Chap. 1, Focal Brain Damage In Early Life, p. 39).

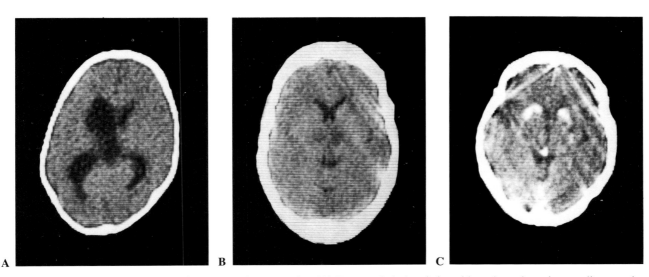

Fig. 10—37 Anoxic lesions revealed by computed tomography. (A) Porencephaly in a baby with prolonged respiratory distress who developed extrapyramidal signs. (B) Bithalamic lucencies in a patient being artifically respired. (C) Post anoxic calcified deposits in the basal ganglia of both hemispheres.

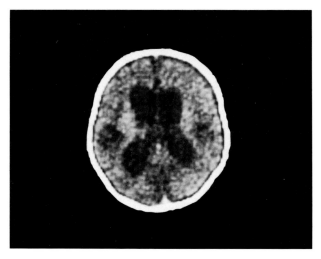

Fig. 10–38 Herpes simplex encephalitis in a 3-month-old baby. Computed tomogram shows symmetrical low-density lesions in the temporal lobes, and the wide lateral ventricles and interhemispherical fissure indicate advanced atrophy.

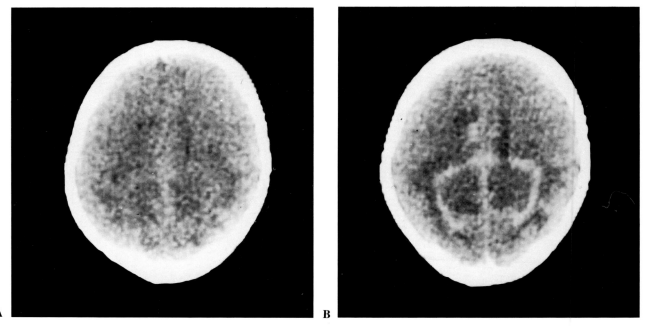

A   B

Fig. 10–39 Adrenal leukodystrophy in a 4-year-old boy with visual loss and increased skin pigmentation. Computed tomogram, vertex views. (A) Unenhanced slice showing extensive bilateral low-density lesions in the parieto-occipital cortex. (B) Same slice with contrast enhancement.

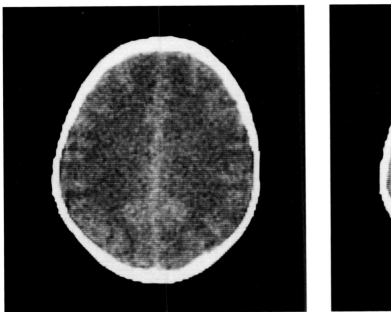
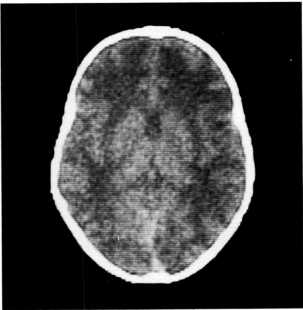

Fig. 10–40 Spongiform leukodystrophy (Canavan's diffuse sclerosis) shown by computed tomography. Involvement of all parts of the white matter of both hemispheres contrasts with sparing of the internal capsules.

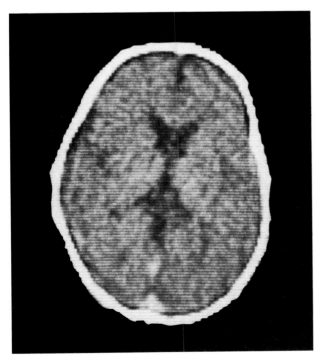
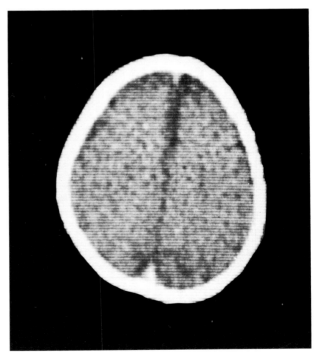

Fig. 10–41 Globoid-cell leukodystrophy (Krabbe's disease). Enhanced computed tomography in this patient revealed only cortical atrophy, especially widening of the interhemispheric fissure.

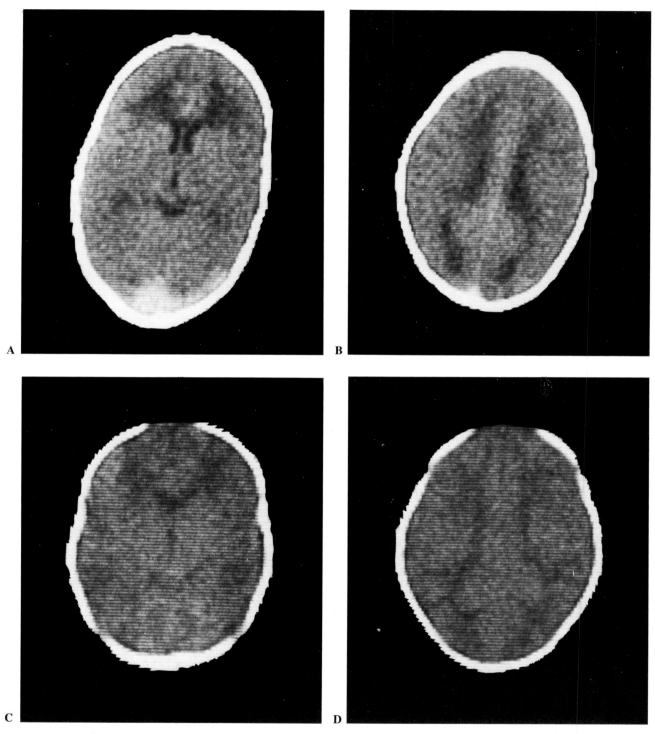

Fig. 10–42 Leukodystrophy, probably metachromatic variety. Computed tomograms of two patient, both showing bilateral low-density, periventricular areas, especially of the frontal lobes. (A and B) A 20-year-old demented epileptic with a peripheral neuropathy. (C and D) A 6-month-old baby.

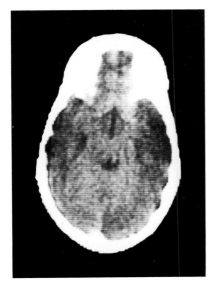
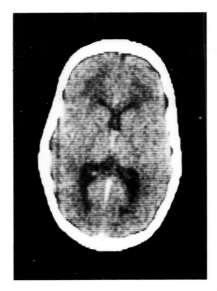
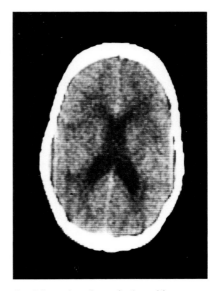

Fig. 10–43 Myotonic muscular dystrophy in a 25-year-old man. Computed tomogram, showing bilateral periventricular white-matter attenuation and enlarged lateral ventricles.

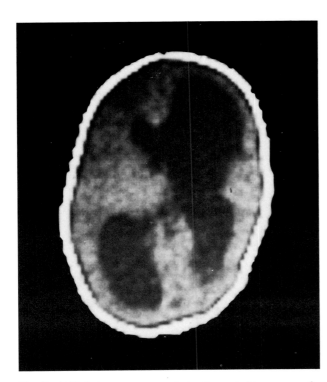

Fig. 10–44 Birth-trauma porencephaly. Computed tomogram of a 3-week-old baby with seizures, showing multifocal porencephaly.

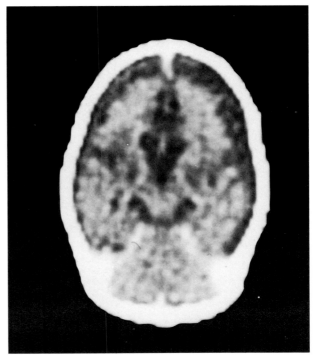

Fig. 10–45 "No-growth" brain associated with hydrocephalus *ex vacuo* and microcephaly. A 3-month-old baby with a history of difficult birth. Repeat examination 6 months later revealed unchanged appearances.

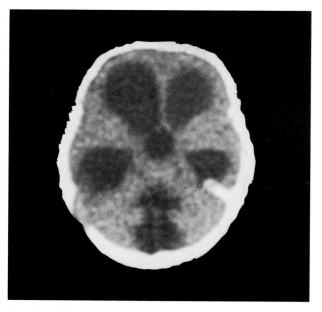

Fig. 10–46 Outlet obstruction, probably due to traumatic subarachnoid hemorrhage at birth. Computed tomogram shows obstructive hydrocephalus, including a large fourth ventricle, vallecula and cisterna magna.

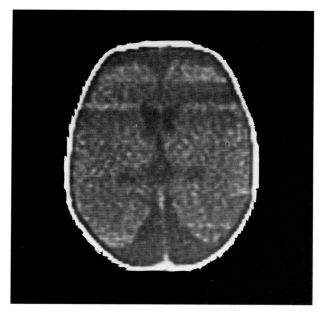 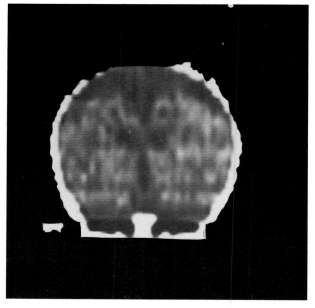

Fig. 10–47 Bilateral subdural collections in a 2-month-old baby with an enlarging head following perinatal injury.

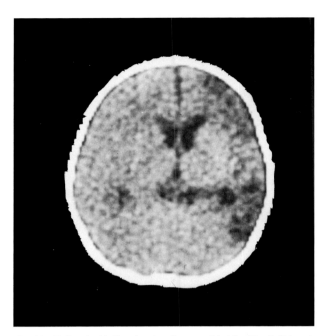

Fig. 10–48 Cortical infarction in a 2-year-old girl with a left hemiplegia from birth. Forceps delivery with bruising of the neck: ? carotid damage.

REFERENCES

Adams, R. D., Fisher, C. M., Hakim, S., Ojemann, R. G. and Sweet, W. H.: Symptomatic occult hydrocephalus with "normal" cerebrospinal-fluid pressure: a treatable syndrome. New England Journal of Medicine, 273, 117–126, 1965.

Allen, J. H., Martin, J. T. and McLain, L. W.: Computed tomography in cerebellar atrophic processes. Radiology, 130, 379–382, 1979.

Antunes, J. L., Schlesinger, E. B. and Michelsen, W. J.: The abnormal brain scan in demyelinating diseases. Archives of Neurology, 30, 269–271, 1974.

Arimitsu, T.,Di Chiro, G., Brooks, R. A. and Smith, P. B.: White-grey matter differentiation in computed tomography. Journal of Computer Assisted Tomography, 1, 437–442, 1977.

Babin, E. and Heldt, N.: Pneumographic findings in infants and children with aqueductal stenosis. Nine cases reviewed, two with anatomical findings. Neuroradiology, 1, 173–178, 1970.

Bannister, R., Gilford, E. and Kocen, R.: Isotope encephalography in the diagnosis of dementia due to communicating hydrocephalus. The Lancet, 2, 1014–1017, 1967.

Benson, D. F., Le May, M., Patten, D. H. and Rubens, A. B.: The diagnosis of normal pressure hydrocephalus. New England Journal of Medicine, 283, 609–615, 1970.

Boltshauser, E. and Isler, W.: Computerised axial tomography in spongy degeneration. The Lancet, 1, 1123, 1976.

Brain, W. R. and Walton, J. N.: Diseases of the Nervous System. 7th Ed. London: Oxford University Press, 1969.

Brett, E. M. and Hoare, R. D.: An assessment of the value and limitations of air encephalography in children with mental retardation and with epilepsy. Brain, 92, 731–742, 1969.

Bruijn, G. W.: Pneumoencephalography in the Diagnosis of Cerebral Atrophy (Academic thesis). Utrecht: Drukkerij H. J. Smits, 1959.

Burhenne, H. J. and Davies, H.: The ventricular span in cerebral pneumography. American Journal of Roentgenology, 90, 1178–1184, 1963.

Cala, L. A., Mastaglia, F. L. and Black, J. L.: Computerized

tomography of brain and optic nerve in multiple sclerosis. Observation in 100 patients, including serial studies in 16. Journal of the Neurological Sciences, 36, 411–426, 1978.

Campbell, A. M. G., Evans, M., Thomson, J. L. G. and Williams, M. J.: Cerebral atrophy in young cannabis smokers. The Lancet, 2, 1219–1224, 1971.

Claveria, L. E., Moseley, I. F. and Stevenson, J. F.: The clinical significance of "cerebral atrophy" as shown by C.A.T. In Du Boulay, G. H. and Moseley, I. F., Ed.: Computerised Axial Tomography in Clinical Practice, 213–216. Berlin: Springer-Verlag, 1977.

Co, B. T., Goodwin, D. W., Gado, M., Mikhael, M. and Hill, S. Y.: Absence of cerebral atrophy in chronic cannabis users. Evaluation by computerized transaxial tomography. Journal of the American Medical Association, 237, 1229–1230, 1977.

Cohan, S. L., Fermaglich, J. and Auth, T. L.: Abnormal brain scans in multiple sclerosis. Journal of Neurology, Neurosurgery and Psychiatry, 38, 120–122, 1975.

Crocker, E. F., Zimmerman, R. A., Phelps, M. E. and Kuhl, D. E.: The effect of steroids on the extravascular distribution of radiographic contrast material and technetium pernechnetate in brain tumors as determined by computed tomography. Radiology, 119, 471–474, 1976.

Cronqvist, S. and Efsing, H. O.: Skull size and ventricular dilatation in subdural hygroma in infants. Acta Radiologica Diagnosis, 10, 11–16, 1970.

Davidoff, L. M. and Epstein, B. S.: The Normal Encephalogram. 3rd Ed. Philadelphia: Lea and Febiger, 1958.

DeMyer, W.: Classification of cerebral malformations. Birth Defects, 7, 78–93, 1971.

Di Chiro, G., Reames, P. M. and Matthews, W. B. Jr.: RISA-ventriculography and RISA-cisternography. Neurology (Minneapolis), 14, 185–191, 1964.

Drayer, B. P., Rosenbaum, A. E. and Higman, H. B.: Cerebrospinal fluid imaging using serial metrizamide CT cisternography. Neuroradiology, 13, 7–17, 1977.

Duda, E. E. and Huttenlocher, P. R.: Computed tomography in adrenoleukodystrophy. Correlation of radiological and histological findings. Radiology, 120, 349–350, 1976.

Eiben, R. M. and Di Chiro, G.: Computer assisted tomography in adrenoleukodystrophy. Journal of Computer Assisted Tomography, 1, 308–314, 1977.

El Gammal, T., Allen, M. B. and Lott, T.: Computed assisted tomography and pneumoencephalography in nontumourous hydrocephalus in infants and children. Computed Tomography, 1, 25–28, 1976.

Engeset, A. and Skraastad, E.: Methods of measurement in encephalography. Neurology (Minneapolis), 14, 381–385, 1964.

Enzmann, D. R., Norman, D., Mani, J. and Newton, T. H.: Computed tomography of granulomatous basal arachnoiditis. Radiology, 120, 341–344, 1976.

Erdohazi, M.: The leukodystrophies. Proceedings of the Royal Society of Medicine, 68, 561–562, 1975.

Evans, W. A.: An encephalographic ratio for estimating ventricular enlargement and cerebral atrophy. Archives of Neurology and Psychiatry (Chicago), 47, 931–937, 1942.

Flament-Durand, J., Ketelbant-Balasse, P., Maurus, R., Regnier, R. and Spehl, M.: Intracerebral calcifications appearing during the course of acute lymphocytic leukemia treated with methotrexate and X rays. Cancer, 35, 319–325, 1975.

Fox, J. H., Ramsey, R. G., Huckman, M. S. and Proske, A. E.: Cerebral ventricular enlargement. Chronic alcoholics examined by computerized tomography. Journal of the American Medical Association, 236, 365–368, 1976.

Fox, J. H., Topel, J. L. and Huckman, M. S.: Use of computerized tomography in senile dementia. Journal of Neurology, Neurosurgery and Psychiatry, 38, 948–953, 1975.

Galera, R. and Greitz, T.: Hydrocephalus in the adult secondary to the rupture of intracranial aneurysms. Journal of Neurosurgery, 32, 634–641, 1970.

Gath, I., Jörgensen, A., Sjaastad, O. and Berstad, J.: Pneumoencephalographic findings in parkinsonism. Archives of Neurology, 32, 769–773, 1975.

Gath, I. and Vinje, B.: Pneumoencephalographic findings in Huntington's chorea. Neurology (Minneapolis), 18, 991–996, 1968.

Gibberd, F. B., Ngan, H. and Swann, G. F.: Hydrocephalus, subarachnoid haemorrhage and ependymomas of the cauda equina. Clinical Radiology, 23, 422–426, 1972.

Gosling, R. H.: The association of dementia with radiologically demonstrated cerebral atrophy. Journal of Neurology, Neurosurgery or Psychiatry, 18, 129–133, 1955.

Granholm, L. and Rådberg, C.: Congenital communicating hydrocephalus. Journal of Neurosurgery, 20, 338–343, 1963.

Granholm, L. and Rådberg, C.: Ventricular diverticulum in infantile hydrocephalus. Acta Radiologica Diagnosis, 3, 156–160, 1965.

Greenberg, H. S., Halverson, D. and Lane, B.: CT scanning and diagnosis of adrenoleukodystrophy. Neurology, 27, 884–886, 1977.

Greitz, T.: Effect of brain distension on cerebral circulation. The Lancet, 1, 863–865, 1969.

Greitz, T., Ekbom, K., Kugelberg, E. and Breig, A.: Occult hydrocephalus due to ectasia of the basilar artery. Acta Radiologica Diagnosis, 9, 312–316, 1969.

Greitz, T. and Grepe, A.: Encephalography in the diagnosis of convexity block hydrocephalus. Acta Radiologica, 11, 232–242, 1971.

Griffith, H. B., Cummins, B. H. and Thomson, J. L. G.: Cerebral arterial spasm and hydrocephalus in leaking arterial aneurysms. Neuroradiology, 4, 212–214, 1972.

Gyldensted, C.: Computer tomography of the cerebrum in multiple sclerosis. Neuroradiology, 12, 33–42, 1976.

Gyldensted, C.: Measurements of the normal ventricular system and hemispheric sulci of 100 adults with computed tomography. Neuroradiology, 14, 183–192, 1977.

Gyldensted, C. and Kosteljanetz, M.: Measurements of the normal hemispheric sulci with computed tomography: a preliminary study on 44 adults. Neuroradiology, 10, 147–149, 1975.

Gyldensted, C. and Kosteljanetz, M.: Measurements of the normal ventricular system with computed tomography of the brain. A preliminary study on 44 adults. Neuroradiology, 10, 205–213, 1976.

Hachinski, V. C., Lassen, N. A. and Marshall, J.: Multi-infarct dementia: A cause of mental deterioration in the elderly. The Lancet, 2, 207–209, 1974.

Hahn, F. J. Y. and Rim, K.: Frontal ventricular dimensions on normal computed tomography. American Journal of Roentgenology, 126, 593–596, 1976.

Harrison, M. J. G., Robert, C. M. and Uttley, D.: Benign aqueduct stenosis in adults. Journal of Neurology, Neurosurgery and Psychiatry, 37, 1322–1328, 1974.

Harwood-Nash, D. C.: Congenital craniocerebral abnormalities and computed tomography. Seminars in Roentgenology, 12, 39–51, 1977.

Haug, G.: Age and sex dependence of the size of normal ventricles on computed tomography. Neuroradiology, 14, 201–204, 1977.

Hauser, S. L., DeLong, C. R. and Rosman, N. P.: Pneumographic findings in the infantile aneurysm syndrome. A correlation with temporal lobe disease. Brain, 98, 667–688, 1975.

Hawkins, T. D., Lloyd, A. D., Fletcher, G. I. C. and Hanka, R.: Ventricular size following head injury in a clinicoradiological study. Clinical Radiology, 27, 279–289, 1976.

Hindmarsh, T.: Computer cisternography for evaluation of CSF flow dynamics. Further experiences. Acta Radiologica Supplementum 355, 269–279, 1977.

Hindmarsh, T. and Greitz, T.: Computer cisternography in the diagnosis of communicating hydrocephalus. Acta Radiologica Supplementum 346, 91–97, 1975.

Hovstad, L., Lochen, E. A. and Sjaastad, O.: Pneumoencephalographic findings in various primary and secondary muscular disorders. Acta Neurologica Scandinavica, 53, 128–136, 1976.

Huang, Y. P., Wolf, B. S., Antin, S. P., Okudera, T. and Kim, I. H.: Angiographic features of aqueductal stenosis. American Journal of Roentgenology, 104, 90–107, 1968.

Huckman, M. S., Fox, J. H. and Ramsey, R. G.: Computed tomography in the diagnosis of degenerative diseases of the brain. Seminars in Roentgenology, 12, 63–76, 1977.

Huckman, M. S., Fox, J. and Topel, J.: The validity of criteria for the evaluation of cerebral atrophy by computed tomography. Radiology, 116, 85–92, 1975.

Hunter, R., Hurwitz, L. J., Fullerton, P. M., Nieman, E. A. and Davies, H.: Unilateral ventricular enlargement. A clinical study of 75 cases. Brain, 85, 295–318, 1962.

James, A. E., DeLand, F. H., Hodges, F. J. and Wagner, H. N.: Normal-pressure hydrocephalus. Role of cisternography in diagnosis. Journal of the American Medical Association, 213, 1615–1622, 1970.

James, A. E., Strecker, E. P., Sperber, E., Flor, W. J., Merz, T. and Burns, B.: An alternative pathway of cerebrospinal fluid absorption in communicating hydrocephalus. Radiology, 111, 143–146, 1974.

Johnstone, E. C., Crow, T. J., Frith, C. D., Husband, J. and Kreel, L.: Cerebral ventricular size and cognitive impairment in chronic schizophrenia. The Lancet, 2, 924–926, 1976.

Kibler, R. F., Couch, R. S. and Crompton, M. R.: Hydrocephalus in that adult following spontaneous subarachnoid haemorrhage. Brain, 84, 45–61, 1961.

Kendall, B. E., Claveria, L. E. and Quiroga, W.: C.A.T. in leukodystrophy and neuronal degeneration. In Du Boulay, G. H. and Moseley, I. F., Ed.: Computerised Axial Tomography in Clinical Practice, 191–202. Berlin: Springer-Verlag, 1977.

Kendall, B. E. and Kingsley, D. P. E.: The value of computerised axial tomography (CT) in cranio-cerebral malformations. British Journal of Radiology, 51, 171–190, 1978.

Kennedy, P., Swash, M. and Wylie, I. G.: The clinical significance of pneumographic cerebellar atrophy. British Journal of Radiology, 49, 903–911, 1976.

Kingsley, D. P. E.: C.A.T. in the phakomatoses. In Du Boulay, G. H. and Moseley, I. F., Ed.: Computerised Axial Tomography in Clinical Practice, 174–181. Berlin: Springer-Verlag, 1977.

Kingsley, D. and Kendall, B. E.: The value of computed tomography in the evaluation of the enlarged head. Neuroradiology, 15, 59–72, 1978.

Kuehnle, J., Mendelson, J. H., Davis, K. R. and New, P. F. J.: Computed tomographic examination of heavy marijuana smokers. Journal of the American Medical Association, 237, 1231–1232, 1977.

Kurlander, G. H., DeMyer, W., Campbell, J. A. and Taybi, H.: Roentgenology of holoprosencephaly. Acta Radiologica Diagnosis, 5, 25–40, 1966.

Lane, B.: Cerebral white matter disease on CT scanning. Proceedings of the 14th Annual Meeting of the American Society of Neuroradiology, 12, 51, 1976.

Lane, B., Carroll, B. A. and Pedley, T. A.: Computerized cranial tomography in cerebral diseases of white matter. Neuroradiology, 28, 534–544, 1978.

La Torre, E. and Occhipinti, E.: Cerebral angiography in hydranencephaly. European Neurology, 2, 184–191, 1969.

Lebow, S., Anderson, D. C., Mastri, A. and Larson, D.: Acute multiple sclerosis with contrast enhancing plaques. Archives of Neurology, 35, 435–439, 1978.

LeMay, M. and Abramowicz, A.: Encephalography in the diagnosis of cerebellar atrophy. Acta Radiologica Diagnosis, 5, 667–674, 1966.

Lorber, J. and Grainger, R. G.: Cerebral cavities following ventricular punctures in infants. Clinical Radiology, 14, 98–109, 1963.

Lux, W. E., Hochwald, G. M., Sahar, A. and Ransohoff, J.: Periventricular water content. Effect of pressure in experimental chronic hydrocephalus. Archives of Neurology, 23, 475–479, 1970.

Lynch, M. J. G.: Brain lesions in chronic alcoholism. Archives of Pathology, 69, 324–353, 1960.

McRae, D. L.: Observations on craniolacunia. Acta Radiologica, 5, 55–64, 1966.

Marions, O. and Lying-Tunell, U.: Constancy of convexity air block on pneumoencephalography. Neuroradiology, 13, 191–193, 1977.

Moseley, I. F. and Sondheimer, F. K.: The twenty-four hour pneumoencephalogram: with particular reference to ventricular size, a series of 150 patients and a review of the literature. Clinical Radiology, 26, 389–405, 1975.

Naidich, T. P., Epstein, F., Linn, J. P., Kricheff, I. I. and Hochwald, G. M.: Evaluation of pediatric hydrocephalus by computed tomography. Radiology, 119, 337–345, 1976.

Newcombe, R. L., Shah, S. H., Hoare, R. D. and Falconer, M. A.: Radiological abnormalities in temporal lobe epilepsy with clinicopathological correlations. Journal of Neurology, Neurosurgery and Psychiatry, 38, 279–287, 1975.

Nielsen, R., Petersen, O., Thygesen, T. and Willanger, R.: Encephalographic ventricular atrophy. Acta Radiologica Diagnosis, 4, 240–256, 1966a.

Nielsen, R., Peterson, O., Thygesen, T. and Willanger, R.: Encephalographic cortical atrophy. Acta Radiologica Diagnosis, 4, 437–448, 1966b.

Northfield, D. W. C.: The Surgery of the Central Nervous System. Oxford: Blackwell Scientific Publications, 1973.

Palmieri, A., Menichelli, F., Pasquini, U. and Salvolini, U.: Role of computed tomography in the post-operative evaluation of infantile hydrocephalus. Neuroradiology, 14, 257–262, 1978.

Poser, C. M., Walsh, F. C. and Scheinberg, L. C.: Hydranencephaly. Neurology, 5, 284–289, 1955.

Rao, K. C. V. G., Brennan, T. G. and Garcia, J. H.: Computed tomography in the diagnosis of Creutzfelt-Jacob disease. Journal of Computer Assisted Tomography, 1, 211–215, 1977.

Ramsey, R. G. and Huckman, M. S.: Computed tomography of porencephaly and other cerebrospinal fluid-containing lesions. Radiology, 123, 73–77, 1977.

Roberts, M. A., Caird, F. I., Grossart, K. W. and Steven, J. L.: Computerized tomography in the diagnosis of cerebral atrophy. Journal of Neurology, Neurosurgery and Psychiatry, 39, 909–915, 1976.

Roberts, M. A., Caird, F. I., Steven, J. L. and Grossart, K. W.: Computerised axial tomography and dementia in the elderly. In Du Boulay, G. H. and Moseley, I. F., Eds.: Computerised Axial Tomography in Clinical Practice, 218–220, Berlin: Springer-Verlag, 1977.

Robertson, W. C., Gomez, M. R., Reese, D. F. and Okazaki, H.: Computerized tomography in demyelinating disease of the young. Neurology, 27, 838–842, 1977.

Russell, D. S.: Observations on the Pathology of Hydrocephalus. Medical Research Council Special Publications Series No. 265. 3rd impression with appendix. HMSO, London, 1966.

Schechter, M. M.: Pneumography in brain atrophy. Seminars in Roentgenology, 5, 196–205, 1970.

Schiersmann, O.: Einführung in die Encephalographie. Stuttgart: George Thieme, 1952.

Sears, E. S., Tindall, R. S. A. and Zernow, H.: Acute multiple sclerosis. Arch Neurology, 35, 426–434, 1978.

Sengupta, R. P. and Hankinson, J.: Extradural haemorrhage – a hazard of ventricular drainage. Journal of Neurology, Neurosurgery and Psychiatry, 35, 297–303, 1972.

Shenkin, H. A., Greenberg, J. O. and Grossman, C. B.: Ventricular size after shunting for idiopathic normal pressure hydrocephalus. Journal of Neurology, Neurosurgery and Psychiatry, 38, 833–837, 1975.

Starer, F.: The radiology of the Sptiz-Holter valve in fifancy. British Journal of Radiology, 46, 485–495, 1973.

Standgaard, L.: The Dandy-Walker syndrome – a case with a patent foramen of the 4th ventricle demonstrated by encephalography. British Journal of Radiology, 43, 734–738, 1970.

Swash, M.: Periaqueductal dysfunction (the sylvian aqueduct syndrome): a sign of hydrocephalus? Journal of Neurology, Neurosurgery and Psychiatry, 37, 21–26, 1974.

Terrence, C. F., Delaney, J. F. and Alberts, M. C.: Computed tomography for Huntington's disease. Neuroradiology, 13, 173–175, 1977.

Thiébaut, F., Wackenheim, A., Vrousos, C. and Subirana, M.: Atrophies du vermis cérébelleux. Acta Radiologica Diagnosis, 5, 716–720, 1966.

Von Gall, M., Becker, H., Artman, H., Lerch, G. and Nemeth, N.: Results of computer tomography in chronic alcoholics. Neuroradiology, 16, 329–331, 1978.

Weinstein, M. A., Duchesneu, P. M. and MacIntyre, W. J.: White and grey matter of the brain differentiated by computed tomography. Radiology, 122, 699–702, 1977.

Weinstein, M. A., Lederman, R. J., Rothner, A. D., Duchesneau, P. M. and Norman, D.: Interval computed tomography in multiple sclerosis. Radiology, 129, 689–694, 1978.

Williams, B.: Is aqueduct stenosis a result of hydrocephalus? Brain, 96, 399–412, 1973.

Wolpert, S. M., Haller, J. S. and Rabe, E. F.: The value of angiography in the Dandy-Walker syndrome and posterior fossa extra-axial cysts. American Journal of Roentgenology, 109, 261–272, 1970.

Yakovlev, P. I. and Wadsworth, R. C.: Schizencephalies. A study of the congenital clefts in the cerebral mantle. II. Clefts with hydrocephalus and lips separated. Journal of Neuropathology and Experimental Neurology, 5, 169–206, 1946.

11 The Spine and Cord

This Chapter deals with the radiological examination and diagnosis of lesions affecting the spinal cord and nerve roots, and their coverings within the spinal canal. Abnormalities of the vertebral column will be discussed only when relevant to neurological diagnosis. Readers seeking a comprehensive account of spinal osteology should consult texts such as Murray and Jacobson's *The Radiology of Skeletal Disorders* (1977).

EXAMINATION OF THE SPINAL CANAL AND ITS CONTENTS

Plain Radiographs: What is Adequate?

Anteroposterior and lateral views, and a chest radiograph, are the basis of any examination of patients suspected of spinal disease, and they should never be omitted before myelography. The extent of the spine to be examined depends on the clinical picture: for example, sciatica calls for careful study of the lumbosacral spine only, and brachialgia or neck pain for detailed examination of the cervical canal. However, patients without a definite clinical level of involvement and all cases of paraplegia require examination of the whole spine. The detection of multiple metastases may alter the surgical approach, and sometimes may eliminate the need for myelography.

Junctional areas may not be well seen due to contrasting tissue densities, and further radiographs may be required if sclerotic or collapsed vertebrae are not to be missed. (1) The craniovertebral junction is best shown on a lateral view of the skull, a film that will also reveal calvarial metastases. (2) The spine at the root of the neck is notoriously difficult to demonstrate: the body of T1 and sometimes C7 vertebra is often invisible on the routine lateral, due to the density of the shoulder girdles, and obliquity of the central ray in the anteroposterior view especially if combined with a round-back kyphosis makes adequate evaluation impossible. A special "through the shoulders" lateral view is necessary. (3) Adequate examination of the conus region may be ensured by overlap radiography, i.e., the use of long-format x-ray films which include the upper lumbar vertebrae on the thoracic radiographs, and the lower thoracic vertebrae on the lumbar radiographs. (4) "Junction shots" of the lumbosacral disc space, beloved of orthopaedists, provide less information to the neuroradiologist, and improved radiographic screens may already have eliminated the need for them.

The capacity and integrity of the spinal canal are the main ingredients of radiological diagnosis of the spine, second only to the importance of ensuring that the vertebral column itself is intact. The size of the canal dictates the significance of osteophytic proliferation and disc degeneration, and it may be directly responsible for the patient's clinical picture. Its front-to-back (sagittal) and side-to-side coronal or interpedicular diameters can be measured in lateral and anteroposterior radiographs, and compared

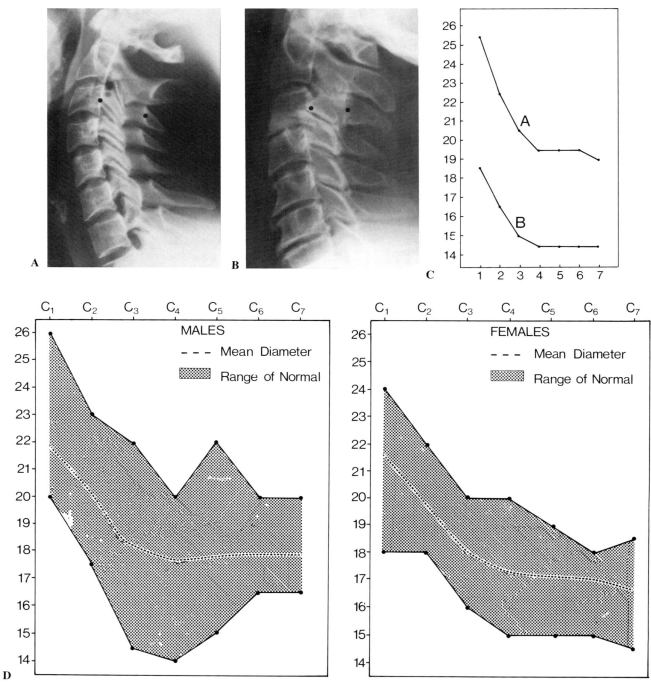

Fig. 11—1 Normal variation in the sagittal diameter of the cervical canal. (A) Wide canal, C3 = 22 mm — note the gap between the apophyseal joints and the roots of the spinous processes. (B) Narrow canal, C3 = 15 mm. — in lateral view, the canal should be as wide as the body. (D, E) Range of normal, based on the measurement of 300 normal adults in Rochester, New York (Burrows, 1963).

to normal tables (Figs. 11–1, 11–2 and 11–3). Typical of all biological measurement, a fairly wide range of normal variation is encountered, depending on factors such as the patient's sex, age and physique.

Pathological narrowing of the canal, like pathological widening, is an important radiological sign.

Before measuring its diameters to reach this diagnosis, the radiologist should pay attention to the shape of the vertebral body in lateral view and to its posterior surface; normally, the body has a greater horizontal than vertical diameter and its posterior surface has the same cortical thickness as the other surfaces. In anteroposterior view, the shape and

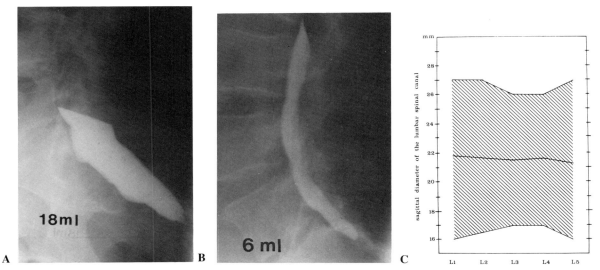

Fig. 11—2 Normal variation in the sagittal diameter of the lumbar canal. (A) Wide canal, L4 = 35 mm. (B) Narrow canal, L4 = 16 mm. (C) Range of normal, based on measurements of 49 normal adults (Hinck, Hopkins and Clark, 1965).

thickness of the pedicles must be taken into account in evaluating the interpedicular measurement. The normal pedicle has an oval medial surface (slightly flattened by rotation of the spine); only dysraphic lesions can show interpedicular widening in the presence of completely normal pedicles.

Other structures to be carefully evaluated at all levels are: vertebra (texture of body, spinous process and transverse processes), disc space (width, ? marginal sclerosis and/or osteophytic proliferation), and paravertebral gutter (pleural reflection, ribs, ? abnormal soft tissue shadow).

Complete examination of the cervical spine requires additional views. These are: (1) Oblique views (45° to median sagittal plane), to see the intervertebral foramina which are invisible on the anteroposterior and lateral views. In a patient with normal anteroposterior and lateral films and a myelographic obstruction in the neck, an oblique view may reveal the cause—a dumbbell neurofibroma of a cervical nerve. "Trauma obliques" (70° to the median sagittal plane, made with the patient supine) are useful in diagnosing fracture-dislocations involving the articular facets (McCall, Park, McSweeney, 1973). (2) Functional examination in lateral projection—either ciné studies or static flexion-extension radiographs—may yield valuable evidence of residual instability after a neck injury.

Oblique views of the lumbar spine are essential to examine completely any patient with backache, especially the nonradiating lower lumbar variety. They reveal the interarticular parts and articular facets of the apophyseal joints on each vertebra. Minor but significant abnormalities of these structures will be missed if these views are omitted. Osteoarthritic changes localized to one apophyseal joint are evidence of lumbosacral instability: in such

a patient, routine anteroposterior and lateral radiographs and lumbar myelography may show no abnormality. If an interarticular part is attenuated or interrupted, the familiar radiological sign, "the broken neck of the scotty dog," will be revealed only in the appropriate oblique projection. The third advantage of oblique views occurs in severe degenerative joint disease. Disc narrowing and marginal osteophytic "beaking" are sometimes—and apophyseal joint sclerosis is always—better demonstrated than in routine anteroposterior or lateral views.

Tomography invariably illuminates lesions that cross a disc space and erode one or adjacent vertebral bodies, and it may provide essential diagnostic information (see Fig. 11-23).

Myelography: Media and Techniques: Errors, Omissions and Artifacts

The ideal contrast medium for myelography must be: (1) nontoxic to the spinal cord, nerves and meninges, ideally, completely absorbable for total excretion, and (2) diagnostically satisfactory, i.e., dense enough but not too dense and usable in volumes that permit sequential study of the full diameter of all parts of the spinal canal. In effect, these criteria refer to hydrosoluble substances, miscible with cerebrospinal fluid.

The first two substances used—gas by Jacobaeus in Stockholm in 1921 and Lipiodol by Sicard and Forestier in Paris in 1921—failed to fulfill either of the above-named criteria. A water-soluble substance, methiodal sodium (Abrodil) introduced in the 1930s by Scandinavian workers, failed to find general acceptance in the English-speaking world, mainly because spinal anesthesia is required to use it. The discovery of iodophendylate (Pantopaque, Myodil) by William Strain (Ramsey, French and

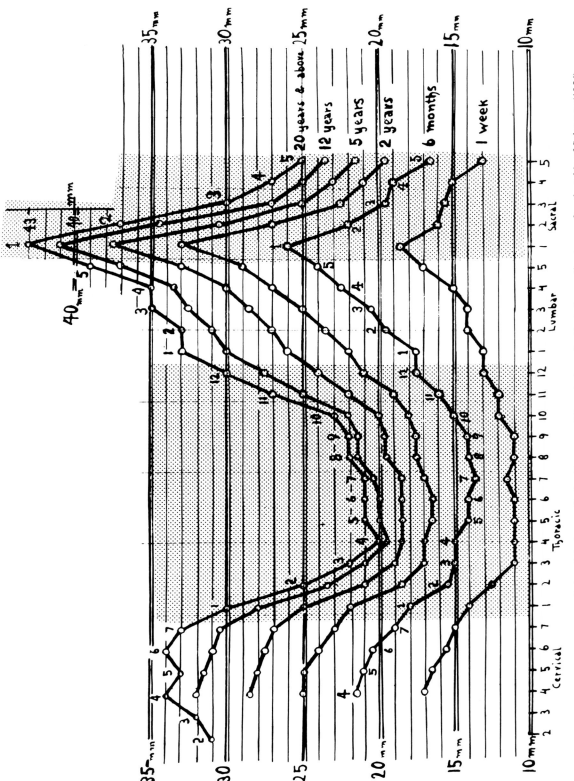

Fig. 11–3 Extreme upper limits of the interpedicular diameters of the spinal canal, adjusted according to age after the table of Schwartz (1956), an elaboration of the original study by Elsberg and Dyke (1934).

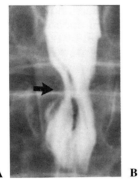
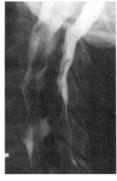

A B

Fig. 11-4 Needle defects and unsatisfactory injection. (A) Hematoma simulating disc prolapse *(arrow)*. Re-examination 12 days later: normal appearances! (B) Partly subdural injection of oil. The well-defined sleeves of contrast medium outline the subdural space, the central column being subarachnoid and moving freely onto the clivus upon tilting. (C) (D) Extra-arachnoid oil, partly subdural and partly extradural. No fluid level could be shown with the patient erect, oil tracking along the nerve root sheaths beyond the vertebral bodies is a feature of contrast medium injected extradurally.

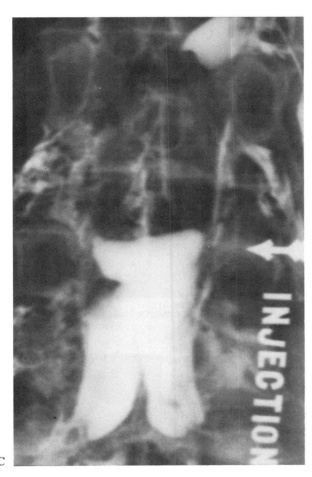

C

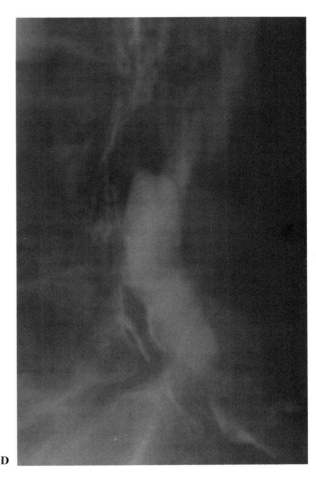

D

Strain, 1944) marked the introduction of myelography as a routine diagnostic investigation in clinical practice. For a quarter of a century, the term "myelography" remained synonymous throughout the English-speaking world with Pantopaque oil myelography (Bull, 1971).

Dissatisfaction with both the poor diagnostic potential of Pantopaque and the high incidence of thecal scarring following its use, led to the introduction in 1965 of meglumine iothalamate (Conray 280) and its dimer, meglumine iocarmate (Dimer-X)

for lumbosacral radiculography. The meglumine salts, while providing far better visualization of the fila radicularia and the entire lumbosacral canal, possess two disadvantages: (1) they are neurotoxic and provoke myoclonic spasms if brought into contact with the spinal cord; and (2) they are just as likely to scar the spinal theca as iophenydylate (Ahlgren, 1973; Johnson and Burrows, 1978).

New Philosophy: Metrizamide (Amipaque), a water-soluble contrast medium introduced in the mid-1970s for whole-spine myelography, appears to

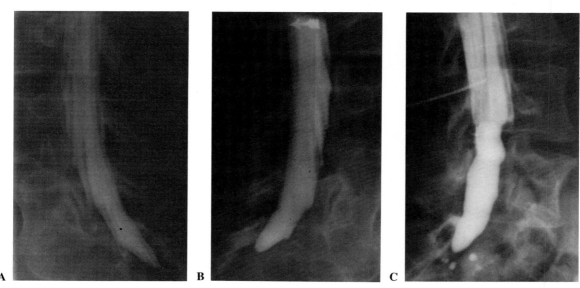

A   B   C

Fig. 11–7 Adhesive arachnoiditis. (A and B) After methylglucamine radiculography. The repeat study 7 months later shows obliteration of the lumbosacral theca and individual nerve roots, due to thecal scarring. (C) Another patient, after laminectomy. Methylglucamine radiculogram reveals normal nerve roots of the cauda equina above the level of L4 vertebra, with thecal constriction and irregularity ("rat's tail") below this level—typical appearances of more advanced scarring.

percent of the Conray patients (Johnson and Burrows, 1978). However, despite this high incidence of scarring it appears that only a relatively small proportion of patients exhibit symptoms that are sufficiently severe to justify repeat myelography—less than 6 percent of this series. Laminectomy also scars the theca, and laminectomy following myelography may produce more arachnoiditis than myelography alone.

THE NEURORADIOLOGY OF THE VERTEBRAL COLUMN

Scoliosis

Radiological evaluation is an essential part of the diagnosis of any case of scoliosis, and such patients should always be subjected to careful neuroradiological examination. The preoperative preparation of severe scoliotic patients should include myelography (preferably gas), in order to exclude neurological causes such as syringomyelia. In infants and young children with severe scoliosis, it is unusual not to find a cause; so-called idiopathic infantile scoliosis may complicate an intraspinal tumor. In the large series reported by Banna and Gryspeerdt (1971), scoliosis was the dominant feature of the four children with extensive lesions—three were intramedullary gliomas and one a voluminous arteriovenous malformation. It does not usually occur in localized tumors or spinal dysraphism. About 10 percent of cases of generalized neurofibromatosis are complicated by scoliosis. Although a sharp-an-

gle curve involving the thoracic spine is said to be characteristic of neurofibromatosis, the degree of scoliotic curvature varies greatly. The scoliosis of this condition is one of two types: (1) neuropathic, caused by intraspinal or paraspinal tumors, or both; or (2) osteopathic, due to a primary developmental mesodermal deficiency of vertebral molding or secondary deformity from an associated thoracic meningocele (Leeds and Jacobson, 1976). Friedreich's ataxia may be complicated by scoliosis, and less often Charcot-Marie-Tooth neuropathy.

Symptomatic Congenital Deformities
Certain congenital deformities of the vertebral column produce neurological deficits that may be halted or reversed by surgical intervention. They comprise a wide variety of conditions which for convenience of discussion are grouped as follows:
1. Bony abnormalities of the craniovertebral angle such as atlanto-occipital assimilation, separate odontoid process and the Klippel-Feil syndrome. These are discussed fully in Chapter 9.
2. Generalized affections, disturbances of the following normal processes:

Intrauterine development: rubella (scoliosis)

Growth of bone, cartilage and/or connective tissue: achondroplasia, mucopolysaccharidosis IV (Morquio-Brailsford's osteochondrodystrophy), dysostosis multiplex (gargoylism), osteopetrosis, osteogenesis imperfecta, generalized neurofibromatosis, idiopathic canal stenosis.

Metabolism: hypophosphatasia, ochronosis.
3. Spinal dysraphism, the term first used by Lich-

tenstein in 1940 to denote those malformations involving any or all of the tissues of the midline of the back.

Textbooks of pediatric and skeletal radiology should be consulted for details of the generalized affections and their differential diagnosis. For a discussion of the way in which they may affect the capacity of the spinal canal, see the section below, Spinal Stenosis.

Generalized Neurofibromatosis: The spinal neurological lesions of this protean congenital abnormality indicate that it is caused by faulty development of mesoderm as well as neuroectoderm. In the past, it has been assumed that the deformities of mesodermal structures encountered in the disease are secondary to neuroectodermal ones, e.g., that the vertebral deformities are always the result of pressure erosion of adjacent neurofibromata. However, it is now clear that the vertebral anomalies may be a true mesodermal dysplasia, occurring in the absence of adjacent neoplasm or meningocele (Laws and Pallis, 1963; Leeds and Jacobson, 1976).

The following signs may be encountered singly, or in various combinations, in the plain radiographs (Hunt and Pugh, 1961). Cutaneous stigmata are not invariably present, therefore these features should always prompt consideration of the diagnosis of generalized neurofibromatosis:

Scoliosis or kyphoscoliosis

Abnormal texture of vertebrae (Murray and Jacobson, 1977)

Scalloped vertebral body: "capstan" deformity (Fig. 10-8)

Enlarged vertebral foramen(ina)

Eroded pedicle(s) (Fig. 11-8).

Paravertebral soft tissue shadow

Associated bone anomalies (spina bifida, vertebral fusion, "ribbon" ribs)

If paraparesis is present, myelography is necessary to explain the causative mechanism of the particular radiological sign. In Figure 11-8 the eroded pedicles and scalloped vertebrae were caused by dural ectasia and a spinal neurofibroma. In Figure 11-9 similar features were due to an associated meningocele. Some authors, including Hilton and McCarthy (1959), believe that in the presence of generalized neurofibromatosis, a thoracic paravertebral shadow is more likely to be a meningocele than a neurogenic tumor. In patients who have no neurological deficit, adjacent vertebral and rib deformities may be sufficiently characteristic of this disease for the correct diagnosis to be made without resorting to myelography (Miles, Pennybacker and Sheldon, 1969).

Spinal Dysraphism: Lichtenstein intended this term to denote those malformations which occur as the result of incomplete fusion of the embryonic structures of the dorsal midline. The term has since been expanded to include the associated abnormalities caused by, or resulting from, this incomplete fusion (Till, 1968). If membranes of the spinal theca protrude beyond the limits of the canal, with or

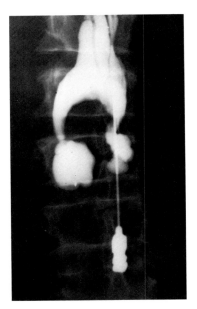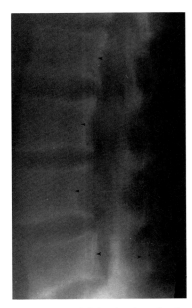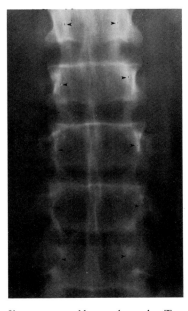

Fig. 11–8 A patient with generalized neurofibromatosis and a high lumbar intradural neurofibroma, proved by myelography. Tomography shows multivertebral posterior scalloping and pedicular erosion *(arrowheads)*. This dural ectasia may be related to a secondary effect of the tumor which, by obstructing the subarachnoid space, produces a chronic hyperpressure system leading to widening of the spinal canal or as a consequence of dural ectasia.

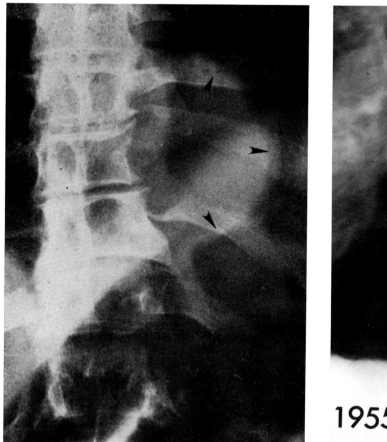

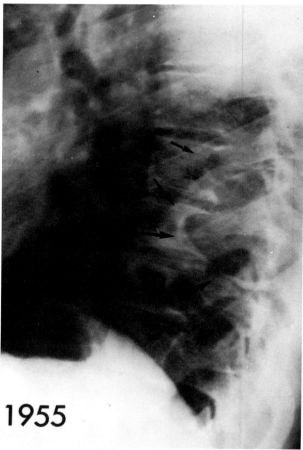

1955

Fig. 11–9 A 24-year-old man with generalized neurofibromatosis. Bone changes are visible similar to those present in Figure 11–8, being associated with a thoracic meningocele. The patient was asymptomatic, and these appearances were discovered in the course of routine chest radiography, viz., a large paravertebral opacity *(arrowheads)* and slight scoliosis concave towards the opacity, erosion of the heads and necks of the 9th and 10th ribs, lateral and posterior scalloping of the bodies of the 8th–12th vertebrae *(arrows)* ("capstan deformity"), erosion of the 10th–12th left pedicles, and widening of the corresponding interpedicular diameters. No intraspinal tumor was found. This case was described and illustrated by J. Miles, J. Pennybacker and P. Sheldon in *The Journal of Neurology, Neurosurgery and Psychiatry, 32,* 99–110, 1969.

without cord or nerve roots, or if the cord lies exposed in the midline of the back, the condition is called *spina bifida cystica.* In this condition, the protruding sac may be filled only with cerebrospinal fluid (meningocele) or it may also contain neural elements (myelomeningocele); a complicating hydrocephalus considerably worsens the prognosis. For the neuroradiologist, the challenge lies in elucidating the nature of the less overt form of congenital deformity, so-called *occult spinal dysraphism.* Under this term are included various anomalies which may cause pes cavus, enuresis or neurological deficits in children. Diagnosis and treatment is only possible with the aid of "dedicated" myelography.

Plain radiographs always reveal some abnormality of the vertebral column. Till (1968) found the following signs: spina bifida (74%), widened vertebral canal (66%), midline bony spur (42%), abnormal laminae (41%) and fused vertebral bodies (21%). The pedicles accompanying the abnormally wide interpedicular diameter are often not deformed (see Fig. 11–15).

Chronic Raised Intraspinal Pressure

An acute pressure syndrome analogous to the "pressure sella" and other radiological signs of raised intracranial pressure does not occur in the spine. However, a chronic hyperpressure state may be produced by intradural and other spinal masses that grow very slowly or by lesions which have been present since birth. The plain-film changes are:

1. Thinning of both pedicles—usually of several adjacent vertebrae—due to pressure erosion of their medial surfaces, with consequent increase in the interpedicular diameter.

2. Smooth excavation of the posterior border of

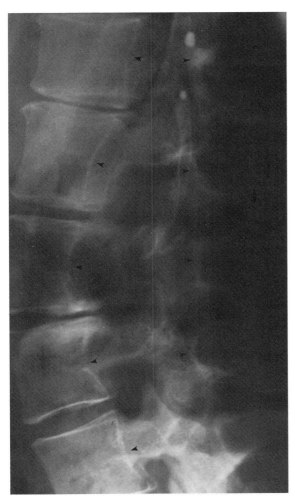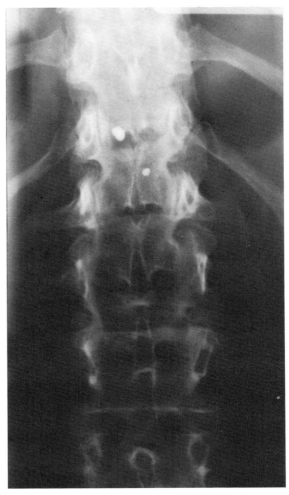

Fig. 11—10 Multivertebral posterior scalloping and interpedicular widening caused by a spinal tumor. The patient was a 50-year-old woman with an ependymoma infiltrating the cauda equina over five segments and exerting direct pressure on the bony walls of the spinal canal. In the lateral radiograph the arrowheads point to erosion of the bases of the spinous processes and posterior scalloping of the vertebral bodies.

the affected vertebrae (posterior scalloping).

3. (Sometimes) excavation of the base of the affected spinous processes, due to pressure erosion of the posterior aspect of the spinal canal.

Although relatively rare, this picture is most frequently produced by an ependymoma of the conus medullaris or cauda equina (Fig. 11 – 10). Very occasionally a solitary neurofibroma (Fig. 11 – 8) or a meningioma may do so. Other space-occupying lesions to be considered are bulky and slow-growing entities such as intraspinal cysts (Murray, 1959; Teng and Papatheodorou, 1966), dermoids, epidermoids and lipomas, and — in the cervical spine — syringomyelia. Several adult cases of multivertebral scalloping associated with uncontrolled communicating hydrocephalus have been reported (Shealy, LeMay and Haddad, 1964).

In the cervical region the sagittal diameter widens ahead of the interpedicular diameter, because of the shape of the spinal canal at this level (Boijsen, 1954; Burrows, 1963). This situation is reversed in the thoracic and lumbar spines where the pedicles erode first. Consequently, the earliest sign of an intraspinal space-occupying lesion at these levels is an increased interpedicular diameter. Posterior vertebral scalloping occurs late, it is believed, as a result of the protective cushion of the posterior longitudinal ligament (Wells, Spillane and Bligh, 1959). Excavation of a single vertebra at any level is probably always caused by tumor (Fig. 11 – 11).

Multivertebral scalloping is a more difficult diagnostic problem. For instance, it is known that a relatively small tumor such as a meningioma may erode the pedicles of bodies of several vertebrae distal to its own level — possibly by causing a closed hyperpressure system through obstruction of cerebrospinal fluid pathway. Secondly, posterior scalloping is not always the result of pressure erosion: Table

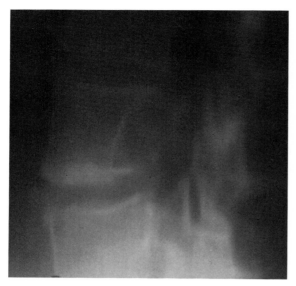
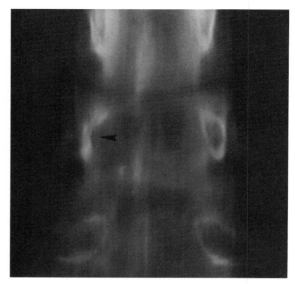

Fig. 11–11 Solitary posterior vertebral scalloping and single pedicular deformity *(arrowhead)* due to direct pressure erosion from a neurofibroma.

Table 11–1 Posterior Vertebral Scalloping

1. Increased intraspinal pressure
    A. Localized – intradural neoplasms, including multiple neurofibromata
    – intraspinal cysts
    – syringomyelia
    B. Generalized – longstanding communicating hydrocephalus
2. Congenital skeletal disorders
    A. Idiopathic (Jefferson, 1955)
    B. Generalized neurofibromatosis
    C. Marfan's syndrome
    D. Ehlers-Danlos's syndrome
    E. Mucoploysaccharidosis IV (Morquio-Brailsford's disease)
    F. Dysostosis multiplex (gargoylism, Hurler's disease)
    G. Osteogenesis imperfecta tarda
3. Small spinal canal – achondroplasia
4. Normal variant – physiological scalloping

Modified from Mitchell, Lourie and Berne, 1967

11–1 lists several generalized skeletal disorders which deform the vertebral bodies and alter the capacity of the spinal canal. As a rule the pedicles retain their normal shape in these disorders — an important radiological feature in the differential diagnosis of intraspinal masses.

Generalized Neurofibromatosis: See previous section, Symptomatic Congenital Deformities.

Marfan's Syndrome: The spinal canal enlarges in both sagittal and coronal planes and involves several vertebrae, sometimes associated with a scoliosis — thus simulating an intraspinal tumor and generalized neurofibromatosis (Nelson, 1958).

Ehlers-Danlos's Syndrome: This is another connective tissue disorder in which the vertebral scalloping is attributed to loss of the protective action of the posterior longitudinal ligament (Mitchell, Lourie and Berne, 1967).

Mucopolysaccharidosis IV (Morquio-Brailsford's Disease): Universal vertebra plana is present, with characteristic deformities of the anterior margins of the bodies. Thorocolumbar scoliosis is a feature.

Dysostosis Multiplex (Gargoylism, Hurler's Disease): "Beaking" of the anteroinferior corner of a deformed thorocolumbar vertebra, with secondary kyphosis, is the typical picture. There is marked scalloping and expansion of the lower lumbar spinal canal.

Achondroplasia: Characteristic is the flattened and triangular appearance of the bodies of T12, L1 and L2 vertebrae, which have concave posterior margins. The extensive vertebral scalloping may be accentuated by the compressed neural tissue — see next section, Spinal Stenosis.

Osteogenesis Imperfecta Tarda: Although not strictly relevant to this section, the adult type of this disease may give rise to differential diagnostic difficulties, e.g., the combination of multivertebral deformity ("fish vertebra" and multiple fractures) and ribbon-like ribs.

Normal Variant: Vertebral scalloping to a minor degree may be a normal variant, and occasionally myelography may be necessary to prove it.

Canal Stenosis

Constitutional or congenital narrowing of the spinal canal is an important concept in neuroradiology. In the cervical and lumbar regions, where degenerative joint disease is prominent in later life, the small spinal canal is of etiological importance. Even without supervening degeneration, however, the capacity of the canal may be too small to avoid compression of the neural tissue — the so-called tight dural canal (Bradley and Banna, 1968).

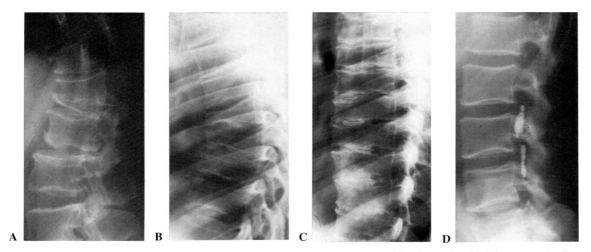

Fig. 11–12 Stenosis of the spinal canal—congenital and developmental causes. (A) Achondroplasia. (B) Scheuermann's disease. (C) Mucopolysaccharidosis IV (Morquio-Brailsford's disease). (D) Congenital constitutional narrowing.

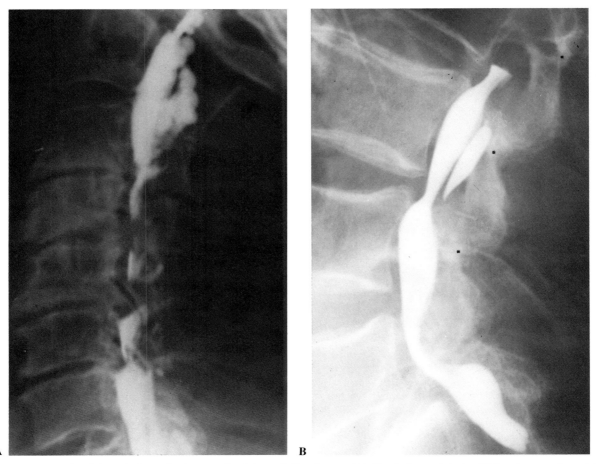

Fig. 11–13 Stenosis of the spinal canal—degenerative joint and disc disease. (A) Cervical spondylosis. (B) Lumbar apophyseal-joint degeneration. Black dots indicate the bases of the spinous processes of the lumbar vertebrae.

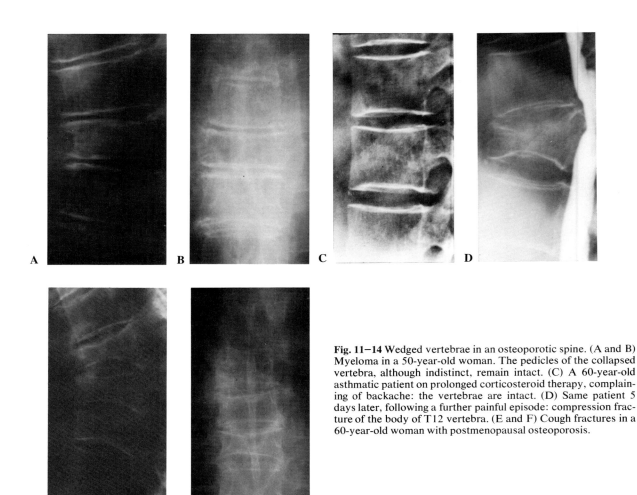

Fig. 11−14 Wedged vertebrae in an osteoporotic spine. (A and B) Myeloma in a 50-year-old woman. The pedicles of the collapsed vertebra, although indistinct, remain intact. (C) A 60-year-old asthmatic patient on prolonged corticosteroid therapy, complaining of backache: the vertebrae are intact. (D) Same patient 5 days later, following a further painful episode: compression fracture of the body of T12 vertebra. (E and F) Cough fractures in a 60-year-old woman with postmenopausal osteoporosis.

1. Primary Congenital Type. This type tends to clinically present in early middle age when aggravated by supervening degenerative changes (Hinck and Sachdev, 1966). It may be related to body habitus, since the victims are often barrel-shaped, short-limbed individuals (Fig. 11−12D).

2. Achondroplasia. The impaired enchondral ossification of this condition gives rise to incomplete development of the neural arches. The spinal canal narrows progressively toward the lumbosacral junction in both its interpedicular and sagittal diameters, in contrast to the increasing diameters normally seen (Fig. 11−12A). The resulting chronic hyperpressure state within the spinal canal produces posterior scalloping of the vertebral bodies. The adult victim is vulnerable to paraplegia due to compression of the spinal cord or cauda equina, resulting from disc prolapse or degenerative disease, or both (Schreiber and Rosenthal, 1952; Epstein and Malis, 1955).

3. Juvenile Discogenic Disorder (Scheuermann's Disease). This self-limiting disorder of adolescence may occasionally be complicated by stenosis of a segment of the thoracic dural tube (Fig. 11−12B, Lindgren, 1941). An association exists between Scheuermann's disease and arachnoid cysts, first reported by Cloward and Bucy (1937).

4. Chronic Fluorine Intoxication: About half of the symptomatic cases of skeletal fluorosis present with neurological deficit − a radiculopathy caused by nerve root compression due to periforaminal bone thickening, or a myelopathy resulting from narrowing of the spinal canal (Siddiqui, 1955; Singh and Jolly, 1961). Canal stenosis is caused by exostoses arising from the posterior surface of the vertebral body, or thickening of the laminae; in the most severe cases, the canal may be almost completely obliterated. Ligamentous calcification may produce the appearance of a "poker spine."

5. Degenerative Joint and Disc Disease: Profound and sometimes obliterating stenosis of the cervical or lumbar spinal canal may be produced by degeneration of the intervertebral joints. Degenerative osteophytosis encroaching upon the canal is far

more likely to arise from the apophyseal joints (= osteoarthritis) than from the intervertebral disc margins (= spondylosis), and both are as frequently encountered by the neuroradiologist as acute disc prolapse (Fig. 11–13).

In the cervical region, the clinical disorder associated with these changes is usually a combination of constitutional narrowing and early osteophytic ingrowth upon the spinal canal (Burrows, 1963; Stoltmann and Blackwood, 1964; Nurick, 1972). Identical pathological mechanisms narrow the lumbar canal, producing intermittent ischemia of the cauda equina or radicular signs (Epstein, Epstein and Lavine, 1962; Joffe, Appleby and Arjona, 1966; Jones and Thomson, 1968; Ramani, 1976; Roberts, 1978).

Generalized Vertebral Involvement
Tables 11–2 and 11–3 list the main lesions that involve more than one vertebra. Certain diseases such as myeloma may present as a solitary focus, possibly as a result of a stress complication, e.g., pathological fracture (Fig. 11–14), before the disease spreads multifocally or diffusely throughout the vertebral column. Such lesions and the tests and criteria for their diagnosis are dealt with in the next two sections, The Solitary Focus and Lesions that Cross the Disc Space.

The Solitary Focus
This section and the next one, Lesions that Cross the Disc Space, deal with the case in which a solitary bone lesion is found in the vertebral column. Myelography usually reveals a total extradural ob-

Table 11–3 Vertebral Porosis

Defective Production of Bone Matrix	
A. Protein intake	Starvation, anorexia nervosa
B. Osteoid	Osteogenesis imperfecta
C. Vitamin C	Scurvy
D. Sex hormones	Postmenopausal (senile)
	Post-castration
E. Physical activity	Disuse, immobilization
Excess Hormone	
A. Thyroid	Thyrotoxicosis
B. Adrenal-cortical	Cushing's syndrome
	Iatrogenic hypercorticism
C. Pituitary	Acromegaly
Neoplastic Infiltration	Metastatic malignancy
	Myelomatosis
	Leukemia

struction at this level, and a skeletal survey shows no other osseous involvement.

Diagnostic interpretation of the plain radiograph is greatly improved by two steps: (1) attention to the clinical findings, which enables the radiologist to focus his attention on the area most likely to contain a lesion, and (2) biplanar tomography of any lesion demonstrated. In this way, minor but significant features, e.g., pedicular deformity and subchondral erosions, will not be missed (Fig. 11–15). Often the pattern of abnormalities involving the spinal canal, vertebral body, pedicles, disc space and paravertebral region is not sufficiently specific to permit firm conclusions, beyond indicating the level of spinal involvement. However, occasionally incontrovertible signs, such as an eroded pedicle or collapse or sclerosis of a vertebral body will confirm the diagnosis of spinal metastases in a patient with cancer.

Table 11–2 Vertebral Sclerosis

Diffuse	Patchy	Solitary ("Ivory Vertebra")
Neoplastic metastases	Neoplastic metastases	Lymphoma
– prostate (common)	– prostate (common)	Paget's disease
– bronchus (rare)	– breast	Mastocytosis
– stomach (rare)	– breast after hormone therapy	Neoplastic metastases, usually prostatic
Paget's disease	– urinary bladder	Primary bone tumor
Fluorosis	– medulloblastoma (children)	
Osteopetrosis	Lymphoma (Hodgkin's disease)	
Idiopathic hypercalcemia	Degenerative disc disease (spondylosis)	
Myeloid metaplasia	Neuropathic disease (Charcot spine)	
Sickle-cell anemia	Paget's disease	
Osteogenesis imperfecta	– multicentric osteosarcoma	
Secondary hyperparathyroidism	Osteomyelitis	
due to chronic renal failure	– low-grade staphylococcal	
Osteomalacia due to hypophosphatasia	– syphilis	
Mast cell disease	– brucellosis	
	– typhoid fever	
	– actinomycosis	
	– coccidiomycosis	
	– chronic pelvic infection	
	Healing states (inflammatory or traumatic)	
	Chronic anemias (sickle-cell, etc.)	
	Mast cell disease	
	Tuberous sclerosis	

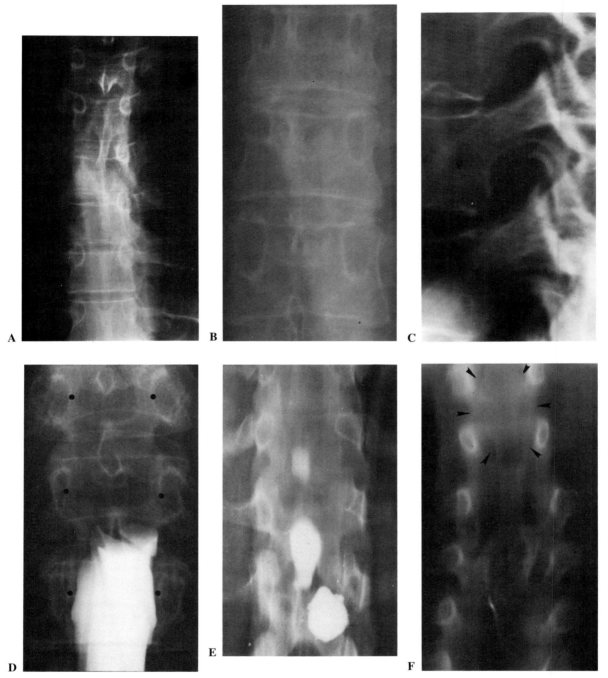

Fig. 11–15 Abnormal pedicles and the interpedicular diameter. (A) Right pedicles of T6 and T7 vertebrae are destroyed by metastatic bronchial cancer. (B and C) Lower half of the right pedicle of T10 vertebra is eroded by a dumbbell neurofibroma. The lateral radiograph shows the enlarged intervertebral foramen. (D) The left pedicle of L1 vertebra has a pointed lower tip, due to erosion of its medial surface by a neurofibroma. This minor bone change might have been dismissed as a normal variant, if measurement *(black dots)* had not revealed interpedicular widening: T12 = 33 mm., L1 = 36 mm., L2 = 34. (E) Bizarre multipedicular scalloping and interpedicular widening due to multiple intradural arachnoid cysts (same case as Fig. 11 – 30). (F) Progressive widening of the lower lumbar canal due to spinal dysraphism, individual pedicles retain their normal shape. This tomogram of the gas myelogram outlines an intradural dermoid at the T12 – L1 level *(arrowheads),* with the cord tethered and reaching below L3.

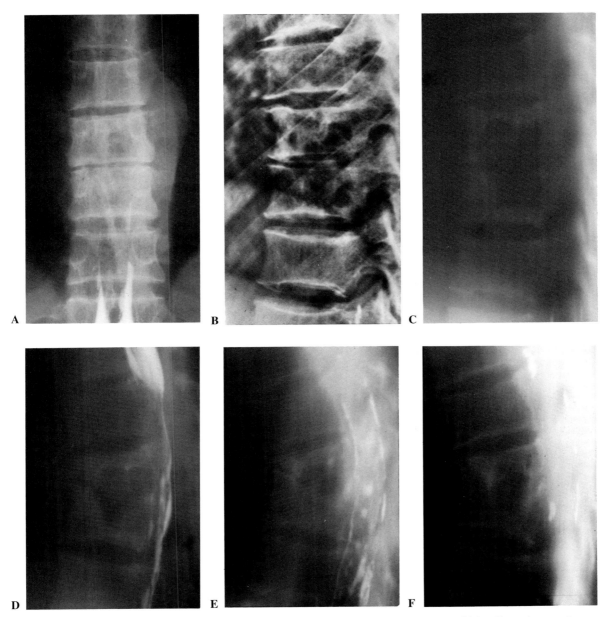

Fig. 11–22 Spinal tuberculosis. A 35-year-old man with paraplegia of sudden onset. (A and B) Initial radiographs reveal a narrowed T8–9 disc space and a prominent paravertebral soft tissue shadow—hallmarks of tuberculous spondylitis. (C) Lateral tomography shows a cavity within the bodies of T8 and T9 vertebrae. (D, E, F) Serial lateral tomograms made over the next 3 years show the changes from destruction to consolidation resulting from therapy. Features to compare: progressive collapse of the vertebral body, reduction in size of the tuberculous cavity, and a theca initially obliterated but with patency later re-established. Reproduced by courtesy of Dr. R. O. Murray, Lord Mayor Treloar's Hospital, Alton.

children and the following in the adult: stress fracture, primary bone tumor such as aneurysmal bone cyst, hemangioma and chordoma, and Paget's disease, in addition to metastatic cancer or myeloma (Fig. 11–24). Partial destruction of adjacent bodies indicates infection, but occasionally neoplastic processes such as myeloma, chordoma and lymphoma may spread across a disc space. The commonest cause of a paravertebral mass is hemorrhage associated with vertebral collapse due to metastatic cancer. Apart from raising the possibility of tuberculous infection, the presence of a paravertebral mass possesses no real value in differential diagnosis.

Ankylosis of a single intervertebral joint is commonly due to previous, healed infection. If the deformity is slight, congenital or postsurgical, fusion should be considered. Multivertebral ankylosis

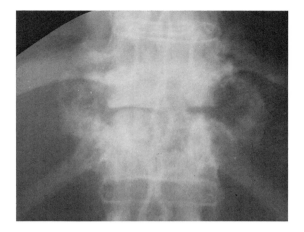

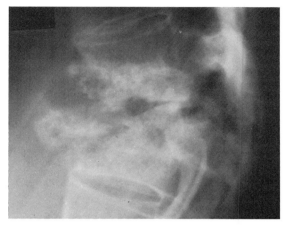

Fig. 11–23 Pyogenic spondylitis complicating corticosteroid therapy in ankylosing spondylitis. Destruction of adjacent parts of the T11 and T12 vertebrae, with florid new bone formation (buttressing).

usually represents end-stage ankylosing spondylitis but congenital and post-rheumatoid fusion must be excluded.

MYELOGRAPHIC DIAGNOSIS AND INTERPRETATION

Topographical Interpretation and Type Diagnosis
Spinal lesions are usually classified according to their anatomical site in relation to the cord and meninges. Using mass lesions as an example, this classification is shown diagrammatically in Figure 11–25. *Intramedullary lesions* lie within the cord and deform its external shape; the majority are gliomas which expand it. *Intradural lesions* lie within the spinal tube but outside the cord, and are usually meningiomas, neurofibromas or arteriovenous malformations. *Extradural lesions* lie completely outside the dural tube which they compress against the walls of the spinal canal; the commonest are degen-

erative joint lesions or neoplastic deposits. Table 11–4 is a comprehensive list of compressive spinal lesions.

Myelography is necessary for differential diagnosis, which consists in providing answers to the following three questions:

What is the level of the lesion?

Is the lesion extradural or intradural? If intradural and above the cauda, is it intramedullary or extramedullary?

What is its likely nature?

Diagnostic accuracy can only be guaranteed if the two criteria of myelography are fulfilled, viz., a full-diameter study is undertaken and at least two radiographic projections of the lesion are obtained. For example, a widened cervical cord in the anteroposterior view, suggesting an intramedullary mass, may be shown in the cross-table lateral view to be the result of a prolapsed cervical disc. See Errors, Omissions and Artifacts, page 486.

Level. The precise level of a myelographic lesion

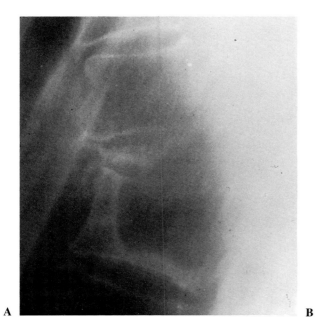

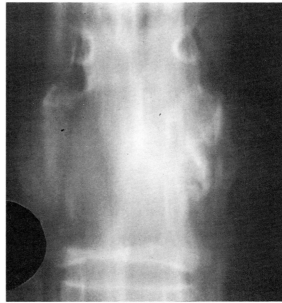

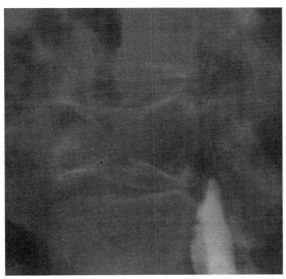

Fig. 11–24 Spinal myeloma. A 48-year-old man complained of girdle pain in the T6 distribution. (A and B) Frontal and lateral tomograms show collapse of the body of T6 and a lytic lesion of the body of T7, with destruction of the posterior elements of the vertebra. (C) Chance finding of an asymptomatic deposit in the body of L3, which is partly collapsed. The disease process, although crossing the T6–7 disc space, has not completely destroyed the epiphyseal plates of the two affected vertebrae. Reproduced by courtesy of Mr. G. Neil-Dwyer, F.R.C.S., The Brook Hospital, London.

and its relationship to the spinal cord and vertebral column, represents information that is even more important to the surgeon in assessing operability than to the radiologist concerned with diagnosis. For this purpose, a lateral (horizontal-ray, cross-table) view is essential, for two reasons: (1) in the absence of plain-film changes, reliance upon the anteroposterior view only may result in erroneous assessment of the level of a total block, which may exceed a vertebra in height; and (2) to assess forward or backward displacement of the cord and/or dural tube within the spinal canal. The anteroposterior view may be unhelpful and even misleading in anterior-lying lesions such as a centrally prolapsed

intervertebral disc: the lateral view will reveal the true nature of the lesion, by showing that the theca is displaced backward at the level of the intervertebral space (Fig. 11–35).

If the block demonstrated following lumbar injection does not correspond to the level of the patient's clinical deficit, a suboccipital injection of contrast medium is necessary to exclude a second lesion, or to reveal its full length.

Topographical Localization. Two myelographic signs indicate whether a lesion is extradural, intradural or intramedullary — the shape of the dural tube and the configuration and position of the cord within it. Topographical diagnosis is explained in Figure

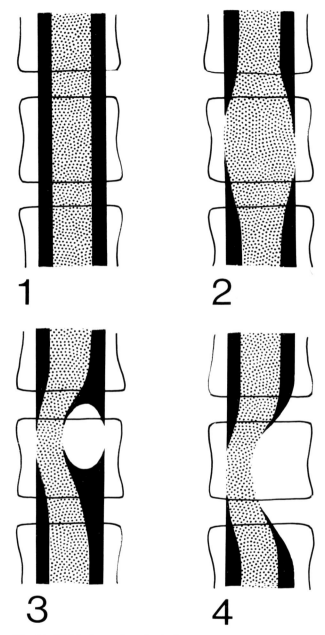

Fig. 11–25 Myelography of spinal tumors. Topographical classification. 1 – Normal anatomy. 2 – Intramedullary. 3 – Intradural. 4 – Extradural. After R. S. C. Couch in the *Proceedings of the Royal Society of Medicine, 55,* 101 – 103, 1962.

11 – 25. The normal cord is seen in anteroposterior, lateral or oblique myelograms as a central filling defect flanked by contrast bands of equal thickness.

(1) Intramedullary tumors widen the cord at the expense of the lateral bands. The bands may be reduced to thin streaks over the segment of the lesion, as in syringomyelia, or they may taper to a complete block; accurate topographical localization is then impossible (Fig. 11 – 26). Widening of the

cord, or of a segment, is not always caused by a glioma-type neoplasm such as ependymoma. In the cervical region, syringomyelia and cervical spondylosis may produce appearances indistinguishable in anteroposterior view from a solid neoplasm of the cord. However, the lateral view will reveal the true state of affairs with disc protrusion. Rare causes of "fat cord" are listed in Table 11 – 5. Focal atrophy of the cord which is usually syringomyelic or post-inflammatory in origin, may be demonstrable only by gas myelography (Fig. 11 – 6).

(2) Intradural extramedullary lesions lie beside, in front or behind the spinal cord. If space-occupying, they will displace it from its central position. The contrast-filled bands on either side of the tumor are altered – one is widened and the other narrowed. The contrast crescent outlining the tumor is sharply defined, so-called "capping" of the tumor (Fig. 11 – 27). If the tumor lies alongside the cord and displaces it sideways, this characteristic appearance will be seen in the anteroposterior view. If the tumor lies in front or behind, the appearance will be visible only in the lateral view. Surgeons who prefer to attack tumors lying anterior to the thoracic cord by lateral costotransversectomy, rather than by conventional laminectomy, can obtain this information only from lateral myelography.

(3) Extradural lesions manifest clinically as paraplegia, by compressing the dural tube. Myelography shows that both tube and cord are displaced and compressed (Fig. 11 – 28). Completely obstructed lesions have a pinched or nondescript appearance and a widened cord shadow in one plane which resembles an intramedullary tumor. Below the conus, the compressed cauda equina often provides a feathered or serrated interface. Topographical localization reduces the diagnostic options. The eight conditions marked in Table 11 – 4 account for the majority of lesions encountered in routine practice. Ten-year totals of the Wessex Neurological Centre, Southampton indicate the following:

Extradural lesions: 850 (discogenic or joint disease, metastases)

Intradural lesions: 125 (neurofibroma and meningioma equally)

Intramedullary: 30 (syringomyelia and gliomas).

Type Diagnosis. Intradural tumors and arteriovenous malformations can usually be recognized from their myelographic characteristics. However, in most extradural and intramedullary lesions, a type diagnosis will depend on the presence of associated plain-film changes. The following advice is helpful in interpretation:

1. Nearly 90 percent of patients with extradural metastases exhibit radiographic evidence of bone destruction, usually involving a pedicle or the vertebral body (Sellwood, 1972).

2. Degenerative joint or discogenic disease is the commonest lesion of the lumbar spine. The neuro-

Table 11–4 Compressive Spinal Lesions

	Extradural	Intradural-Extramedullary	Intradural-Intramedullary
Congenital	Craniovertebral-angle lesions Achondroplasia Mucopolysacchoridosis IV Meningocele Arachnoid cyst		Arachnoid cyst Dermoid Epidermoid Lipoma Hamartoma Teratoma Neurenteric cyst
Traumatic	Arachnoid cyst Fracture/dislocation Hematoma		Syringomyelia Hematomyelia
Inflammatory	Abscess (pyogenic, etc.) Granuloma (tuberculoma, etc.) Echinococcosis	Arachnoiditis	Granuloma Abscess Myelitis Schistosomiasis
Neoplasms	**Secondary deposits** Hemopoietic and reticuloendothelial lesions (myeloma, leukemia, lymphoma, etc.) Primary vertebral tumors (sarcomas, giant cell tumor of bone, aneurysmal bone cyst, benign osteoblastoma, chondromyxoid fibroma, hemangioma, chondroma, osteoma. Intraspinal tumors (neuroblastoma, sarcoma, hemangioblastoma, hemangiopericytoma, meningioma (rare), neurofibroma.	Neoplastic metastases (rare) Cauda equina deposits (cancer, leukemia, lymphoma and CNS seedlings) **Meningioma** Meningeal sarcoma **Neurofibroma** Sarcoma Ependymoma	**Glioma-type tumors** (ependymoma, astrocytoma) Capillary hemangioblastoma Lipoma
Miscellaneous	Sarcoidosis Fluorosis Urate deposits (gout) Paget's disease Arteriovenous malformation Extradural hemorrhage Extramedullary hemopoiesis	**Arterovenous malformation** Arachnoid cyst	**Syringomyelia** Hydromyelia Hematomyelia Transverse myelitis in multiple sclerosis
Degenerative	**Spondylosis** **Disc prolapse**		

Note: The 8 commonest lesions are printed in bold type.

radiologist's duty is to search for an alternative cause of the myelographic abnormality, e.g., neurofibroma, metastatic cancer, myeloma.

3. Irregular pattern or poor flow of the contrast medium. Firstly, verify by erect screening that the contrast medium has not been injected subdurally or epidurally. Secondly, search for the serpiginous vessels of an arteriovenous malformation. Thereafter consider causes of adhesive arachnoiditis and conus infiltration.

4. Dilated and tortuous vessels often accompany total myelographic obstructions caused by neoplastic or disc disease (Fig. 11–10). Arteriovenous malformations infrequently produce total obstruction.

Compressive Lesions

Neoplastic Metastases

A. Extradural: Of all cases of metastatic cancer that present with neurological signs, 40 percent involve the extracranial nervous system; 70 percent of these arise from bronchus, breast or prostate. The vast majority of deposits are extradural (Fig. 11–28). Nearly 90 percent of these have plain-film changes: vertebral body altered (83%), pedicle destroyed (30%) or paravertebral soft tissue shadow (15%) (Sellwood, 1972). Diagnosis is usually difficult only in the 10 percent in whom no plain-film evidence is present. Especially if there are no signs of a primary tumor, non-neoplastic causes of extradural obstruction must be considered (see below).

In lymphoma the axial skeleton is involved in 10 to 20 percent of patients, but only a small proportion of these develop paraplegia. The bone changes in Hodgkin's lymphoma are sclerotic or mixed, while those in the non-Hodgkin's types (giant follicular lymphoma, reticulum-cell and lymphomatous sarcoma) are usually lytic (Ngan and Preston, 1975).

B. Intradural: Pathologists not infrequently find cytological or autopsy evidence of seedling spread of intracranial tumors to the spinal canal and cauda equina. The majority are malignant glioblastomas but a greater proportion of medulloblastomas, ependymomas and choroid plexus papillomas exhibit this type of metastasis — probably about 50 percent. The diagnosis is usually made clinically. Oil myelography using a conventional technique rarely reveals the lesion: Bryan (1974) found that the metastases had been shown in only three out of 22 instances revealed by autopsy. With full-diameter myelography the yield is higher (Fig. 11–29). Three patterns

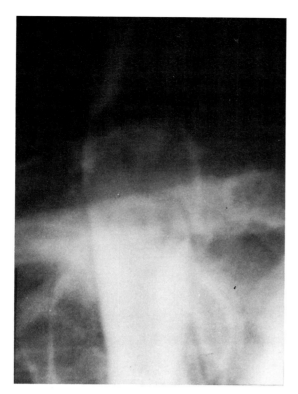 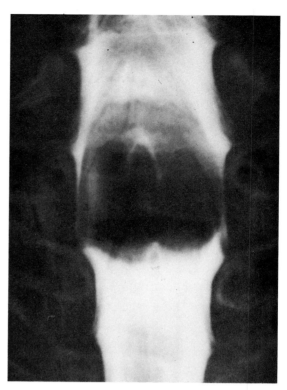

Fig. 11–26 Intramedullary cyst at the T1 level, shown by full-diameter (metrizamide) myelography. Note nodular enlargements of the nerve roots. The cord is widened in both its sagittal and coronal diameters.

are found: (1) Discrete nodular implants upon the spinal cord and cauda equina. The nodules are usually on the posterior aspect of the cord, suggesting that gravity plays a part in their distribution. They vary in size, and if sufficiently large may cause a total obstruction. (2) Diffuse meningeal involvement produces a picture indistinguishable from adhesive arachnoiditis. (3) Diffuse infiltration of individual roots of the cauda equina. This type of intradural infiltration may also complicate extraneurological diseases such as bronchial carcinoma (Guyer, Westbury, and Cook, 1968), lymphoma, leukemia or sarcoidosis (Wood and Bream, 1959).

Table 11–5 The Widened Spinal Cord

Intramedullary	– Ependymoma
	– Astrocytoma
	– Hemangioblastoma
	– Lipoma
	– Hydrosyringomyelia
	– Hematomyelia
	– Cyst
	– Myelitis (postinflammatory or due to demyelinating disease)
	– Schistosomiasis
	– Sarcoidosis
	– Radiation myelopathy
Extramedullary	pressure may cause radiological cord widening:
	– Congenital narrowing of the spinal canal
	– Acquired extradural masses, e.g., arachnoid cyst, hemorrhage, disc prolapse

The myelographic differential diagnosis includes multiple tumors (neurofibromata or ependymomata) artifact (gas bubbles) and—if thickened cords are present—arteriovenous malformation and enlarged nerves, e.g., hypertrophic interstitial polyneuritis (Lewtas and Dimant, 1957) and Charcot-Marie-Tooth's disease (Kremeinitzer, Ager and Zingesser, 1976).

Primary Spinal Tumors
The following groups are included in the Cleveland Clinic series reported by Tucker and his colleagues (1962), who also reviewed the work of Rasmussen, Kernohan and Adson (1940)—a total of nearly 800 spinal tumors:

Primary osteogenic (aneurysmal bone cyst, giant cell tumour, osteoblastoma, chordoma etc.): 12%

Neurofibroma: 28%

Meningioma: 26%

Intramedullary (ependymoma, astrocytoma, "cyst," miscellaneous): 34%

About 50 percent occur in the thoracic spine. Neurofibromata and meningiomas are found in patients aged 50 to 60 years, the remainder are tumors of childhood or adolescence.

Meningioma and Neurofibroma. These benign neoplasms together constitute the largest and surgically most important group of spinal tumors. Traditionally both are described as intradural tumors, but

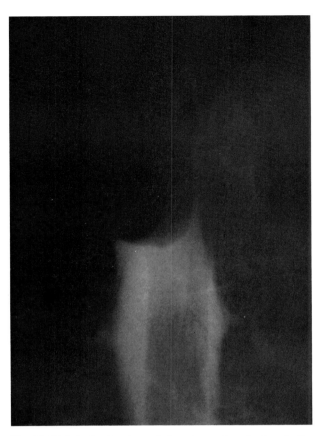

Fig. 11–27 Intradural extramedullary tumor (meningioma), displacing the spinal cord to the left side, and showing the typical sharp "cut-off" of a spinal meningioma or neurofibroma.

10 percent of spinal meningiomas and 30 percent of neurofibromas are extradural (Bull, 1953; Hallpike and Stanley, 1968). Nearly all meningiomas occur in the thoracic spine, and the majority in middle-aged women. Plain-film changes are unusual: meningiomas frequently contain histological deposits of calcium but these are seldom visible radiologically—and only uniquely to the extent shown in Figure 11–16; Pear and Boyd, 1974). By contrast, neurofibromas occur at all levels of the spine. Lumbar extradural neurofibromas may mimic a totally extruded lumbar intervertebral disc. Thoracic and cervical intradural neurofibromas are often dumb-bell tumors, one part of which lies in the spinal canal and the other part in the paravertebral gutter of the thorax or in the soft tissues of the neck. Such a tumor enlarges the intervertebral foramen through which it grows and may deform the pedicle. About 50 percent of spinal neurofibromas show pressure erosion of the adjacent pedicle or posterior scalloping of the vertebral body (Figs. 11–11 and 11–15).

Intramedullary and Other Rare Tumors. Most swellings of the spinal cord are caused by syringomyelia or hydromyelia, usually unassociated with neoplasms—see the Syringomyelia Syndrome, be-low. The commonest true intramedullary neoplasms are ependymomas and astrocytomas. They may produce diffuse widening of the cord over as many as ten segments ("giant tumors of the spinal cord"—Elsberg and Dyke, 1934), or they may be relatively localized (Fig. 11–26). Typically ependymomas of the conus and filum terminale are large and bulky (Fig. 11–10), filling the thecal tube and producing plain-film changes of chronic raised pressure; while those above the filum are often small and show no plain-film changes.

Other excessively rare intramedullary tumors are lipomas, dermoid and epidermoids (pearly tumors) and hemangioblastomas. Spinal hemangioblastomas are encountered as isolated lesions or as part of the Von Hippel-Lindau syndrome (Kendall and Russell, 1966).

Non-Neoplastic Masses
The commonest causes of non-neoplastic compression are degenerative joint disease and prolapsed intervertebral discs, which are discussed below in a separate section. The variety of other non-neoplastic lesions are shown in Table 11–4, and only three individual entities will be dealt with here.

(1) Spontaneous Epidural Hematoma. This rare cause of sudden paraplegia, which often follows unaccustomed exertion, has been attributed to

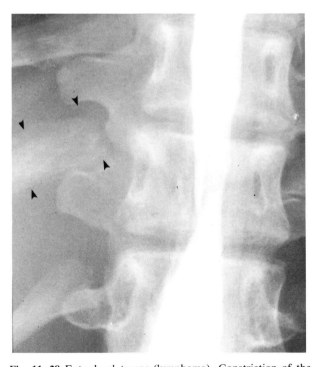

Fig. 11–28 Extradural tumor (lymphoma). Constriction of the dural tube with spinal cord compression at the level of the T11 vertebra. No abnormality of the vertebrae is visible, but the right 11th rib is infiltrated with lymphomatous tumor (arrowheads) and surrounded by a soft-tissue mass.

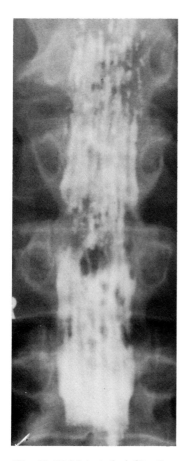

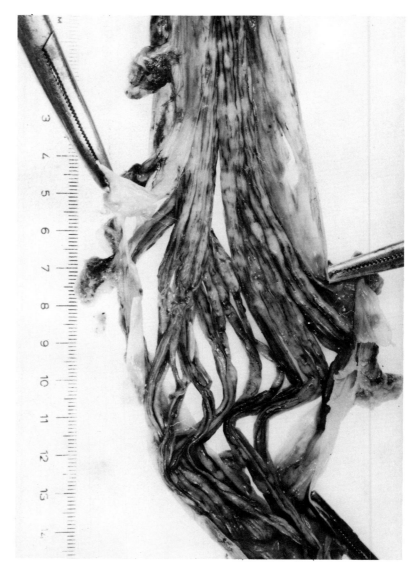

Fig. 11–29 Metastatic infiltration of the cauda equina, in a 72-year-old man with bronchial cancer. This case was published and illustrated by P. B. Guyer, H. Westbury and P. L. Cook in *The British Journal of Radiology, 41,* 615–619, 1968.

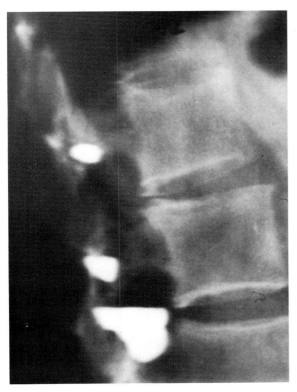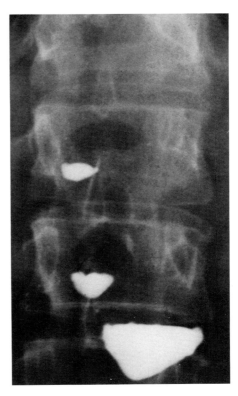

Fig. 11–30 Intradural arachnoid cysts causing intermittent conus and cauda compression. Myelogram with the patient erect demonstrates fluid levels and posterior situation of the cysts in the spinal theca. Same case as in Figure 10–15E.

hemorrhage from an unidentified arteriovenous malformation hypertension, or a coagulation defect; as a rule no cause can be found (Tsai, Popp and Waldman, 1975; Grollmus and Hoff, 1975).

(2) Epidural Granuloma, including Tuberculosis and Pyogenic Abscess. This lesion may follow hematogenous infection from a remote focus or there may be recognizable disc-space changes from an adjacent osseous focus (Robinson and Shapiro, 1967).

(3) Arachnoid Cyst. These cystic pouches which exert their compressive effect through being distended with fluid, may be extradural or intradural, congenital or acquired. Teng and Papatheodorou (1966) compared the intradural variety which lie on the posterior wall of the theca, to the pockets of a jacket which fill only in the erect position, and fail to fill if the patient is first placed head-down and supine. Acquired cysts are post-traumatic in origin, and acquired intradural cysts may complicate arachnoiditis and ankylosing spondylitis. Most arachnoid cysts occur in the thoracic region and a distinct variety is the large sausage-shaped bag of fluid compressing the spinal cord, which is found in kyphoscoliotic young men (Dastur, 1963; Raja and Hankinson, 1970). A wide variety of myelographic deformities is found, often associated with plain-

film changes (Fig. 11–30). The diagnosis may be missed without full-diameter or supine oil myelography.

Degenerative Joint and Disc Diseases
The neurological complications of lumbar disc disease were widely recognized after 1940 when Mixter and Barr confirmed a causal relationship between sciatica and prolapse of a lower lumbar intervertebral disc. Less well established is the concept introduced by Verbiest (1954), of cauda equina compression caused by degenerative encroachment of the posterior articular processes upon the diameter of the spinal canal. It is logical to the neuroradiologist to discuss the appearances of these two disease processes under the same heading, not only because of the overlap in signs and symptoms but also because of the identical and demonstrable mechanical effect produced by both conditions, viz., spinal stenosis.

Clinical Aspects. Both at the cervical and lumbar levels, two clinical patterns are found: cord compression and nerve root irritation. Combined pictures also occur, and if the cauda equina is involved sphincteric disturbances may be prominent. The signs and symptoms exhibited by a particular patient will depend largely on the level of the com-

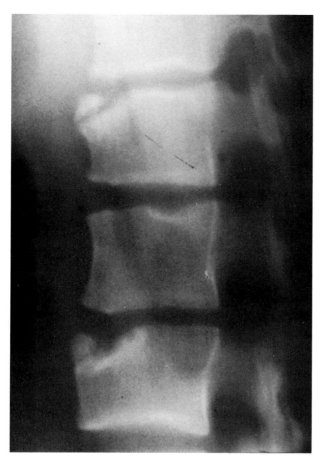

Fig. 11–31 Juvenile discogenic disorder in a youth with backache. Lateral tomograms, showing irregular contours of the anterior one-third of the disc margins of two vertebral bodies caused by fragmentation of the "ring" epiphyses. A Schmorl node is present on the vertebra between. Permanent deformity of the vertebral body may result from this self-limiting disease.

pression. Prolapse of the lumbosacral disc produces sciatica and sensory changes over the dorsum of the foot, while compression of the cauda equina or conus medullaris causes more complex neurological syndromes. One of these is the exercise-related syndrome of "intermittent claudication of the cauda equina" (Blau and Logue, 1961), for which a variety or combination of mechanical factors may be responsible.

It is usually impossible to predict the causal mechanism of compression from the clinical presentation alone, i.e., whether disc prolapse or hypertrophic changes in the apophyseal joints, or rarely, another cause such as spinal neoplasm, is responsible. The correct etiological diagnosis of degenerative disc or joint disease can be provided only by radiological examination.

Radiographic Appearances. Plain radiography is usually more useful in excluding congenital or neoplastic lesions which produce back pain or root

signs, than in contributing materially to the diagnosis of degenerative disc or joint disease. In the latter condition, moreover, the osteophytes that obliterate the intervertebral foramina and/or spinal canal may have a cartilaginous content, therefore only myelography will indicate their true extent.

The following signs indicate disc degeneration: (1) Loss or reversal of the normal cervical or lumbar lordosis. (2) Disc space narrowing. These two signs, with or without associated marginal osteophytosis or sclerosis, may be the only evidence of acute prolapse. Herniation of the nucleus pulposus through the annulus causes neurological signs only if the disc protrusion compresses the neural tube, i.e., if it extends directly backward, or backward and to one side. (3) Schmorl's node. Fissures in the articular plate lead to herniation of the nucleus pulposus into the vertebral body. Although common in autopsy material, relatively few Schmorl's nodes are visible radiographically (Fig. 11–31) and few have any clinical relevance. (4) Ballooning of all the discs in bone-softening diseases such as osteomalacia or osteoporosis, producing biconcave vertebral bodies ("fish spine"). (5) Calcification. Asymptomatic calcification of a solitary disc space in an adult denotes degenerative disease in the nucleus pulposus or annulus fibrosus. More than one disc calcifies in ochronosis. In children, disc space calcification may be painful but reversible: usually, as the calcium is resolved, the pain disappears. (6) Chronic degeneration of a disc causes dehydration and therefore narrowing of the disc space, reactive sclerosis of the marginal bone, and occasionally a partial vacuum may produce gas within it. The reactive bone sclerosis may be gross and appear to involve entire vertebral bodies, deforming the lower cervical spine ("crumbling spine") or lumbar spine and resembling osteoblastic metastases. Excessive disorganization of the lumbar articulations should prompt suspicion of syphilis (Charcot spine — Ramani and Sengupta, 1973).

Degenerative changes in the apophyseal joints, best portrayed in the oblique views (see Fig. 11–37) may be florid and widespread or confined to one joint. Osteophytic proliferation may significantly reduce the cross-sectional area of the neural tube, altering its shape and compressing its contents. The combination of marginal osteophytic beaking, disc narrowing and posterior-joint degeneration was present in 85 percent of Roberts' (1978) 92 patients with end-stage lumbar spondylosis, and in none of these were the radiographs completely normal. A less frequent cause of compression is spondylolisthesis due to degenerative slippage of the apophyseal joints.

The critical factor in degenerative spinal compression is the constitutional diameter of the canal. Figure 11–32 illustrates the effect of the same degenerative changes in two patients: in the patient

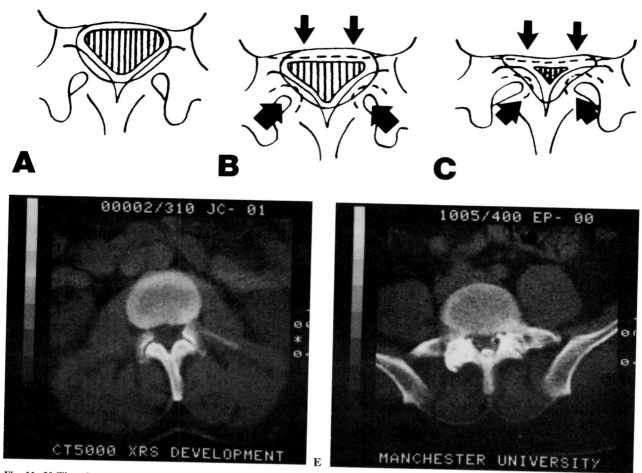

Fig. 11–32 Thecal constriction in lumbar stenosis. (A–C) Diagrammatic representation of three different spinal canals. (A) Normal canal, no spondylosis. (B) Normal canal with spondylosis; slight constriction. (C) Stenotic canal with comparable degree of spondylosis; marked constriction. Reproduced by courtesy of Dr. G. Roberts, The University Hospital of Wales, Cardiff. (D) Computed tomogram of the lumbar spine at the level of an intervertebral disc: normal spinal canal. (E) Computed tomogram made at the same level in a patient with severe spinal stenosis caused by osteophytic hypertrophy of the apophyseal joints. Residual thecal contrast medium is present. Reproduced by courtesy of Professor I. Isherwood, University of Manchester, Manchester.

with the "wide" canal they scarcely deform the thecal tube, while in the patient with the "narrow" canal, they obliterate it.

Myelography. Degenerative disc and joint lesions represent the commonest indications for myelography. The neuroradiologist should practice a contrast technique which includes the following: (1) Provocative myelography, i.e., careful study of the effect of posture upon the level of the suspected lesion. In cervical problems a pillow under the chest of the supine patient will enable him to flex and extend his neck in the course of the examination (Fig. 11–33). In lumbar spondylosis or disc prolapse, the full extent of the lesions may only be shown by weight-bearing or flexion-extension views (Fig. 11–34). (2) Full-diameter studies including lateral and oblique views to demonstrate the entire circumference of the neural tube. (3) Lumbar myelography includes examination of the conus medullaris, be-

cause neoplasms arising from it may mimic disc prolapse clinically. (4) Cervical myelography includes examination of the craniovertebral angle with the patient supine (see Chap. 9). Cervical spondylosis is a normal ageing phenomenon, like gray hair, and its presence in an older patient should prompt a careful examination to exclude another cause of the patient's symptoms and signs.

Lumbar Differential Diagnosis. A nucleus pulposus herniating backward either in the middle of the spinal canal (central prolapse) or to one side (lateral prolapse) appears as a filling defect behind the disc space (Fig. 11–35). Total disc prolapse may produce complete myelographic obstruction. Differentiation between acute disc prolapse and chronic disc degeneration may be possible, in that acute disc prolapse is usually confined to one disc space (sometimes two), while degeneration involves all the lumbar spaces.

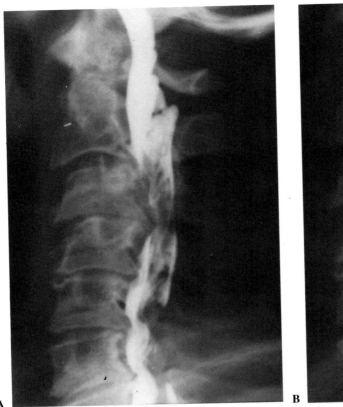
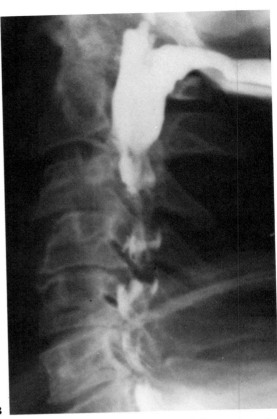

Fig. 11–33 Cervical spondylosis aggravating spinal stenosis. The "pinching" effect of degenerative disease of disc spaces and apophyseal joints compromises the spinal theca between the C2 and C7 vertebrae. (A) Flexion encourages contrast flow. (B) Extension almost obliterates the tube below the C2 level.

Sclerosis of the apophyseal joints distorts the straight posterior aspect of the tube (best seen in oblique lumbar myelograms, Fig. 11–37). Initially the hypertrophied joint masses indent the theca at the level of each intervertebral space; the lower two spaces are most often and severely affected. If associated disc degeneration is present, the dural tube is compressed from in front as well as behind, giving a multiple "pinching" appearance (Fig. 11–36). Florid lumbar degenerative disease ("end-stage spondylosis"—Roberts, 1978) may completely obliterate the lumbar theca in the L3–5 segment (Fig. 11–37). Lumbar injection of the contrast medium may then fail, and cisternal injection will be necessary—it is indicated by the presence of florid lumbar spondylosis.

Over 90 percent all abnormal lumbar myelograms are the result of disc or degenerative joint disease. Therefore the question to be answered, in respect of any lumbar myelographic abnormality demonstrated, is: Why is this lesion not disc and/or joint degenerative disease? Total obstructions may be caused by spinal tumors such as neurofibromas, metastatic cancer or myeloma and the plain radiographs may contain clues to the correct diagnosis,

e.g., posterior scalloping, pedicular deformity or destruction and collapse of vertebral body. Spinal arachnoiditis following laminectomy and/or myelography may produce bizarre deformities of the lumbosacral theca, and anatomical variations such as a shallow sacral pouch or a wide lumbosacral gap may be misdiagnosed as disc prolapse.

Cervical Differential Diagnosis. Apparent widening of the spinal cord shown by myelography poses the question: Intramedullary or extradural (Fig. 11–38)? Flexion of the neck tends to relieve a spondylotic obstruction, and the lateral view may indicate this cause. Intramedullary masses are probably 100 times as infrequent as cervical spondylosis. Acute disc prolapse is relatively uncommon, and may complicate traffic and other injuries.

Non-compressive Lesions

Spinal Dysraphism

Myelography is an essential guide for the surgeon, who may be able to alleviate neurological symptoms by releasing a tethered conus, bands or adhesions. Although oil myelography performed with

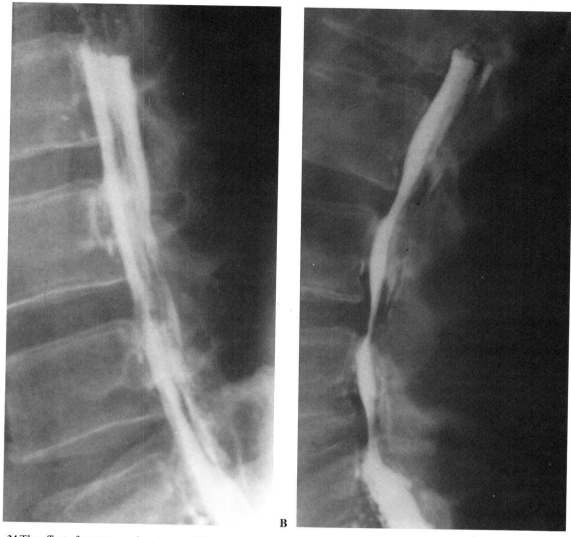

A   B

Fig. 11−34 The effect of posture on thecal constriction. A 63-year-old patient with end-stage lumbar spondylosis examined by erect full-diameter myelography. (A) Flexion. (B) Extension. Extension accentuates thecal constriction, while flexion relieves it.

the child supine as well as prone (Gryspeerdt, 1963; Burrows, 1968) proved satisfactory, examinations with gas injected suboccipitally under general anesthesia or metrizamide are more rewarding in their yield of diagnostic information (Roth, 1965; Cook, 1976).

In Till's (1968) operative series, myelography revealed the following:

Low and tethered conus, bands: 79% (Fig. 11−39)

Diastematomyelia or "split spinal cord": 47% (Fig. 11−40)

   Intraspinal lipoma: 20%

   Dermoid cyst: 9%

   Hamartoma: 3%

   Angioma: 1%

   Neurenteric cyst: 1% (Fig. 11−41)

The diagnosis is synthesized from the following in-

formation: (1) Level of termination of the conus medullaris. (2) Mobility of the lower end of the spinal cord—tethering by bands or cords abolishes the "floppy" characteristic of the normal cord. (3) The relationship of the conus and nerve roots to the abnormality in the bony neural arch, which is technically useful preoperative information for the surgeon.

The Syringomyelia Syndrome

Longitudinal cavitation of the spinal cord is a nosological entity with a well-defined clinical picture. Most cases appear to arise *de novo* in early life, but a cystic cord may complicate spinal trauma, inflammation or neoplasm. Several causative mechanisms have been suggested. The most credible to the neuroradiologist is probably the hydrodynamic theory of Gardner (1965) who postulated a mechanical

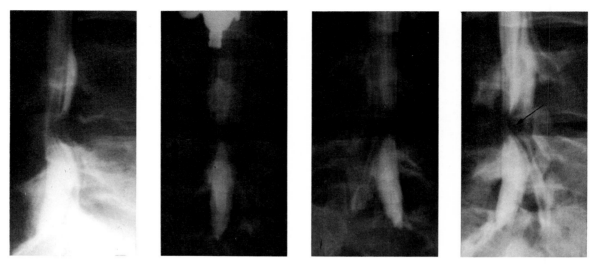

Fig. 11–35 Acute central prolapse of L4–5 disc. In addition to complaining of backache and bilateral sciatica, the patient exhibited bilateral sensory changes in the L5 dermatome, caused by compression of the L5 nerve roots within the spinal canal one level higher (*arrows*).

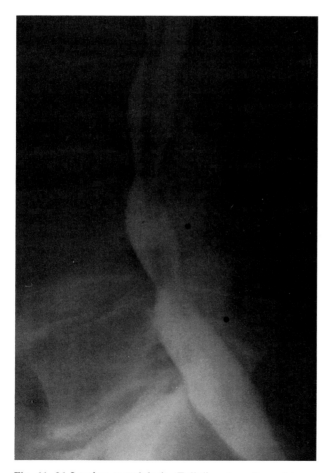

Fig. 11–36 Lumbar spondylosis. Full-diameter oil myelogram with the patient erect showing thecal constriction caused by posterior indentation of the dural tube. Black dots indicate the bases of spinous processes.

basis for the cystic cavitation. Two factors are involved: (1) developmental obstruction of the outlet of the fourth ventricle; and (2) transmission of the normal pulsation of the cerebrospinal fluid in the fourth ventricle resulting from the intracranial arterial pulse wave. Gardner believes that the outflow obstruction is caused by the cerebellar tonsils, which, being arrested in a descended position in the course of development, plug the foramen magnum during cardiac systole. This leads to secondary dilatation of the central canal of the spinal cord, thus establishing a direct communication between the fourth ventricle and the maze of cavities which replace the solid tissue of the cord. Gardner's theory was successfully used by Appleby and his colleagues (1969) to explain cases of "secondary" syringomyelia in which the outlet obstruction is caused by arachnoid adhesions. However, the theory does not explain the existence of cord cavitation which does not communicate with the cerebrospinal fluid pathway.

For radiological purposes, two types of syringomyelia are found: (1) communicating or typical syringomyelia, and (2) non-communicating or secondary syringomyelia, which may complicate traumatic paraplegia, tuberculosis or pyogenic spinal or intracranial infection, or spinal tumors.

Radiological Aspects: The neuroradiologist should regard widening of the spinal cord as a diagnostic sign that needs to be explained, and he must provide the answers to two questions: (1) Is the expansion solid or cystic? (2) If cystic, are there other features indicating the type of syringomyelia present, such as tonsillar ectopia or intramedullary neoplasm?

Cyst Demonstration. Computed tomography of the spinal canal promises to oust myelography and cyst visualization ("endomyelography" — Westberg,

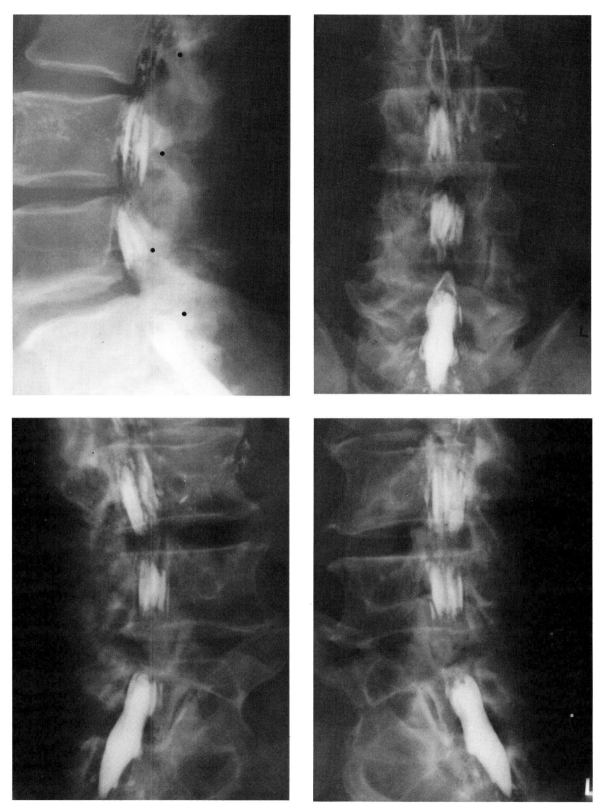

Fig. 11–37 End-stage lumbar spondylosis aggravating spinal stenosis. The degenerative changes at the disc spaces are overshadowed by florid overgrowth of the apophyseal joints, which is best seen in the oblique views. The canal is reduced to slit-like segments. Lumbar puncture may be impossible. Black dots indicate the bases of spinous processes.

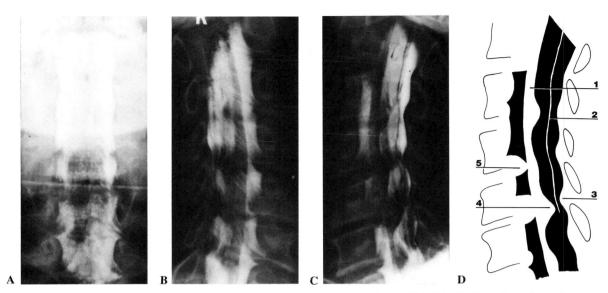

Fig. 11-38 Cervical spondylosis. Full-diameter metrizamide myelogram, illustrating the "pinching" effect of anterior and posterior indentation on the contours of the dural tube. (A, B and C) Anterior and both oblique views. (D) Explanatory diagram of oblique C. 1 – Spinal cord. 2 – Dentate ligament. 3 – Posterior protrusion (*left* apophyseal joint). 4 – Anterior protrusion (*left* side of disc space). 5 – Anterior protrusion (*right* side of disc space). Indentations from the right apophyseal joints are hidden from view; they are seen in oblique B.

1966; Kendall and Symon, 1973) in the diagnosis of cystic tumors of the spinal cord. Di Chiro and his colleagues (1975) and more recently Forbes and Isherwood (1978), using the computed tomographic method, have been able to demonstrate longitudinal cavitation in patients with surgically verified syringomyelia. Figure 11-42 illustrates the dynamic changes that occur in the caliber of the cord when

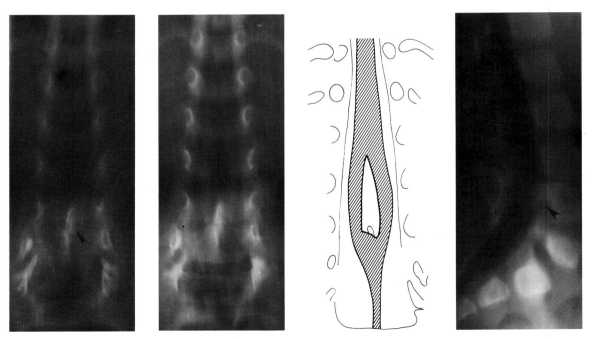

Fig. 11-39 Spinal dysraphism — split spinal cord. Frontal and lateral tomograms of a lumbar gas myelogram of a 2-year-old girl. The cord is widely split and transfixed by a bony spur *(arrowhead)* which was shown to form part of a malformation of the laminar arches. Below the spur the two components reunite in a mass. Operation: complete diplomyelia, the mass was a mixed tangle of nerves and blood vessels. This case was described and illustrated by P. L. Cook in *The British Journal of Radiology, 49*, 502 – 515, 1976.

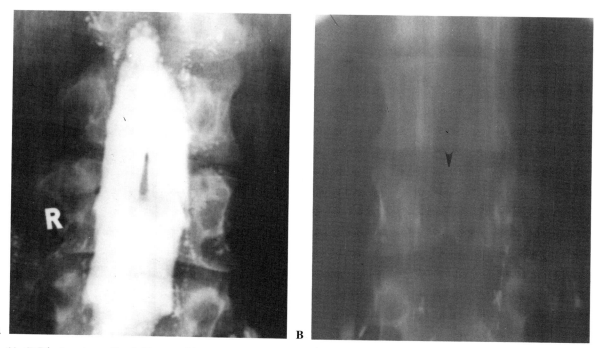

Fig. 11–40 Diastematomyelia. A 39-year-old woman with increasing difficulty in walking due to weakness of the hip and thigh muscles. (A) Oil myelogram, showing a midline filling defect at the level of the L3 vertebra, a bony spur which tethered the conus. (B) Tomogram showing the bifid body of L3 vertebra *(arrowhead)* from which the bony spur arose.

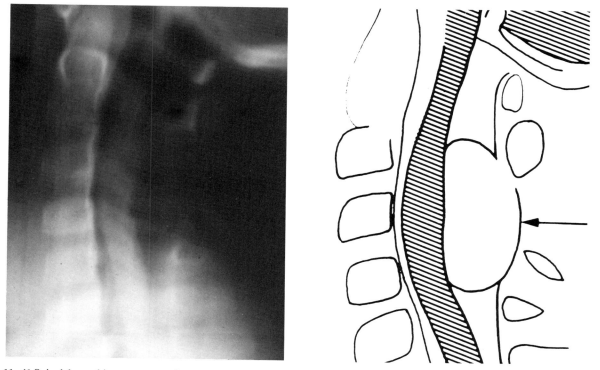

Fig. 11–41 Spinal dysraphism—neurenteric cyst. Lateral tomogram of cervical gas myelogram. The cervical cord is displaced by a mass lying behind it within the subarachnoid space. The spinal canal is widened and the laminae of C3 and C4 vertebrae are ununited. Operation: enteric cyst containing gastric mucosal elements. This case was described and illustrated by P. L. Cook in *The British Journal of Radiology, 49*, 502–515, 1976.

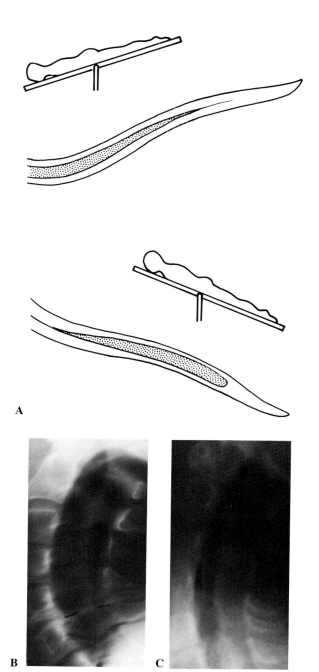

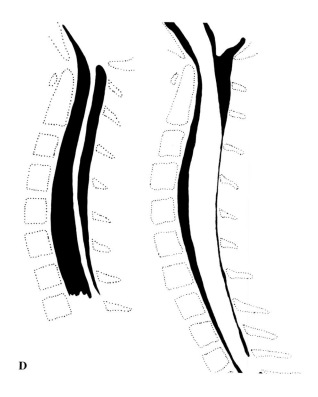

Fig. 11–42 Syringomyelia. (A) Diagram to illustrate "collapse" of the cystic, partly fluid-filled spinal cord within the spinal theca, when the patient is tilted from the head-down to the head-up position. This diagram explains why oil myelography, performed with the patient head-down, may sometimes reveal a widened cord. (B–D) Gas myelography performed by Bradac's technique reveals widening and collapse of the cervical spinal cord. (B) Patient in head-up position, showing collapsed cord *(arrows)*. (C) Patient in head-down position, depicting a wide cord. (D) Line drawing of B and C. This case was described and illustrated by G. B. Bradac in *Neuroradiology, 4,* 41–45, 1972.

tilting the patient. These changes depend on the spinal cord being sufficiently thin-walled, so that it can distend and collapse, also on the length of the cyst and whether the spinal cerebrospinal fluid can escape via the central canal into the fourth ventricle (Logue, 1971). Total replacement of the cerebrospinal fluid in the spinal canal during gas myelography results in the cord being completely surrounded by air, and its dimensions can then be accurately delineated by tomography (Figs. 11–42, 11–43). Conventional oil myelography, made with the patient prone, demonstrates a wide cord in about half

of patients with clinical signs of syringomyelia. The fluid content of the cystic lesion is best revealed by computed tomography of the spinal canal and cord (Fig. 11–44). Previously, Greitz and Ellertsson (1969) developed a technique of combining cyst puncture with the injection of radioisotope. Within a few hours in cases of communicating syringomyelia, the radioisotope can be detected in the basal cisterns—thus confirming Gardner's theory. Injection into a non-communicating cyst, on the other hand, shows no passage into the fourth ventricle.

Craniovertebral Angle Lesion. The majority of patients with communicating syringomyelia have tonsillar ectopia. All 35 patients in Logue's (1971) operated series showed an obstructive lesion at the craniovertebral angle—tonsillar plugging, outlet adhesions or cyst formation. The radiologist's most important task in investigating a case of syringo-

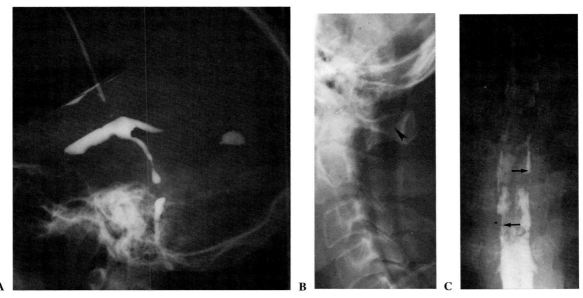

Fig. 11–43 Syringomyelia secondary to tuberculous meningitis in a 34-year-old man. He had suffered from tuberculous meningitis at the age of 8 years and developed shoulder pains, limb signs and visual difficulties at 16 years. (A and B) Combined oil and gas studies showing partly obliterated 4th ventricle, hydrocephalus and herniated cerebellar tonsils *(arrowhead)*. (C) Oil myelogram, showing adhesive arachnoiditis and some widening of the thoracic spinal cord *(arrows)*. Diagnosis: Syringomyelia and convexity-block hydrocephalus secondary to tuberculous meningitis.

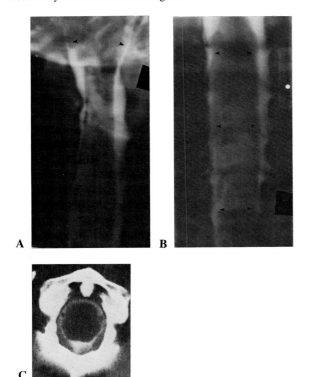

Fig. 11–44 Combined syringomyelia and syringobulbia. (A and B) Oil myelogram made with the patient in the prone position shows an enlarged spinal cord and medulla *(arrowheads)*. (C) Computed tomogram made after enhancement with intrathecal metrizamide reveals the lesion to be a hollow tube, filled with fluid of the density of cerebrospinal fluid. Reproduced by courtesy of Professor Ian Isherwood, University of Manchester, Manchester, England.

myelia is to demonstrate the presence and nature of any such obstruction, because surgical treatment will succeed only if it can be removed. Gas myelography is not completely reliable for this purpose, and an injection of oil may be unavoidable.

Plain-Film Evidence: (1) Scoliosis: 85 percent (McRae and Standen, 1966). (2) Abnormally wide cervical spinal canal (Fig. 11–45): in 25 to 50 percent of patients, but only in those in whom the signs and symptoms appear before the age of 30 years (Boijsen, 1954; Wells, Spillane and Bligh, 1959). (3) Bony abnormality of the craniovertebral angle. Despite the incidence of tonsillar ectopia, only about 25 percent show skeletal abnormalities (atlanto-occipital assimilation, basilar impression). (4) Arrested hydrocephalus. (5) Neuropathic joints, usually in the upper limbs (Fig. 11–45). The humeral head may disappear, also terminal phalanges of the fingers.

Non-Communicating Syringomyelia: Cord cavitation frequently accompanies spinal tumors: 16 percent of the large series of syringomyelic patients reported by Poser (1956) had intramedullary tumors, and 31 percent of the Mayo Clinic series of 205 intramedullary tumors showed syringomyelia.

The differential diagnosis between solid intramedullary tumors and syringomyelia will remain difficult without the benefit of computed tomography of the spine. Myelographic features favoring the solid tumor are: irregularity of the cord outline, worm-like blood vessels on the cord's surface, an eccen-

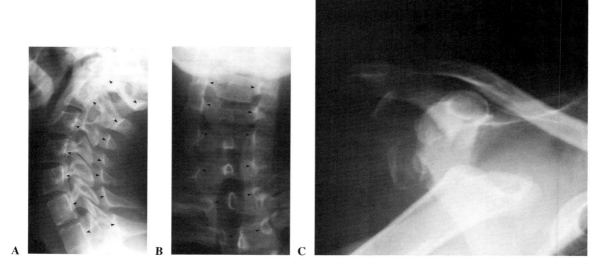

Fig. 11–45 Plain-film evidence of syringomyelia. (A and B) Widened cervical spinal canal *(arrowheads)*. (C) Neuropathic joint of the upper limb. The head of the humerus has been destroyed and the shoulder is dislocated.

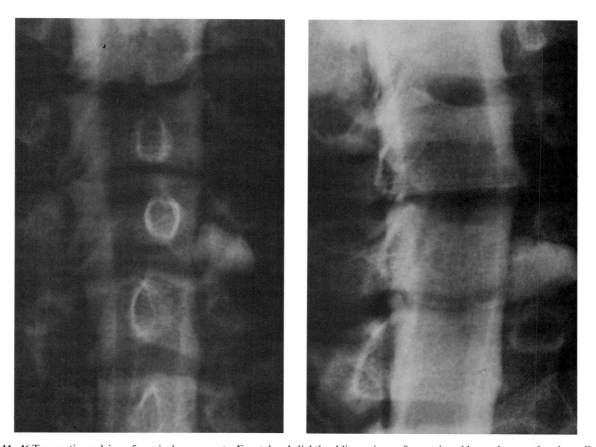

Fig. 11–46 Traumatic avulsion of cervical nerve roots. Frontal and slightly oblique views of a metrizamide myelogram showing a diverticulum corresponding to the left 7th cervical root. There is no diverticulum at the level of the 6th root but the root itself is pathological, compared to the one above and the opposite roots. Metrizamide, due to its lesser density than Pantopaque, may be able to reveal root lesions even if they have not ruptured the root sheaths with diverticulum formation. Reproduced by courtesy of Professor Per Amundsen, Ullevål Hospital, Oslo.

tric position of the intramedullary mass, a complete myelographic block and the absence of congenital skeletal anomalies (McRae and Standen, 1966).

Injury Patterns

Post-traumatic complications and distant sequelae are more likely to concern the neuroradiologist than the acute spinal injury, in which the indications for myelography are controversial.

Nerve Root Damage. *(1) Brachial plexus:* postnatal tearing or avulsion of the lower roots of the brachial plexus may follow traffic or industrial accidents in which sudden traction is applied to the abducted arm. Irregular pouches form almost im-

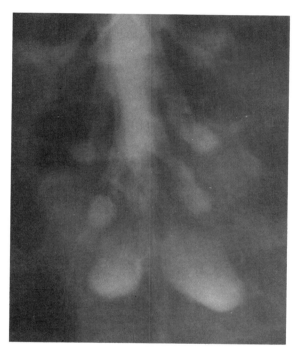

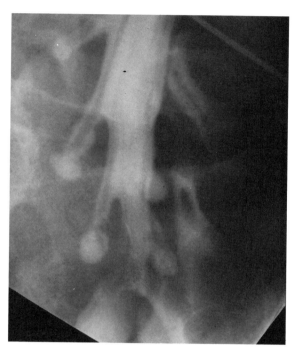

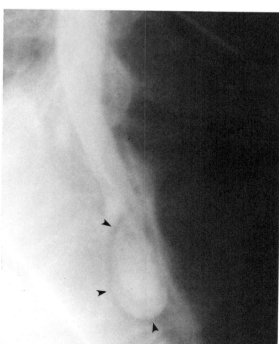

Fig. 11–47 Perineurial cysts on the lumbosacral nerve roots. They are multiple and symmetrical and can erode the walls of the lumbosacral canal *(arrowheads)*. The cysts fill better with water-soluble contrast media which are less viscous than oil.

mediately around the torn root, and they may extend laterally beyond the spinal canal. These characteristic lesions were first shown myelographically in 1947 by Murphey, Hartung and Kirklin, who named them traumatic meningoceles (Fig. 11–46). Features that distinguish them from congenital root-pouch cysts are their unilaterality and the fact that they are only rarely found on nerve roots other than C7, C8 or T1. Subsequent healing may obliterate the pouch and leave a contrast-filled cyst in the paravertebral area (Davies, Sutton and Bligh, 1966; Yeoman, 1968). Another myelographic sign of plexus damage is displacement of the contrast column away from one or more pedicles, with consequent loss of the normal symmetrical appearance, due to an intraspinal extradural hematoma.

(2) Lumbosacral Plexus: Only a few cases have been described in the world literature, nearly all following severe traffic accidents in which the pelvis was fractured and a sacroiliac joint diastased (Alker, Glasauer, Zoll and Schlagenhauff, 1967; Payne and Thomson, 1969). In acutely injured patients with neurological deficit in the appropriate limb, the myelographic demonstration of dural sacs is diagnostic of nerve root damage.

Other sacral diverticula that may give rise to confusion are perineural cysts (Fig. 11–47). These cysts, first described by Tarlov in 1938 (Tarlov, 1970), may cause sciatica, and their surgical removal may be curative. They lie laterally along the nerve roots and their communication with the subarachnoid space may be so narrow, that they fail to fill immediately upon myelography. But radiographs exposed several days after the injection of oil will demonstrate the cysts filled with contrast medium (Sutton, 1963).

Spinal Cord Compression An immediate neurological deficit is usually caused by extradural compression due to hematoma and/or vertebral fractures, or hematomyelia. The masterly review of penetrating spinal injuries produced at the end of World War II by Hinkel and Nichols (1946) remains a valuable source of reference. See also Laasonen (1977). Two important neurological complications may occur after a symptom-free interval — recorded in one case as long as 37 years after the injury (Pye and Hickey, 1975). These are: (1) Extradural cysts within the spinal canal produced by adhesions. Called traumatic arachnoid diverticula, they compress the spinal cord by exerting a ball-valve action when the patient is erect (Fig. 11–48). Similar cysts may complicate disc operations (Shahinfar and Schechter, 1966). (2) A progressive myelopathy may be a sequel to traumatic paraplegia, which Barnett and his colleagues have proved to be caused by syringomyelic longitudinal cavitation of the spinal cord (Barnett, Botterell, Jousse and Wynn-Jones, 1966).

Angioma of the Spinal Canal

Spinal arteriovenous malformations are similar to intracranial angiomas in their relationships to the meninges and neural tissue. Application of the technique of selective spinal angiography developed by

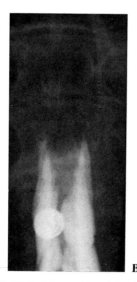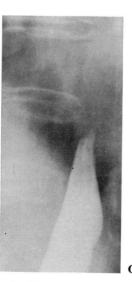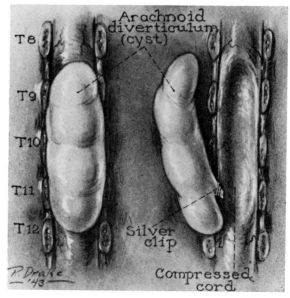

Fig. 11–48 Post-traumatic subdural arachnoid cyst. (A and B) Complete obstruction to lumbar-injected oil. In the anterior view the cyst simulates an intramedullary tumor (metal ball = skin marker), but the lateral views shows the spinal cord to be displaced forward by a sausage-shaped mass. No oil enters the cyst. (C) Diagram used by C. A. Good, A. W. Adson and K. H. Abbott to illustrate a similar case, reported in © 1944, *The American Journal of Roentgenology, 52,* 53–56, 1944.

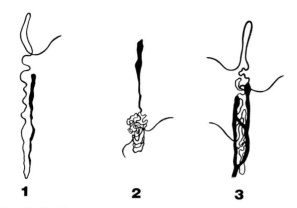

Fig. 11–49 Diagrammatic representation of the three types of arteriovenous malformation of the spinal cord. *(Left)* Type 1, plain arteriovenous fistula. *(Center)* Type 2, glomus. *(Right)* Type 3, juvenile. Classification proposed and illustrated by G. Di Chiro and L. Wener in *The Journal of Neurosurgery, 39,* 1–29, 1973.

Djindjian in Paris and Di Chiro in Bethesda permits the following morphological classification (Fig. 11–49).

1. Plain arteriovenous fistula: one or two tightly coiled continuous vessels extending longitudinally over several segments.
2. Glomus type: a localized plexus of tightly packed vessels with one or a few feeding arteries and localized to one segment.
3. Juvenile type: a voluminous malformation supplied by many large feeding arteries and often filling the spinal canal. This type is encountered almost exclusively in children.

A small proportion of arteriovenous malformations develop in the extradural space, and usually present as cases of sudden spinal cord compression ("spontaneous epidural hemorrhage"). The majority occupy a wholly intradural situation. The hypertrophic vascular elements may lie behind or in front of the spinal cord, or envelop it, and they may penetrate into the cord substance. Hematomyelia or subarachnoid hemorrhage is the precipitating event in the sudden-onset cases, but more characteristic clinical features are the long duration and variable intensity of symptoms. Di Chiro and Wener (1973) claim that subarachnoid hemorrhage in a case of spinal arteriovenous malformation is nearly always caused by an associated berry aneurysm. The true incidence of spinal arteriovenous malformation is difficult to estimate because spinal angiography, essential for complete diagnosis, remains a specialized procedure performed in relatively few centres. Lombardi and Migliavacca (1959) treated 18 spinal angiomas in the same period as they operated upon 200 spinal neoplasms.

Selective Angiography. The definitive method of diagnosing spinal angiomas is angiography. It is essential, not only for identifying the 25 percent of angiomas that are missed by oil myelography (Djindjian, 1968), but also in preoperative assessment. The site and origin of the arterial feeders can be demonstrated, as well as the extent of the malformation and its position relative to the spinal cord, and the presence of any associated aneurysm.

Selective catheterization and injection of each lumbar and intercostal artery may reveal the greater radicular artery (artery of Adamkiewicz, see Doppman and Di Chiro, 1968), the main source of arterial blood of the spinal cord. Usually this artery arises from an intercostal or lumbar artery between T8 and L1 on the left side. It makes a characteristic "hairpin bend" to become the anterior spinal artery in the anterior median sulcus. Arteriovenous malformations may be irrigated by this artery and/or other hypertrophied feeders. The subtraction technique reveals these arteries and the extent of the angioma (Fig. 11–50).

Oil Myelography. Prior to spinal angiography, the diagnosis of spinal angiomas rested upon the demonstration of serpiginous negative filling defects in an oil myelogram (Fig. 11–51). However, even the most spectacular appearances may provide only an incomplete picture of the extent of the lesion, due to the fact that the superficial vessels may not be outlined, nor those that disappear into the substance of the spinal cord. The irregular filling defects are not specific: it is impossible to distinguish between dilated veins and hypertrophied arteries, and similar appearances may represent adhesive arachnoiditis, metastases or other intradural lesions (Lombardi and Migliavacca, 1959). An essential part of adequate myelographic technique is examination of the patient supine, since this position occasionally reveals small angiomas that are invisible in the prone position. Of the 53 patients reported by Aminoff and Logue (1974), six had "normal" myelograms.

Other myelographic features of spinal angioma are total obstruction to contrast flow or expansion of the spinal cord, due to intradural hematoma or hematomyelia.

Plain Radiographs. Dorsal scoliosis is a frequent accompaniment of the juvenile voluminous type of arteriovenous malformation. Occasionally pedicular erosion or widening of the interpedicular diameter may occur (Fig. 11–51).

Ankylosing Spondylitis
This curious collagenous disease of joints is important to the neuroradiologist because of its neurological complications. The typical clinical problem is that of a young man, with back pain and a stiff spine, who is found to have a low-grade fever and a raised erythrocyte sedimentation rate. Although the boundary between ankylosing spondylitis and rheumatoid arthritis is imprecise, no serological evidence of such association exists.

The destructive changes in the axial skeleton fol-

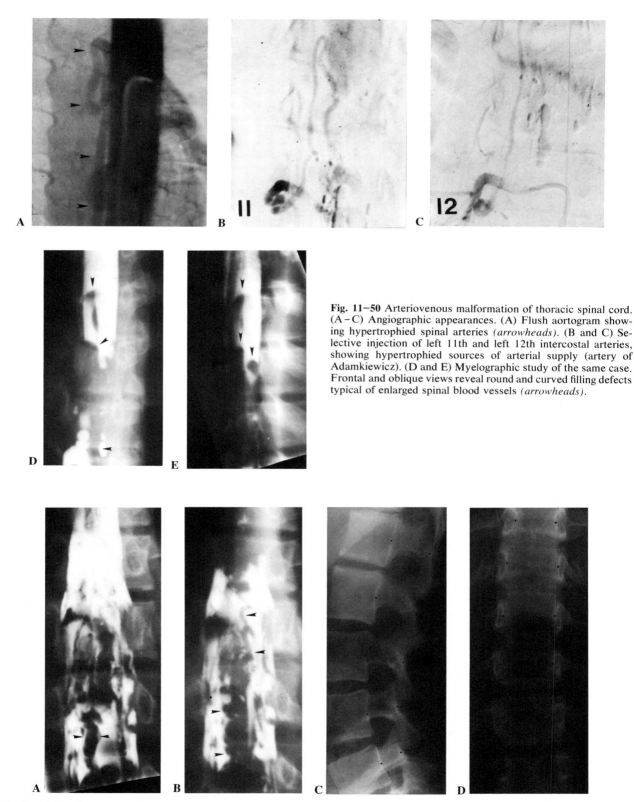

Fig. 11–50 Arteriovenous malformation of thoracic spinal cord. (A–C) Angiographic appearances. (A) Flush aortogram showing hypertrophied spinal arteries *(arrowheads)*. (B and C) Selective injection of left 11th and left 12th intercostal arteries, showing hypertrophied sources of arterial supply (artery of Adamkiewicz). (D and E) Myelographic study of the same case. Frontal and oblique views reveal round and curved filling defects typical of enlarged spinal blood vessels *(arrowheads)*.

Fig. 11–51 Arteriovenous malformation of the spinal cord shown by oil myelography. (A) Voluminous angioma (type 3), which fills the conus-cauda part of the spinal canal. (A and B) Prone and supine examination reveals abnormal serpiginous vessels on the posterior and anterior surfaces of the spinal canal. (C and D) Plain radiographs show widening of the interpedicular and sagittal diameters of the spinal canal.

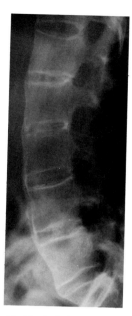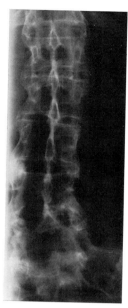

Fig. 11–52 Ankylosing spondylitis. Classical appearances of established disease, the "bamboo spine": calcification of the interspinous and longitudinal ligaments and the disc spaces and reshaping ("squaring") of the vertebral bodies. Less well known is attenuation of the laminar arches through pressure erosion by thecal diverticula, causing apparent enlargement of the intervertebral foramina and some pedicular deformity—note the left laminae of the L3, L4 and L5 vertebrae. For water-soluble lumbar radiculogram of this case, see Figure 11–53.

low a recognizable radiological pattern. The disease starts as an inflammatory synovitis in the lower two-thirds of the sacroiliac joints. The margins become blurred, then sclerotic and finally the joints are obliterated by fibrous and bony union. As the process ascends to involve the synovial (apophyseal) joints of the vertebral column, the vertebral

bodies become immobilized and altered in shape ("squared"). The anterior and posterior longitudinal ligaments calcify and calcium is also deposited in the disc spaces—imparting the characteristic appearance of ankylosing spondylitis, viz., "bamboo spine" (Fig. 11–52).

The clinical features of ankylosing spondylitis as described originally by Von Bechterew in 1893 embodied complex neurological abnormalities. He claimed that these were caused by degeneration of the posterior nerve roots and dorsal columns of the spinal cord, and at the level of the cauda equina by meningeal erosions. Matthews (1968) reported a case complicated by the cauda equina syndrome, in which large arachnoid cysts were shown at autopsy to have eroded the laminae and spinous processes of the lower lumbar vertebrae. Full-diameter myelography reveals the excessive expansion of the theca that may occur, and supine oil myelography may show oil residues trapped in the dorsal cystic spaces (Fig. 11–53). The pathogenesis of the cauda equina syndrome in ankylosing spondylitis is not clear: although the sagittal diameter of the spinal canal is abnormally large, other radiological features of raised intraspinal pressure such as interpedicular widening or posterior scalloping are absent. Thus the origin or role of the cysts in causing signs of cauda equina irritation in this condition remains speculative (Hassan, 1976).

In the cervical spine, atlantoaxial dislocation may occasionally complicate ankylosing spondylitis although not as frequently as rheumatoid arthritis (Sharp and Purser, 1961). Fractures also aggravate the condition, and occur through the line of a cervical disc space. End-stage ankylosing spondylitis of the cervical spine resembles the Kippel-Feil syndrome and long-standing Still's disease.

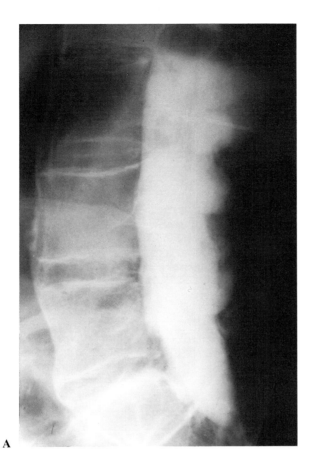

A

Fig. 11–53 Ankylosing spondylitis. (A) Water-soluble lumbar radiculogram showing extensive thecal ectasia and diverticular formation at the expense of the posterior longitudinal ligament and the laminar walls of the spinal canal. Same case Figure 11–52. This case was described and illustrated by I. Hassan in *The Journal of Neurology, Neurosurgery and Psychiatry, 39,* 1172–1178, 1976. (B and C) Another patient examined supine by oil myelography, showing posterior thecal diverticula.

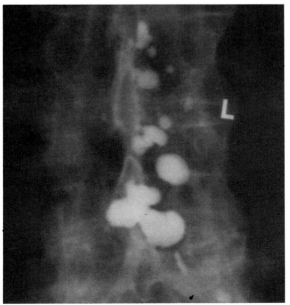

B

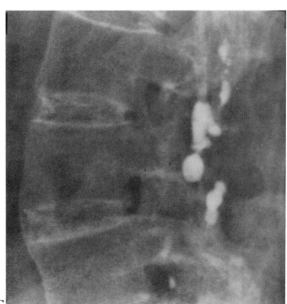

C

REFERENCES:

Ahlgren, P.: Longterm side effects after myelography with water-soluble contrast media. Conturex, Conray meglumine 282, and Dimer-X. Neuroradiology, 6, 206–211, 1973.

Alker, G. J., Glasauer, F. E., Zoll, J. G. and Schlagenhauff, R.: Myelographic demonstration of lumbosacral nerve root avulsion. Radiology, 89, 101–104, 1967.

Aminoff, M. J. and Logue, V.: Clinical features of spinal vascular malformations. Brain, 97, 197–210, 1974.

Amundsen, P.: Metrizamide in cervical myelography. Survey and present state. Acta Radiologica Supplementum 355, 1977.

Appleby, A., Bradley, W. G., Foster, J. B., Hankinson, J. and Hudgson, P.: Syringomyelia due to chronic arachnoiditis at the foramen magnum. Journal of the Neurological Sciences, 8, 451–464, 1969.

Banna, M. and Gryspeerdt, G. L.: Intraspinal tumours in children (excluding dysraphism). Clinical Radiology, 22, 17–32, 1971.

Barnett, H. J. M., Botterell, E. H., Jousse, A. T. and Wynn-Jones, M.: Progressive myelopathy as a sequel to traumatic paraplegia. Brain, 89, 159–174, 1966.

Blau, J. N. and Logue, V.: Intermittent claudication of the cauda equina. The Lancet, 1, 1081–1086, 1961.

Boijsen, E.: The cervical spinal canal in intraspinal expansive masses. Acta Radiologica, 42, 101–115, 1954.

Bradac, G. B.: The value of gas myelography in the diagnosis of syringomyelia. Neuroradiology, 4, 41–45, 1972.

Bradley, W. G. and Banna, M.: The cervical dural canal. A study of the "tight dural canal" and of syringomyelia by prone and supine myelography. British Journal of Radiology, 41, 608–614, 1968.

Bryan, P.: CSF seeding of intra-cranial tumours: A study of 96 cases. Clinical Radiology, 25, 355–360, 1974.

Bull, J. W. D.: Spinal meningiomas and neurofibromas. Acta Radiologica, 40, 283–300, 1953.

Bull, J. W. D.: Myelography. Neuroradiology, 2, 1–2, 1971.

Burrows, E. H.: The sagittal diameter of the spinal canal in cervical spondylosis. Clinical Radiology, 14, 77–86, 1963.

Burrows, F. G. O.: Some aspects of occult spinal dysraphism. A study of 90 cases. British Journal of Radiology, 41, 496–507, 1968.

Cashion, E. L.: Cervical intervertebral disc space infection following cerebral angiography. Neuroradiology, 2, 176–178, 1971.

Cloward, R. B. and Bucy, P. C.: Spinal extradural cyst and kyphosis dorsalis juvenilis. American Journal of Roentgenology, 38, 681–706, 1937.

Cook, P. L.: Gas myelography in the investigation of occult spinal dysraphism. British Journal of Radiology, 49, 502–515, 1976.

Couch, R. S. C.: Tumours of the spinal canal. Proceedings of the Royal Society of Medicine, 55, 101–103, 1962.

Danziger, J., Jackson, H. and Bloch, S.: Congenital absence of a pedicle in the cervical vertebra. Clinical Radiology, 26, 53–56, 1975.

Dastur, H. M.: The radiological appearances of spinal extradural arachnoid cysts. Journal of Neurology, Neurosurgery and Psychiatry, 26, 231–235, 1963.

Davies, E. R., Sutton, D. and Bligh, A. S.: Myelography in brachial plexus injury. British Journal of Radiology, 39, 362–371, 1966.

Di Chiro, G., Axelbaum, S. P., Schellinger, D., Twigg, H. L. and Ledley, R. S.: Computerized axial tomography in syringomyelia. New England Journal of Medicine, 292, 13–16, 1975.

Di Chiro, G. and Wener, L.: Angiography of the spinal cord. A review of contemporary techniques and applications. Journal of Neurosurgery, 39, 1–29, 1973.

Djindjian, R.: Technique de l'arteriographie de la moelle épiniére par aortographie sélective. La Presse Medicale, 76, 159–162, 1968.

Doppman, J. and Di Chiro, G.: The arteria radicularis magna: radiographic anatomy in the adult. British Journal of Radiology, 41, 40–45, 1968.

Elsberg, C. A. and Dyke, C. G.: The diagnosis and localization of tumors of the spinal canal by means of measurements made on the x-ray films of the vertebrae. Correlation of clinical and x-ray findings. Bulletin of the Neurological Institute of New York, 3, 359–394, 1934.

Epstein, J. A., Epstein, B. S. and Lavine, L.: Nerve root compression associated with narrowing of the lumbar spinal canal. Journal of Neurology, Neurosurgery and Psychiatry, 25, 165–176, 1962.

Epstein, J. A. and Malis, L. I.: Compression of spinal cord and cauda equina in achondroplastic dwarfs. Neurology, 5, 875–881, 1955.

Forbes, W. St. C. and Isherwood, I.: Computed tomography in syringomyelia and the associated Arnold-Chiari type 1 malformation. Neuroradiology, 15, 59–72, 1978.

Gardner, W. J.: Hydrodynamic mechanisms of syringomyelia. Journal of Neurology, Neurosurgery and Psychiatry, 28, 247–259, 1965.

Good, C. A., Adson, A. W. and Abbott, K. H.: Spinal extradural cysts (diverticulum of spinal arachnoid): report of a case. American Journal of Roentgenology, 52, 53–56, 1944.

Greitz, T. and Ellertsson, A. B.: Isotope scanning of spinal cord cysts. Acta Radiologica Diagnosis, 8, 310–320, 1969.

Grollmus, J. and Hoff, J.: Spontaneous spinal epidural haemorrhage: good results after early treatment. Journal of Neurology, Neurosurgery and Psychiatry, 38, 89–90, 1975.

Gryspeerdt, G. L.: Myelographic assessment of occult forms of spinal dysraphism. Acta Radiologica Diagnosis, 1, 702–717, 1963.

Guyer, P. B., Westbury, H. and Cook P. L.: The myelographic appearances of spinal cord metastases. British Journal of Radiology, 41, 615–619, 1968.

Hadley, L. A.: Congenital absence of pedicle from the cervical vertebra. Report of three cases. American Journal of Roentgenology, 55, 193–197, 1951.

Hallpike, J. and Stanley, P.: A case of extradural spinal meningioma. Journal of Neurology, Neurosurgery and Psychiatry, 31, 195–197, 1968.

Hassan, I.: Cauda equina syndrome in ankylosing spondylitis: a report of six cases. Journal of Neurology, Neurosurgery and Psychiatry, 39, 1172–1178, 1976.

Hilton, M. D. and McCarthy, H. H.: Intrathoracic meningocele. Journal of Thoracic Surgery, 37, 261–268, 1959.

Hinck, V. C., Hopkins, C. E. and Clark, W. M.: Sagittal diameter of the lumbar spinal canal in children and adults. Radiology, 85, 929–937, 1965.

Hinck, V. C. and Sachdev, N. S.: Developmental stenosis of the cervical canal. Brain, 89, 27–37, 1966.

Hinkel, C. L. and Nichols, R. L.: Opaque myelography in penetrating wounds of the spinal canal. American Journal of Roentgenology, 55, 689–709, 1946.

Hunt, J. C. and Pugh, D. G.: Skeletal lesions in neurofibromatosis. Radiology, 76, 1–20, 1961.

Hurteau, E. F., Baird, W. C. and Sinclair, E.: Arachnoiditis following the use of iodised oil. Journal of Bone and Joint Surgery, 36, 393–400, 1954.

Jacobaeus, H. C.: On insufflation of air into the spinal canal for diagnostic purposes in cases of tumors of the spinal canal. Acta Medica Scandinavica, 55, 555–564, 1921.

Jacobsen, H. H. and Hyllested, K.: Localised atrophy of the spinal cord. Acta Radiologica, 50, 211–261, 1958.

Jefferson, A.: Localized enlargement of the spinal canal in the absence of tumour: a congenital abnormality. Journal of Neurology, Neurosurgery and Psychiatry, 18, 305–309, 1955.

Joffe, R., Appleby, A. and Arjona, V.: Intermittent ischaemia of the cauda equina due to stenosis of the lumbar canal. Journal of Neurology, Neurosurgery and Psychiatry, 29, 315–318, 1966.

Johnson, A. J. and Burrows, E. H.: Thecal deformity after lumbar myelography with iophendylate (Myodil) and meglumine iocarmate (Conray 280). British Journal of Radiology, *51*, 196–202, 1978.

Jones, R. A. C. and Thomson, J. L. G.: The narrow lumbar canal. Journal of Bone and Joint Surgery, *50-B*, 595–605, 1968.

Kendall, B. and Russell, J.: Haemangioblastomas of the spinal cord. British Journal of Radiology, *39*, 817–823, 1966.

Kendall, B. and Symon, L.: Cyst puncture and emdomyelography in cystic tumours of the spinal cord. British Journal of Radiology, *46*, 198–204, 1973.

Kremenitzer, M., Ager, P. J. and Zingesser, L. H.: Myelographic evidence for nerve root enlargement in a case of Charcot-Marie-Tooth disease. Neuroradiology, *11*, 165–167, 1976.

Laws, J. W. and Pallis, C.: Spinal deformities in neurofibromatosis. Journal of Bone and Joint Surgery, *45*, 674–862, 1963.

Laasonen, E. M.: Myelography for severe thoracolumbar injuries. Neuroradiology, *13*, 165–168, 1977.

Leeds, N. E. and Jacobson, H. G.: Spinal neurofibromatosis. American Journal of Roentgenology, *126*, 617–623, 1976.

Lewtas, N. A. and Dimant, S.: The diagnosis of hypertrophic interstitial polyneuritis by myelography. Journal of the Faculty of Radiologists, *8* 276–277, 1957.

Lichtenstein, B. W.: "Spinal dysraphism"; spina bifida and myelodysplasia. Archives of Neurology and Psychiatry (Chicago), *44*, 792–810, 1940.

Lindgren, E.: Myelographic changes in kyphosis dorsalis juvenilis. Acta Radiologica, *22*, 461–470, 1941.

Logue, V.: Syringomyelia: A radiodiagnostic and radiotherapeutic saga. Clinical Radiology, *22*, 2–17, 1971.

Lombardi, G. and Migliavacca, F.: Angiomas of the spinal cord. British Journal of Radiology, *32*, 810–814, 1959.

Lombardi, G. and Passerini, A.: Spinal cord diseases. A radiologic and myelographic review. Baltimore: Williams and Wilkins, 1964.

McCall, I. W., Park, W. M. and McSweeney, T.: The radiological demonstration of acute lower cervical injury. Clinical Radiology, *24*, 235–240, 1973.

McLeod, R. A., Dahlin, D. C. and Beabout, J. W.: The spectrum of osteoblastoma. American Journal of Roentgenology, *126*, 321–335, 1976.

McRae, D. L. and Standen, J.: Roentgenologic findings in syringomyelia and hydromyelia. American Journal of Roentgenology, *98*, 695–703, 1966.

Matthews, W. B.: The neurological complications of ankylosing spondylitis. Journal of the Neurological Sciences, *6*, 561–573, 1968.

Miles, J., Pennybacker, J. and Sheldon, P.: Intrathoracic meningocele. Its development and association with neurofibromatosis. Journal of Neurology, Neurosurgery and Psychiatry, *32*, 99–110, 1969.

Mitchell, G. E., Lourie, H. and Berne, A. A.: Various causes of scalloped vertebrae with notes on their pathogenesis. Radiology, *89*, 67–74, 1967.

Mixter, W. J. and Barr, J. S.: Protrusion of the lower lumbar intervertebral disks. New England Journal of Medicine, *223*, 523–529, 1940.

Murphey, F., Hartung, W. and Kirklin, J. W.: Myelographic demonstration of avulsing injury of the brachial plexus. American Journal of Roentgenology, *58*, 102–105, 1947.

Murray, R. O.: Intradural arachnoid cyst of the lumbar spinal canal. British Journal of Radiology, *32*, 689–692, 1959.

Murray, R. O. and Jacobson, H. H.: The radiology of skeletal disorders. Edinburgh: Churchill Livingstone, 1977.

Nelson, J. D.: The Marfan syndrome, with special reference to congenital enlargement of the spinal canal. British Journal of Radiology, *31*, 561–570, 1958.

Ngan, H. and Preston, B. J.: Non-Hodgkin's lymphoma presenting with osseous lesions. Clinical Radiology, *26*, 351–356, 1975.

Payne, R. F. and Thomson, J. L. G.: Myelography in lumbosacral plexus injury. British Journal of Radiology, *42*, 840–845, 1969.

Pear, B. L. and Boyd, H. R.: Roentgenographically visible calcifications in spinal meningioma. American Journal of Roentgenology, *120*, 32–45, 1974.

Peterson, H.: The hazards of myelography. Radiology, *115*, 237–239, 1975.

Poser, C. M.: The relationship between syringomyelia and neoplasm. Springfield: Charles C Thomas, 1956.

Prakash, B., Banerji, A. K. and Tandon, P. N.: Aneurysmal bone cyst of the spine. Journal of Neurology, Neurosurgery and Psychiatry, *36*, 112–117, 1973.

Pye, I. F. and Hickey, M. C.: Traumatic arachnoid diverticula: a report of two cases causing spinal cord compression. British Journal of Radiology, *48*, 889–893, 1975.

Raja, I. A. and Hankinson, J.: Congenital spinal arachnoid cysts. Report of two cases and review of the literature. Journal of Neurology, Neurosurgery and Psychiatry, *33*, 105–110, 1970.

Ramani, P. S.: Variations in size of the bony lumbar canal in patients with prolapse of lumbar intervertebral discs. Clinical Radiology, *27*, 301–307, 1976.

Ramani, P. S. and Sengupta, R. P.: Cauda equina compression due to tabetic arthropathy of the spine. Journal of Neurology, Neurosurgery and Psychiatry, *36*, 260–264, 1973.

Ramsey, G. H., French, J. D. and Strain, W. H.: Iodinated organic compounds as contrast media for radiographic diagnoses: Pantopaque myelography. Radiology, *43*, 236–240, 1944.

Rasmussen, T. B., Kernohan, J. W. and Adson, A. W.: Pathologic classification, with surgical consideration of intraspinal tumors. Annals of Surgery, *111*, 513–530, 1940.

Roberts G. M.: Lumbar stenosis. The significance of the narrow lumbar spinal canal and its diagnosis in spondylotic cauda equina syndrome. M.D. Thesis, University of London, 1978.

Robinson, F. and Shapiro, R.: Chronic non-specific spinal epidural granuloma. Clinical Radiology, *18*, 166–172, 1967.

Roth, M.: Caudal end of the spinal cord. Acta Radiologica Diagnosis, *3*, 177–187, 1963.

Roth, M. and Hanak, L.: Atrophie de la moelle épinière. Étude clinique et radiologique. Revue Neurologique, *113*, 171–182, 1965.

Schimmel, D. H., Newton, T. H. and Mani, J.: Widening of the cervical intervertebral foramen. Neuroradiology, *12*, 3–10, 1976.

Schreiber, F. and Rosenthal, H.: Paraplegia from ruptured lumbar discs in achondroplastic dwarfs. Journal of Neurosurgery, *9*, 648–651, 1952.

Schwartz, G. S.: The width of the spinal canal in the growing vertebra with special reference to the sacrum. American Journal of Roentgenology, *76*, 476–481, 1956.

Sellwood, R. B.: The radiological approach to metastatic cancer of the brain and spine. British Journal of Radiology, *45*, 647–651, 1972.

Shahinfar, A. H. and Schechter, M. M.: Traumatic extradural cysts of the spine. American Journal of Roentgenology, *98*, 713–719, 1966.

Sharp, J. and Purser, D. W.: Spontaneous atlanto-axial dislocation in ankylosing spondylitis and rheumatoid arthritis. Annals of the Rheumatic Diseases, *20*, 47–77, 1961.

Shealy, C. N., LeMay, M. and Haddad, F. S.: Posterior scalloping of vertebral bodies in uncontrolled hydrocephalus. Journal of Neurology, Neurosurgery, and Psychiatry, *27*, 567–573, 1964.

Sicard, J. A. and Forestier, J. E.: Méthode générale d'exploration radiologique par l'huile iodeé (Lipiodol). Bulletin et memoires de la Société de médicine de Paris, *46*, 463–469, 1922.

Siddiqui, A. H.: Fluorosis in Nalgonda district, Hyderabad-Deccan. British Medical Journal, *2*, 1408–1413, 1955.

Singh, A. and Jolly, S. S.: Endemic fluorosis. Quarterly Journal of Medicine, *30*, 357 – 372, 1961.

Skalpe, I. O. and Amundsen, P.: Lumbar radiculography with metrizamide, a non-ionic water-soluble contrast medium. Radiology, *115*, 91 – 95, 1975.

Stoltmann, H. F. and Blackwood, W.: The role of the ligamenta flava in the pathogenesis of cervical myelopathy. Brain, *87*, 45 – 50, 1964.

Sutton, D.: Sacral cysts. Acta Radiologica Diagnosis, *1*, 787 – 795, 1963.

Tarlov, I. M.: Spinal perineural and meningeal cysts. Journal of Neurology, Neurosurgery and Psychiatry, *33*, 833 – 843, 1970.

Teng, P. and Papatheodorou, C.: Spinal arachnoid diverticula. British Journal of Radiology, *39*, 249 – 254, 1966.

Till, K.: Spinal dysraphism: A study of congenital malformations of the back. Developmental Medicine and Child Neurology, *10*, 471 – 478, 1968.

Tsai, F. Y., Popp, A. J. and Waldman, J.: Spontaneous spinal epidural hematoma. Neuroradiology, *10*, 15 – 30, 1975.

Tucker, A. S., Aramsri, B. and Gardner, W. J.: Primary spinal tumours: a seven-year study. American Journal of Roentgenology, *87*, 371 – 374, 1962.

Verbiest, H.: Radicular syndrome from developmental narrowing of lumbar vertebral canal. Journal of Bone and Joint Surgery, *36B*, 230 – 237, 1954.

Wells, C., Spillane, J. and Bligh, A.: The cervical canal in syringomyelia. Brain, *82*, 23 – 39, 1959.

Westberg, G.: Gas myelography and percutaneous puncture in the diagnosis of spinal cord cysts. Acta Radiologica Supplementum 252, 1966.

Wood, E. H. and Bream, C. A.: Spinal sarcoidosis. Radiology, *73*, 226 – 233, 1959.

Yeoman, P.: Cervical myelography in traction injuries of the brachial plexus. Journal of Bone and Joint Surgery, *50B*, 253 – 260, 1968.

I

N

O

T